D1746259

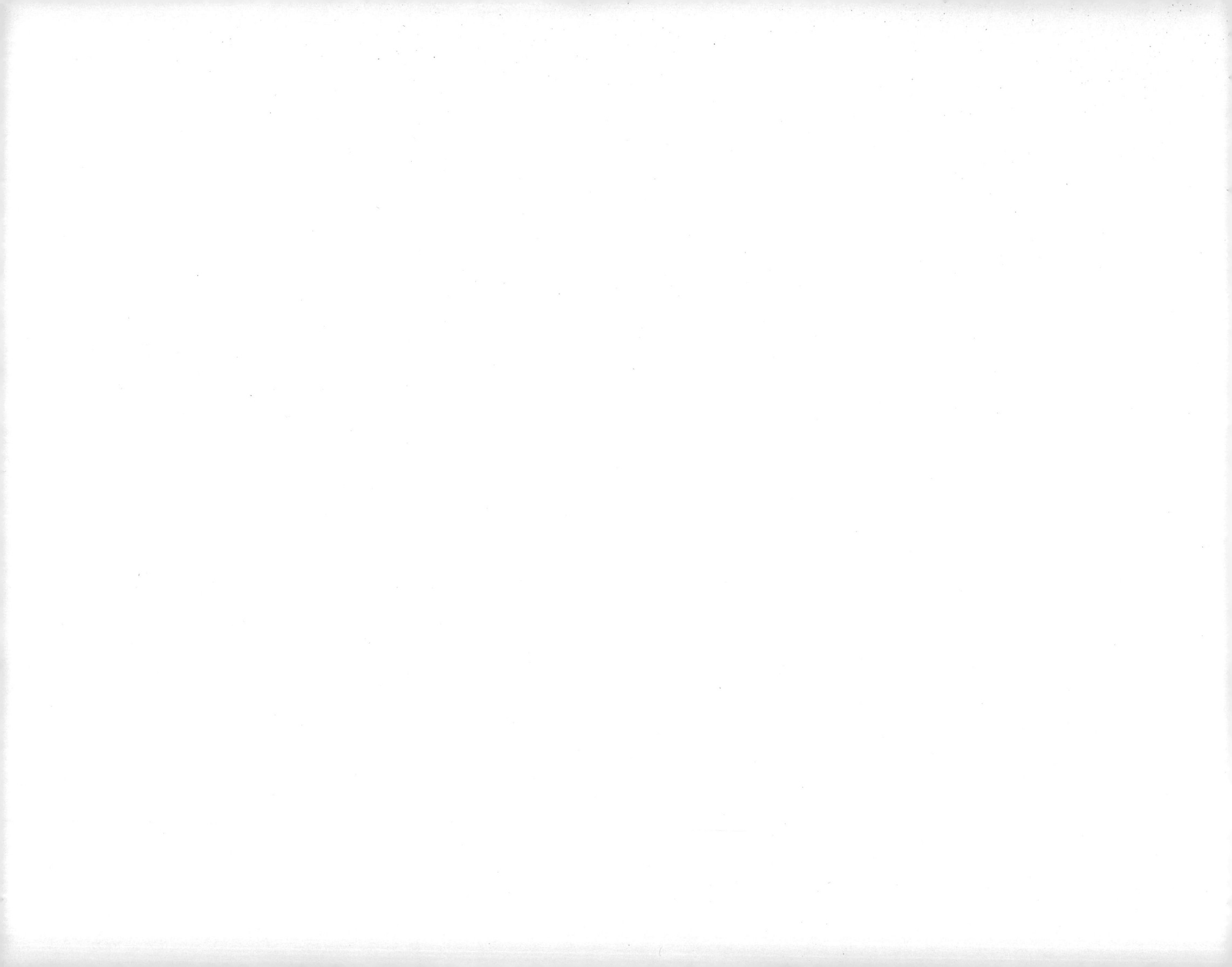

MAMMOGRAPHY
GUIDE TO INTERPRETING, REPORTING AND AUDITING MAMMOGRAPHIC IMAGES
Re.Co.R.M.
(from italian Reporting and Codifying the Results of Mammography)

V. LATTANZIO G. SIMONETTI

Mammography

Guide to Interpreting, Reporting and Auditing Mammographic Images – Re.Co.R.M

Preface by Cosimo Di Maggio

Springer

Vincenzo Lattanzio
Director, Breast Imaging Unit
Azienda Policlinico
Bari, Italy

Giovanni Simonetti
Head, Department of Imaging and Interventional Radiology
Azienda Policlinico Università Tor Vergata
Rome, Italy

The Authors wish to thank KODAK for the support and help in the realization and distribution of this volume

Originally published as:
Mammografia
Guida alla refertazione e alla codifica dei risultati Re.Co.R.M
Vincenzo Lattanzio and Giovanni Simonetti
© 2002 Gruppo Editoriale IDELSON-GNOCCHI srl dal 1908
All Rights Reserved

Translation by Athina Papa, Lorena Rossi, Tiziana Turzi, Bari, Italy

Library of Congress Control Number: 2004115462

ISBN 3-540-20018-5 Springer Berlin Heidelberg New York

This work is subject to copyright. All rights are reserved, whether the whole or part of the material is concerned, specifically the rights of translation, reprinting, reuse of illustrations, recitation, broadcasting, reproduction on microfilm or in any other way, and storage in data banks. Duplication of this publication or parts thereof is permitted only under the provisions of the Copyright Law of September 9, 1695 in its current version, and permission for use must always be obtained from the Publisher and the author. Violations are liable to prosecution under the Copyright Law.

© Vincenzo Lattanzio 2005
Printed in Italy

The use of general descriptive names, registered names, trademarks, etc. in this publication does not imply, even in the absence of a specific statement, that such names are exempt from the relevant protective laws and regulations and therefore free for general use.
Product liability: The publishers cannot guarantee the accuracy of any information about dosage and application contained in this book. In every individual case the user must check information by consulting the relevant literature.

Worldwide distribution rights: Springer-Verlag Berlin Heidelberg New York

Springer is a part of Springer Science+Business Media
springeronline.com

Cover design: Vincenzo Lattanzio

Typesetting and printing: Italgrafica Sud, Bari, Italy

in collaboration with
S I R M
Società Italiana di Radiologia Medica
Senology Section
(in office 2000-2004)

President
Giovanni Simonetti

Board of Directors
Roberta Chersevani
Alfonso Frigerio
Angela Maria Guerrieri
Pietro Panizza

Secretary
Elsa Cossu

CONTENTS

Foreword IX

Preface XIII

Part 1 **MAMMOGRAPHY TERMINOLOGY** 1

    THE NORMAL BREAST 3
        Radiological anatomy of the breast 4
        Variations of normal 11
    MAMMOGRAPHIC SIGNS 23
        Opacity 25
            Circumscribed opacity 27
            Stellate opacity 55
            Diffuse opacity 75
        Architectural distortion 81
        Calcifications 97
            Probably benign calcifications 129
            Doubtful or indeterminate calcifications 179
            Probably malignant calcifications 203
        Radiolucency 227
        Asymmetry 235
        Focal asymmetric density 239
        Skin thickening and retraction 243
        Oedema 247
        Asymmetrically dilated ducts 253

Part 2	**INTERPRETING AND REPORTING**	255
	Interpretation	256
	Communication and language	260
	The Re.Co.R.M. Diagnostic assessment categories	266

Part 3	**MAMMOGRAPHY AUDIT**	269

FOREWORD

When Enzo Lattanzio showed me his book and asked me to write the foreword for it, I took one look and said: "It's too big. It won't fit into a regular bookcase." Enzo looked me straight in the eye and replied: "It doesn't belong in a bookcase, it belongs on a desk, where it can be delved into constantly."

Senology is not a branch of medicine like ophthalmology, rheumatology or cardiology: it is a discipline that centres around a single organ and involves a slew of specialists, including radiologists, surgeons, pathologists, oncologists, gynaecologists, and more. Each is called upon to contribute special skills and they must indeed have very special skills in their own particular area. Thus, though senology can and does exist, there is no such thing as a "senologist." Senology is a highly complex discipline but still, when there is no disease, or where there are only benign lesions, imaging techniques can answer virtually all questions.

An hourglass is a good metaphor for describing how breast disease is tackled from many different quarters. The lower part of the glass represents the preclinical investigations, functional tests and epidemiological analyses. Diagnostic imaging occupies the "waist", and all the other specialties are in the top half. Breast imaging takes up little space, but it is fundamental: without it the top half of the hourglass will collapse and the bottom cannot hold it up and prevent disease taking over. Diagnostic imaging can detect lesions small enough to be successfully treated, and has given extraordinary impetus to the fight against breast cancer. It has also contributed significantly toward making senology a recognized discipline. It was mammography that brought it to the forefront: when Charles M. Gros realized that a dedicated instrument was required to explore the breast, mammography became the driving force behind senology. The quality of mammograms has gradually improved and the radiation doses are now smaller. The art of interpreting these images has become increasingly refined and we can now characterize even the tiniest lesions.

Senology is becoming increasingly complex: though many other techniques have challenged mammography, some providing both morphological and functional information, none have yet matched its ability to offer diagnostic hypotheses of sufficiently high predictive value, and it is still the only technique that can detect lesions only a few hundred microns in diameter.

However, science marches on relentlessly. Molecular biology will surely sooner or later completely solve breast problems upstream of the diagnostic stage, but in the meantime other diagnostic approaches focussing more on the functional side such as MRI, contrast-enhanced US and PET, are starting to reveal the limits of mammography, which, despite the advent of digital systems, is still based on morphology. In addition, the spread of methods involving needle biopsies for cytology or histological examinations might suggest that the careful analysis of subtle mammographic findings of small lesions is redundant – considering mammography as a technique belonging more to the field of perception than to the field of diagnosis and characterization. Nothing could be further from the truth. If every lesion – small or large – were biopsied, women might be reluctant to agree to regular check-ups and all our efforts to promote prevention would be in vain.

So much has been learnt over recent years that radiologists can no longer afford to regard mammograms with the cocksure diagnostic certainty of the past. Until science discovers the secret of preventing cells from turning malignant, and can offer truly effective therapy at any stage of the disease, and until new diagnostic techniques are developed that can supply accurate, repeatable and affordable functional or morpho-functional information, mammography remains the only viable method for detecting most tumours early enough for effective treatment, without unnecessary biopsies or other invasive procedures.

Therefore it is still essential to distinguish between what is decidedly negative on a mammogram, as opposed to what needs regular monitoring, and what requires a needle biopsy. The secret of making such distinctions accurately is to understand and learn to interpret the most subtle signs typical of breast lesions, thus acquiring knowledge and skills. This book provides all the necessary resources.

The American College of Radiology's BI-RADS® (Breast Imaging Reporting and Data System) and the ANAES (Agence Nationale d'Accréditation et d'Evaluation de la Santé) guidelines have shown the way, emphasizing the validity and importance of mammography, but many practitioners are still unfamiliar with breast imaging techniques. This book will undoubtedly provide valuable support for physicians everywhere: it practically ensures success.

It goes without saying that this is more than just a collection of images; contributions from many sources have been welcomed, used and improved. All the images have been painstakingly selected and reproduced to the highest standards to make then as easy as possible to consult and memorize.

I was delighted to accept the invitation to write this foreword because it obliged me to read the book thoroughly, and I am happy I did because it gave me a chance to put my knowledge to the test and acquire valuable new insights. All too often people of my age and position believe that textbooks like this are for younger colleagues, or newcomers venturing into this area the first time. We often leaf quickly through the pages and take it for granted that we already know all there is to know. But that is certainly not the case: this book offers a method of interpreting mammograms that older practitioners may never have learned, having received their training long before the advent of "evidence-based medicine", back when this approach was still in its infancy.

This book is a valuable learning tool and is of course primarily aimed at the younger, less experienced practitioner. There is therefore really no need to recommend to such that they read it, as the humble learner will undoubtedly jump at the chance to enrich his or her education with such a store of valuable knowledge.

However, I do recommend that senior practitioners like myself who are already familiar with mammograms, and may indeed have even contributed to the birth and development of diagnostic senology, consult this book with the attention it deserves. It will help them learn the difference between culture and erudition, between presumption and knowledge.

Cosimo di Maggio
Professor of Radiology, University of Padova

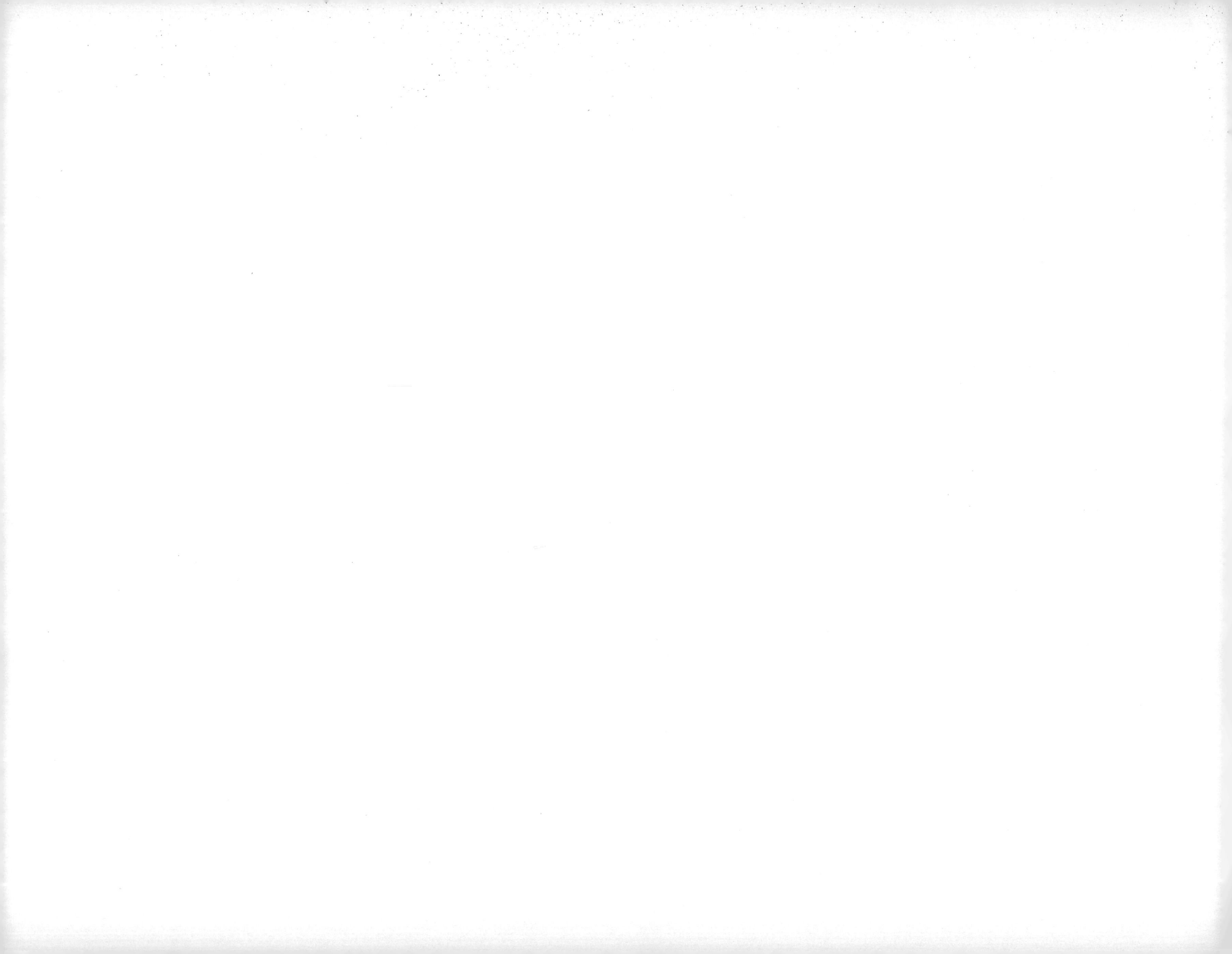

PREFACE

The terminology currently used in mammography is by no means uniform and clear-cut, and may frequently even be inappropriate for describing mammographic findings from a semiological and semantic point of view. Moreover, the natural evolution of language has added to the confusion. In view of the extensive use of mammography and the innumerable exams performed every day, mostly on asymptomatic individuals, there is an urgent need to standardize the language used to describe elementary mammographic abnormalities.

There have already been attempts to adopt a common, standardized, appropriate terminology to describe mammographic findings and establish a logical link between their diagnostic meaning, and clinical recommendations for the patient in order to suggest the proper action to be taken.

The American College of Radiology BI-RADS® (Breast Imaging Reporting and Data System) is the first example of a system adopted by a scientific society nationwide, followed by ANAES (Agence Nationale d'Accréditation et d'Evaluation de la Santé). The terminology proposed in this volume aims to identify simple, logical and intuitive morphological mammographic categories and their main features, to help define and interpret the different findings more easily for diagnostic assessment along a coherent path that leads to the clinical recommendations directing the patient towards the most appropriate decision and treatment. Every effort has been made to ensure the language used here is in line with accepted international terminology. Of course there is bound to be some overlap between categories of signs that have similar characteristics. It will be up to the individual radiologist to choose the appropriate terms on a case-by-case basis.

The adoption and dissemination of a common language is a cultural and professional necessity for the individual radiologist, as well as a conditio sine qua non for the successful fulfillment of everyday duties and the ability to share experiences with others.

The images in this atlas were chosen on the basis of the quality of the original documents: only those best illustrating the various anatomical situations and mammographic categories were selected, to permit a ready understanding and exhaustive analysis of the various characteristic signs and findings. The artwork and page layouts, often deliberately repetitive in respect of both texts and images, are designed to encourage the radiologist to follow an "automatic" process starting with perception and leading through analysis to the final diagnosis.

The majority of the mammograms are set out with the lefthand image showing the almost exact dimensions of the breast – as they usually appear in the radiologist's routine work, and the righthand page depicting details or magnification views that guide the radiologist towards the final evaluation.

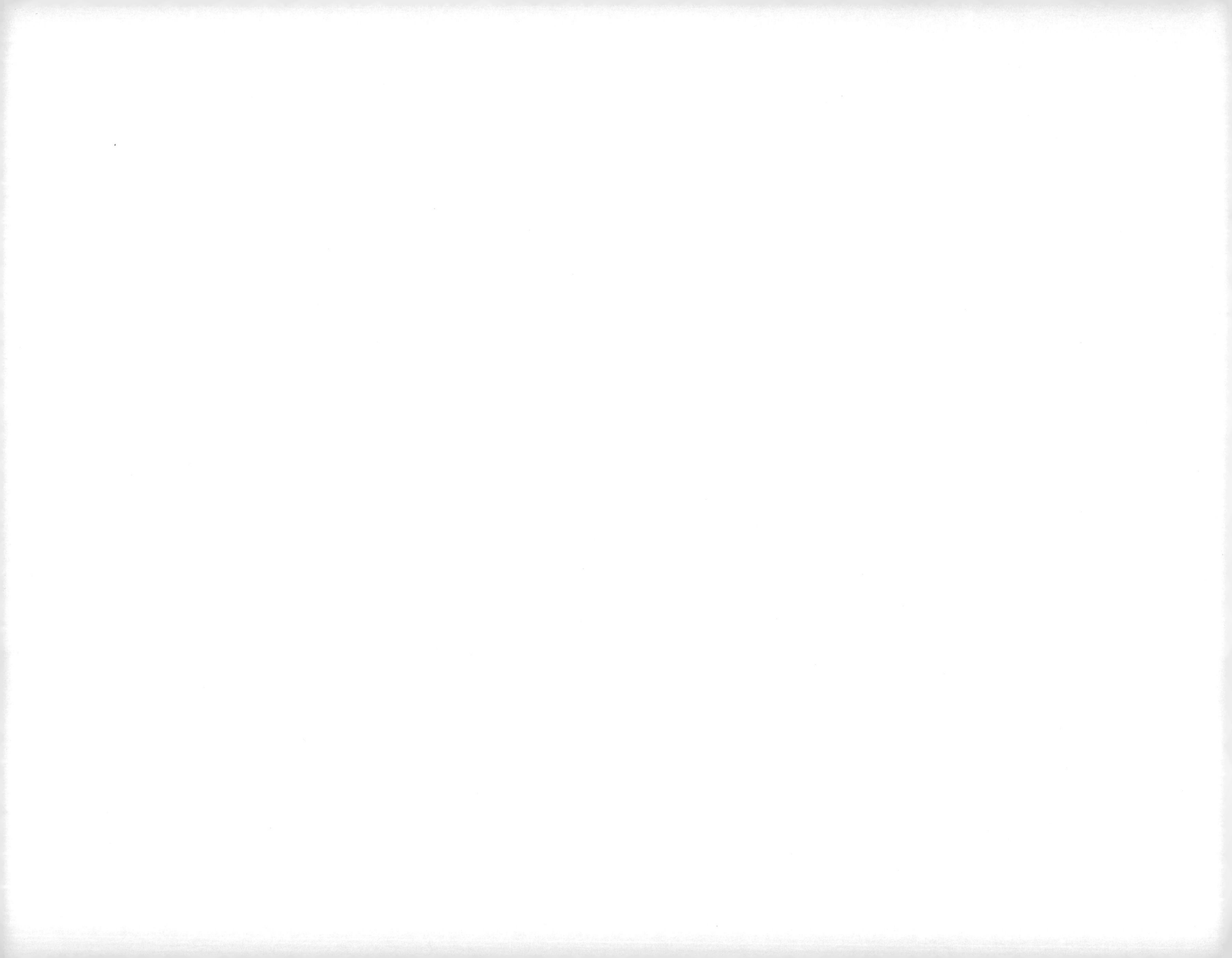

PART 1

MAMMOGRAPHY: TERMINOLOGY

THE NORMAL BREAST

To correctly approach and interpret breast pathologies, it is essential to understand the normal anatomy. Although this concept obviously applies to all organs, it is particularly relevant to the breast, where there is such extensive morphological and functional variability; the radiological image reflects the degree to which the radiation is absorbed by the different anatomical structures and their different quantitative proportions and spatial arrangement.

The tissues primarily appearing in a mammogram are fibrous-connective and adipose tissue and, to a lesser extent, ductal epithelium. The density of the fibroglandular and stromal architecture and, consequently, the overall radiological appearance is related to the degree of hydration of the connective tissue, determined by hormonal stimuli. It is therefore impossible to establish a single, unique "standard" normal radiological anatomy. It is, however, possible to agree that there are many different patterns of normal anatomy, depending on the individual fibroglandular tissue, and that the same individual may present physiological and functional variations within the range of normality.

When there are no patent signs of focal or diffuse lesions, the radiologist can inform the patient that her exam is "normal", implying that there is a normal pattern of different mammary structure types detected at mammography. This allays anxiety caused by the possibility of disease, and enables the patient to avoid further unnecessary exams and useless follow-up.

Radiological anatomy of the breast

Schematically, the radiological examination may show the following normal anatomical structures:
- skin
- nipple and areola
- fatty tissue
- the breast tissue proper, or corpus mammae
- blood vessels

Skin

The skin appears as a thin, continuous, radiopaque rim homogeneous in density, approximately 1 mm thick and readily visible against the radiolucency of the underlying subcutaneous premammary fatty tissue. If the breast is very dense because of the higher density of the underlying parenchymal structure, however, the skin may occasionally not show up clearly even on a correctly exposed mammogram.

Nipple and areola

The skin surrounding the nipple – the areola – can be up to 3-5 mm thick, with a central opacity, roughly cylindrical in shape and of variable size and density, corresponding to the nipple. Posteriorly there is a generally triangular, heterogeneous trabecular area, the retroareolar region, which is of particular interest on account of the difficulty of detecting any focal abnormalities that may be there.
Under normal conditions, the lactiferous ducts and sinuses are not seen. If they are enlarged they resemble ribbon-like opacities of varying thickness, running in parallel or divergent lines.

Fatty tissue

Varying amounts of fatty tissue may be present, forming anything from a thin subcutaneous layer to "islets" of various sizes that may occupy the whole breast, depending on the characteristics and age of the individual woman.
The parenchymal cone is surrounded by fatty tissue which constitutes the premammary fat anteriorly and the retromammary fat posteriorly. Anteriorly, subcutaneous fat appears as a radiolucent layer of variable thickness, traversed by planar sheets of fibrous tissue, the crests of Duret, which accommodate Cooper's ligaments. The superficial extensions of Cooper's ligaments come to peaks attached to the skin, which anchor the body of the breast to the subcutaneous tissues, known as retinacula cutis.
Posteriorly, adipose tissue outlines the retromammary space (the bursa of Chassaignac), which separates the breast from the prepectoral fascia overlying the pectoralis major muscle.

NORMAL

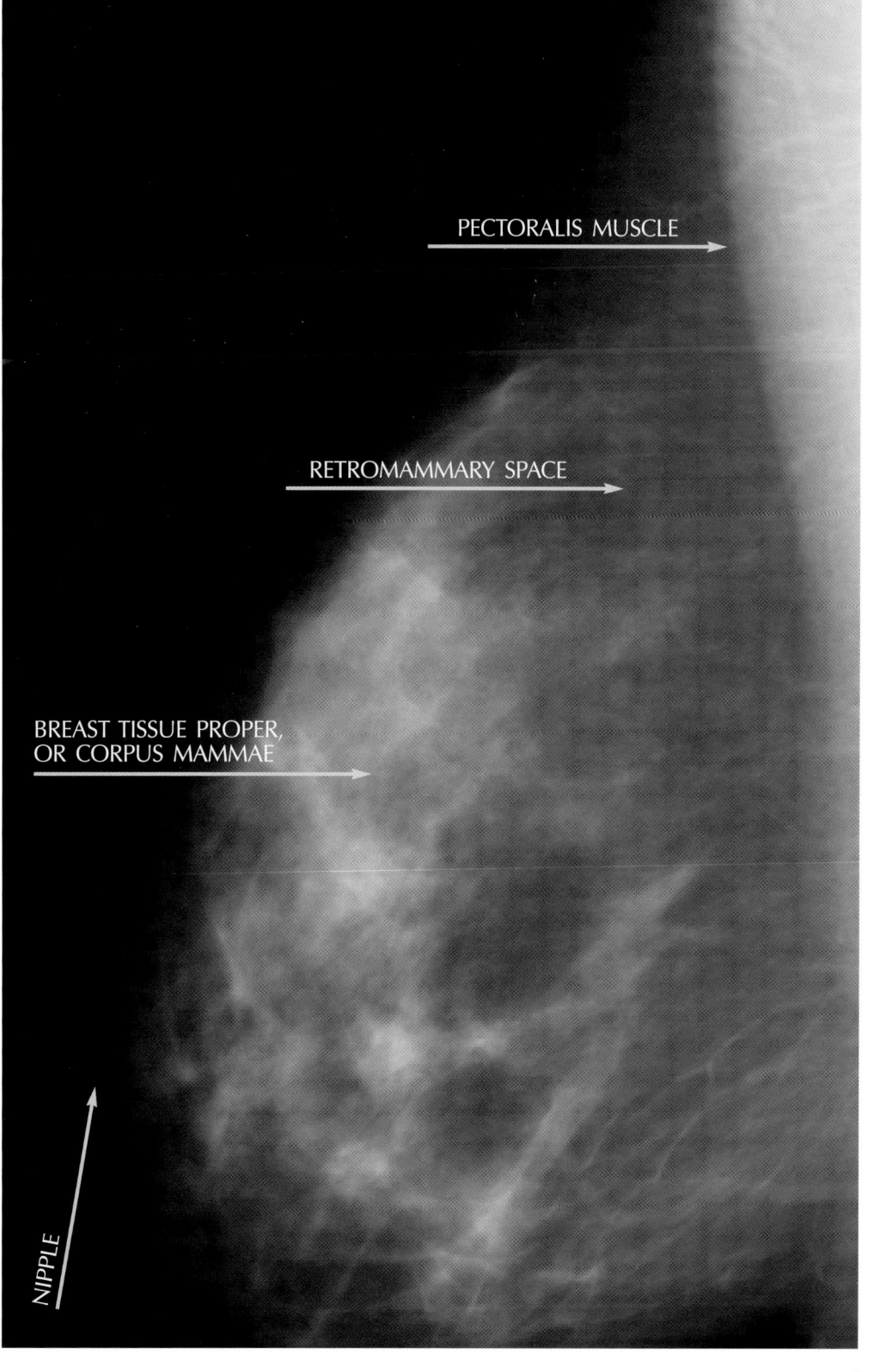

NORMAL

Breast tissue proper, or corpus mammae

The body of the mammary gland is roughly cone-shaped with the floor resting on the chest wall and the tip projecting towards the nipple. The shape and density of breast structures vary from individual to individual, and are influenced by specific sensitivity to hormonal stimuli, which affect relations between the various tissue components and hence the morphology of the breast.

The concept of mammographic "density" as being strictly related to advancing age is obsolete, so adipose tissue is not synonymous with a senile breast, and, similarly, the so-called "dense breast" is not necessarily a young breast. Nor is it possible to establish a link, in terms of pathogenesis and symptoms, between breasts that are patchy and dense at mammography and conditions such as dysplasia or fibrocystic breast disease. These terms have given rise to much confusion among clinicians and radiologists; not only are they well and truly outdated but they are in fact inappropriate with modern radiology, since they belong to the realm of pathology.

The variety in the mammographic appearance of the "individual" types of mammary structures is in all likelihood related to differences in the normal processes of development and involution, more than to pathological conditions.

For teaching purposes, it may be useful to classify mammographic structures into six main groups reflecting the most frequently encountered breast tissue patterns, as shown on the opposite page.

Pectoralis muscle

The pectoralis muscle is homogeneously radiopaque; it is located in front of the chest wall and is shaped like an upside-down triangle in the lateral and mediolateral oblique views. In the craniocaudal view it is crescent-shaped and variably visible depending on the anatomy of the chest and the position and compression of the breast. In a very small proportion of cases (1%) one can see medially a small triangular or flame-shaped portion of muscle adjacent to the sternum, which must not be misinterpreted as a mass.

Generally, a correctly executed mediolateral oblique projection shows the lower margin of the pectoralis muscle following an imaginary line that runs anteriorly through the nipple.

Blood vessels

Vessels are more readily visible in breasts that contain plentiful fatty tissue, and appear as thin ribbon-like opacities that may be more or less tortuous; vessel walls may be calcified, in which case they give typical "railwayline" images. In the early stages of calcification, only scattered elongated "casts" are seen, in a linear pattern, reflecting partial, fragmentary calcification of the vascular wall.

NORMAL

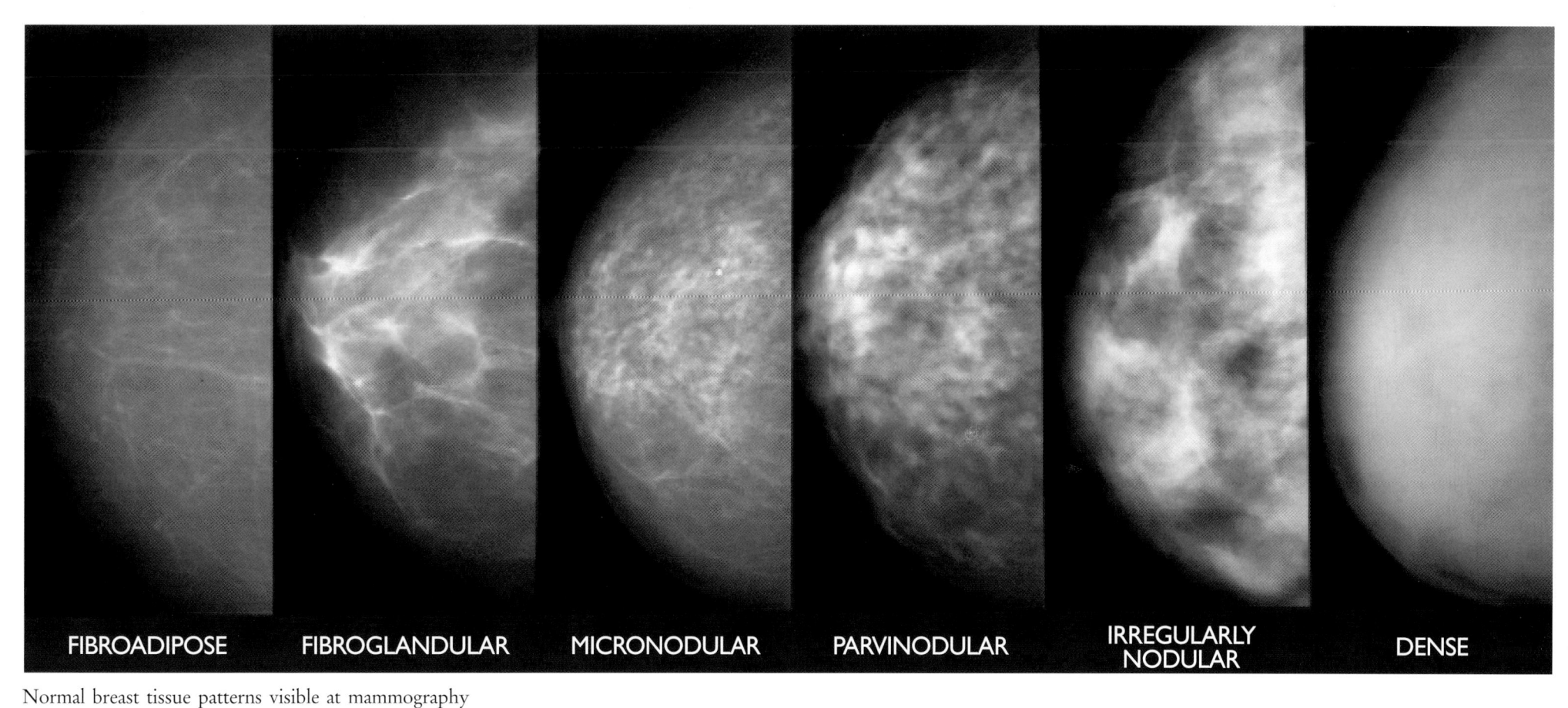

| FIBROADIPOSE | FIBROGLANDULAR | MICRONODULAR | PARVINODULAR | IRREGULARLY NODULAR | DENSE |

Normal breast tissue patterns visible at mammography

NORMAL

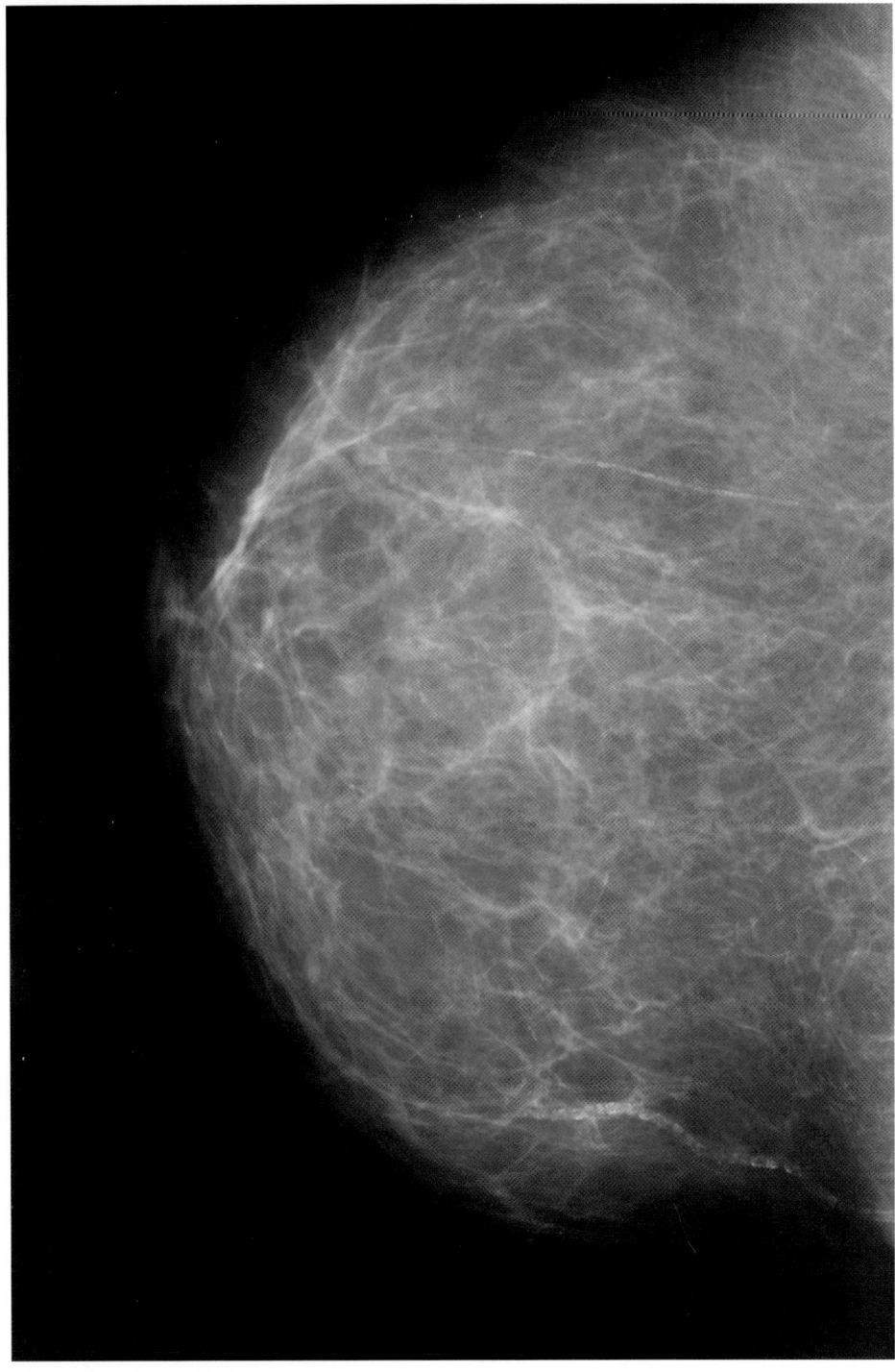

Fibroadipose structure
Total absence of fibroglandular tissue. Only traces of the stromal network may remain.

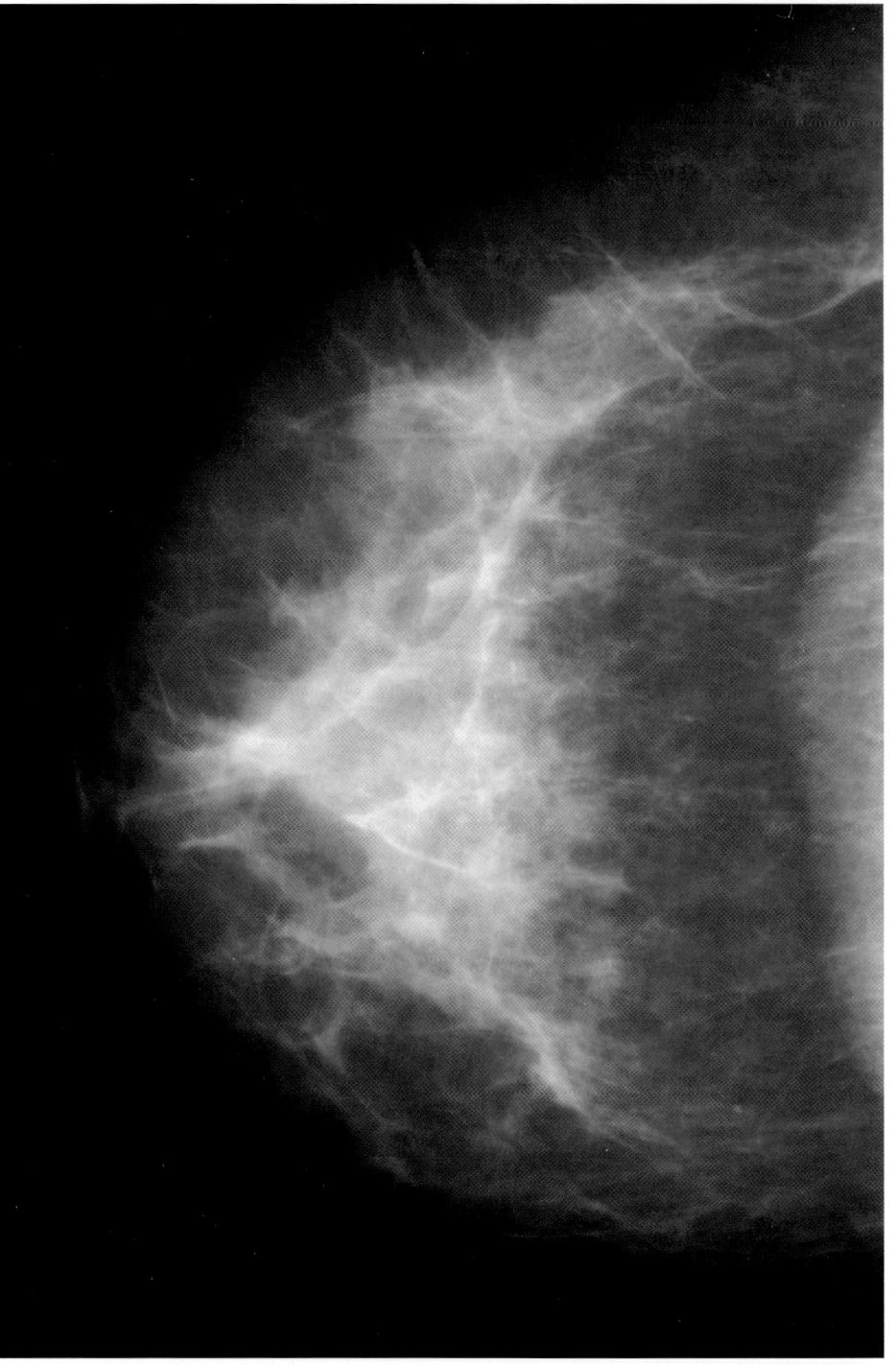

Fibroglandular structure
Typical triangular fibroglandular configuration, clearly showing the tip of the triangle in the retroareolar region and the perimammary fatty spaces. The parenchymal component is prevalently planar in appearance, or slightly nodular. The texture of the stroma is readily recognized, with the crests of Duret outlining the adipose areas between the retinacula cutis.

NORMAL

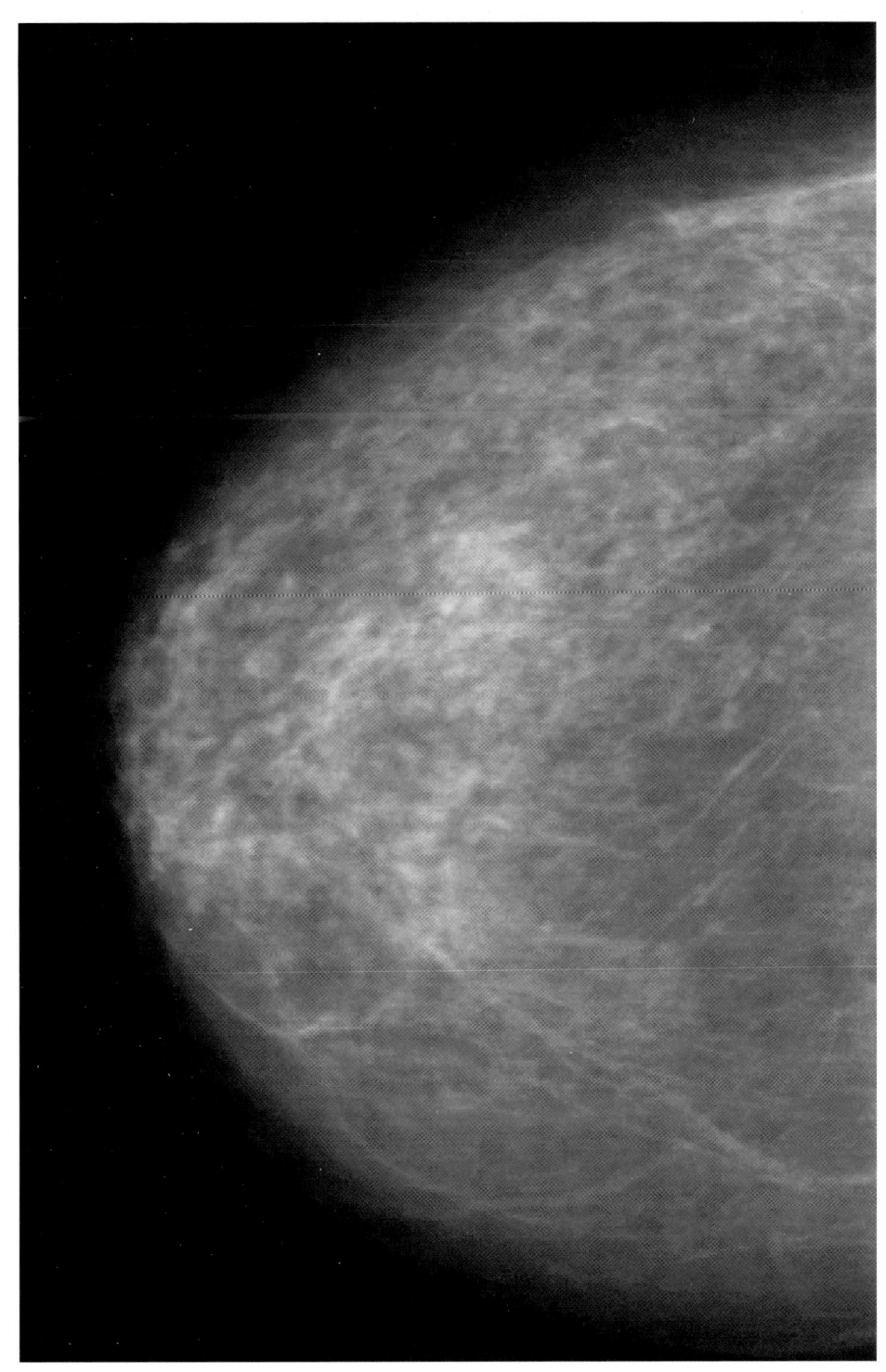

Micronodular structure
Less adipose tissue is seen. The fibroglandular component is abundant, most of it forming a "cobblestone" effect made up of small radiopaque nodular opacities measuring up to 3 mm in diameter.

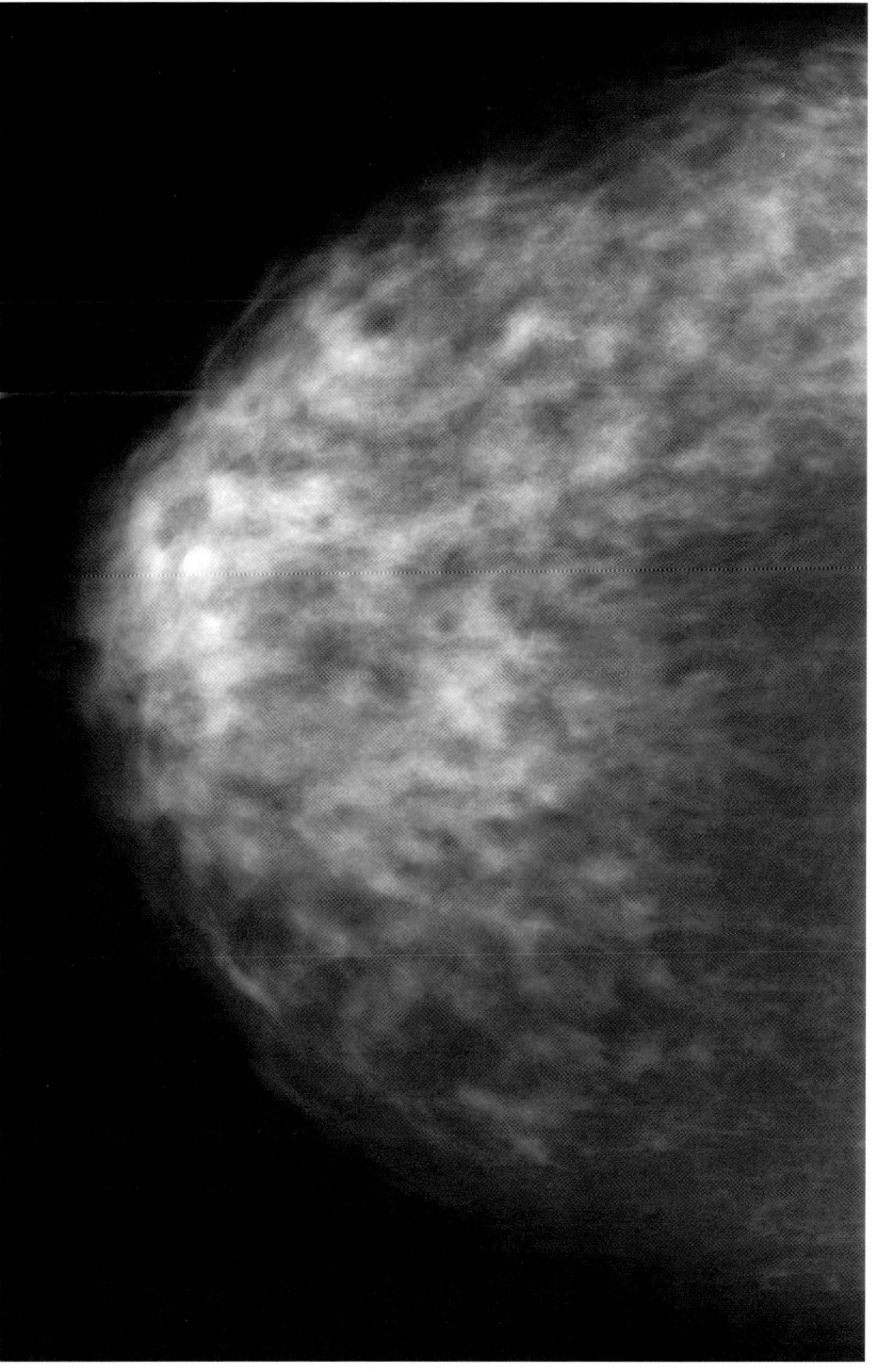

Parvinodular structure
Similar to the previous. The elementary radiopaque nodules are larger, some reaching 6-7 mm in diameter.

NORMAL

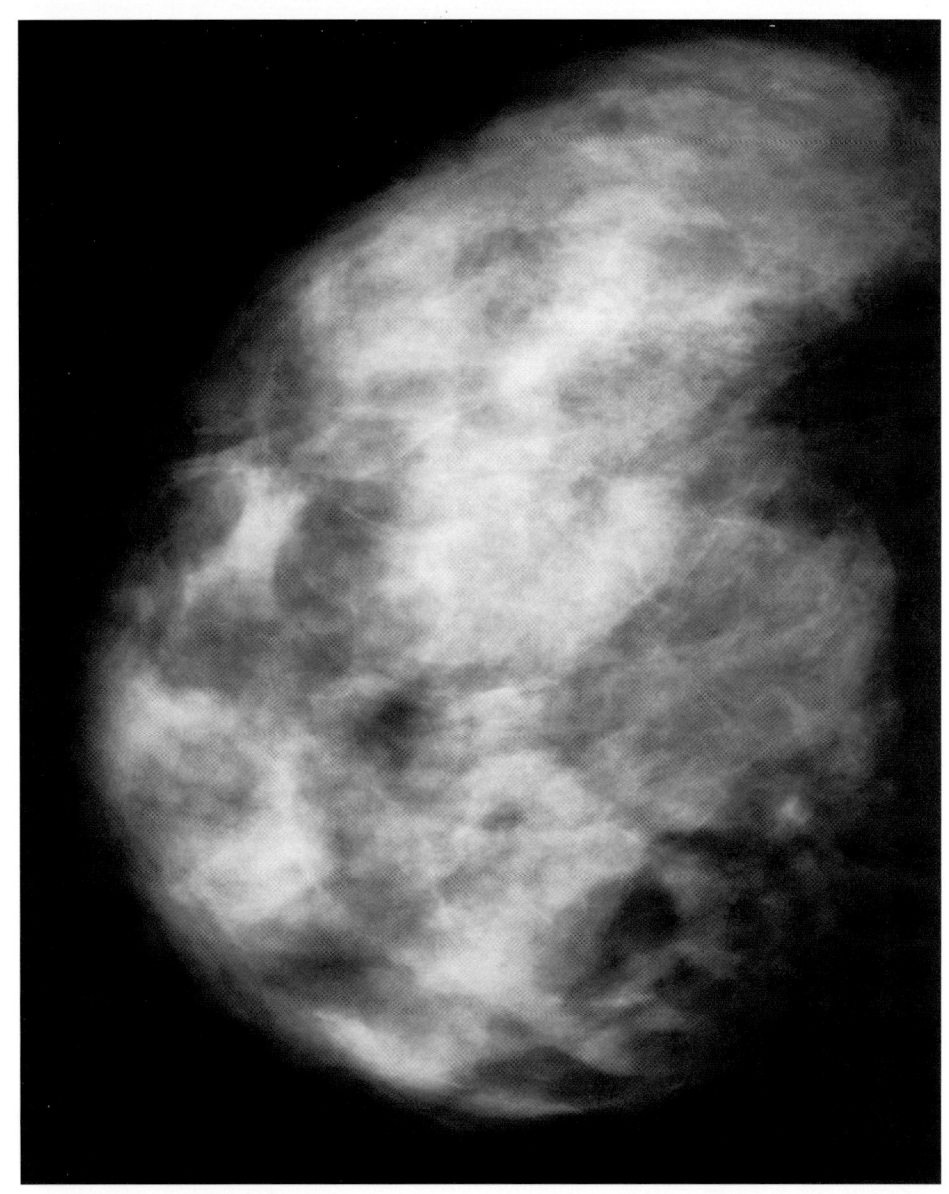

Irregularly nodular structure
Generally little fatty tissue present. The fibroglandular component is heterogeneous, featuring nodules of various sizes, either solitary or clustered in "patches". The stroma may be more or less marked.

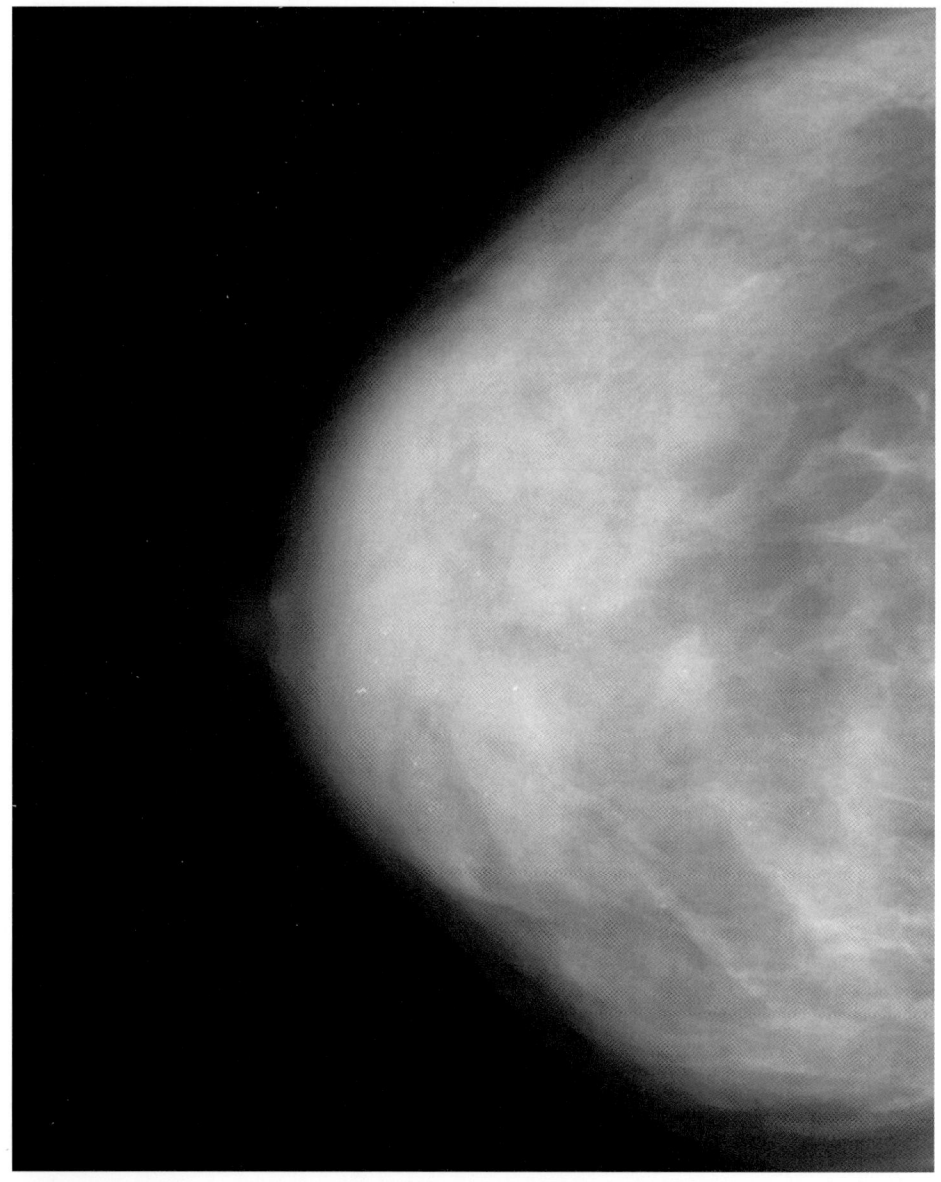

Dense structure
Virtually no fatty tissue is present. The mammogram shows an intensely and uniformly radiopaque glandular and stromal "block" in which the structures of the breast cannot be distinguished.

In terms of difficulties for the radiologist in reading and interpreting mammograms, the spectrum ranges from fatty structures, which are the easiest to interpret, to dense ones, which are the hardest, and in which it is virtually impossible to define the morphological features or to distinguish normal structures from pathological ones. In between lie structures that may present varying degrees of interpretative difficulty.

# VARIATIONS OF NORMAL

NORMAL

Accessory breast tissue
Bilateral fibroglandular structures are present in the axilla, mostly to the left.

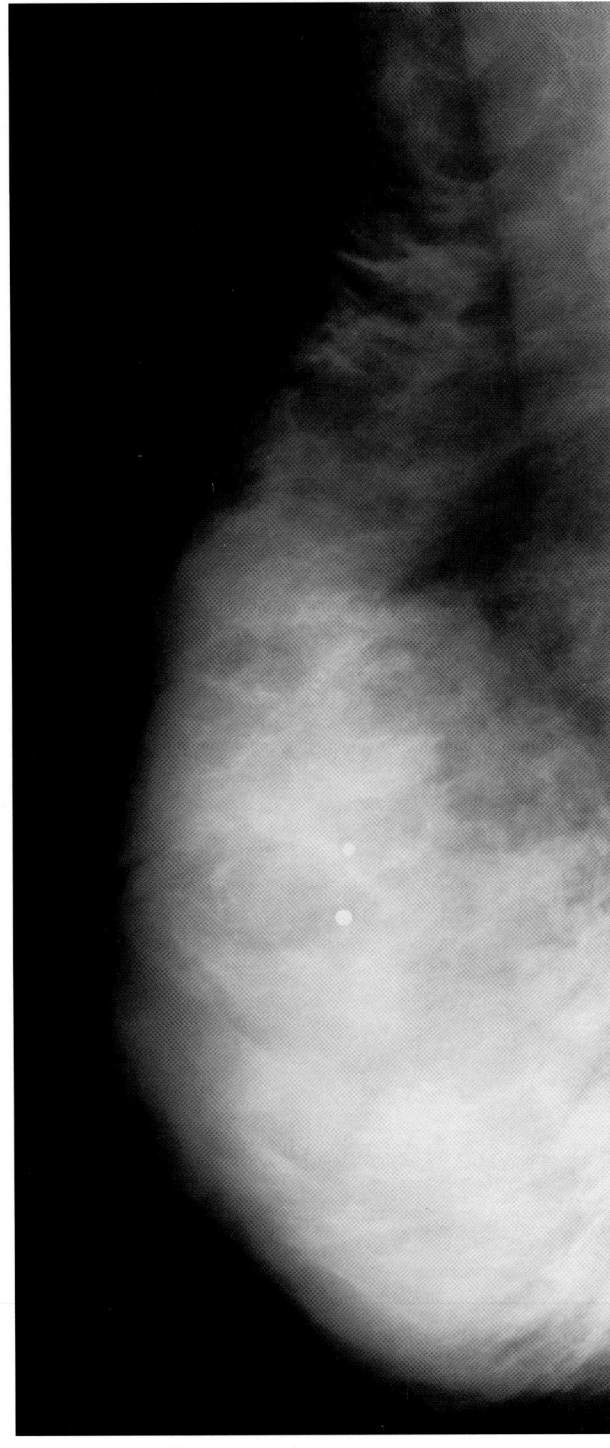

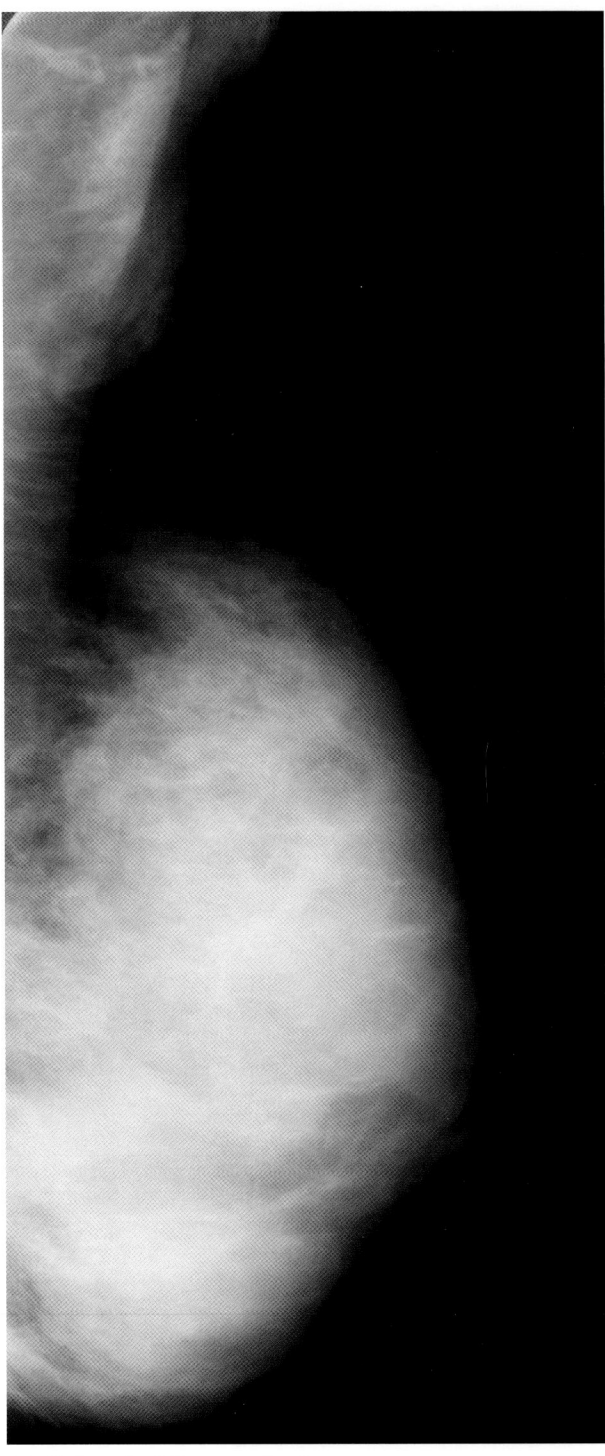

Mediolateral oblique projection

Mediolateral oblique projection

Accessory breast tissue

Bilateral fibroglandular structures are present in the axilla, mostly to the left. The areas of accessory fibroglandular tissue, which may contain a pathological focal mass, require close examination and an ultrasound scan may be helpful.

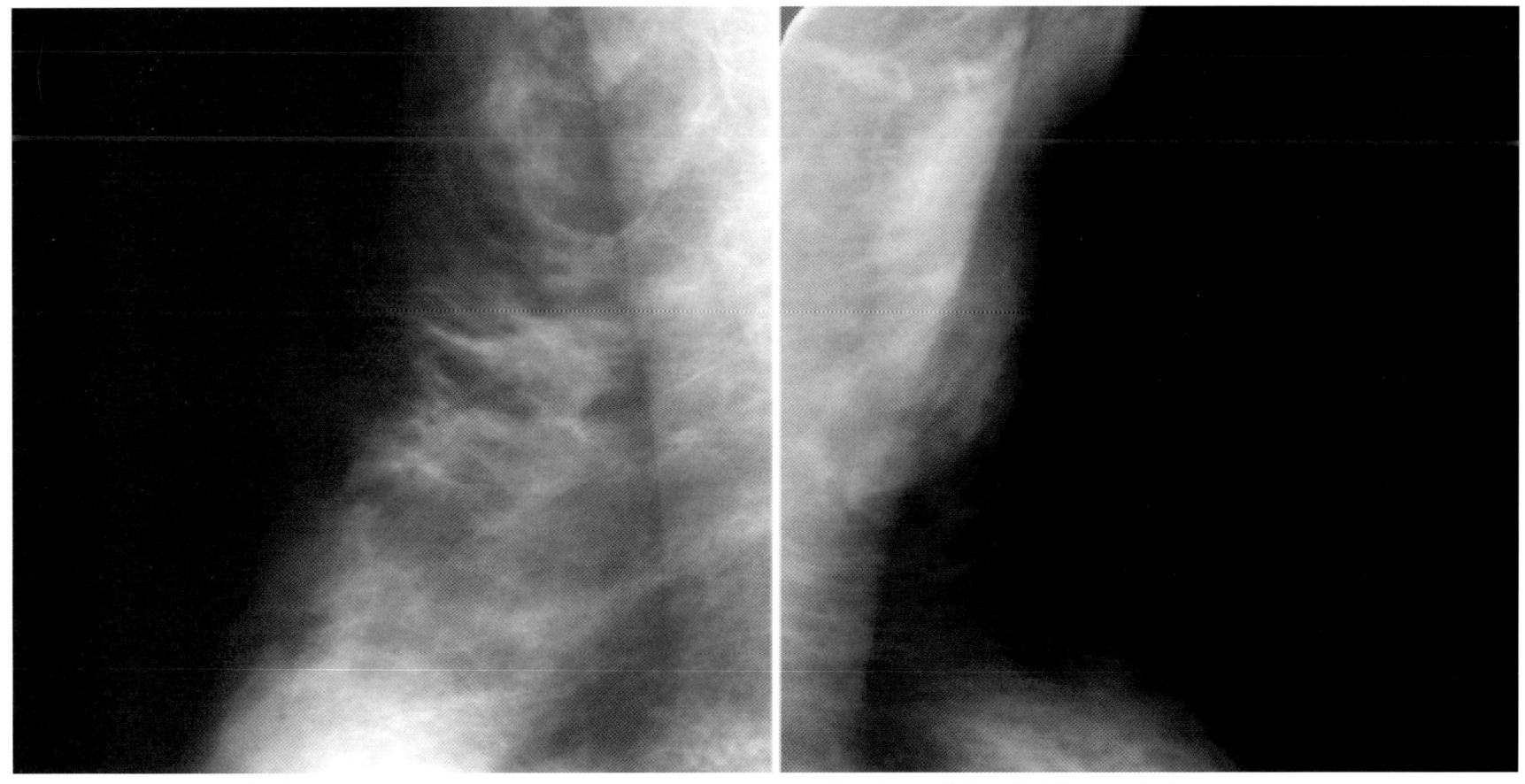

Detail of the mediolateral oblique projection

Detail of the mediolateral oblique projection

NORMAL

Accessory breast tissue

On the right, there is an oval-shaped opacity in the axilla, with partially defined margins and the same density as the underlying fibroglandular tissue. Bilaterally there are multiple circumscribed opacities of different sizes, with regular margins and uniformly high density. The finding is compatible with bilateral aspecific adenopathies and an area of accessory breast tissue on the left.

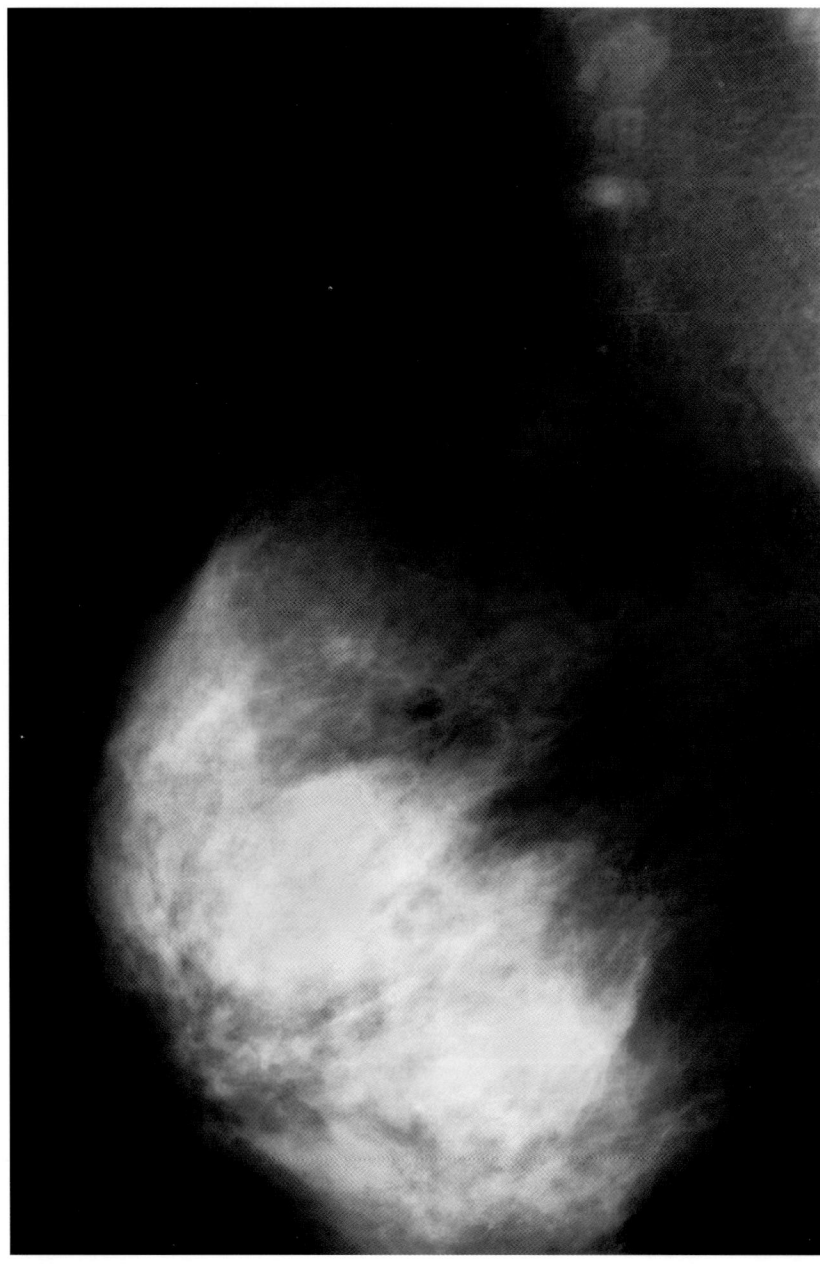

Mediolateral oblique projection

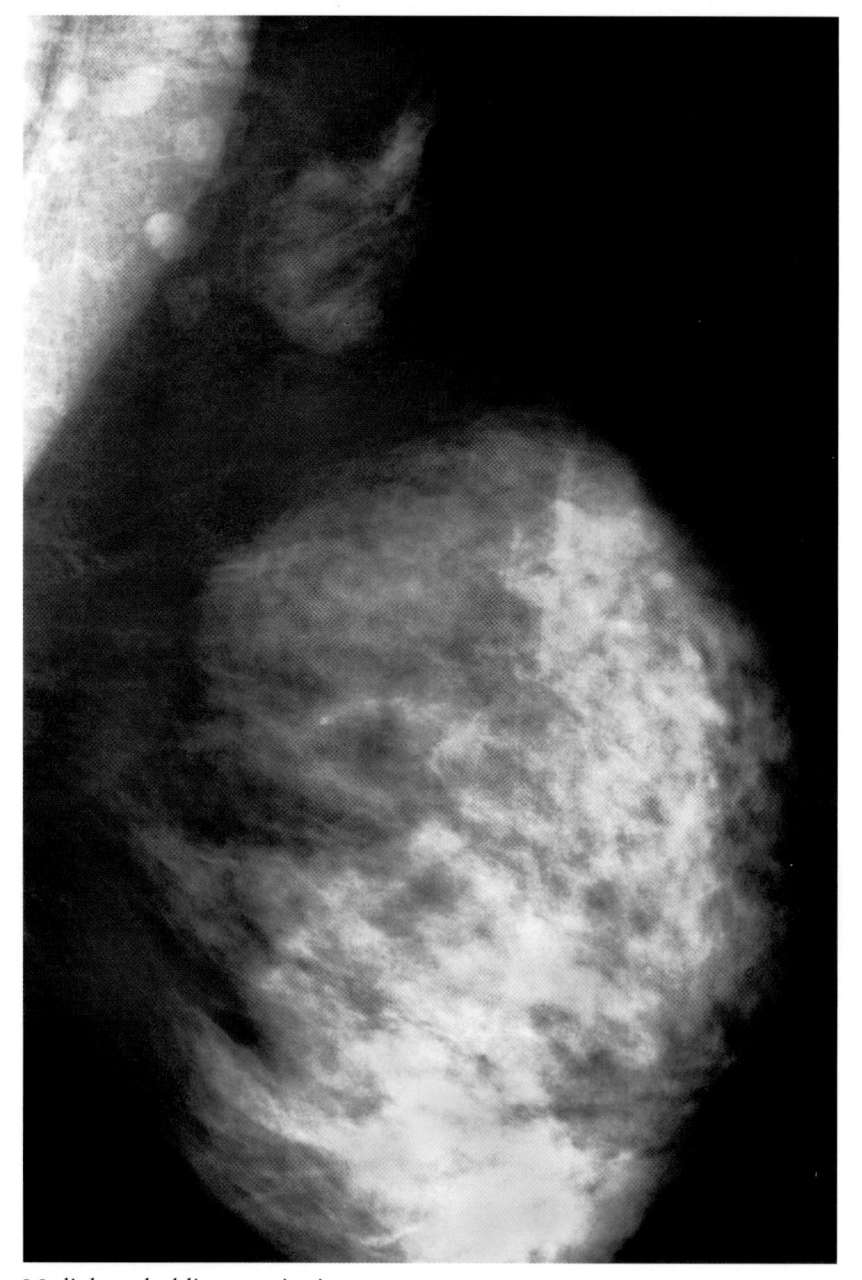

Mediolateral oblique projection

Accessory breast tissue

On the right, there is an oval-shaped opacity in the axilla, with partially defined margins and the same density as the underlying fibroglandular tissue. Bilaterally there are multiple circumscribed opacities of different sizes, with regular margins and uniformly high density. The finding is compatible with bilateral aspecific adenopathies and an area of accessory breast tissue on the left.

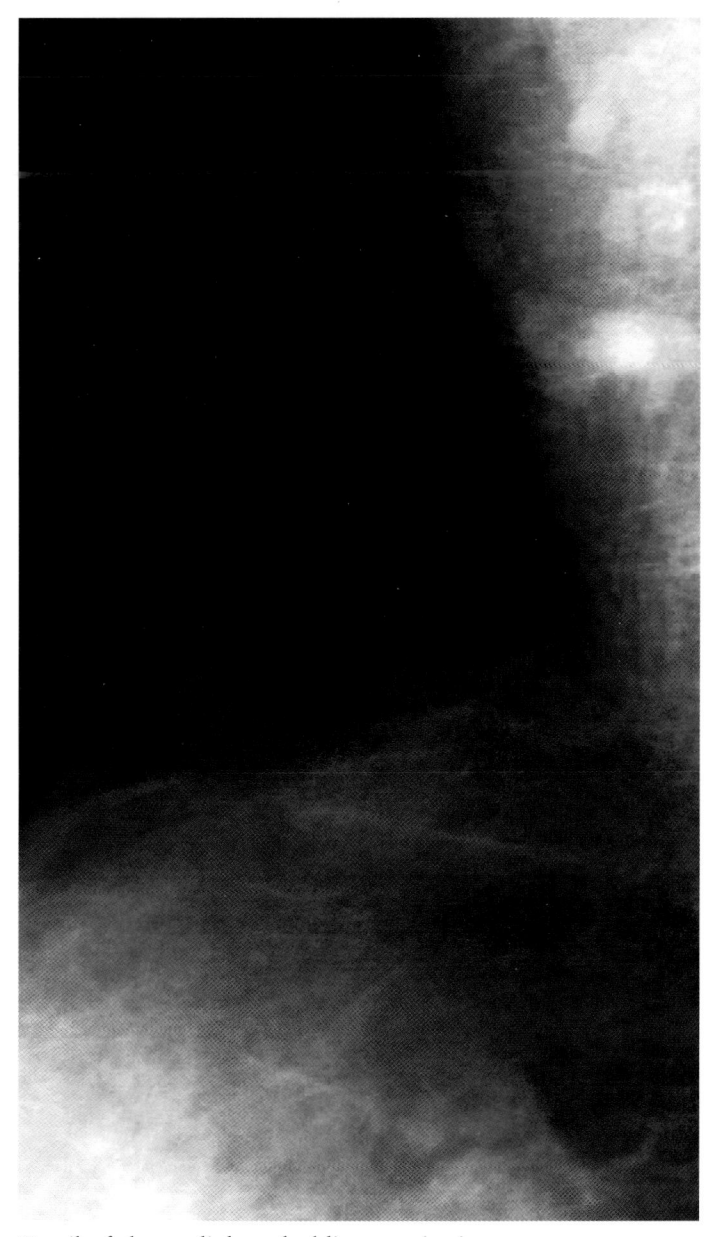

Detail of the mediolateral oblique projection

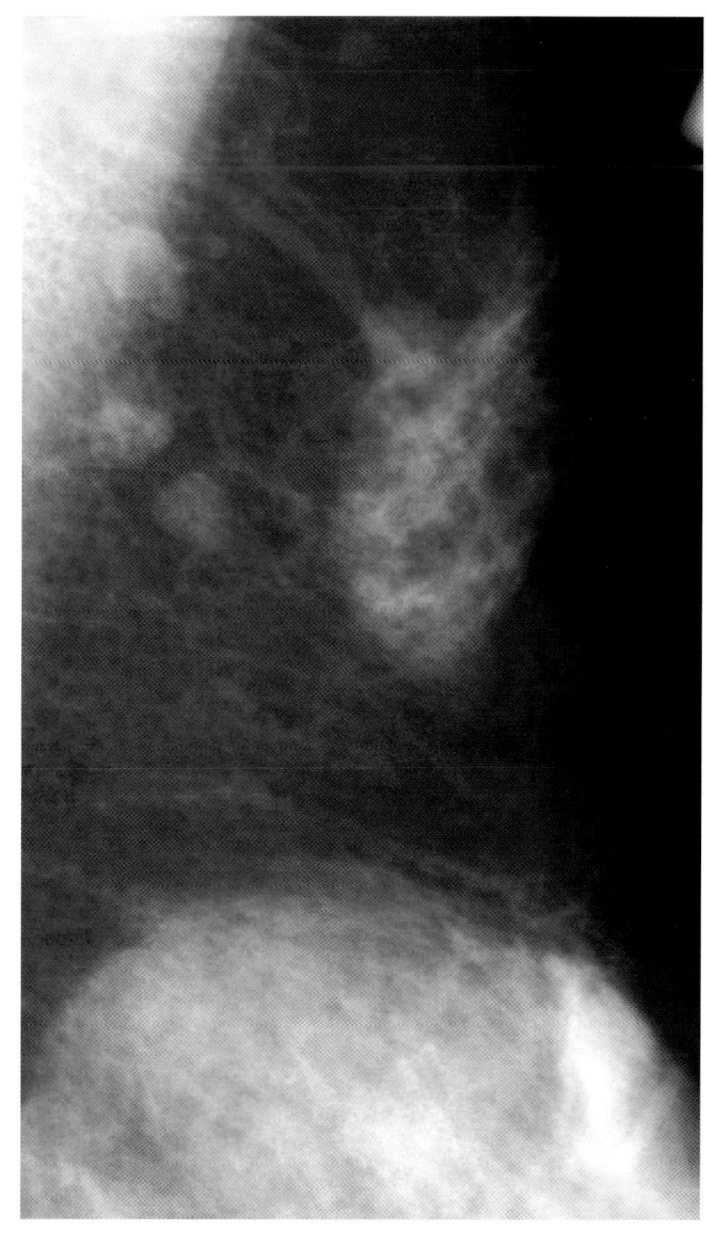

Detail of the mediolateral oblique projection

NORMAL

Intramammary lymph node

An oval opacity is seen in a para-equatorial position deep in the upperouter quadrant, with sharp margins and an eccentric radiolucent area, corresponding to the intramammary lymph node. The finding of one or more low-density circumscribed round or oval opacities, usually not bigger than 1 cm, occasionally with a "lucent" centre, in the upperouter quadrant or external equatorial region, is consistent with intramammary lymph nodes and is a normal variant in approximately 5% of all mammograms.

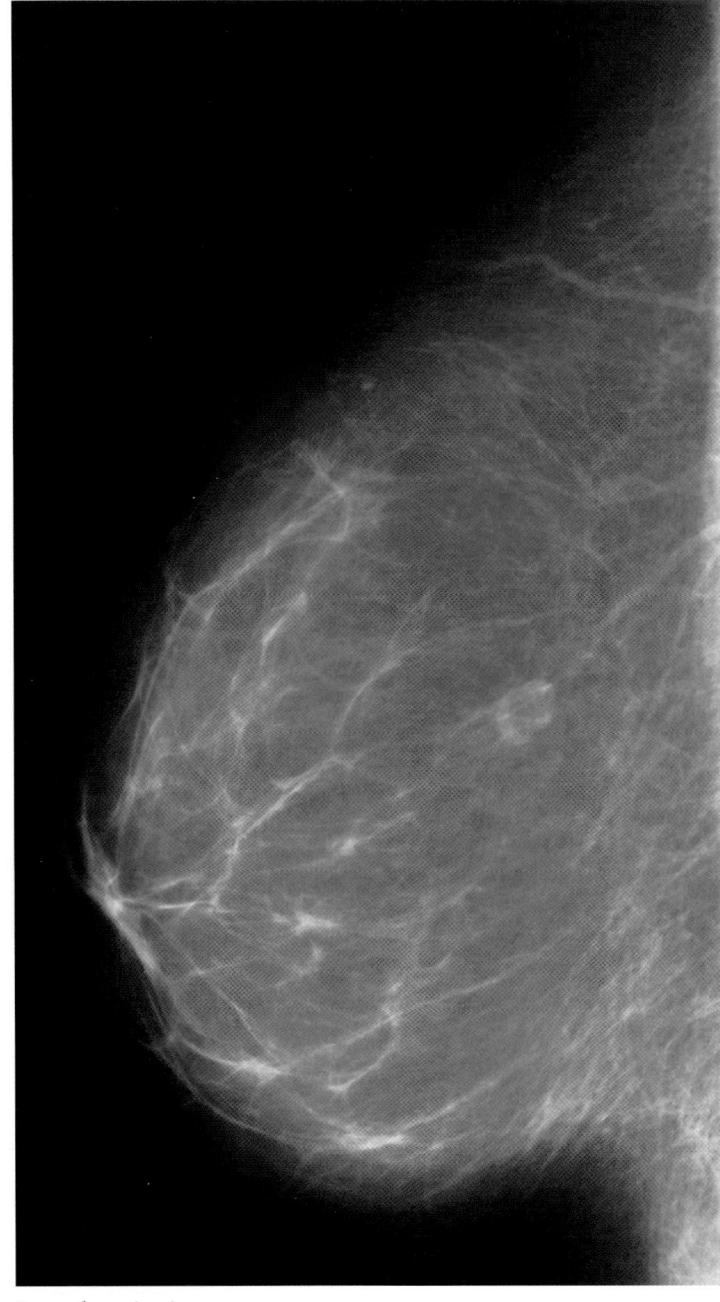

Lateral projection

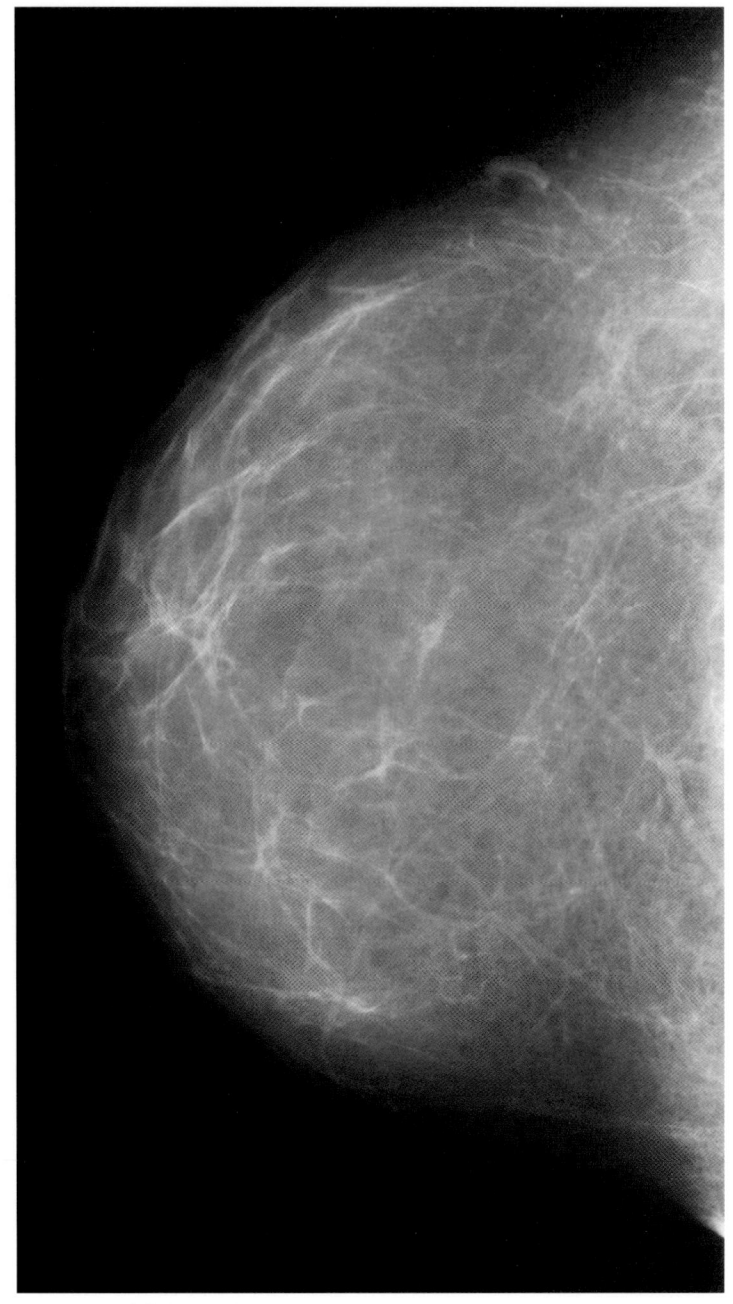

Craniocaudal projection

Intramammary lymph node

An oval opacity is seen in a para-equatorial position deep in the upperouter quadrant, with sharp margins and an eccentric radiolucent area, corresponding to the intramammary lymph node. The finding of one or more low-density circumscribed round or oval opacities, usually not bigger than 1 cm, occasionally with a "lucent" centre, in the upperouter quadrant or external equatorial region, is consistent with intramammary lymph nodes and is a normal variant in approximately 5% of all mammograms.
In the close-up, the lymph node shows an eccentric hilar notch, a fairly typical feature.

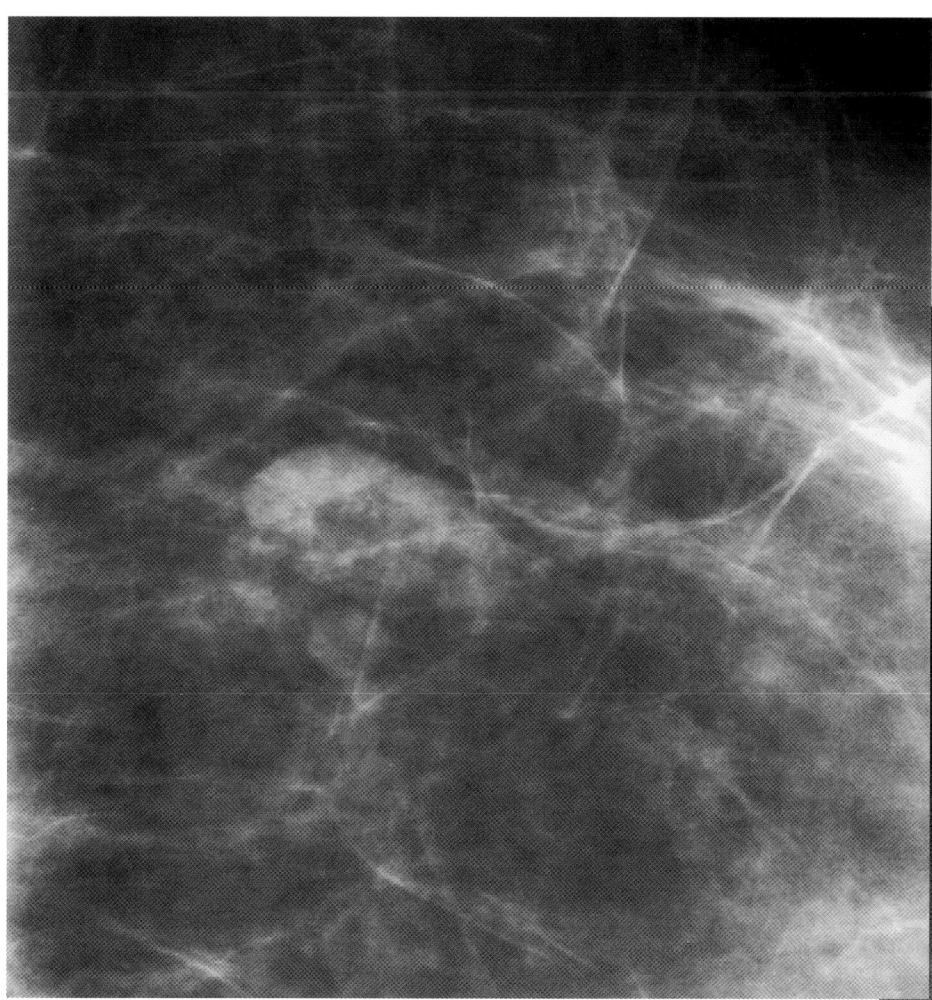

Magnification view

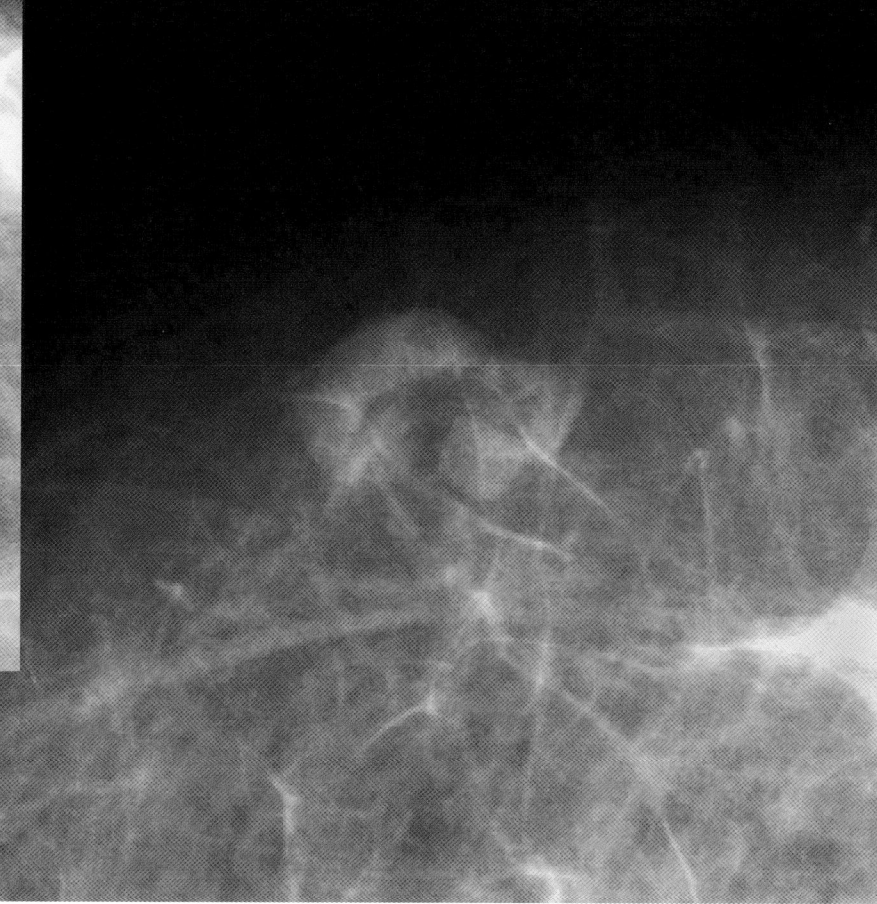

Magnification view

NORMAL

Intramammary lymph node

Small bilateral circumscribed multiple opacities, with sharp margins. On the right, the largest opacity has an eccentric pattern of radiolucency. The finding of one or more low-density circumscribed round or oval opacities, usually not bigger than 1 cm, occasionally with a "lucent" centre, in the upperouter quadrant or external equatorial region, is consistent with intramammary lymph nodes and is a normal variant. Intramammary lymph nodes in the central or medial portion of the breast are extremely uncommon, occurring in less than 1% of cases.

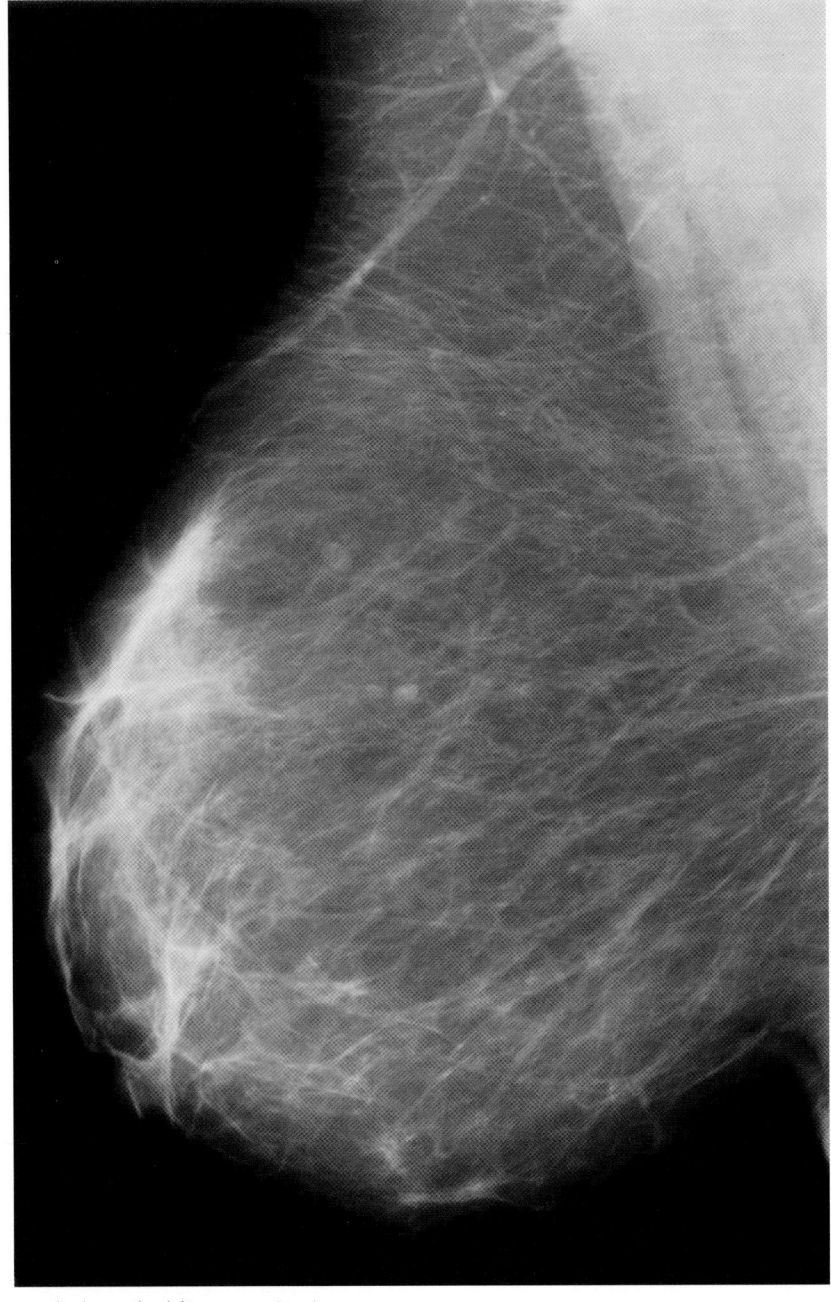

Mediolateral oblique projection

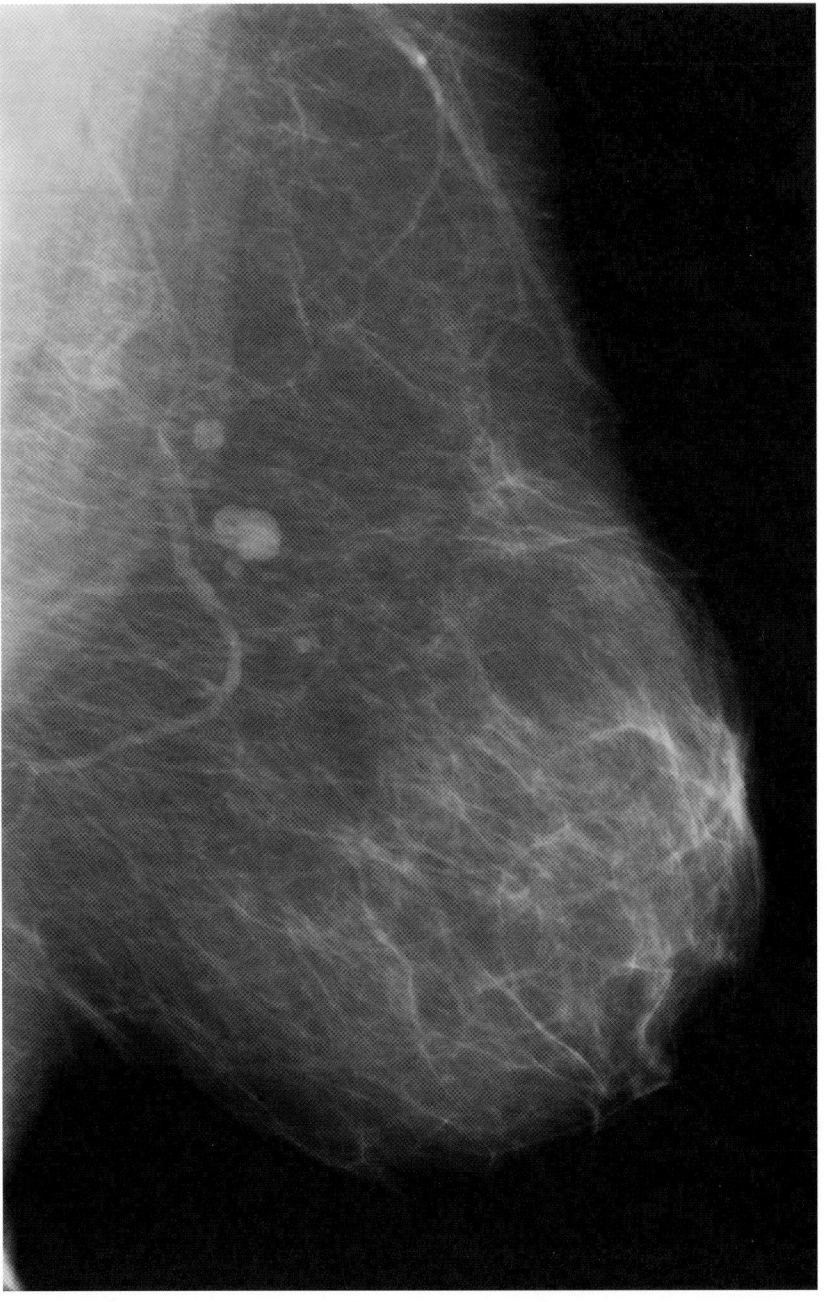

Mediolateral oblique projection

Intramammary lymph node

Small bilateral circumscribed multiple opacities, with sharp margins. On the right, the largest opacity has an eccentric pattern of radiolucency. The finding of one or more low-density circumscribed round or oval opacities, usually not bigger than 1 cm, occasionally with a "lucent" centre, in the upperouter quadrant or external equatorial region, is consistent with intramammary lymph nodes and is a normal variant.

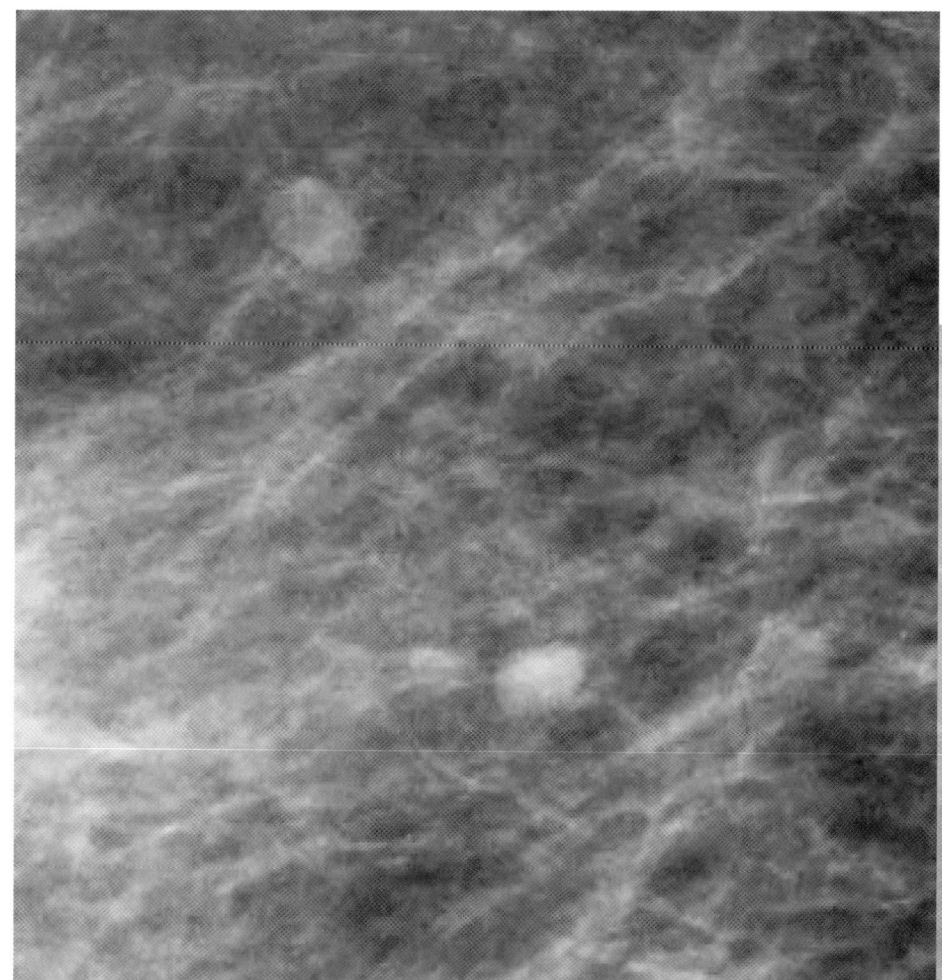

Magnification view

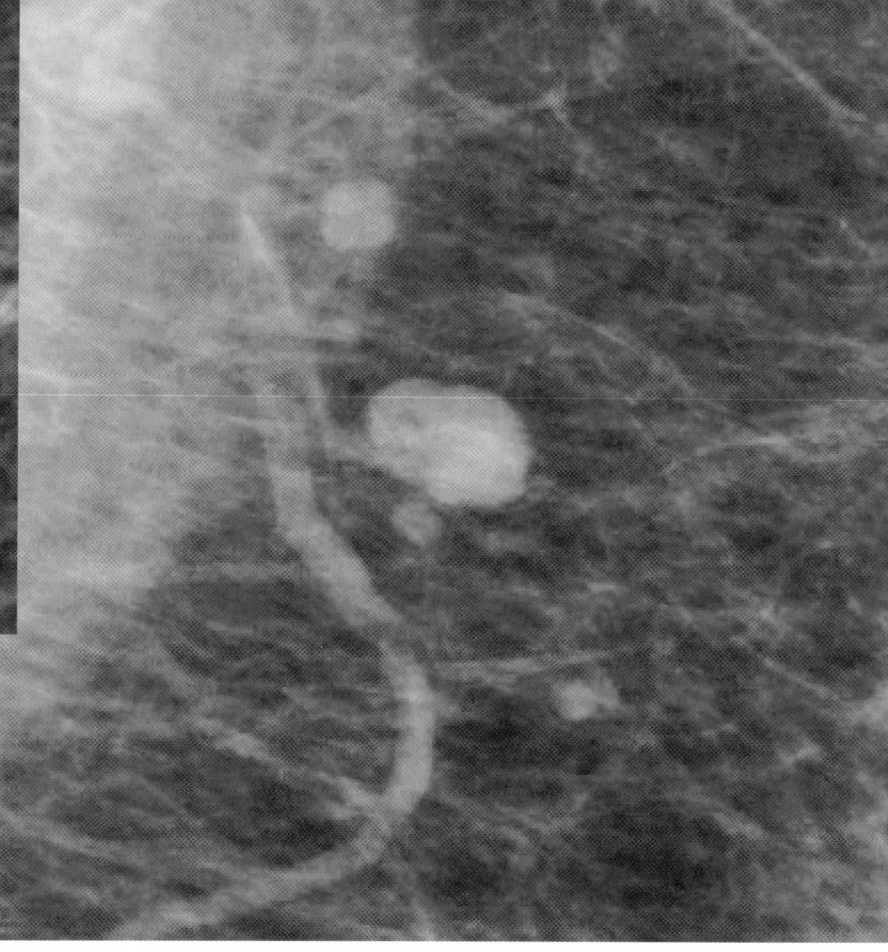

Magnification view

NORMAL

Lipomatosis of the axillary cavity
Bilaterally, the axillary profile has lost its concavity, as if the subcutaneous tissue had become slack or relaxed, due to hyperplasia of the fatty tissue, also causing deep skin folds. Multiple aspecific, non pathologic adenopathies are seen, some apparently made up entirely of a "radiolucent" hilus.

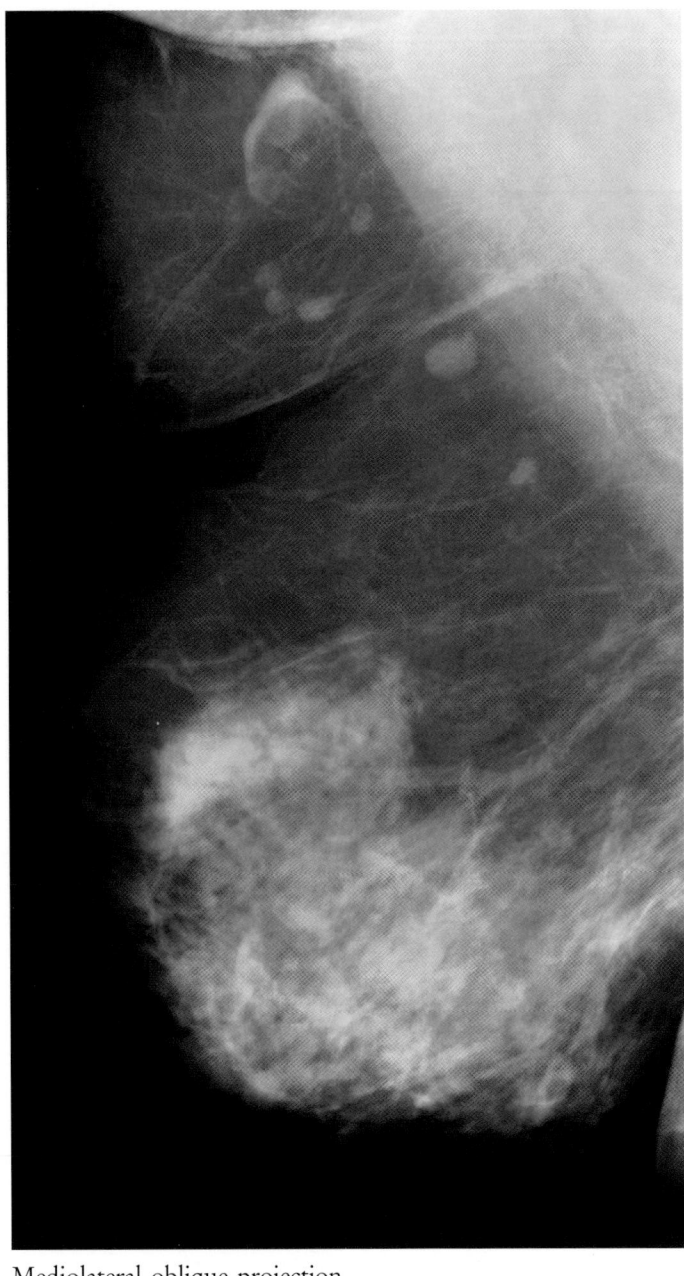

Mediolateral oblique projection

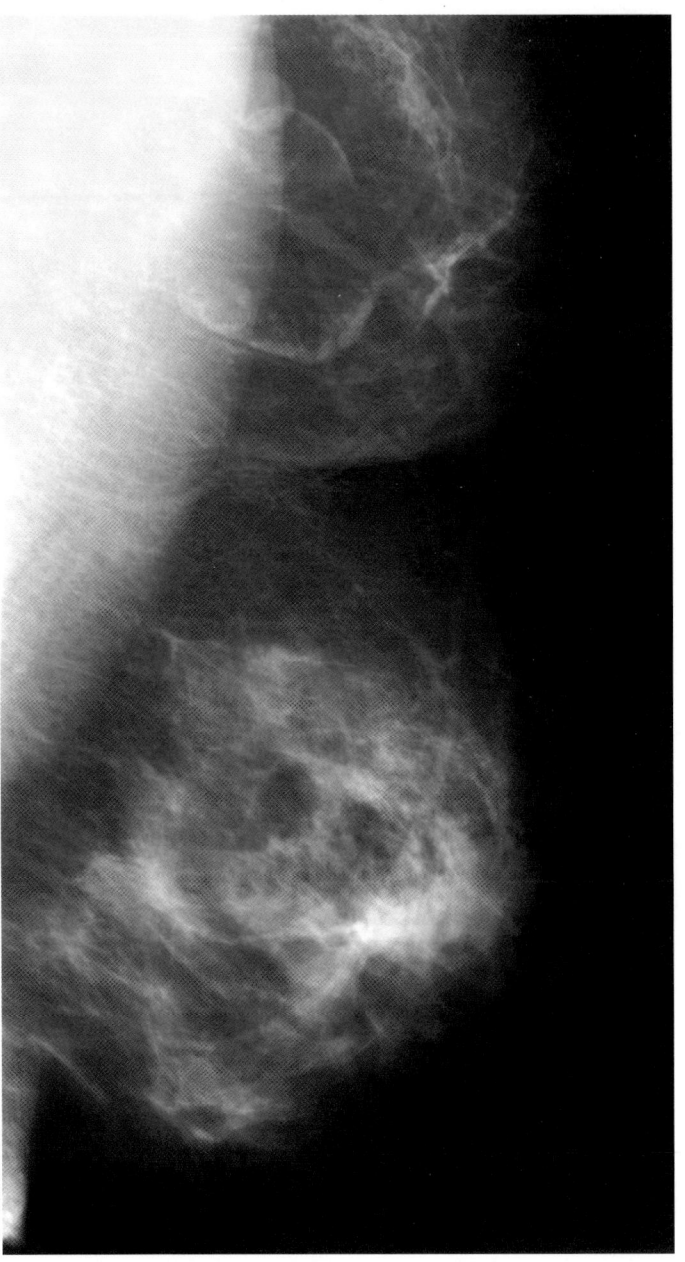

Mediolateral oblique projection

Axillary lymph nodes

Circumscribed sharp-edged mono- or bilateral opacities, varying in density and volume, are commonly observed in the armpit; some have a lucent centre and may become slivers of tissue due to marked fatty infiltration. These are caused by aspecific adenopathies and are not a sign of malignancy.

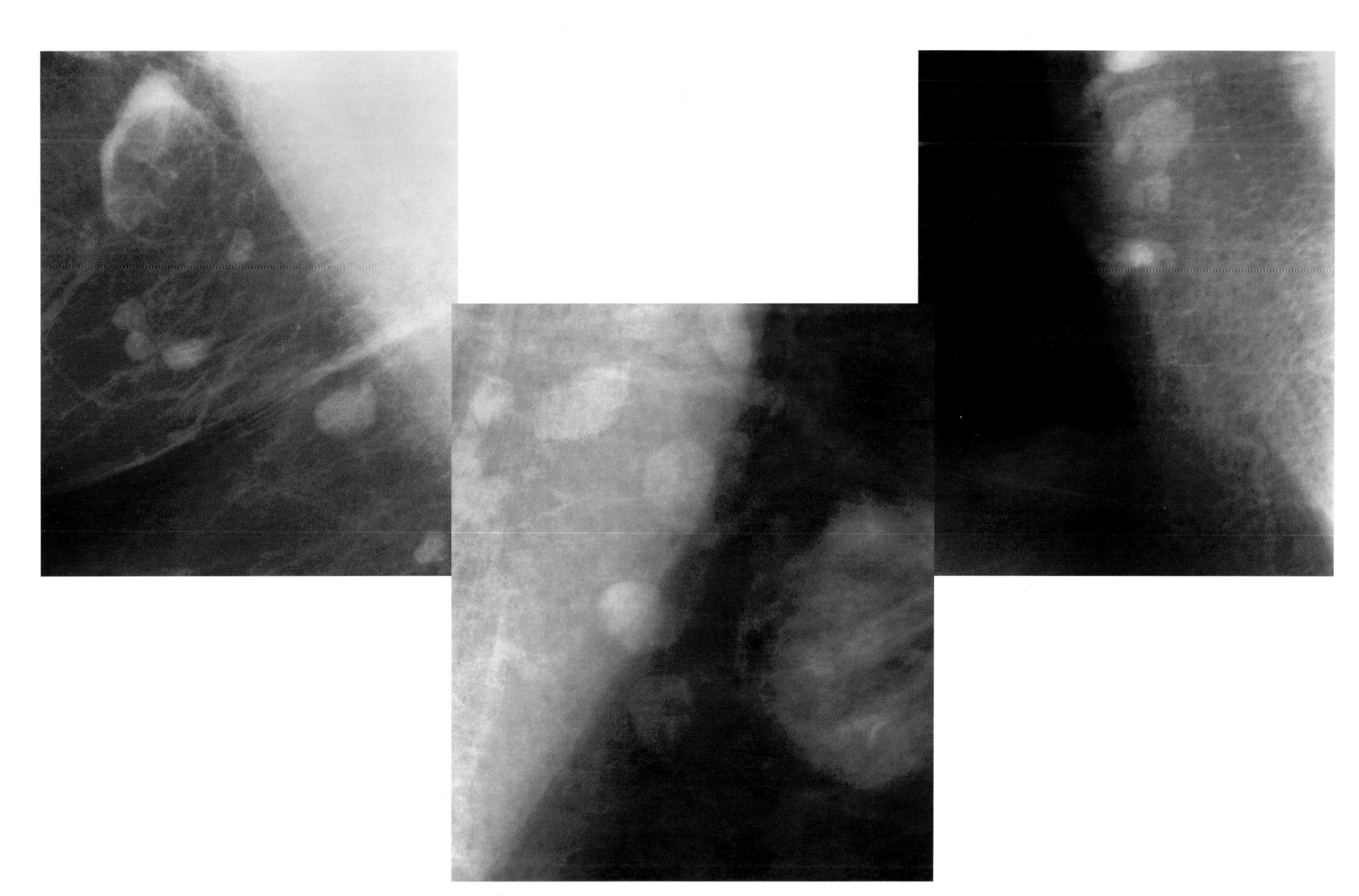

Magnification views

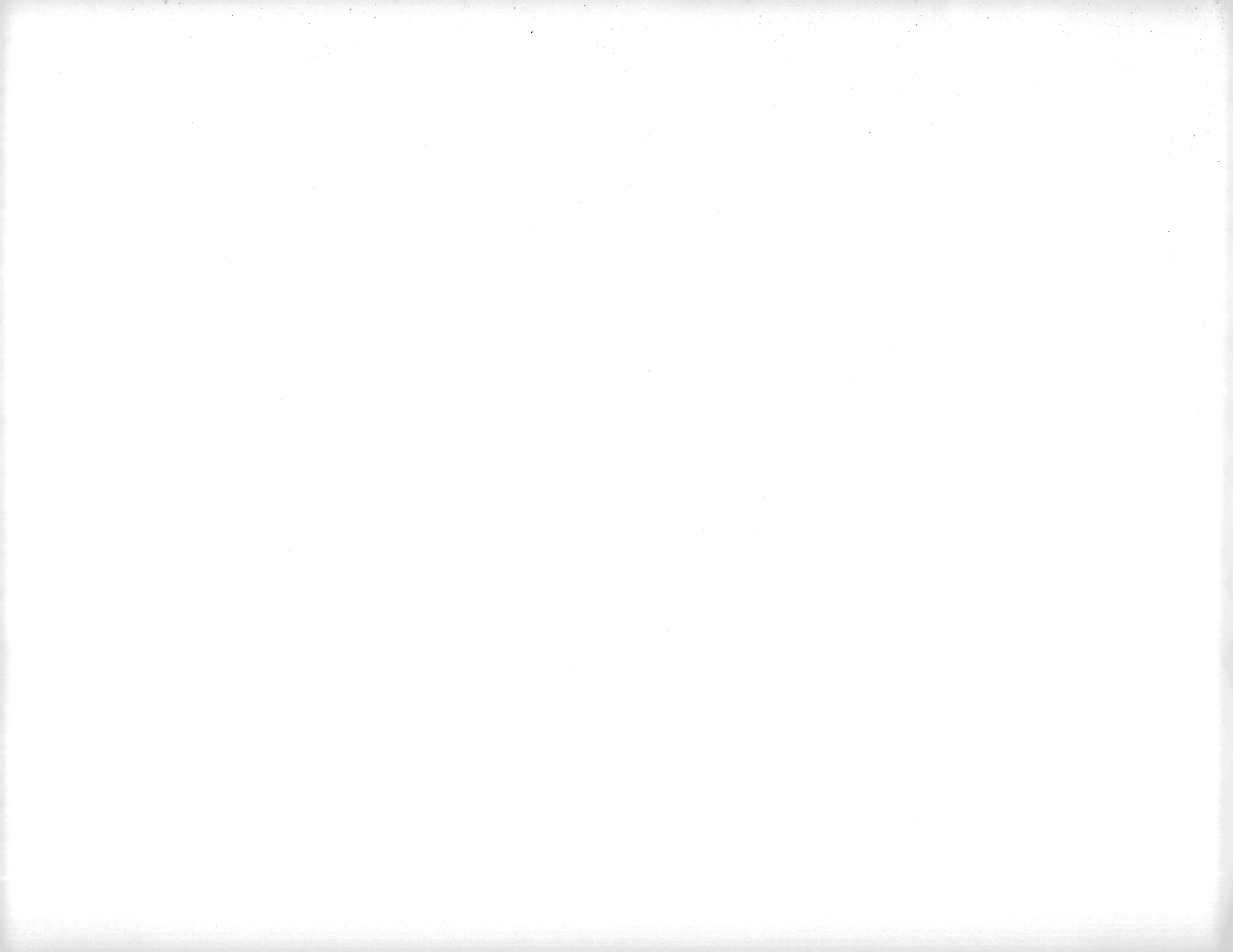

MAMMOGRAPHIC SIGNS

The detection and identification of elementary mammographic signs form the basis for correctly interpreting breast pathologies and describing them accurately in the mammographic report. The specific features are the basis for classifying the lesions as either benign or malignant. These features define the positive predictive value (PPV), i.e. the odds that a mammographic sign is associated with or actually shows a cancerous lesion.

Mammographic signs can be described in terms of:

- *Opacity (mass)*
- *Architectural distortion*
- *Calcifications*
- *Radiolucency*
- *Asymmetry*
- *Focal asymmetry*
- *Skin thickening and retraction*
- *Oedema and trabecular thickening*
- *Asymmetrically dilated ducts*

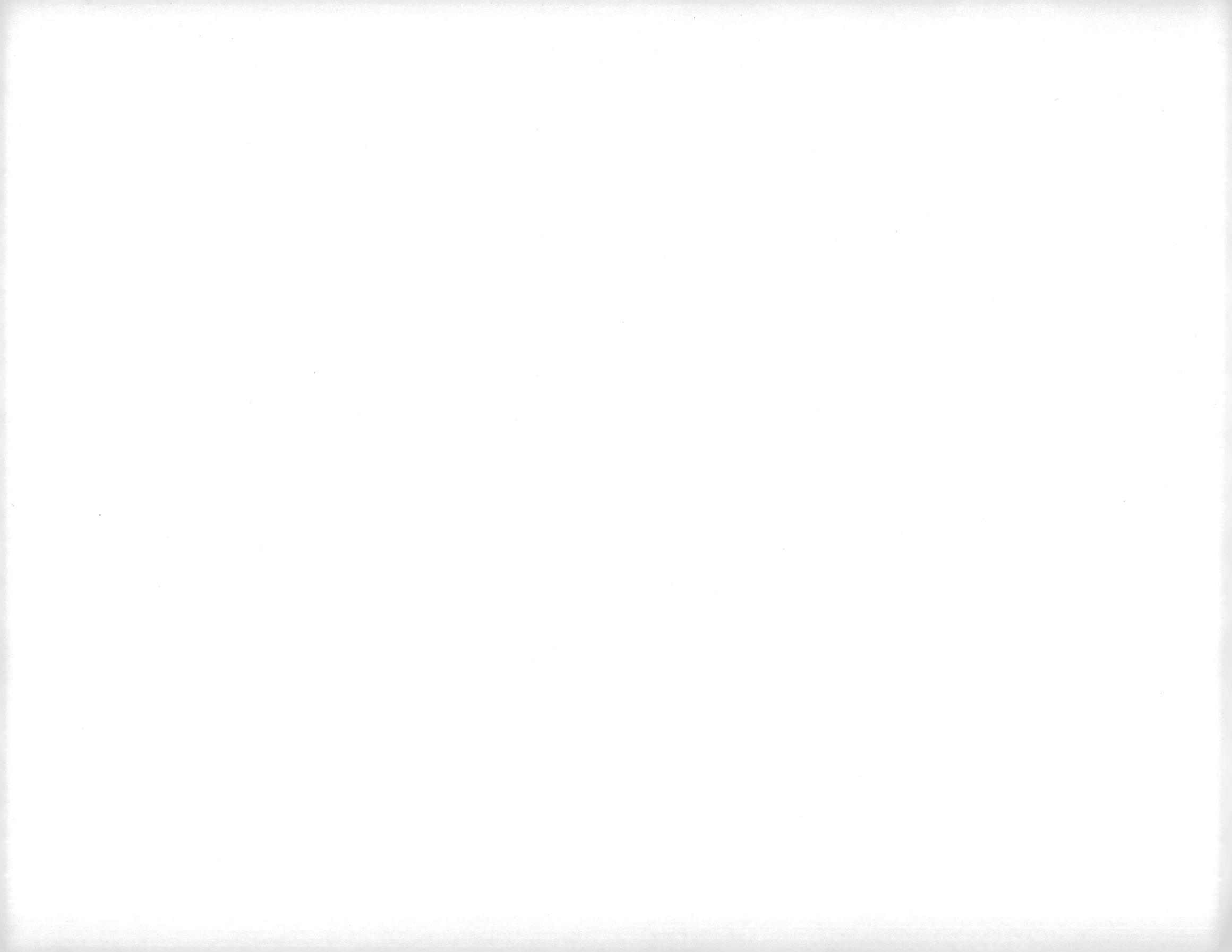

OPACITY

Definition
A space-occupying lesion visible in two projections, implying the concept of mass and volume. An alteration visible in just one projection can be described as a density or focal asymmetry.

Classification
Opacities may be circumscribed, stellate or diffuse.

Evaluation
Analysis of an opacity must evaluate:
its shape, margins, density, diameter, site and position, associated microcalcifications, number (one or more), mono- or bilaterality, correlation with patient's history and physical examination.

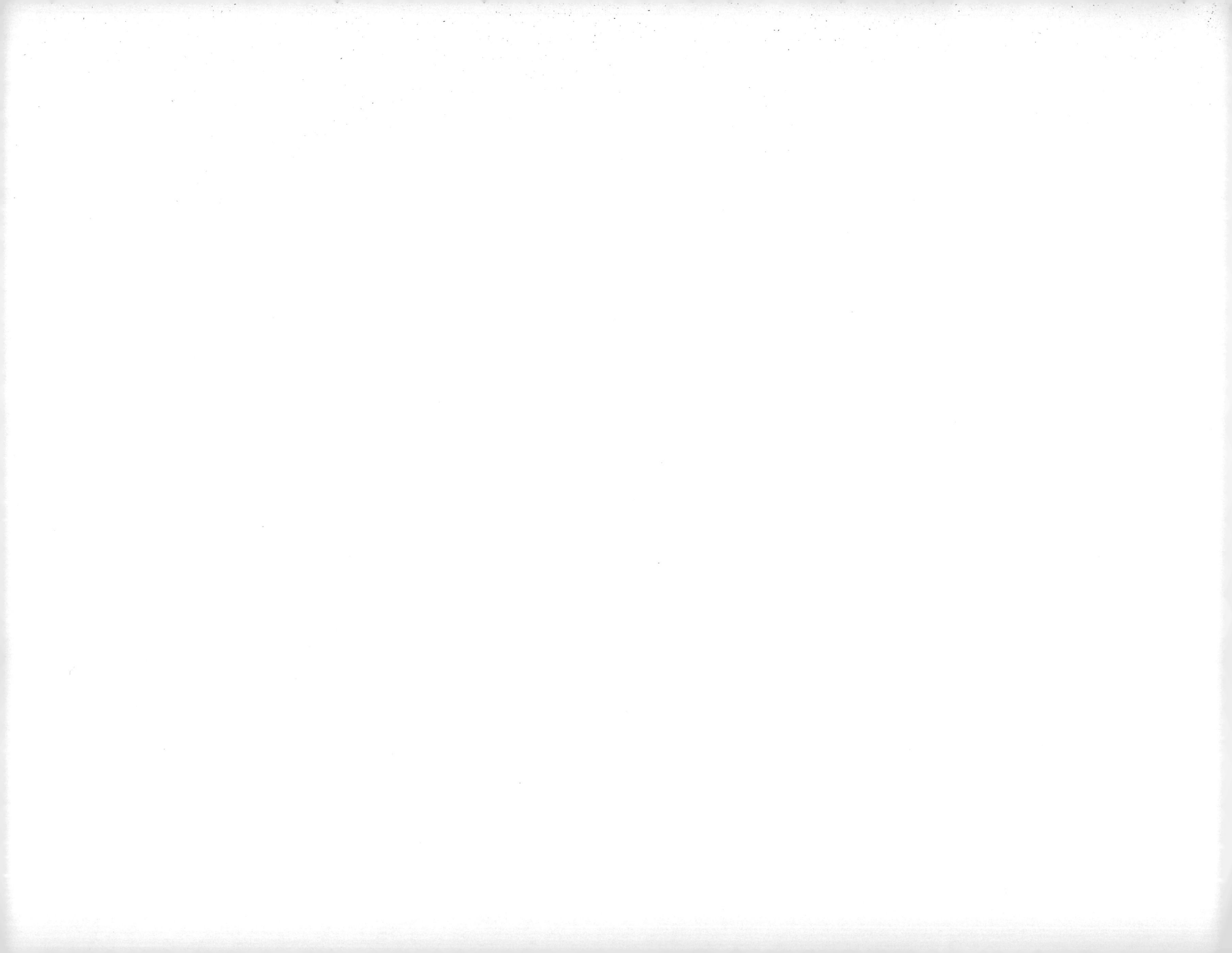

Circumscribed opacity

Definition
A morphologically well-defined opacity with a curved shape, either round or oval.

Shape
Circumscribed opacities may be round, oval, lobulated or irregular.

Margins
Margins may be sharp, blurred, ill-defined or spiculated.

Density
The density of an opacity may be the same as or higher than that of the surrounding tissue. The opacity may contain fatty tissue, giving mixed images with alternating dense and radiolucent areas.

CIRCUMSCRIBED OPACITY

Round shape
Round opacity with sharp margins. A radiolucent rim almost completely encloses the mass. Density is homogeneous and markedly higher than the surrounding tissue.

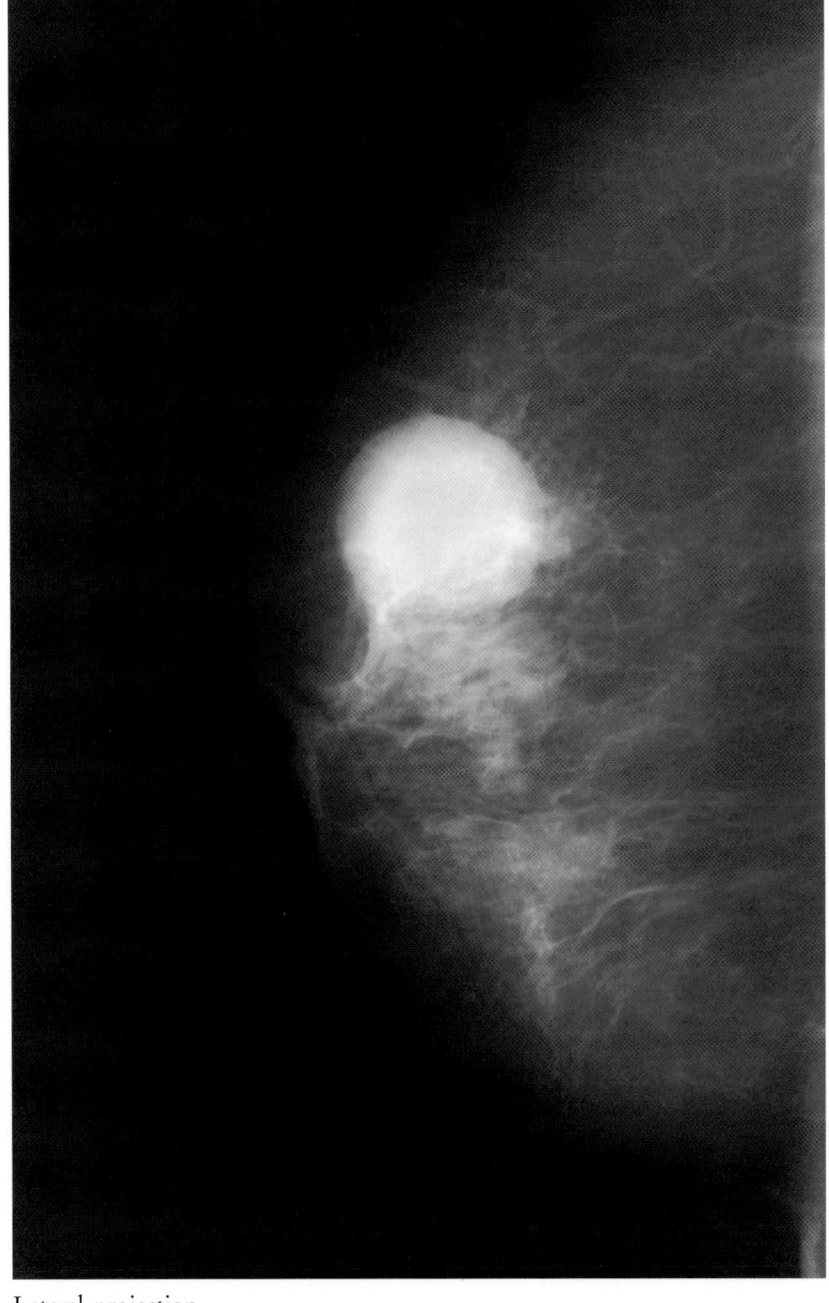

Lateral projection

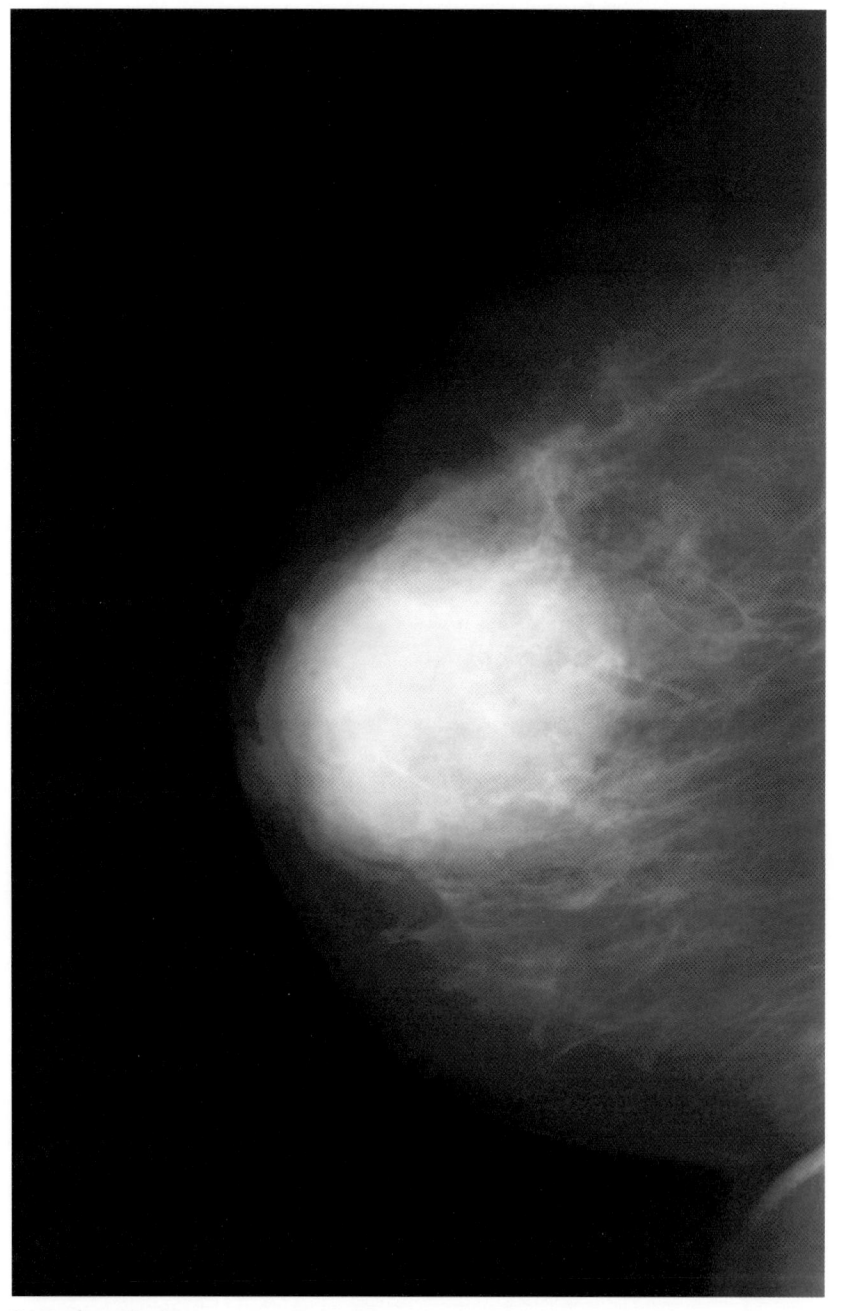

Lateral projection

Round shape

Round opacity with sharp margins. A radiolucent rim almost completely encloses the mass.
Density is homogeneous and markedly higher than the surrounding tissue (A, B).
Multiple circumscribed opacities, varying in volume, are disseminated throughout the breast.

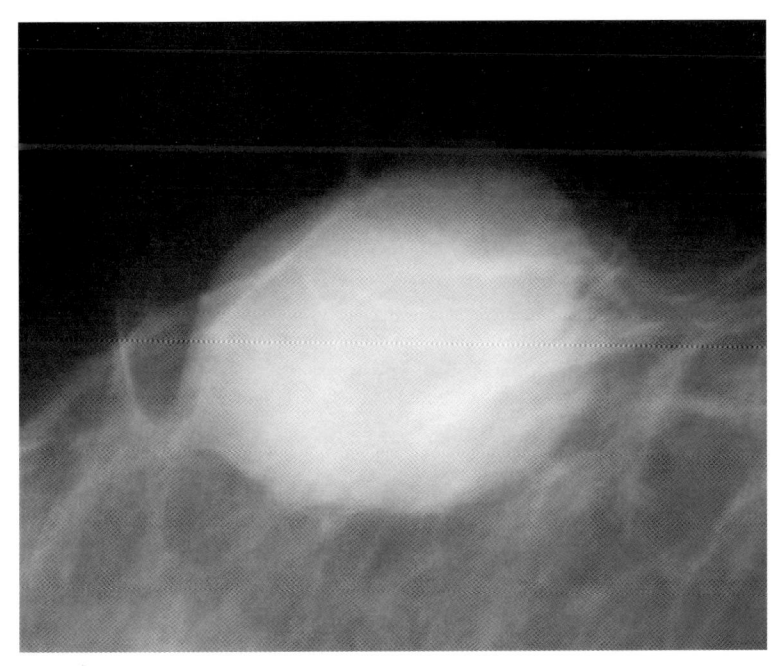

Detail of the craniocaudal projection (A)

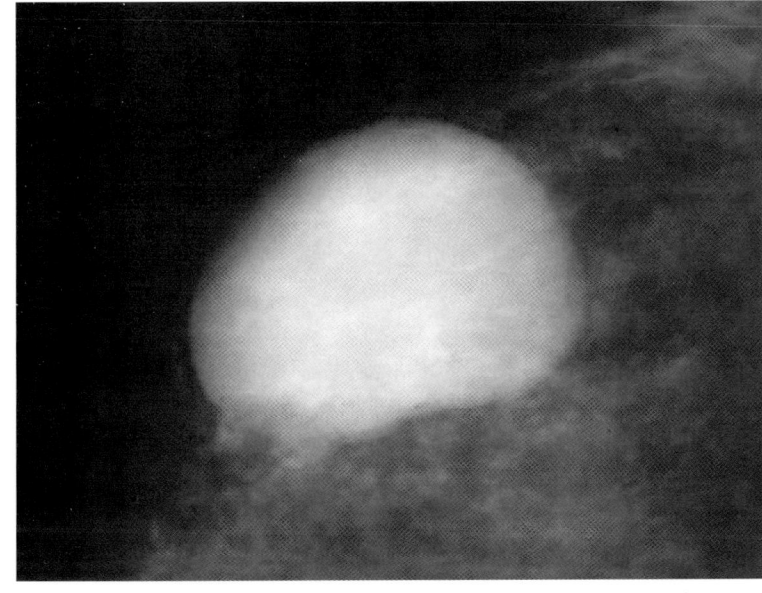

Detail of the craniocaudal projection (B)

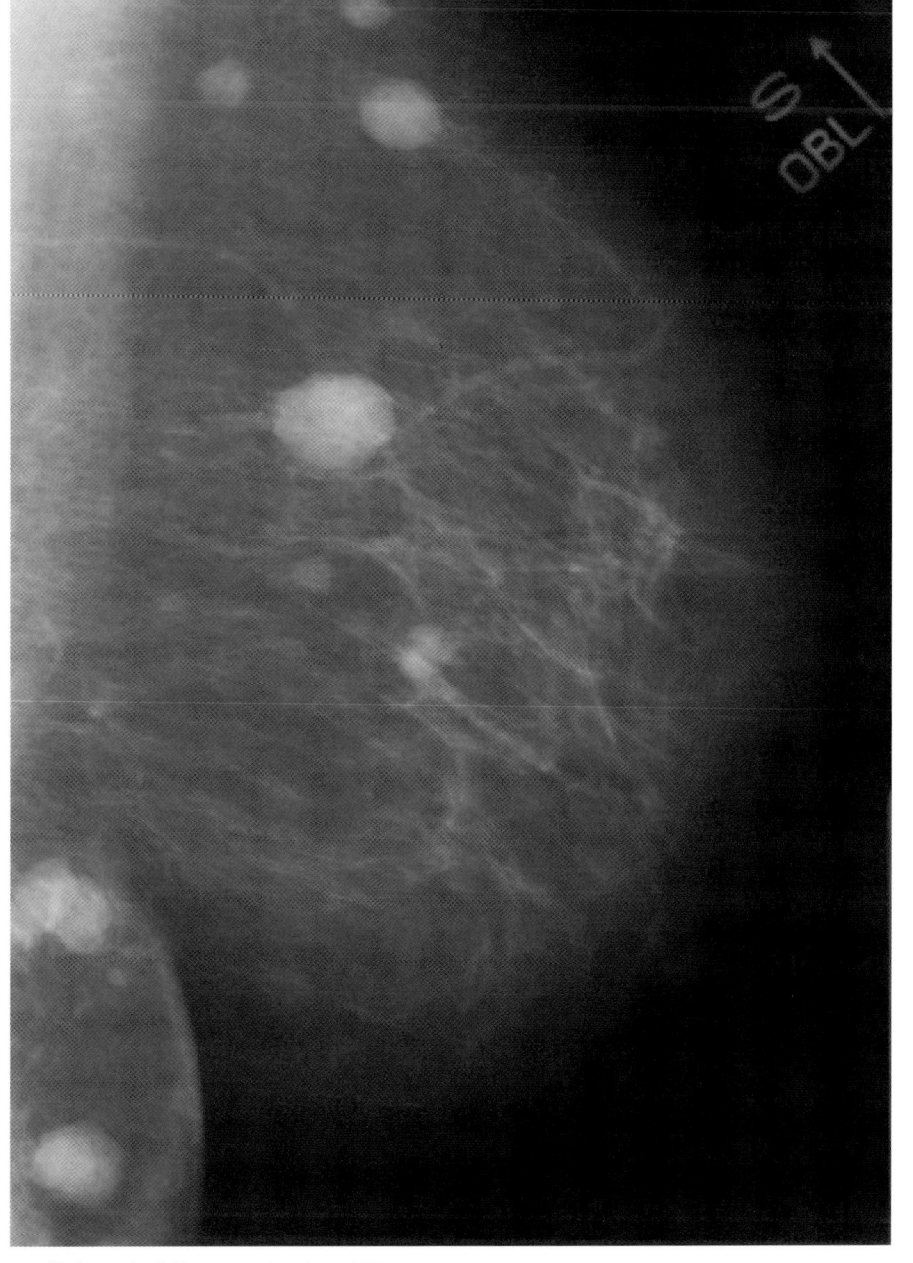

Mediolateral oblique projection (C)

CIRCUMSCRIBED OPACITY

Oval shape
Circumscribed retroareolar oval opacity with well-defined margins. Radiolucent rim completely surrounding the mass.

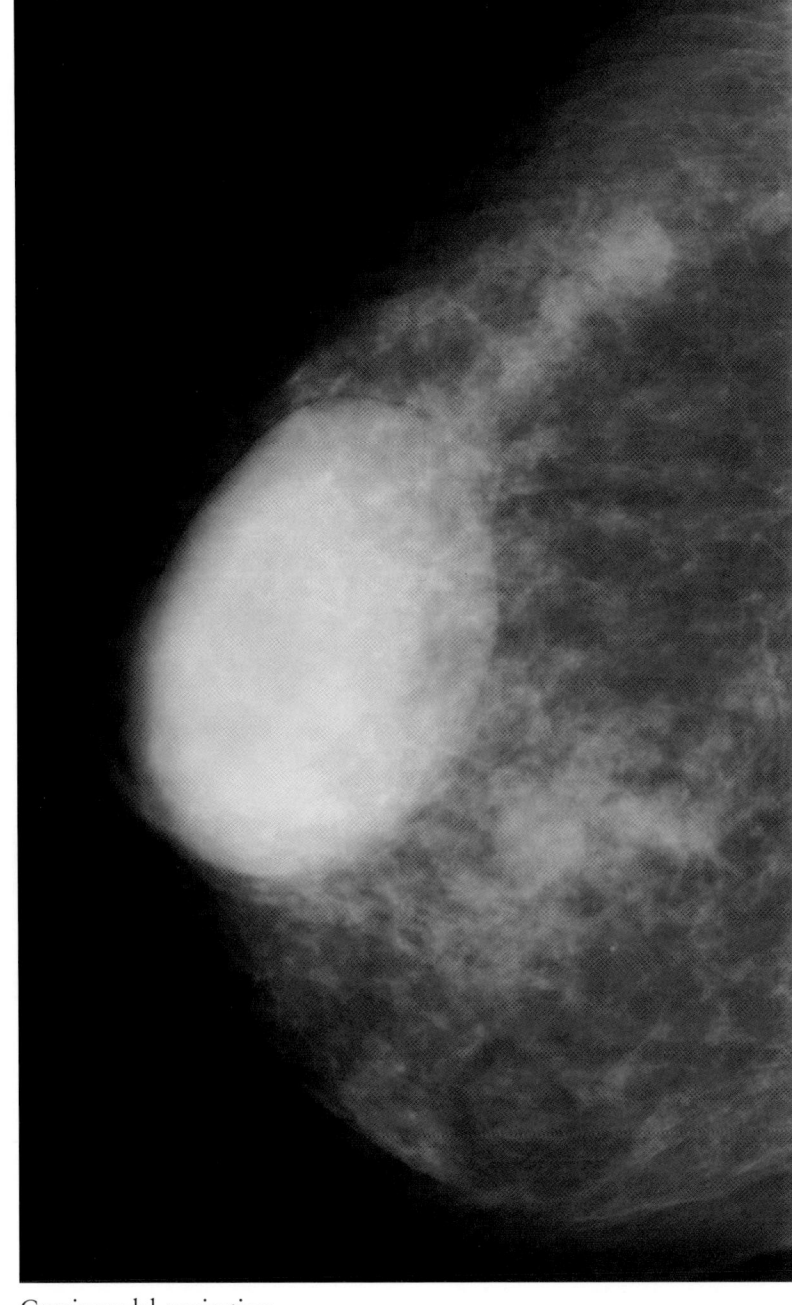

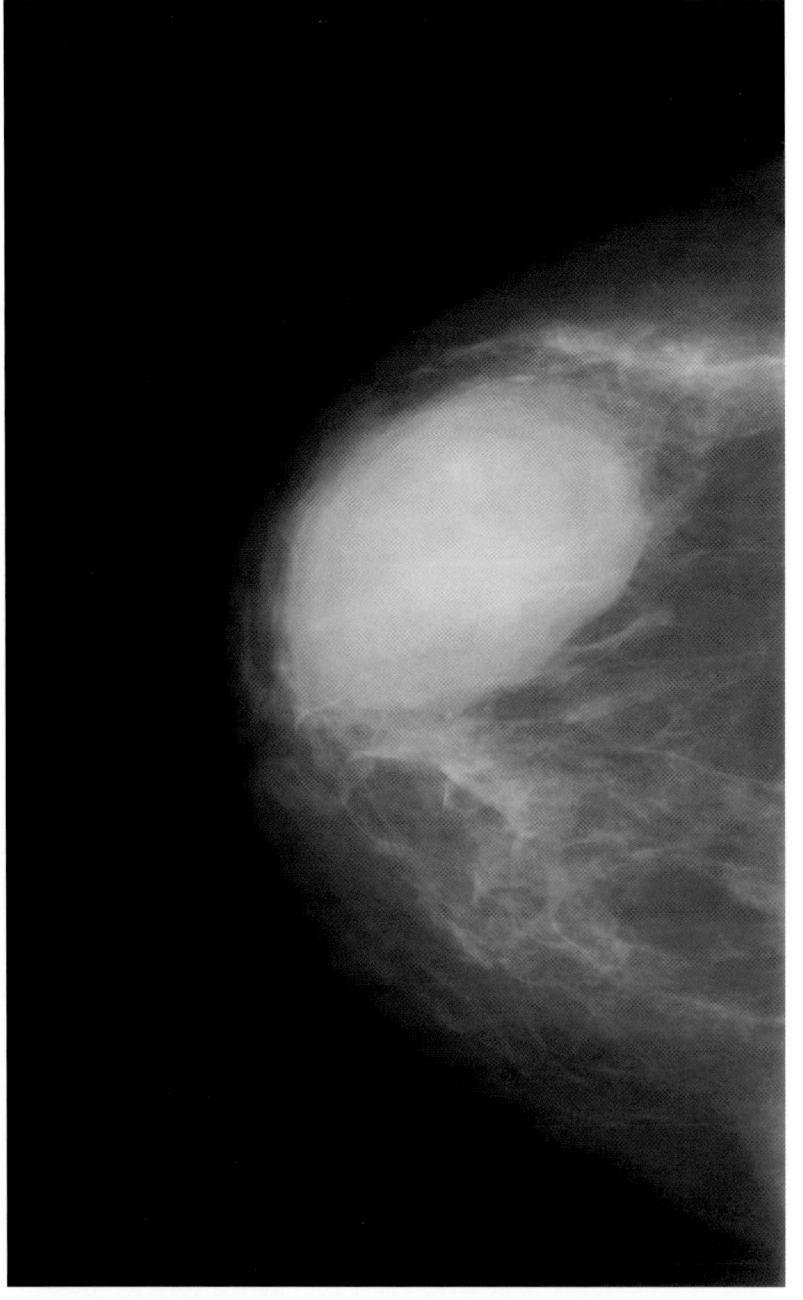

Craniocaudal projection

Craniocaudal projection

Oval shape

Elliptical opacity, with sharp margins. Radiolucent rim almost completely enclosing the mass. Density is homogeneous and markedly higher than the surrounding tissue.

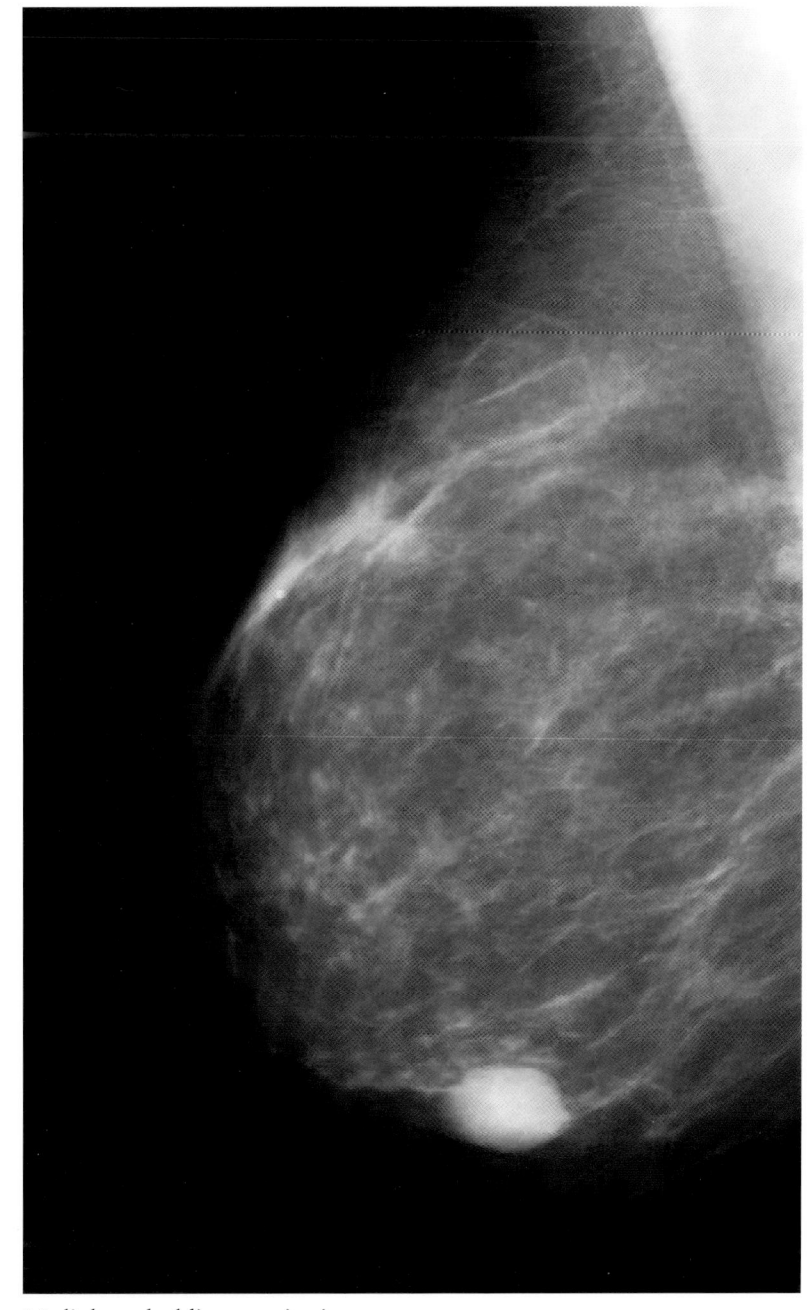

Mediolateral oblique projection

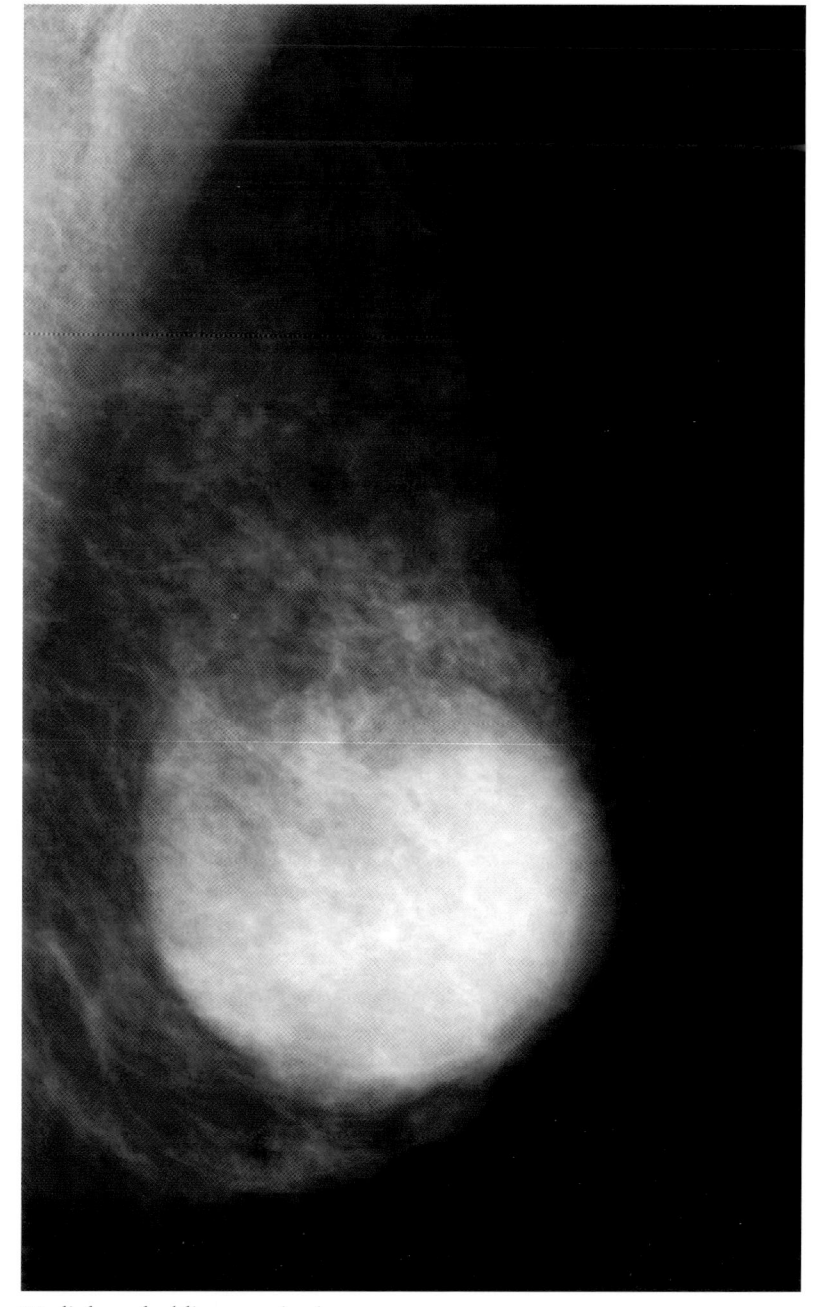

Mediolateral oblique projection

CIRCUMSCRIBED OPACITY

Lobulated shape

A circumscribed, retroareolar lobulated opacity is visible, with sharp margins, and a radiolucent rim clearly seen posteriorly. Density markedly higher than the surrounding tissue.

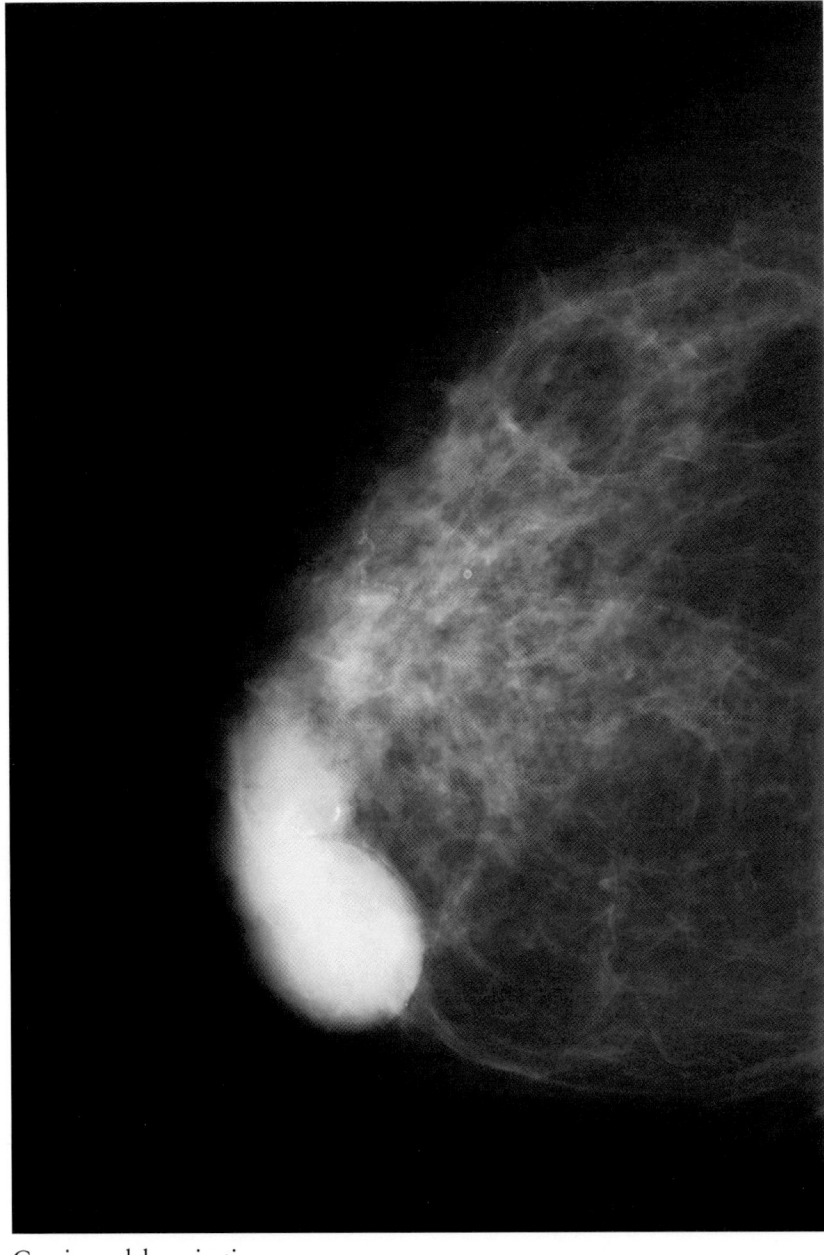

Craniocaudal projection

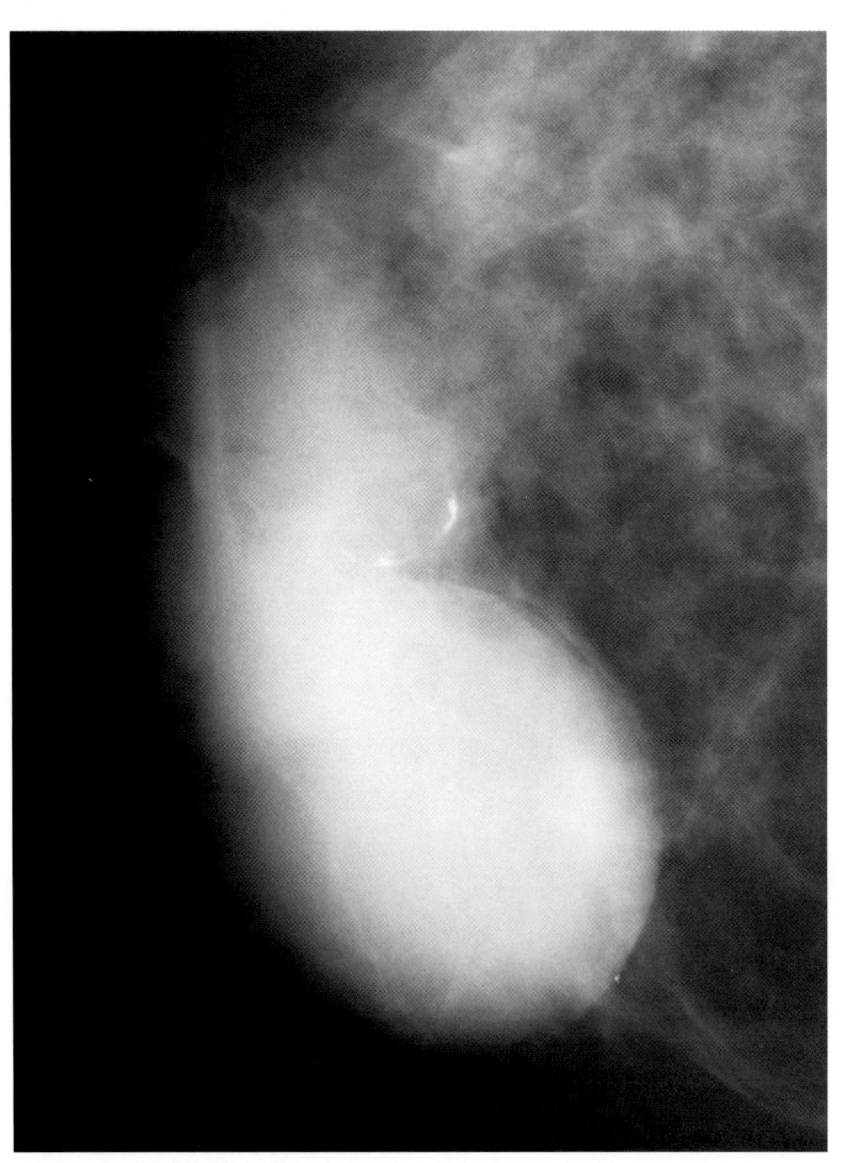

Craniocaudal projection, close-up

Lobulated shape

A circumscribed, retroareolar lobulated opacity is visible, with sharp margins, and a radiolucent rim clearly seen posteriorly. Density markedly higher than the surrounding tissue.

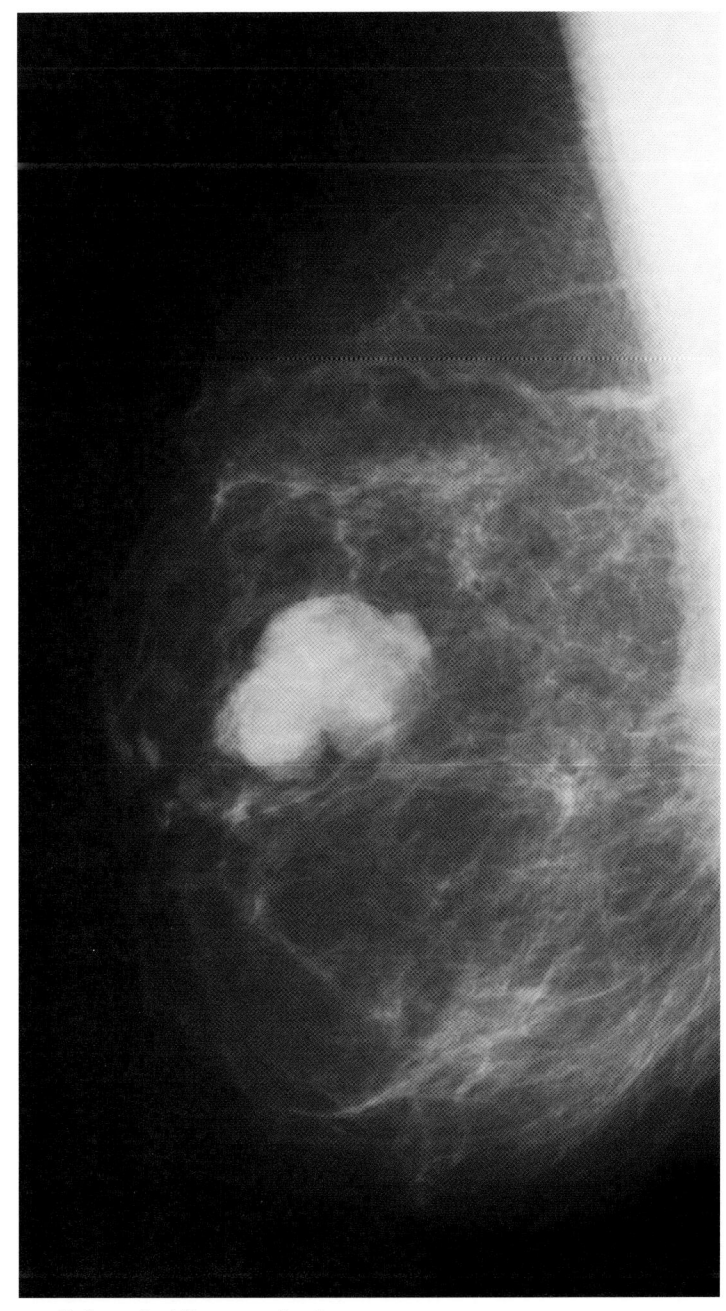

Mediolateral oblique projection

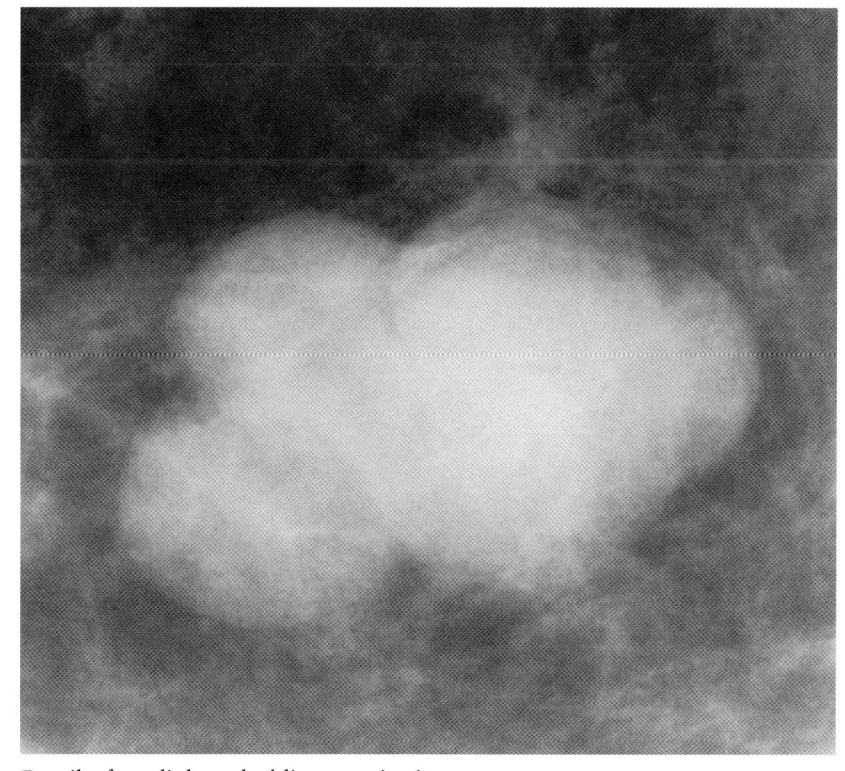

Detail of mediolateral oblique projection

CIRCUMSCRIBED OPACITY

Lobulated shape

This spot compression view shows a circumscribed lobulated opacity with sharp margins and high density.

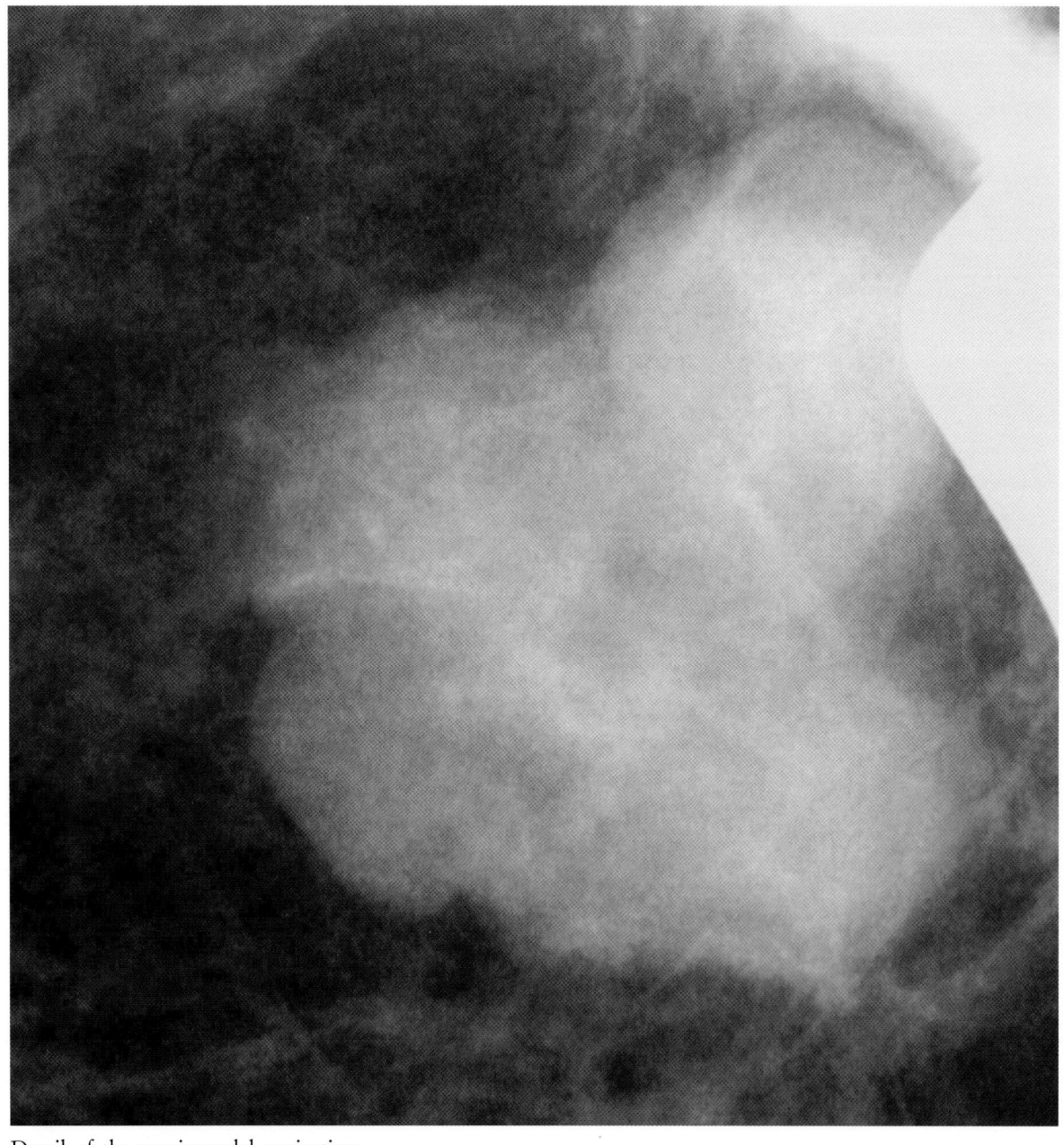

Detail of the craniocaudal projection

Lobulated shape

This spot compression view shows two circumscribed lobulated opacities with sharp margins and high density.

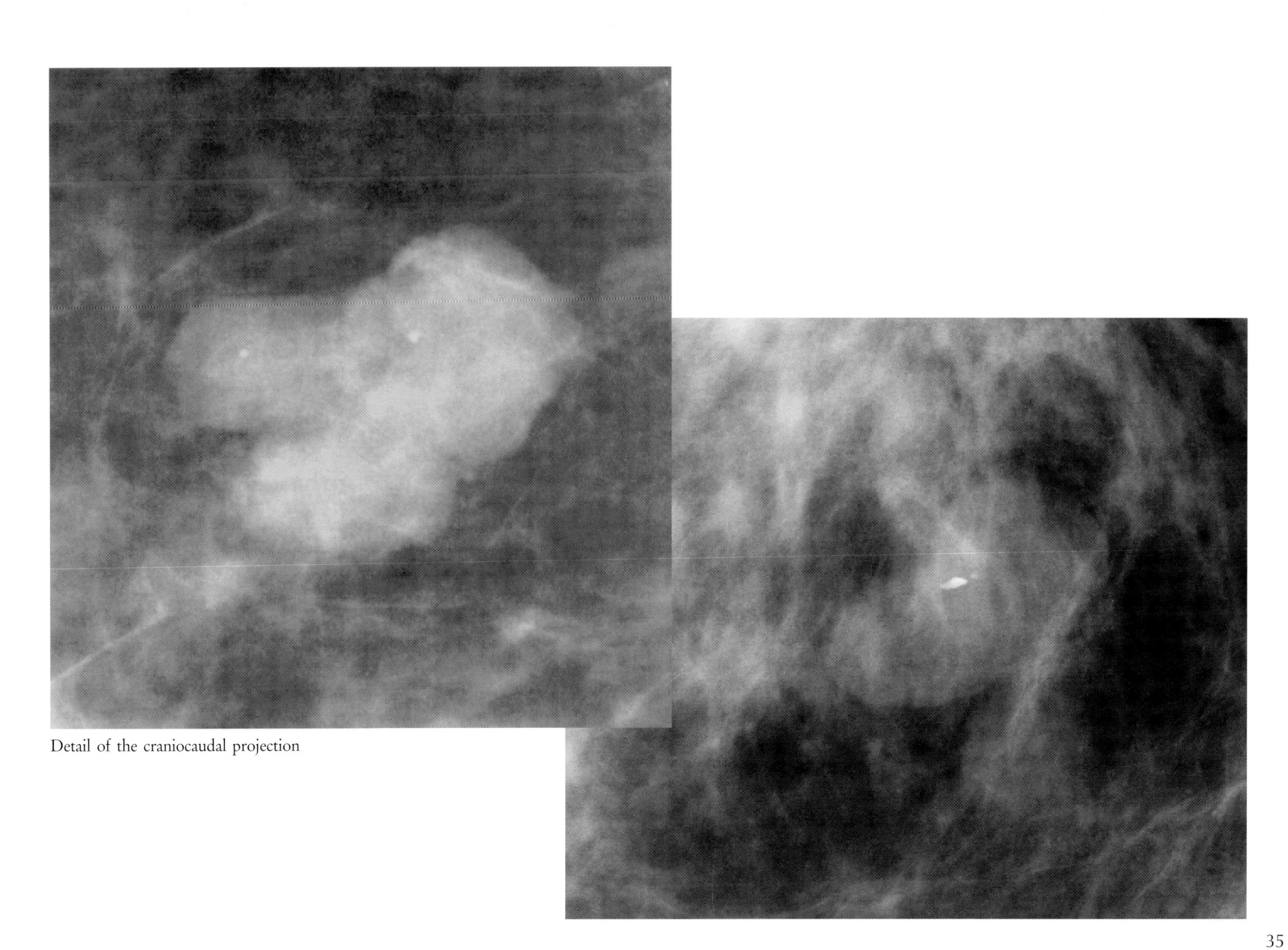

Detail of the craniocaudal projection

CIRCUMSCRIBED OPACITY

Irregular shape

Deep in the centre is a circumscribed low-density opacity, irregular in shape, with margins ill defined posteriorly and blurred anteriorly by breast tissue (A). Behind the areola is a circumscribed high-density opacity, irregular in shape, with moderately thickened and retracted areolar skin (B).

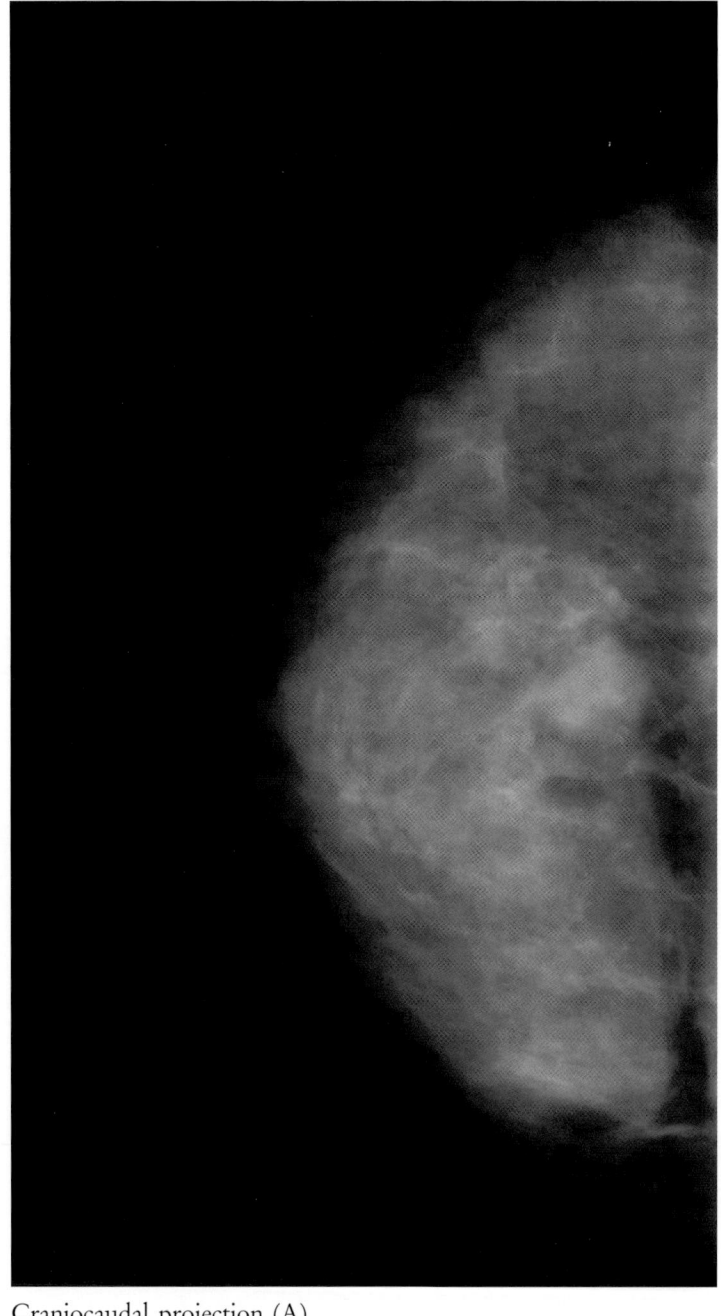

Craniocaudal projection (A)

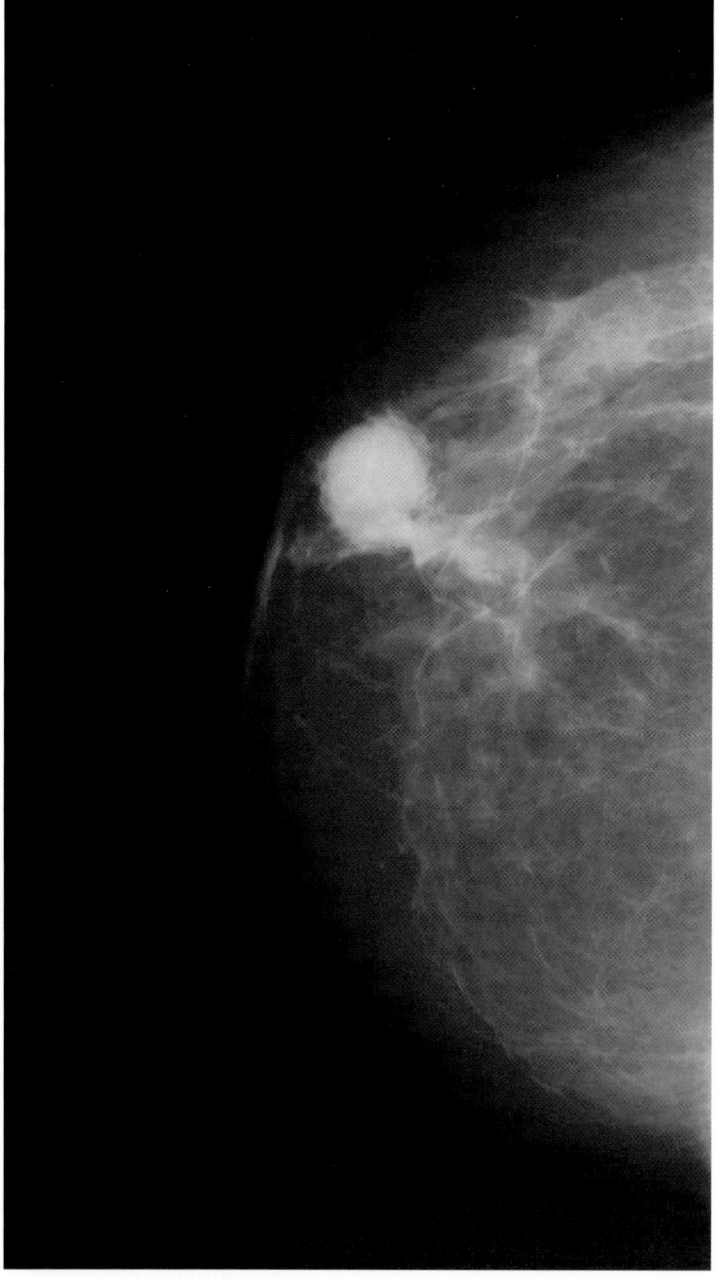

Craniocaudal projection (B)

Irregular shape

An irregularly shaped, circumscribed, low-density opacity, with margins ill defined posteriorly and blurred in the fibroglandular tissue anteriorly (A). Behind the areola is an irregularly shaped, circumscribed, high-density opacity, with moderately thickened and retracted areolar skin (B). The spot compression clearly shows the irregular margins.

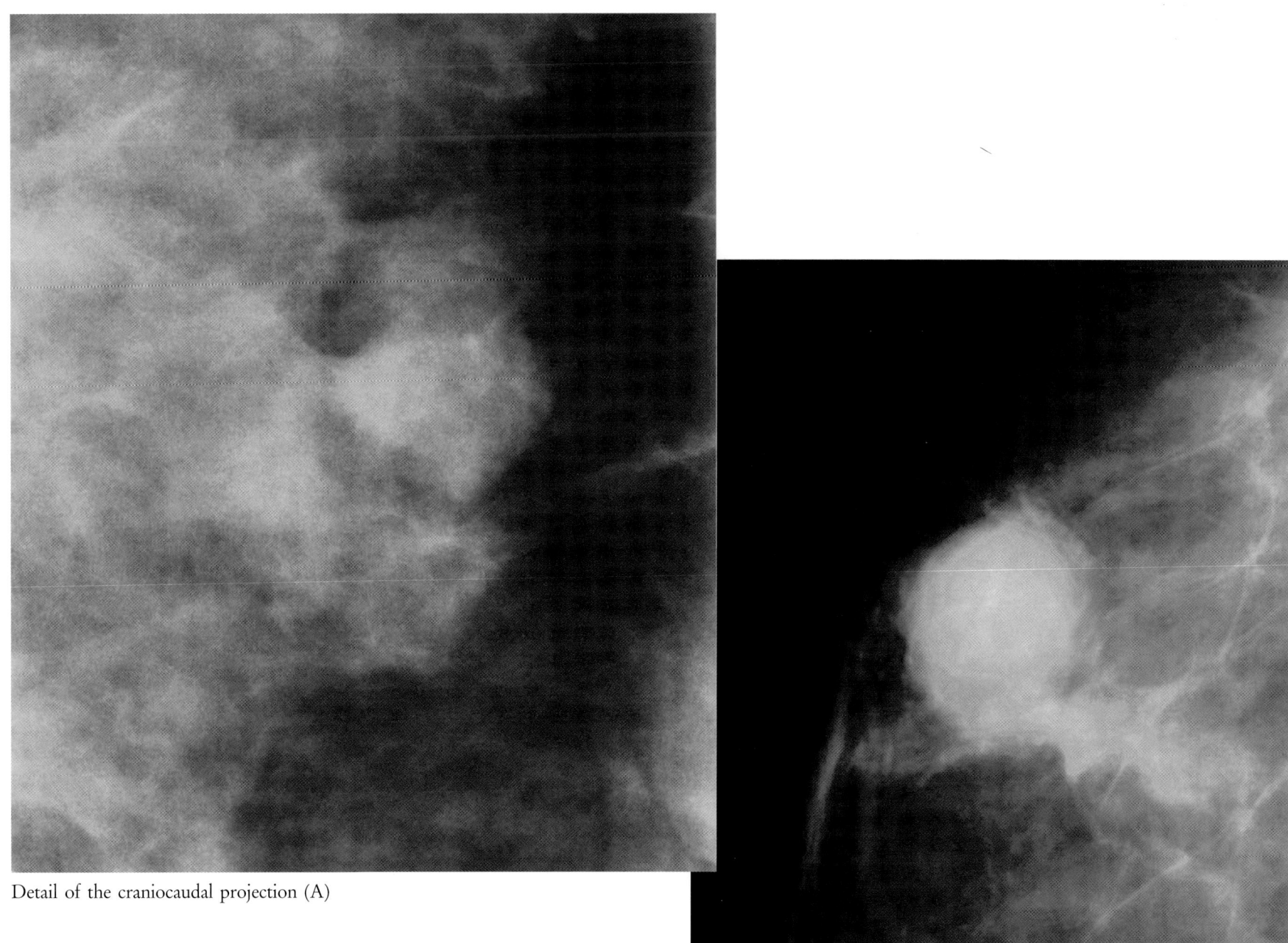

Detail of the craniocaudal projection (A)

Detail of the craniocaudal projection (B)

CIRCUMSCRIBED OPACITY

Irregular shape

In an outer central position, there is an irregularly shaped circumscribed opacity of higher density than the surrounding fibroglandular tissue, with ill-defined margins (A). In a central location, an irregularly shaped circumscribed opacity with ill-defined margins is visible, of the same density as the surrounding tissue (B).

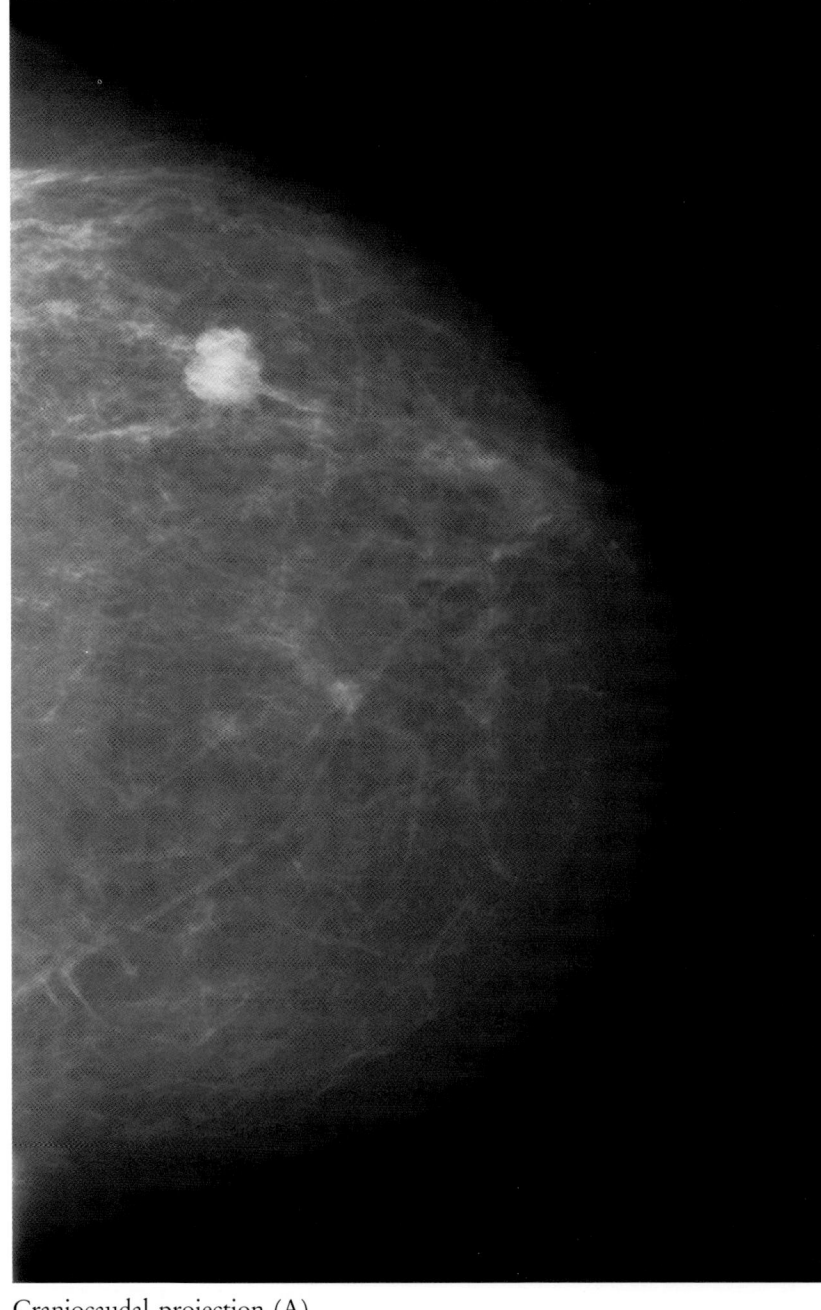

Craniocaudal projection (A)

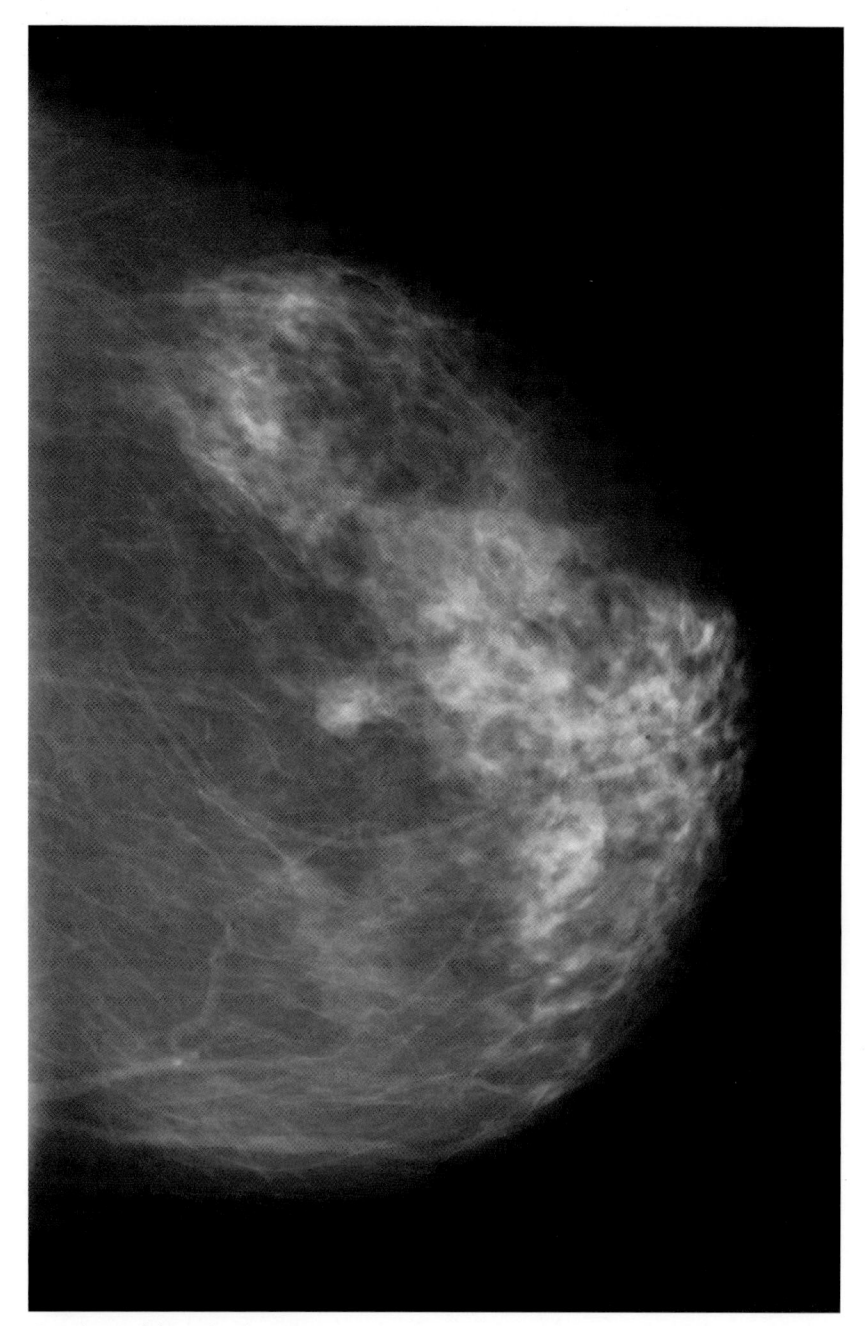

Craniocaudal projection (B)

CIRCUMSCRIBED OPACITY

Irregular shape
The spot compression views show intralesional granular calcifications (A) (C), and the irregular margins are easier to see (A) (B) (C).

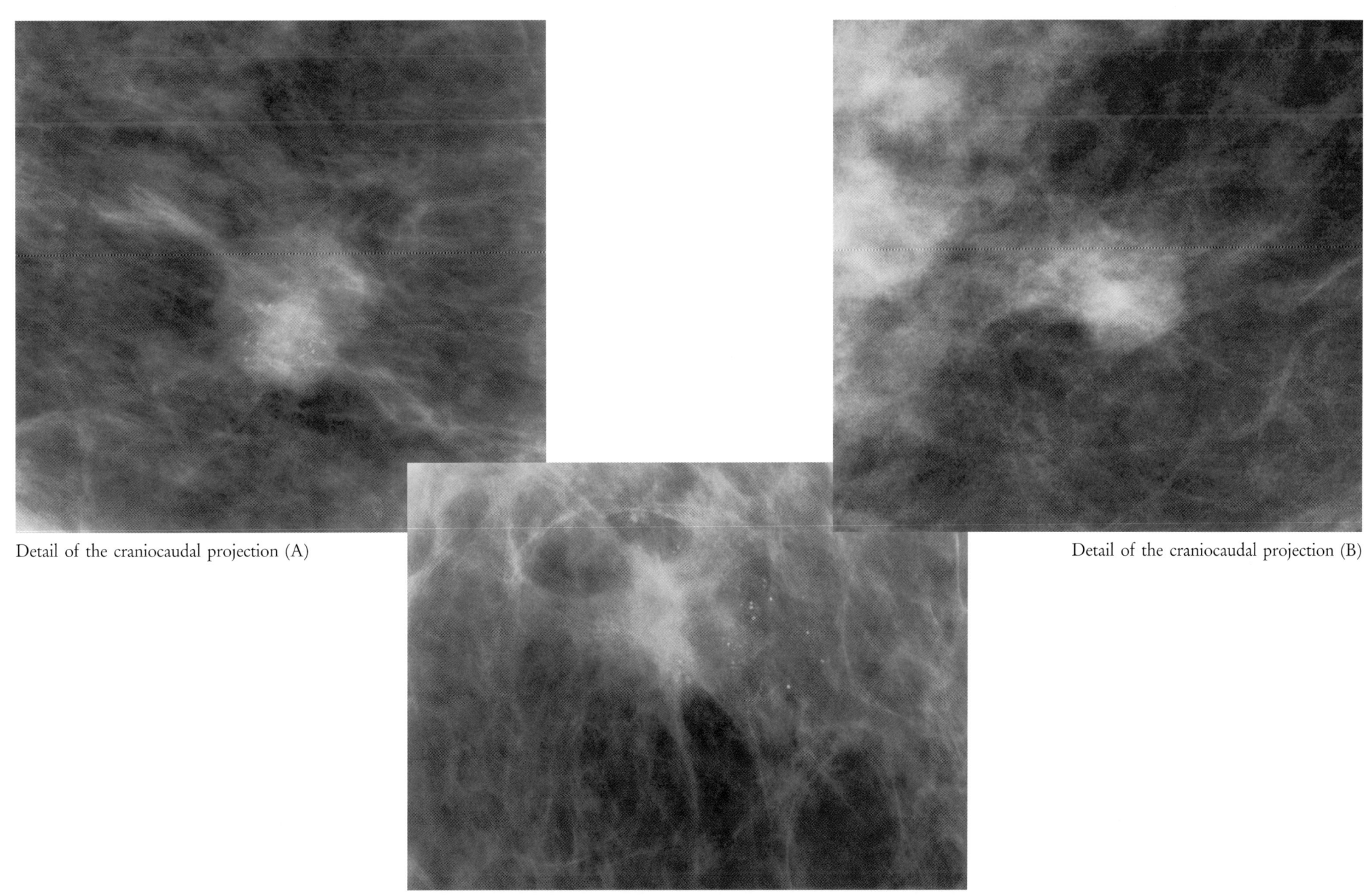

Detail of the craniocaudal projection (A)

Detail of the craniocaudal projection (B)

Detail of the craniocaudal projection (C)

CIRCUMSCRIBED OPACITY

Sharp margins

The spot compression views show examples of circumscribed opacities with sharp margins; the radiolucent rim is readily identified. Density higher than the surrounding fibroglandular tissue.

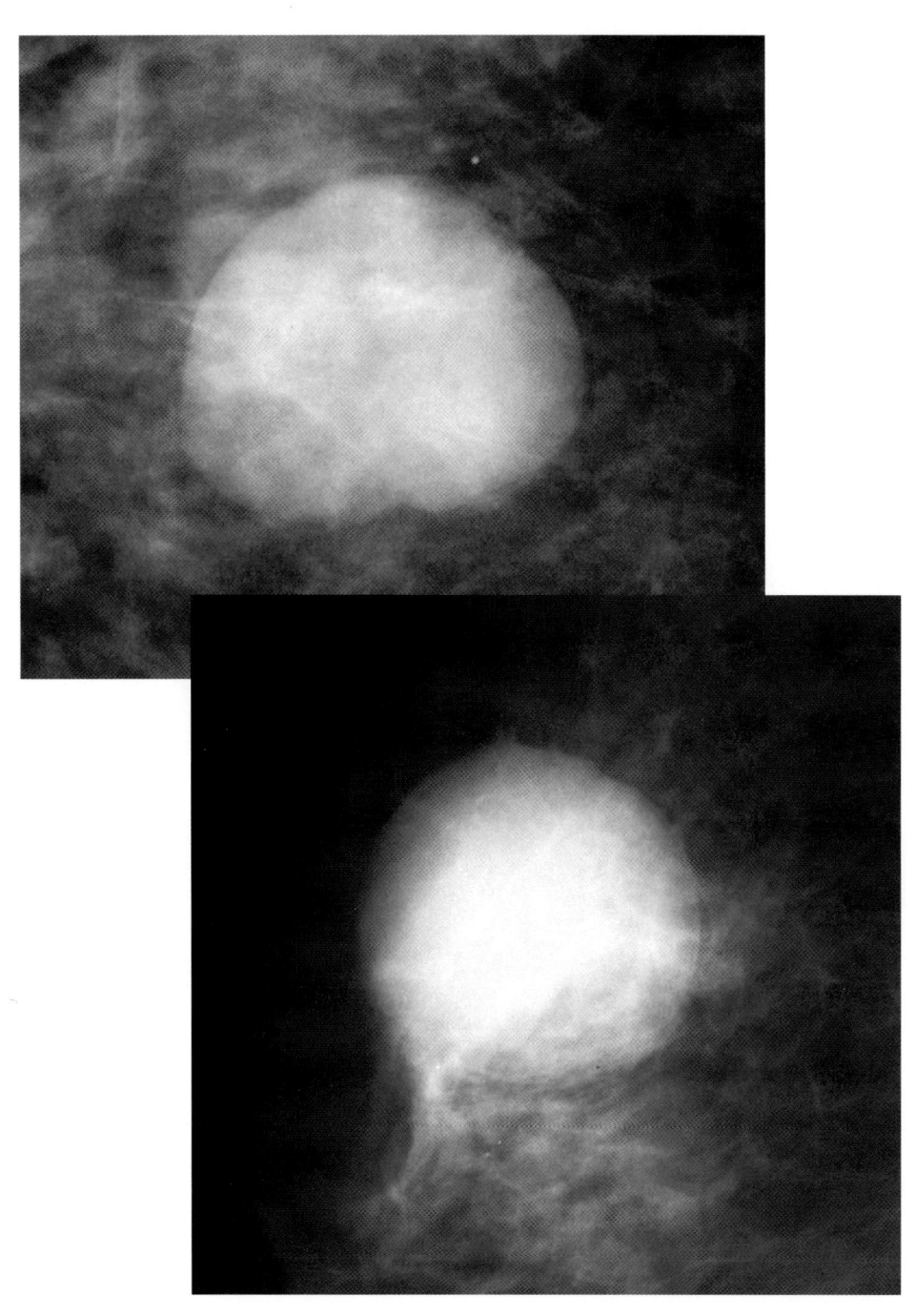

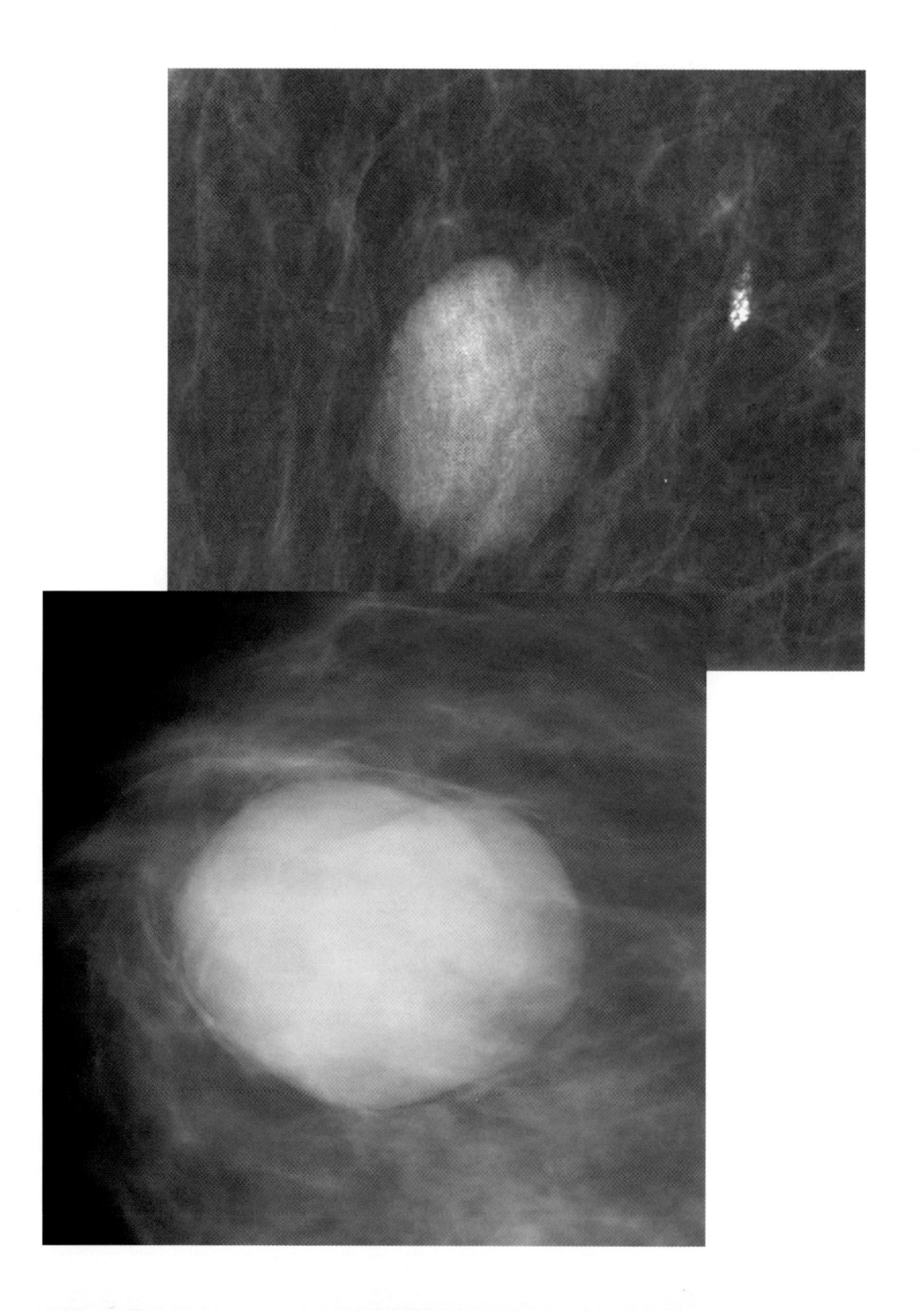

CIRCUMSCRIBED OPACITY

Blurred margins
The spot compression views show circumscribed opacities of different density, with completely or partially blurred margins.

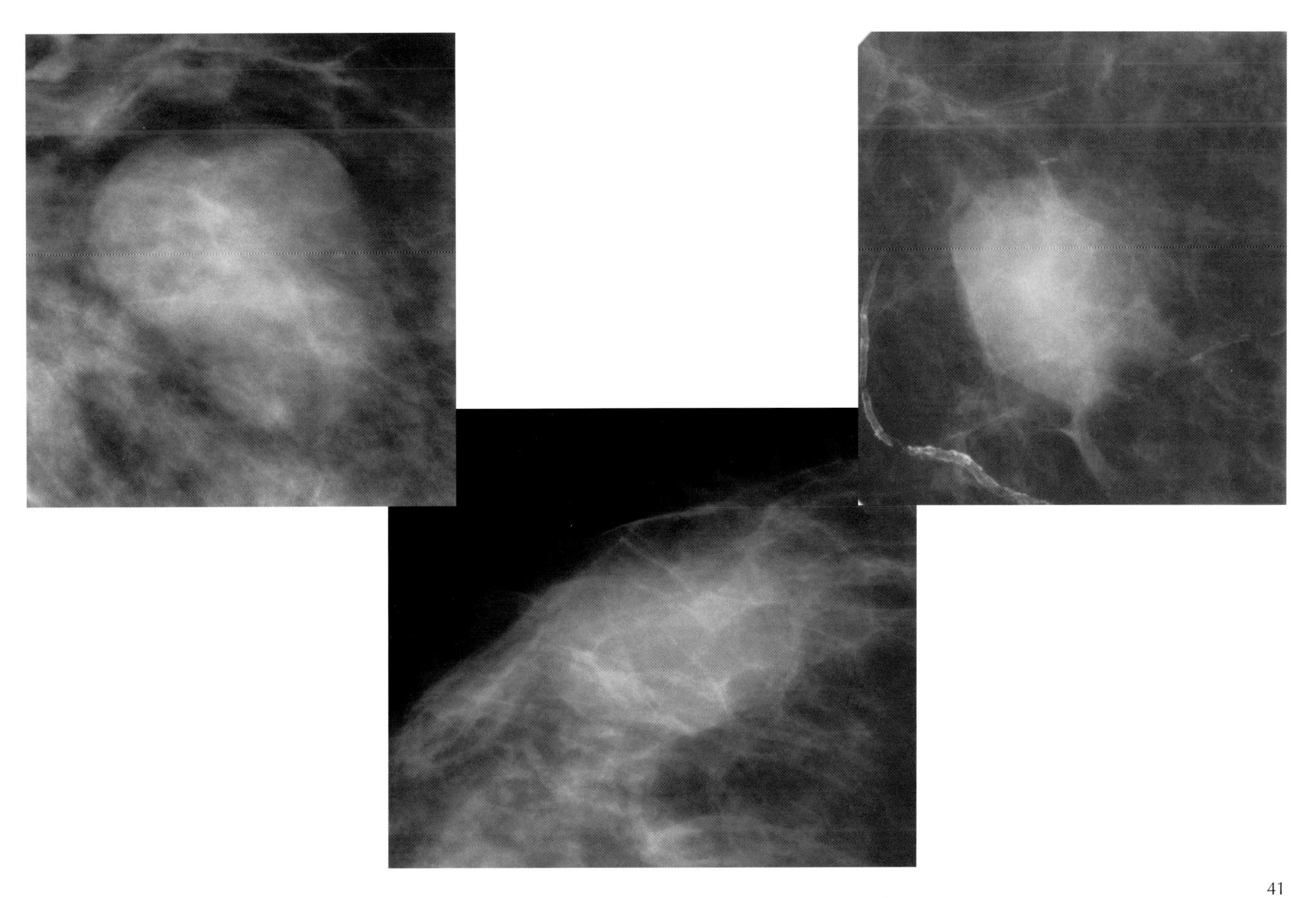

CIRCUMSCRIBED OPACITY

Blurred margins

An ovalish circumscribed opacity with blurred margins is seen in an upper position behind the areola, with the same density as the surrounding fibroglandular tissue; equal density and blurred margins make detection very difficult in either projection.

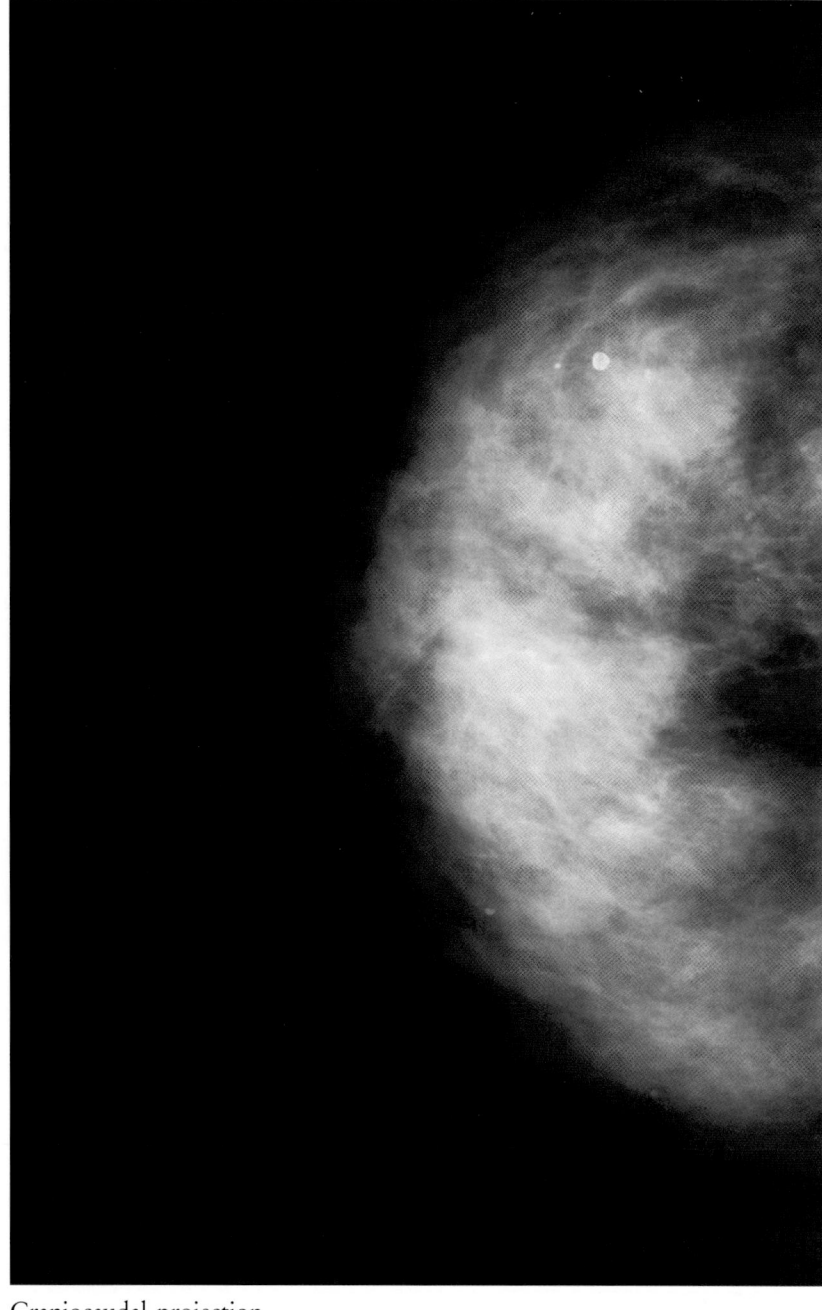

Craniocaudal projection

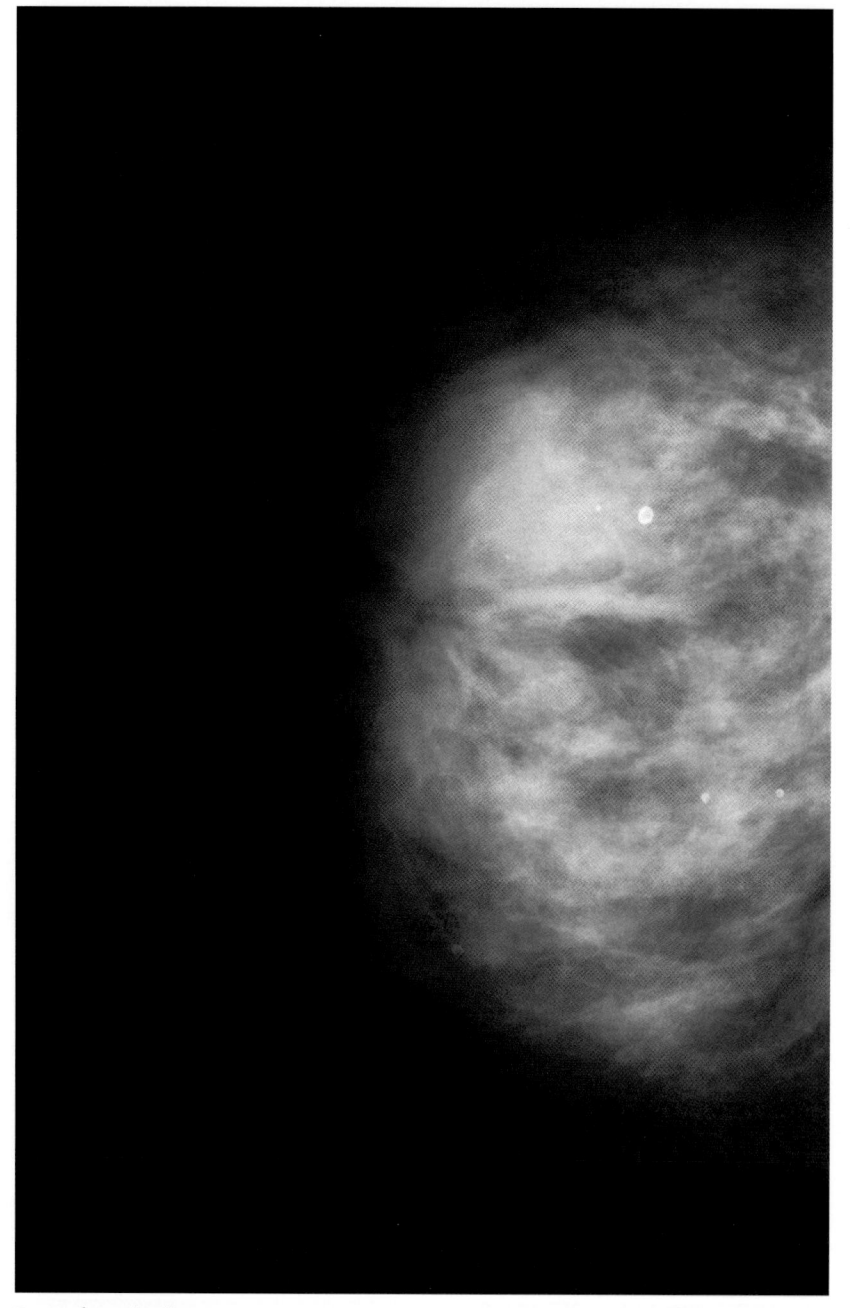

Lateral projection

Blurred margins

An ovalish circumscribed opacity with blurred margins is seen in an upper position behind the areola, with the same density as the surrounding fibroglandular tissue. Posteriorly and inferiorly, a partial radiolucent rim is barely visible.

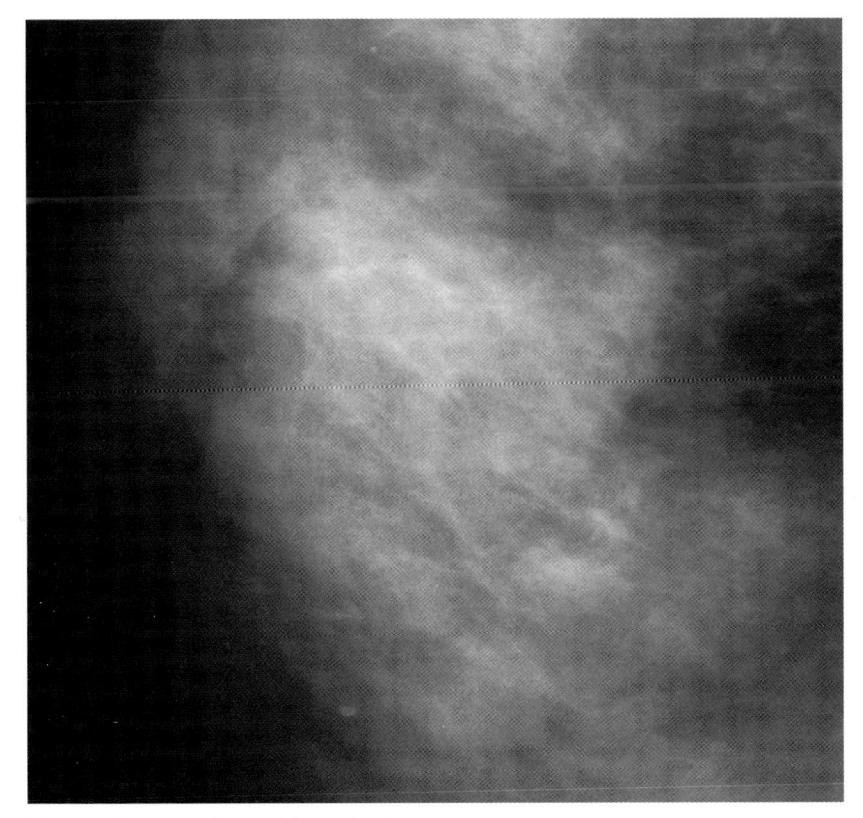

Detail of the craniocaudal projection

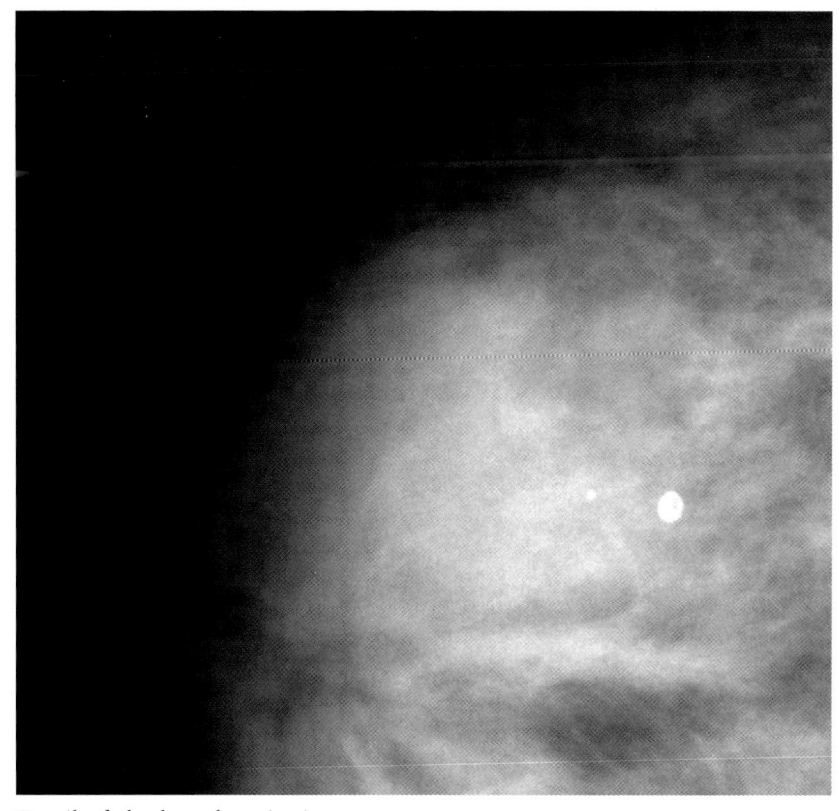

Detail of the lateral projection

CIRCUMSCRIBED OPACITY

Ill-defined margins

In an outer posterior location there are two opacities with ill-defined margins, with the same density as the surrounding fibroglandular tissue. In the spot compression view the ill defined margins appear more clearly.

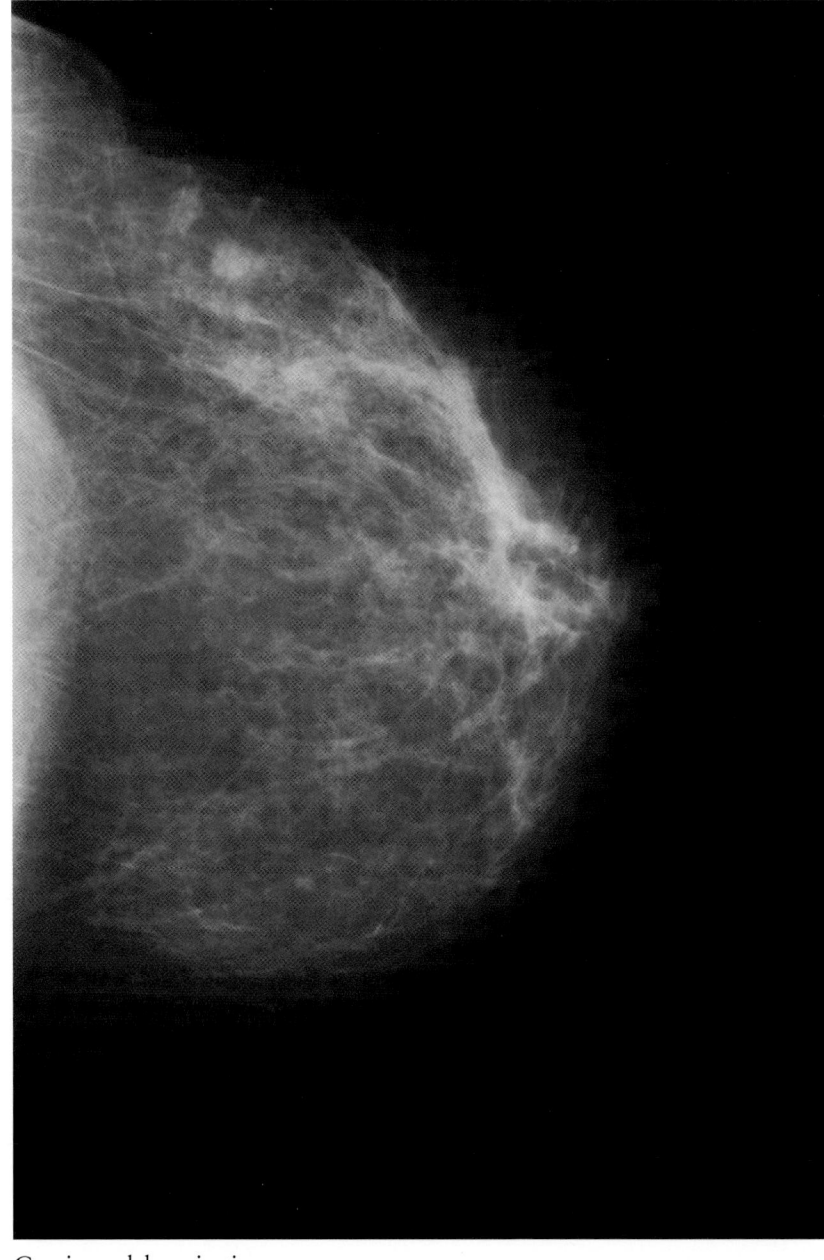

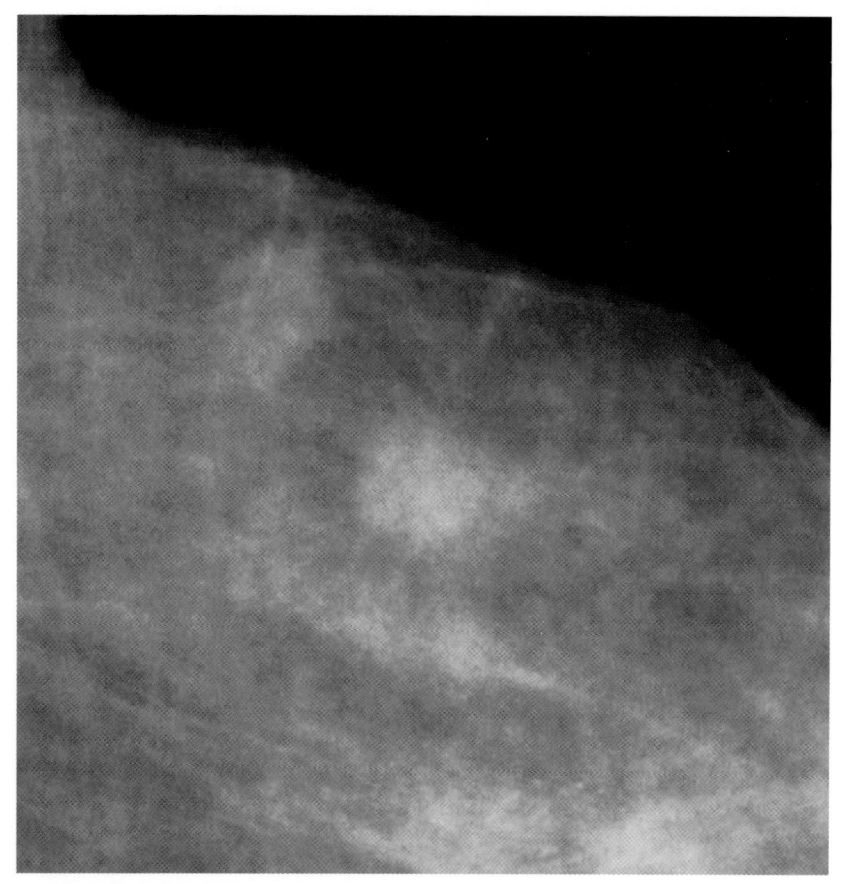

Detail of the craniocaudal projection

Craniocaudal projection

Ill-defined margins

The spot compression views show several opacities with ill-defined margins and more or less marked irregularities.

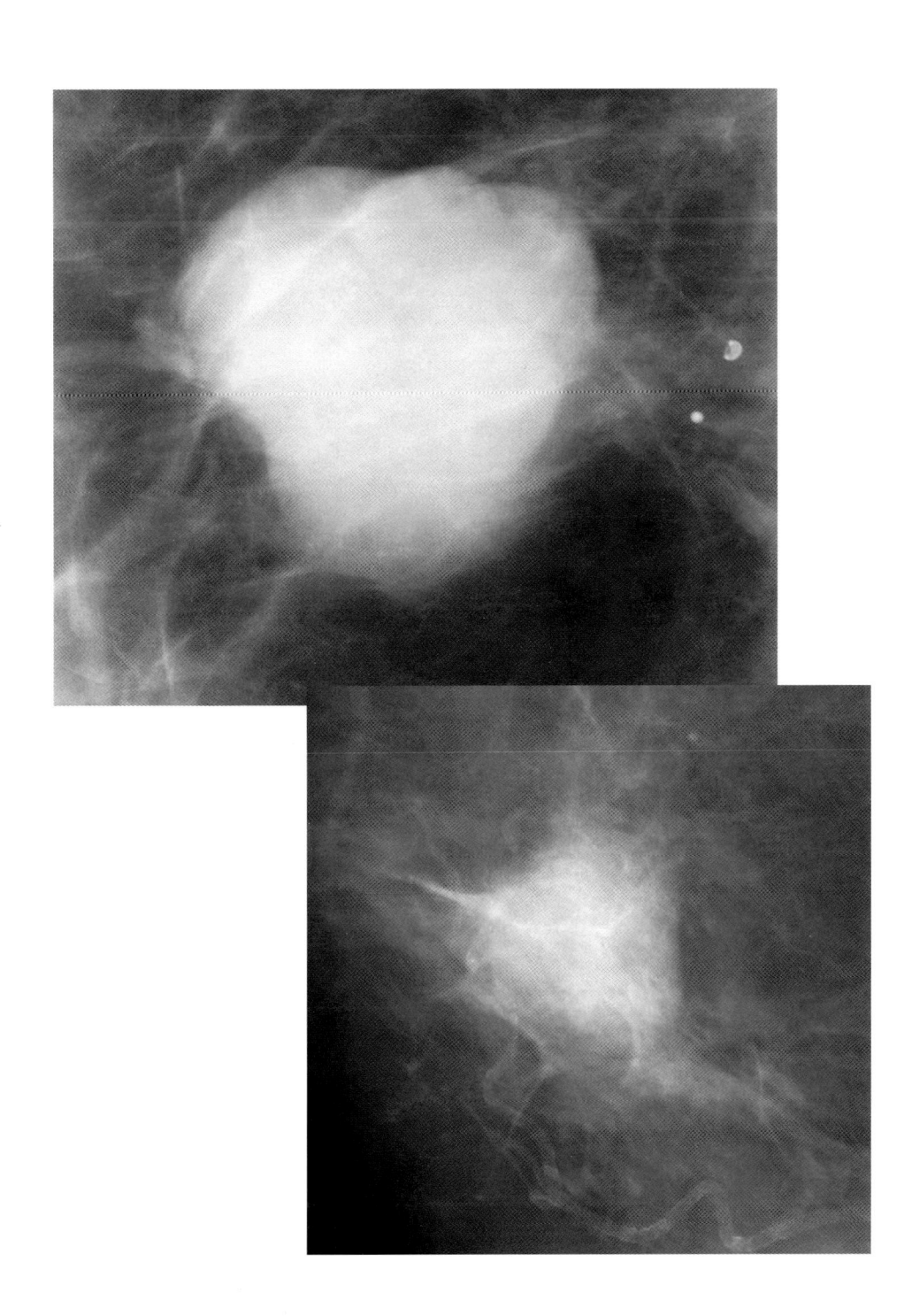

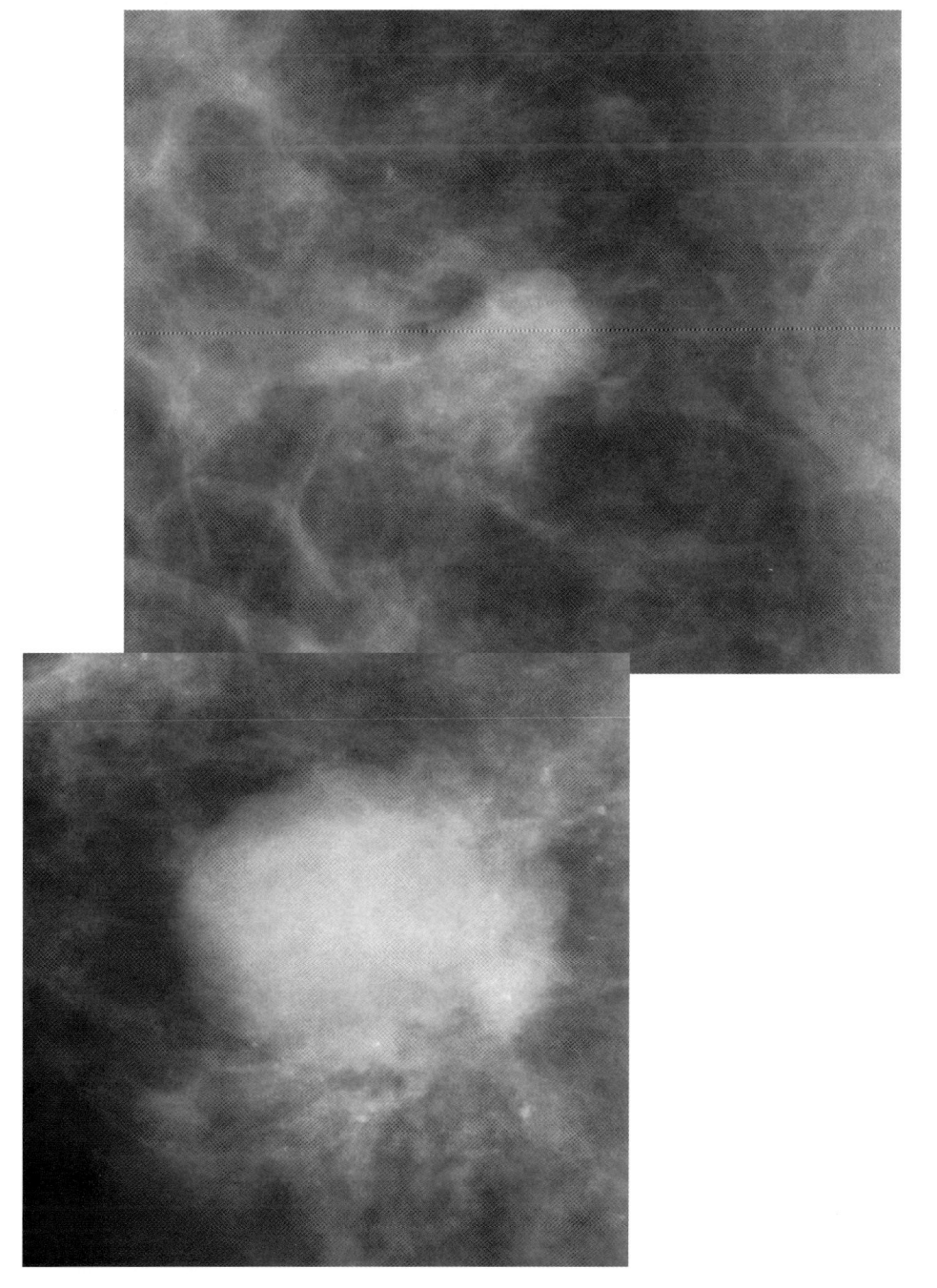

CIRCUMSCRIBED OPACITY

Spiculated margins
Examples of circumscribed opacities with spiculated margins, the spot compression views showing a finely serrated or scalloped appearance.

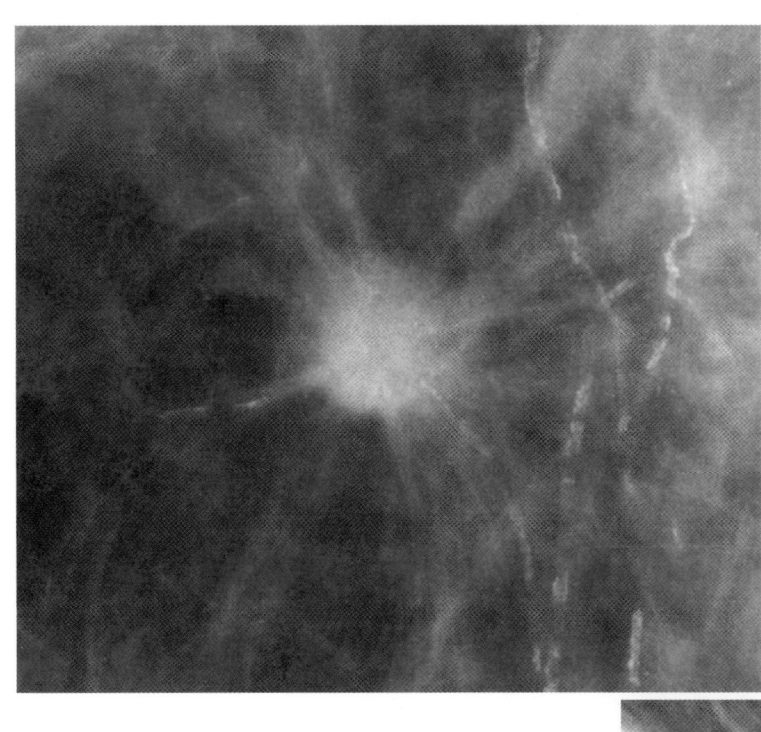

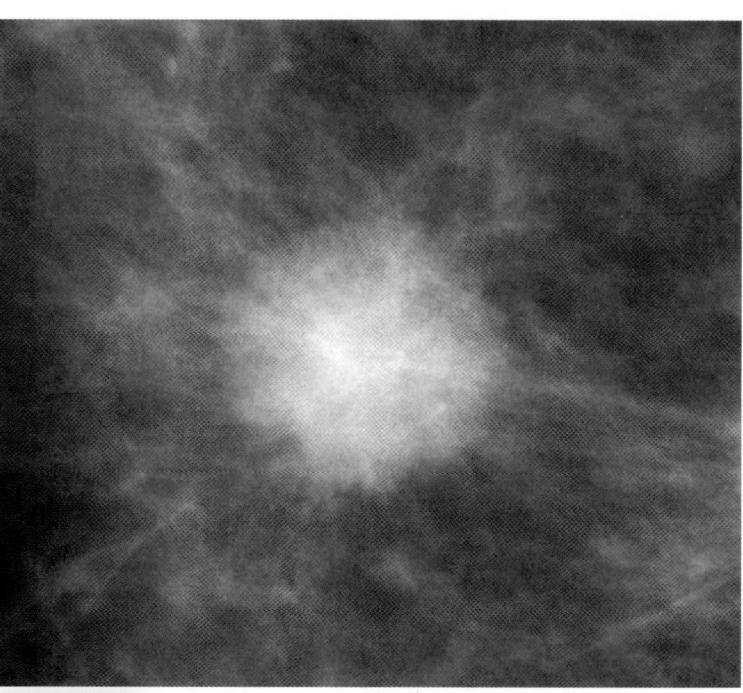

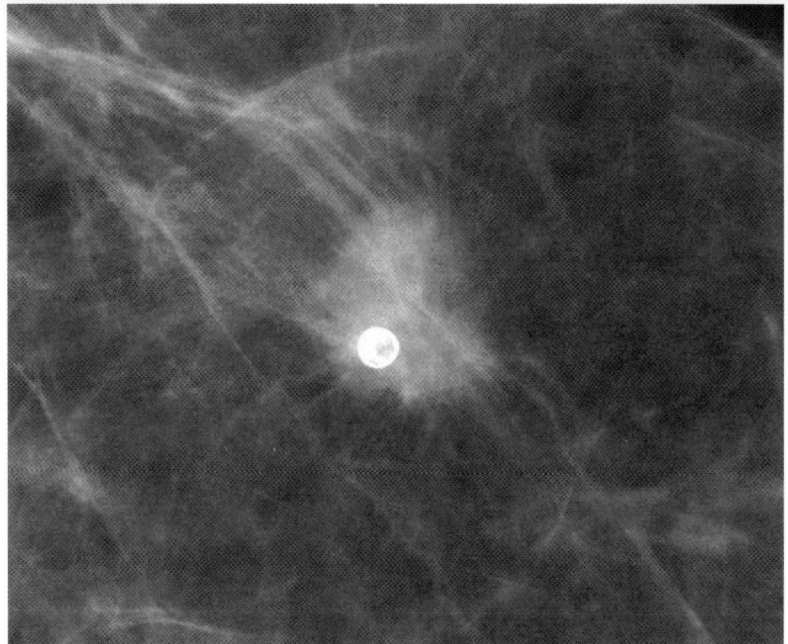

Spiculated margins

Examples of circumscribed opacities with spiculated margins, showing a finely serrated or scalloped appearance in the spot compression views.

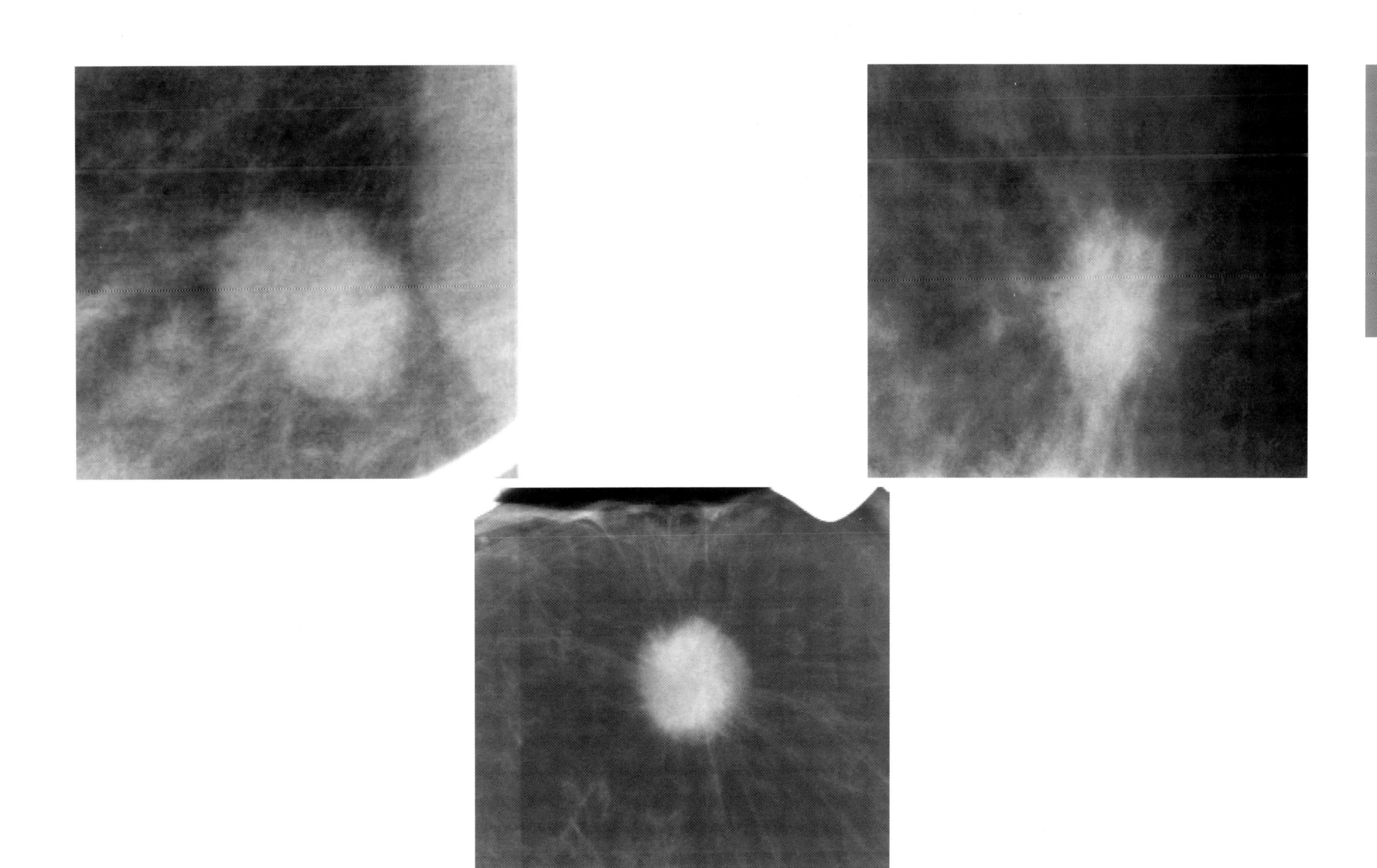

CIRCUMSCRIBED OPACITY

High density

Ovalish, elliptical opacity with sharp, regular margins and a radiolucent rim almost completely enclosing it. Homogeneous density, distinctly higher than the surrounding fibroglandular tissue.

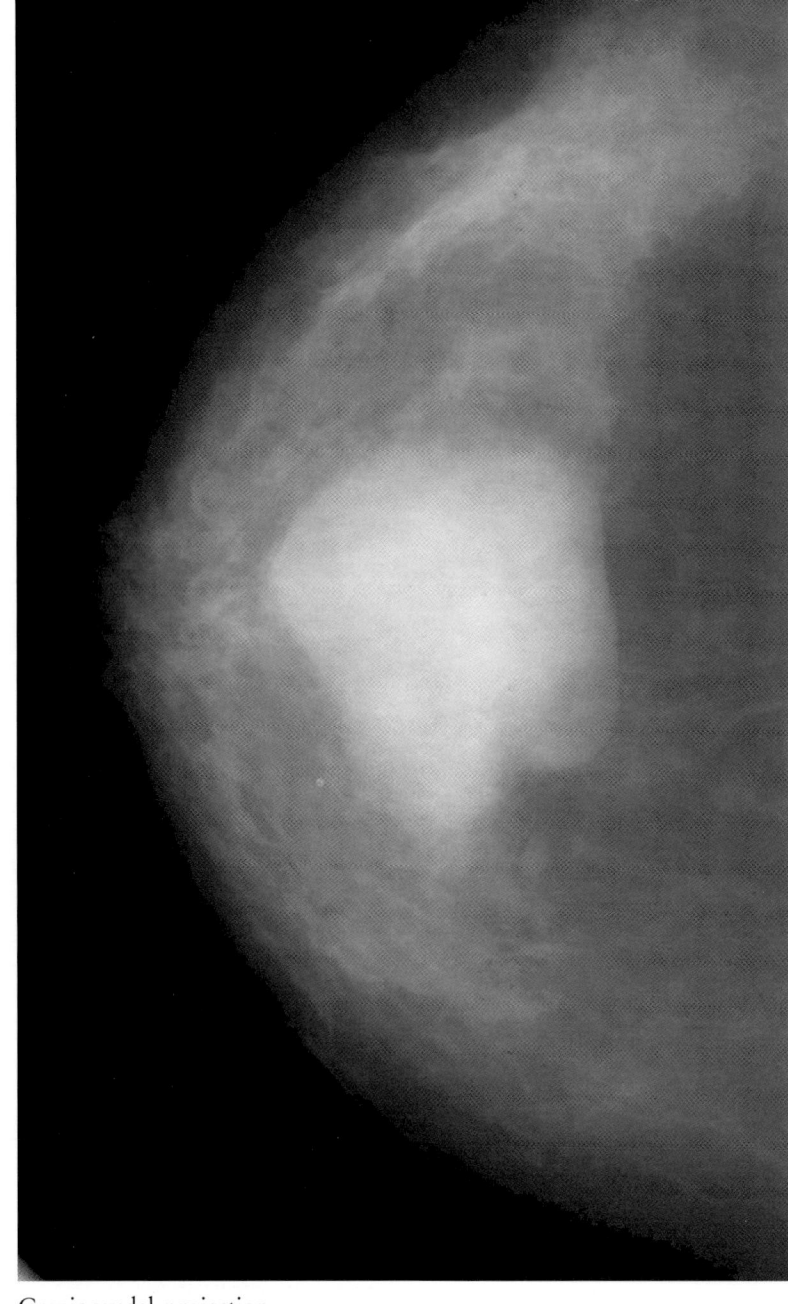

Craniocaudal projection

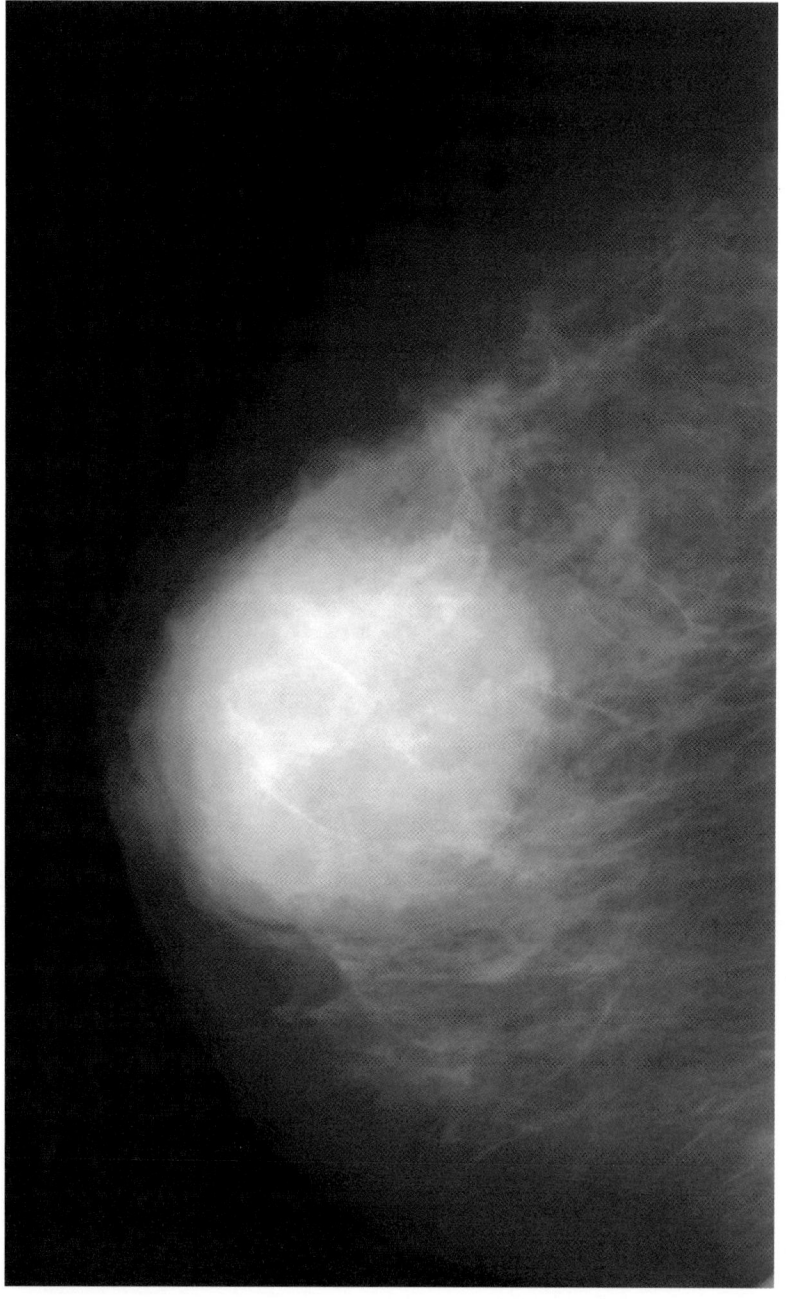

Lateral projection

Equal density

An ovalish opacity behind the areola, with blurred margins and low density, the same as the surrounding fibroglandular tissue, which can be seen "through" it. This pattern is highly predictive of a benign lesion.

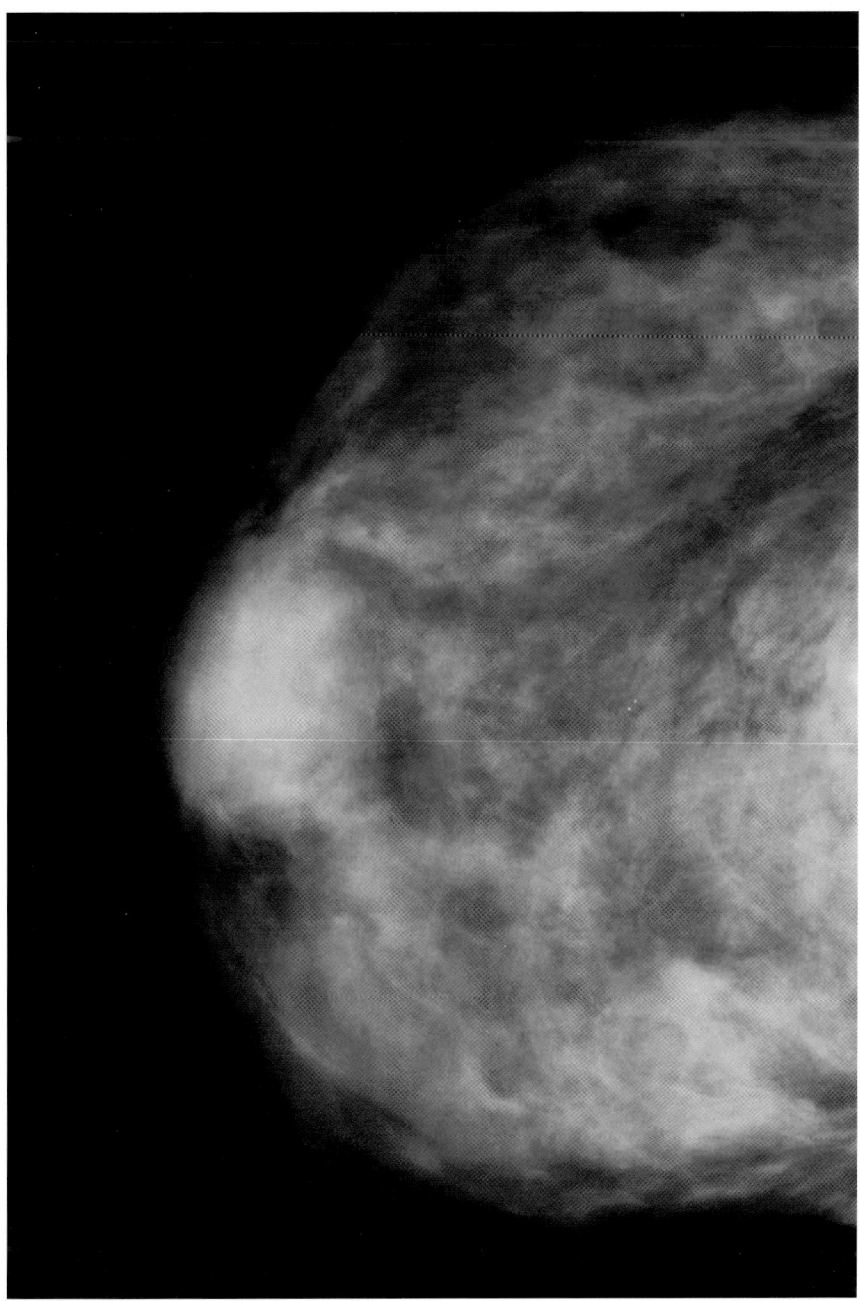

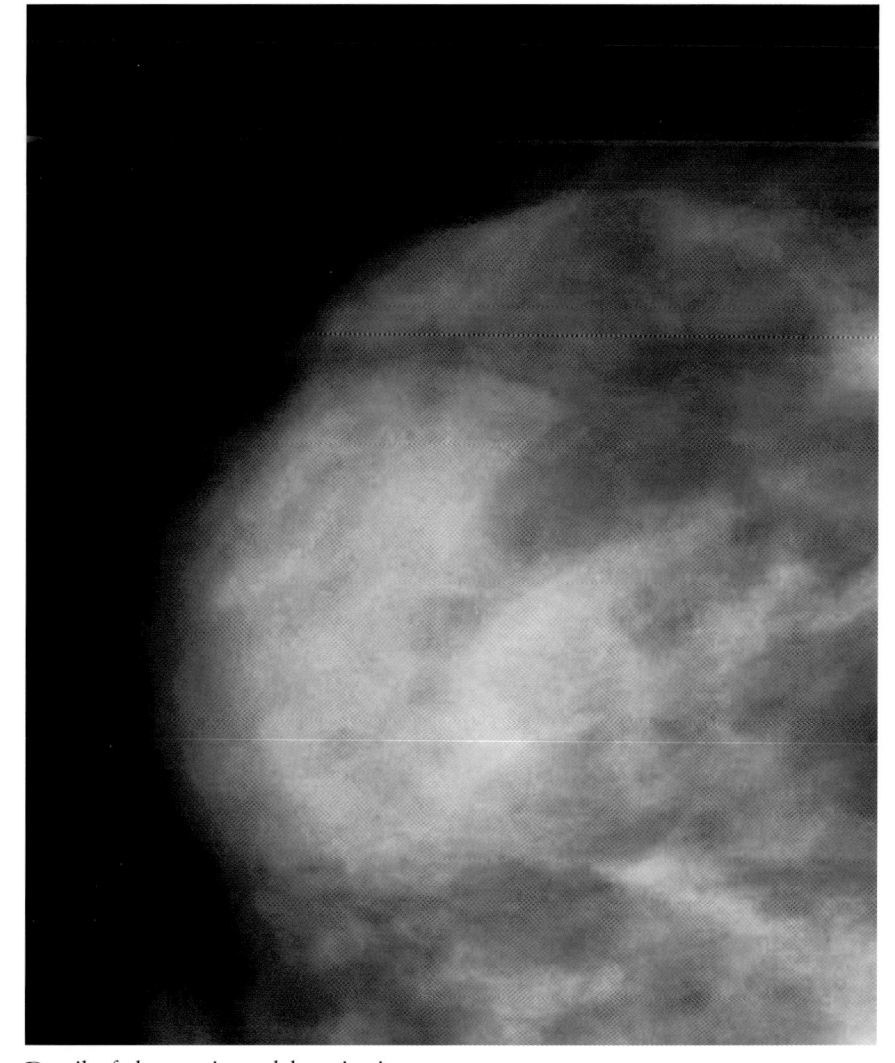

Craniocaudal projection

Detail of the craniocaudal projection

CIRCUMSCRIBED OPACITY

Equal density
Bilateral ovoid opacities, in different quadrants; blurred margins, similar density to the adjacent fibroglandular tissue. Some seem denser because they overlap one another, not because they are structurally different.

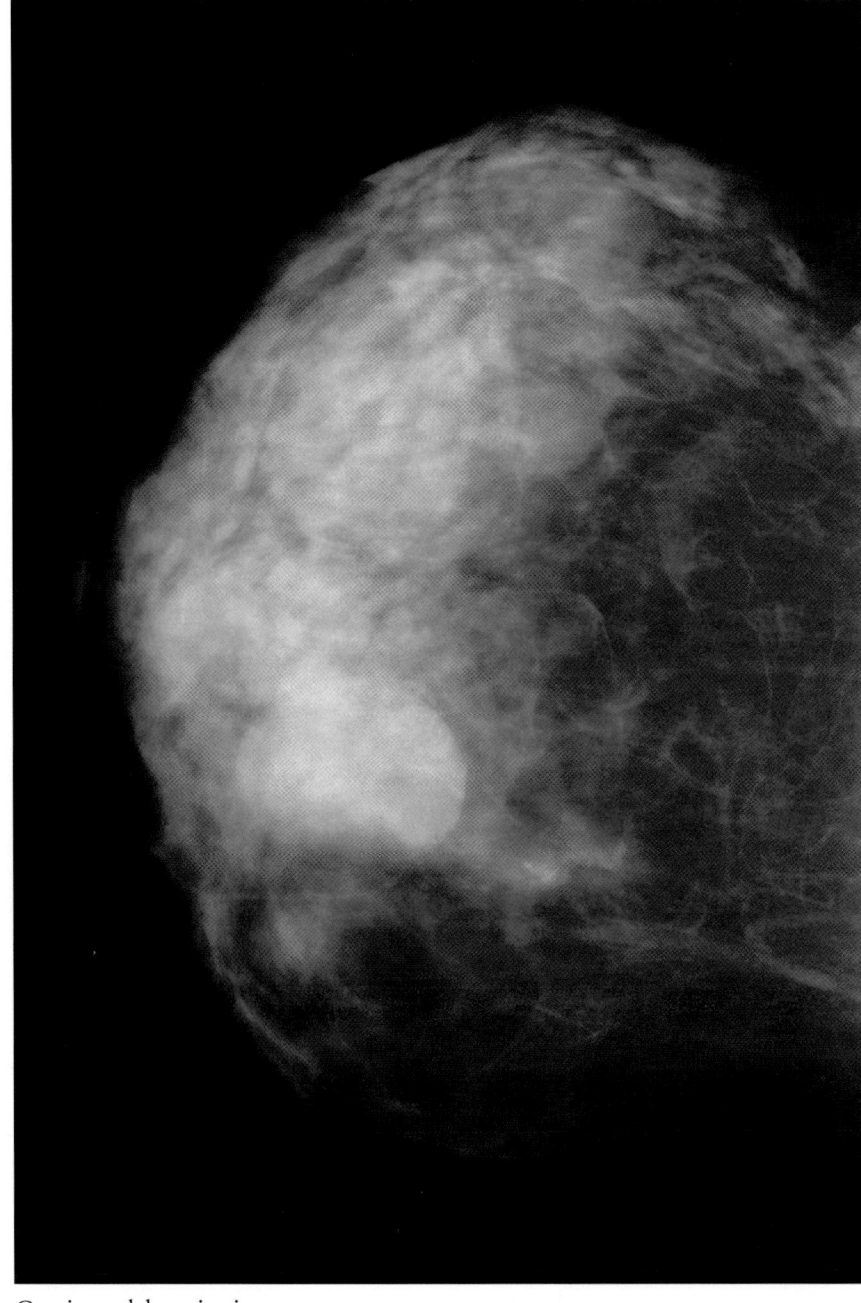

Craniocaudal projection

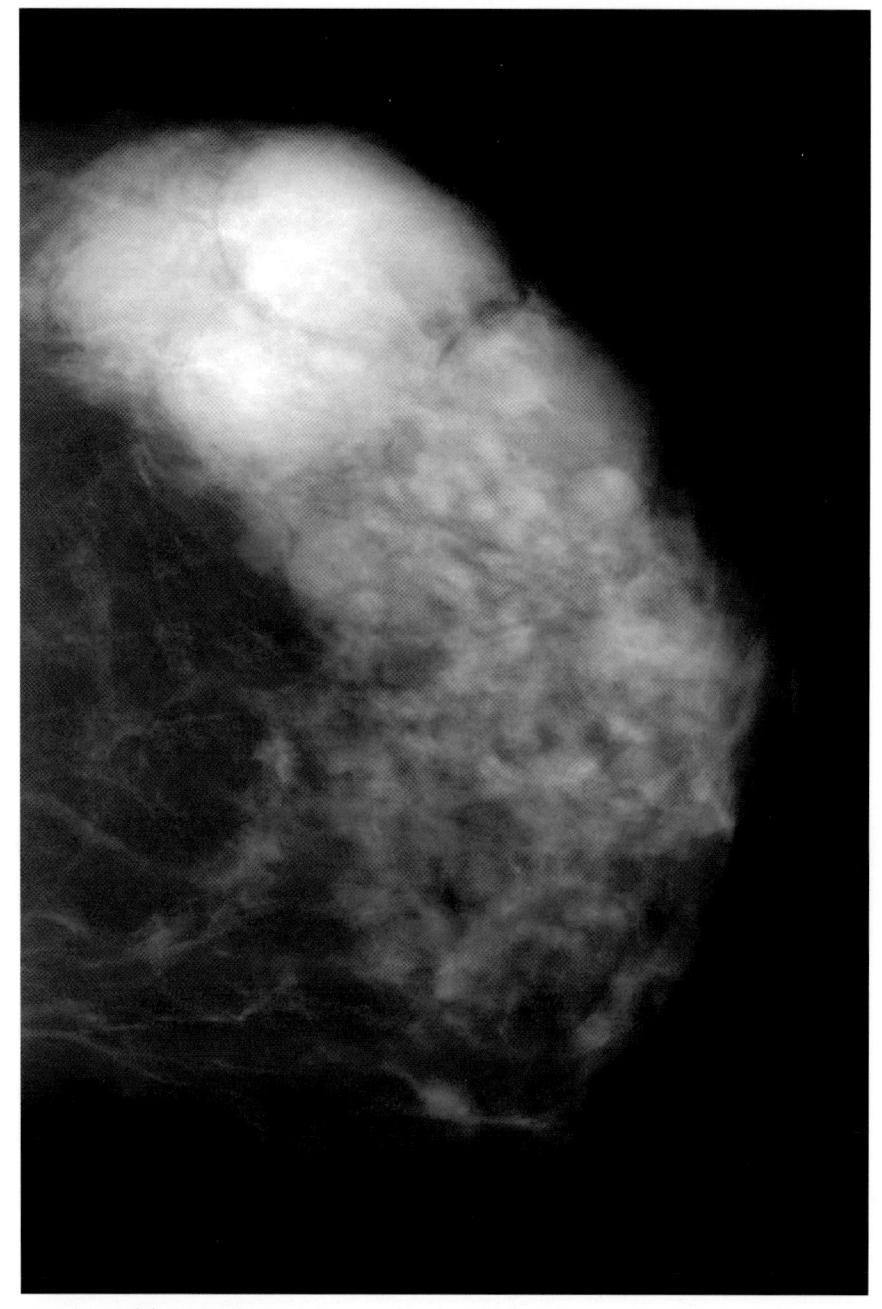

Craniocaudal projection

Equal density

Bilateral ovoid opacities, in different quadrants; blurred margins, similar density to the adjacent fibroglandular tissue. Some seem denser because they overlap one another, not because they are structurally different. The spot compression view shows the radiolucent rim around some of the lesions.

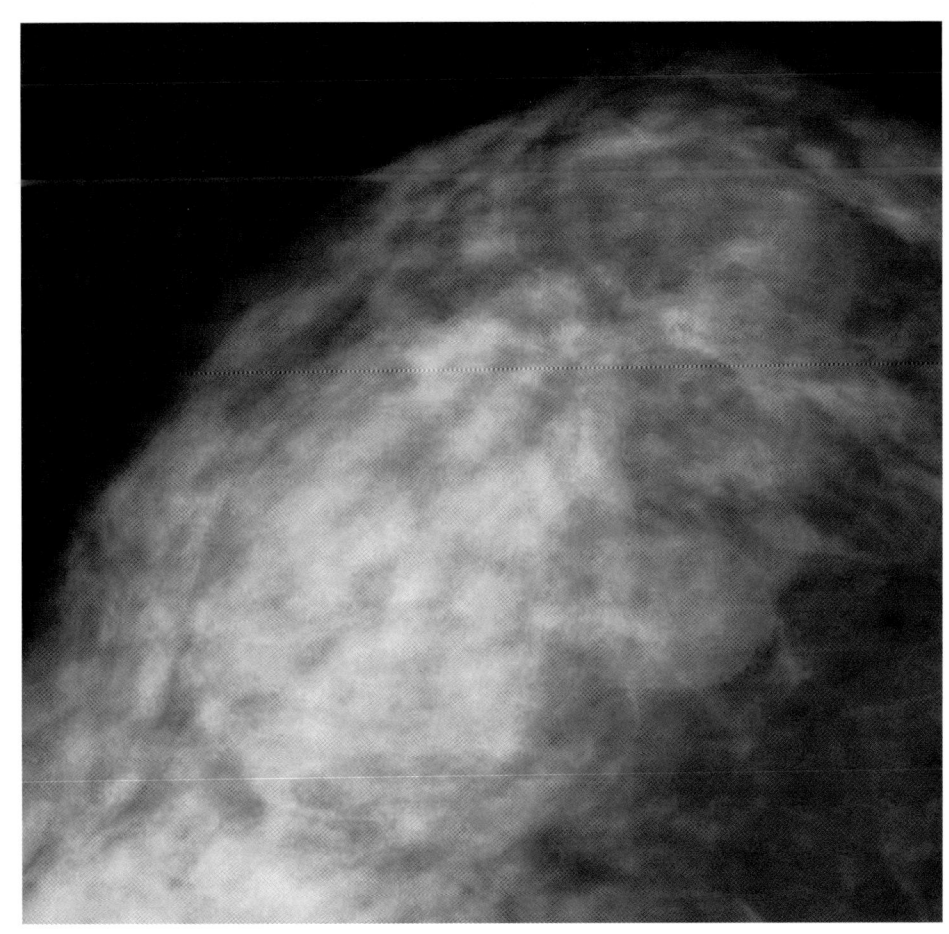

Detail of the craniocaudal projection

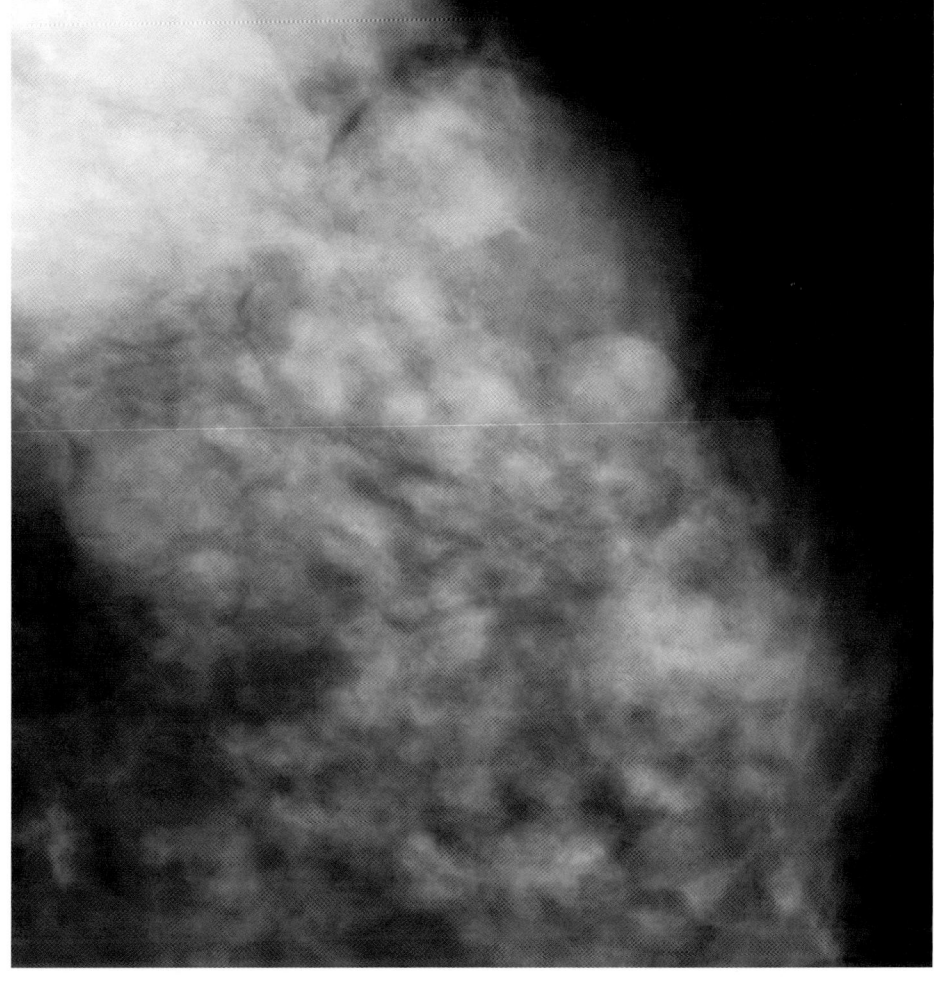

Detail of the craniocaudal projection

CIRCUMSCRIBED OPACITY

Mixed density

An oval mass lesion is seen superiorly; regular margins, mixed density, and an eccentric radiolucent notch due to fat at the hilum (axillary lymph node).

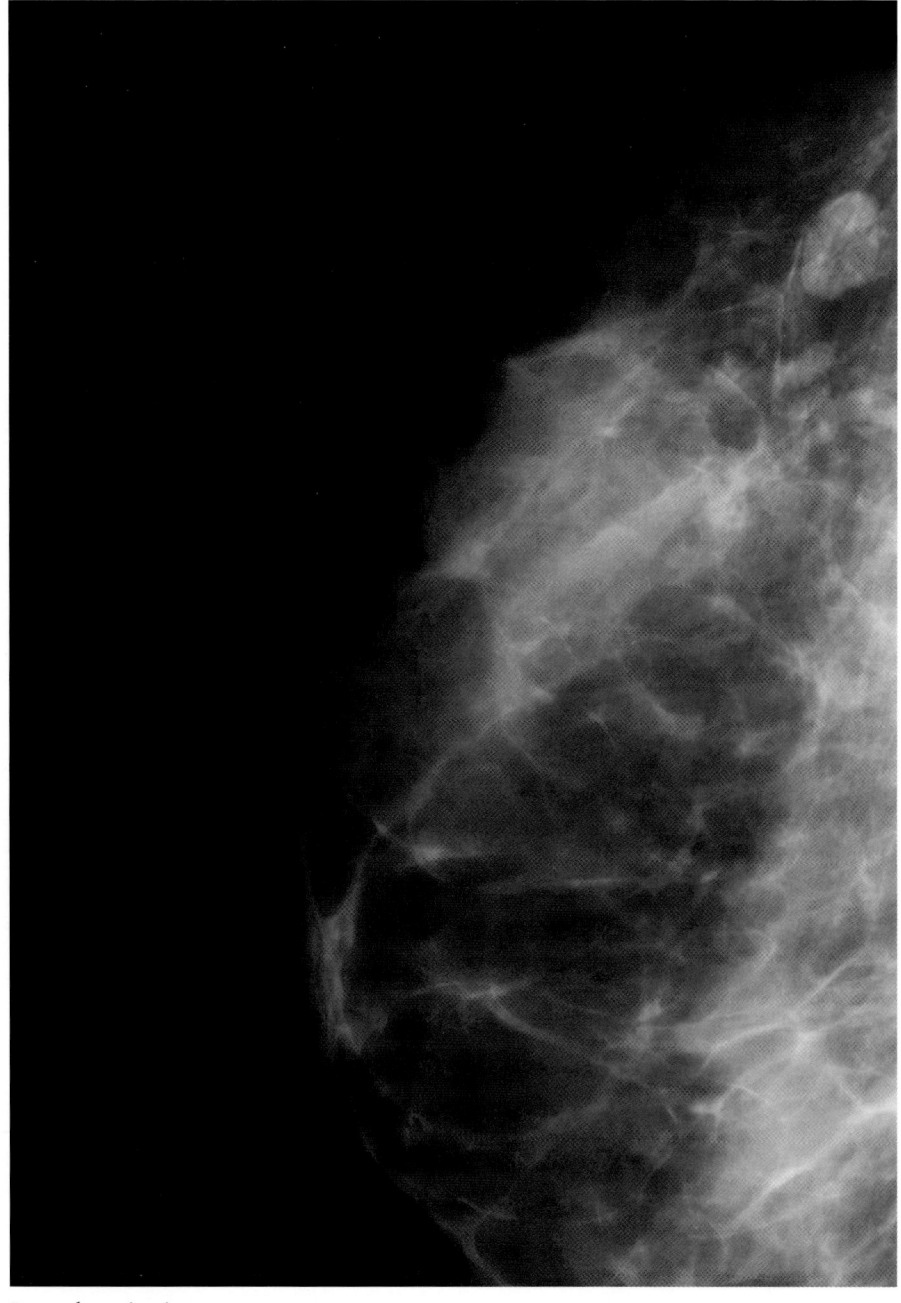

Lateral projection

Magnification view

Mixed density

An oval fat-containing mass lesion with sharp, regular margins and a radiolucent rim almost entirely enclosing it. Inside it, radiolucent areas are mixed with circumscribed opacities, looking like a "slice of salami" (fibroadenolipoma or hamartoma).

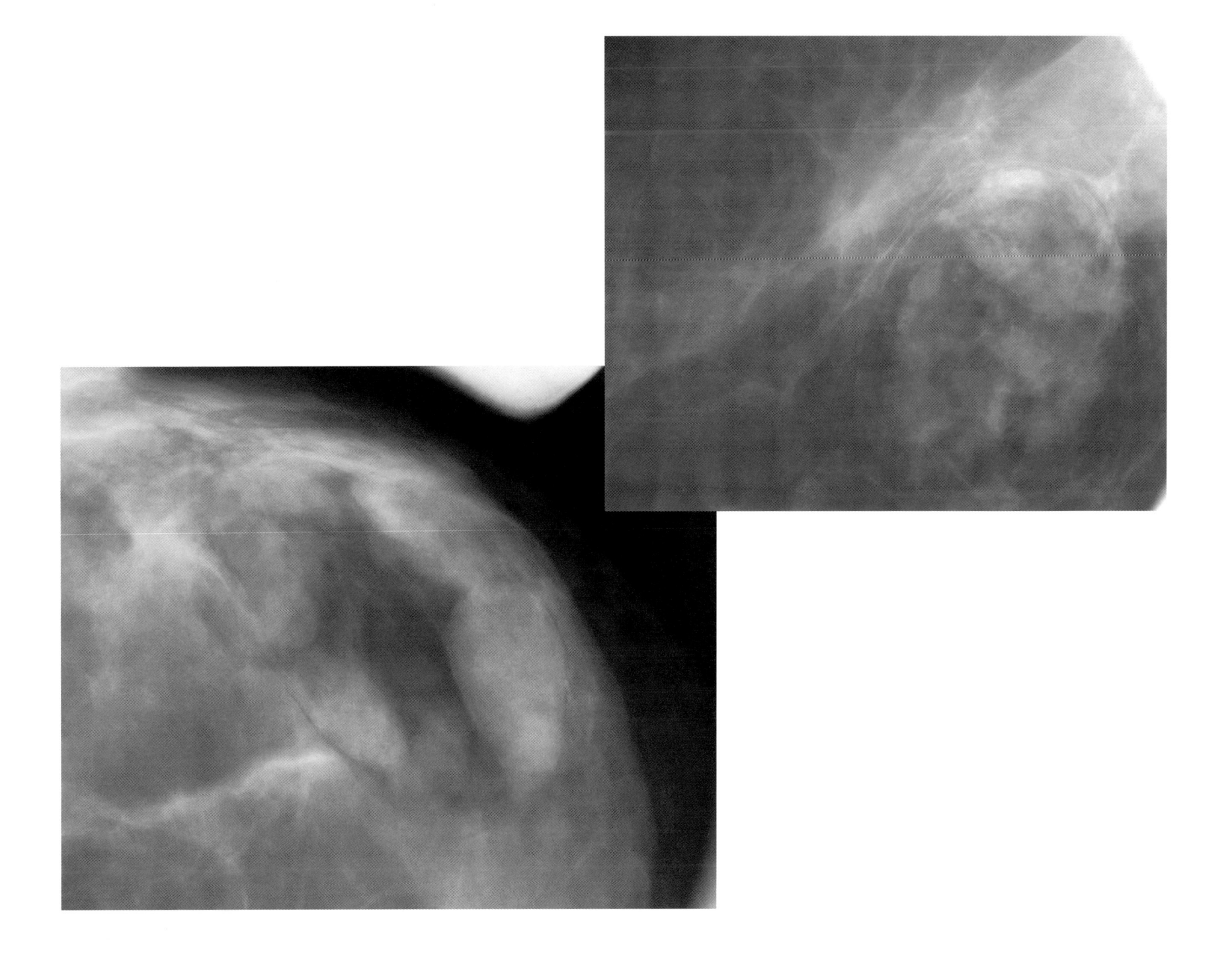

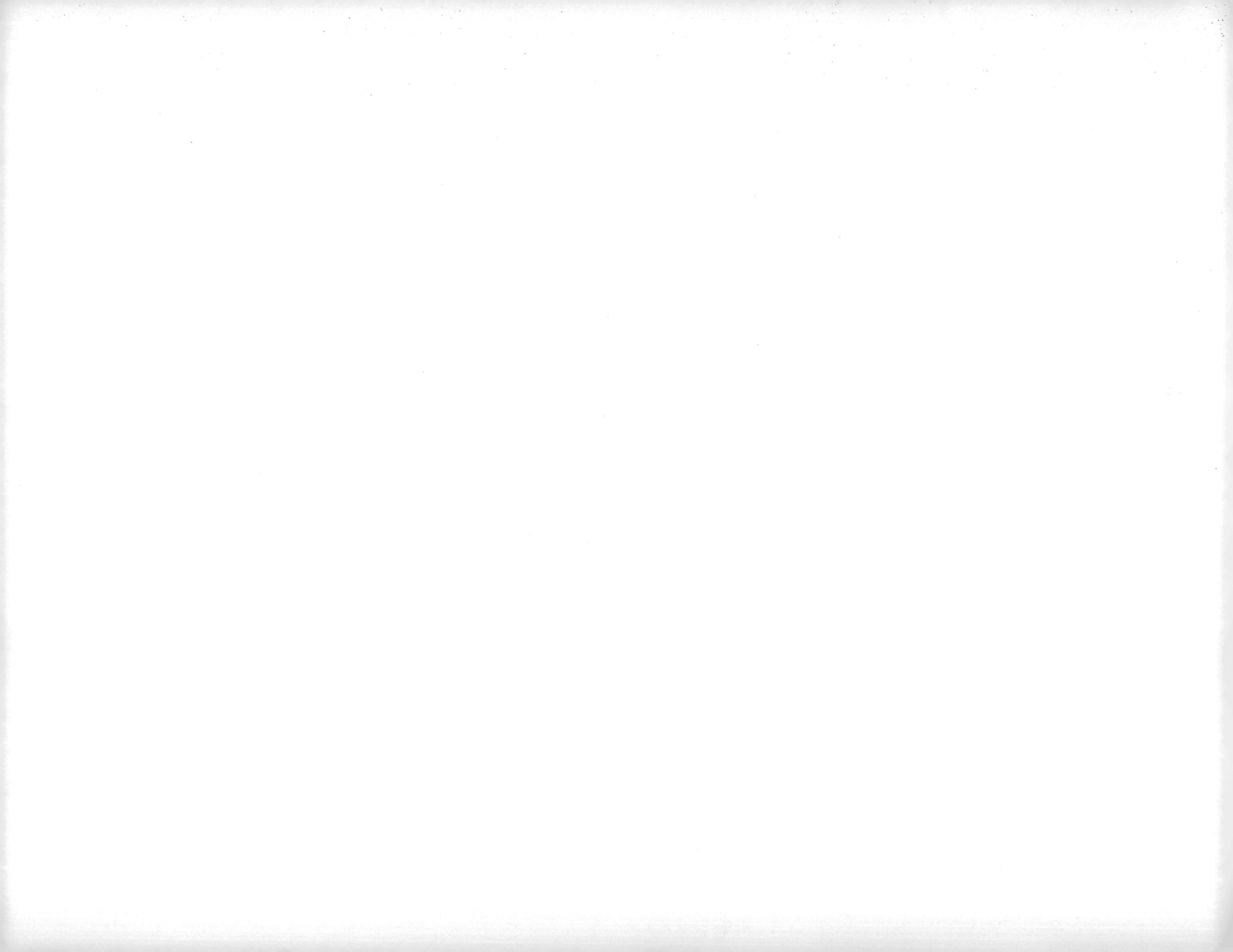

Stellate opacity

Definition
Opacity with irregular margins, with the pattern of a stellate lesion.

Margins
Opacity with more or less homogeneous short spicules, their length proportionate to the size of the tumour centre from which they originate, in a classic stellate pattern; or else non-homogeneous, elongated and markedly asymmetrical, alternating with hyperlucency and a "rosette"-like appearance.

Density
The opacity is sometimes denser than the surrounding parenchyma, relatively homogeneous, with a tumour centre, or else it may be non-homogeneous, with hyperlucent areas and no central nucleus.

STELLATE OPACITY

A non-homogeneous stellate opacity with irregular margins, distinctly hyperdense, with fibrous lines radiating in the surrounding parenchyma. The tumour centre is well defined. The oblique projection shows thick, retracted skin.

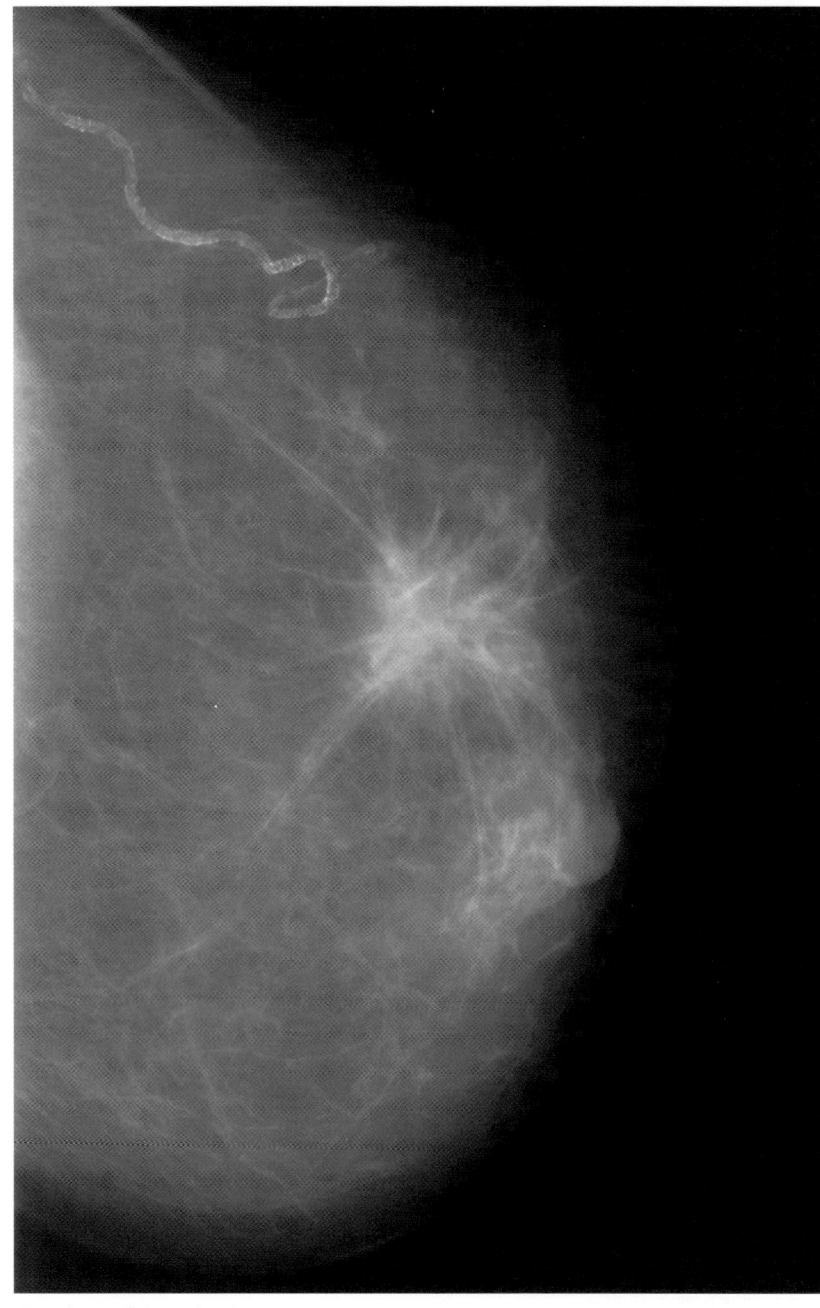

Craniocaudal projection

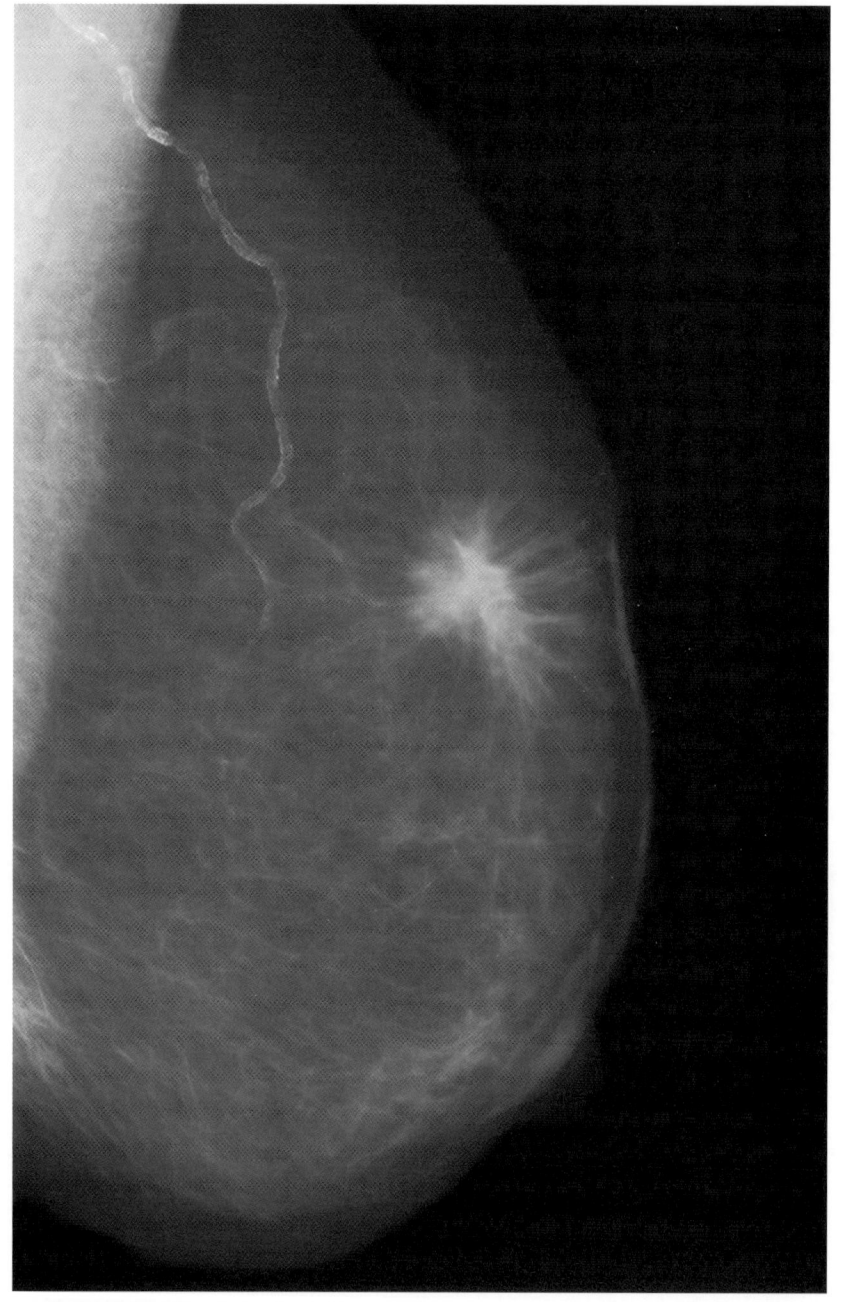

Mediolateral oblique projection

STELLATE OPACITY

A non-homogeneous stellate opacity with irregular margins, distinctly hyperdense, with fibrous lines radiating in the surrounding parenchyma. The fibrous strands look relatively homogeneous and their length is proportionate to the size of the nucleus. The oblique projection shows thick, retracted skin.

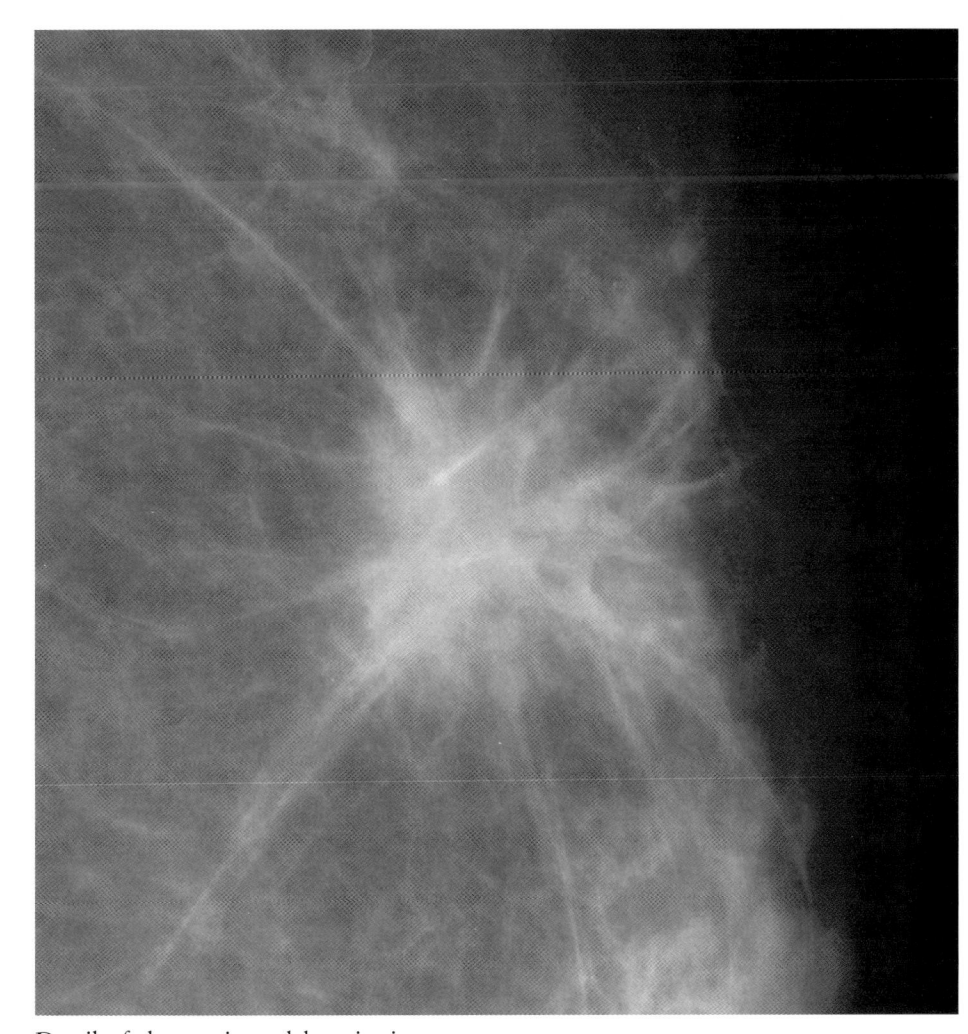

Detail of the craniocaudal projection

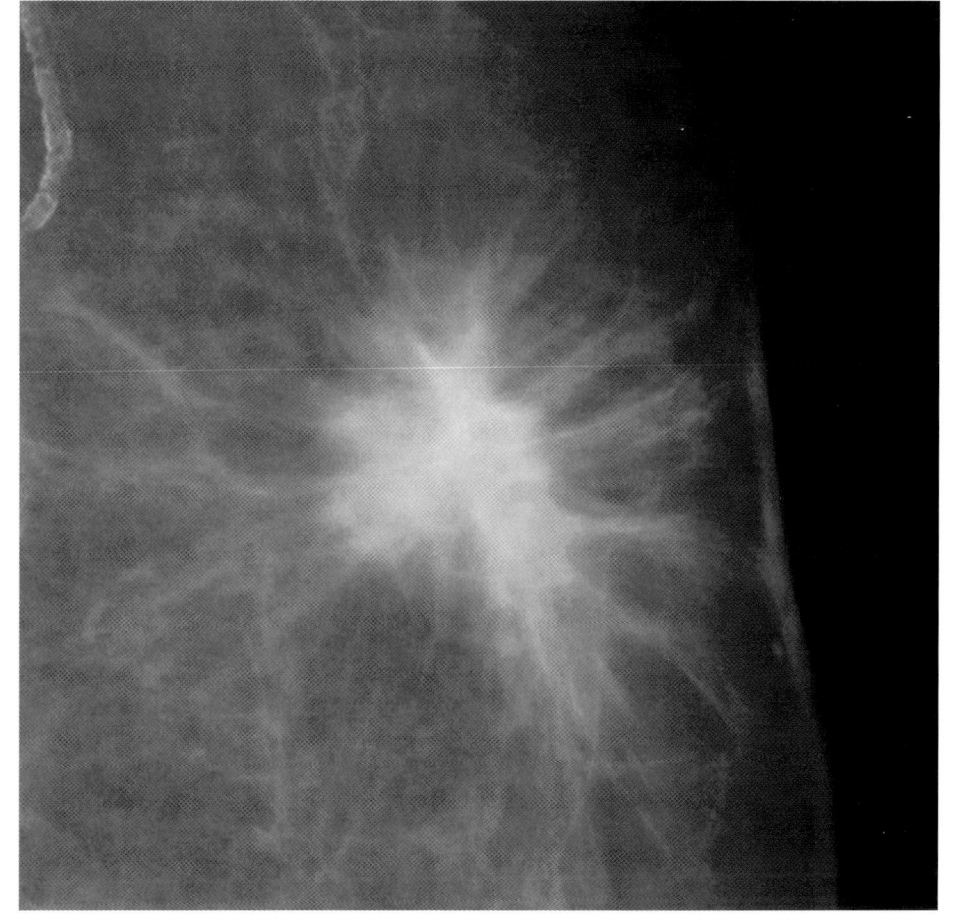

Detail of the oblique projection

STELLATE OPACITY

Deep in the upper region a stellate opacity is visible. It is denser than the surrounding parenchyma and has short, homogeneous spicules around the margins; their length is proportionate to the size of the clearly visible tumour centre.

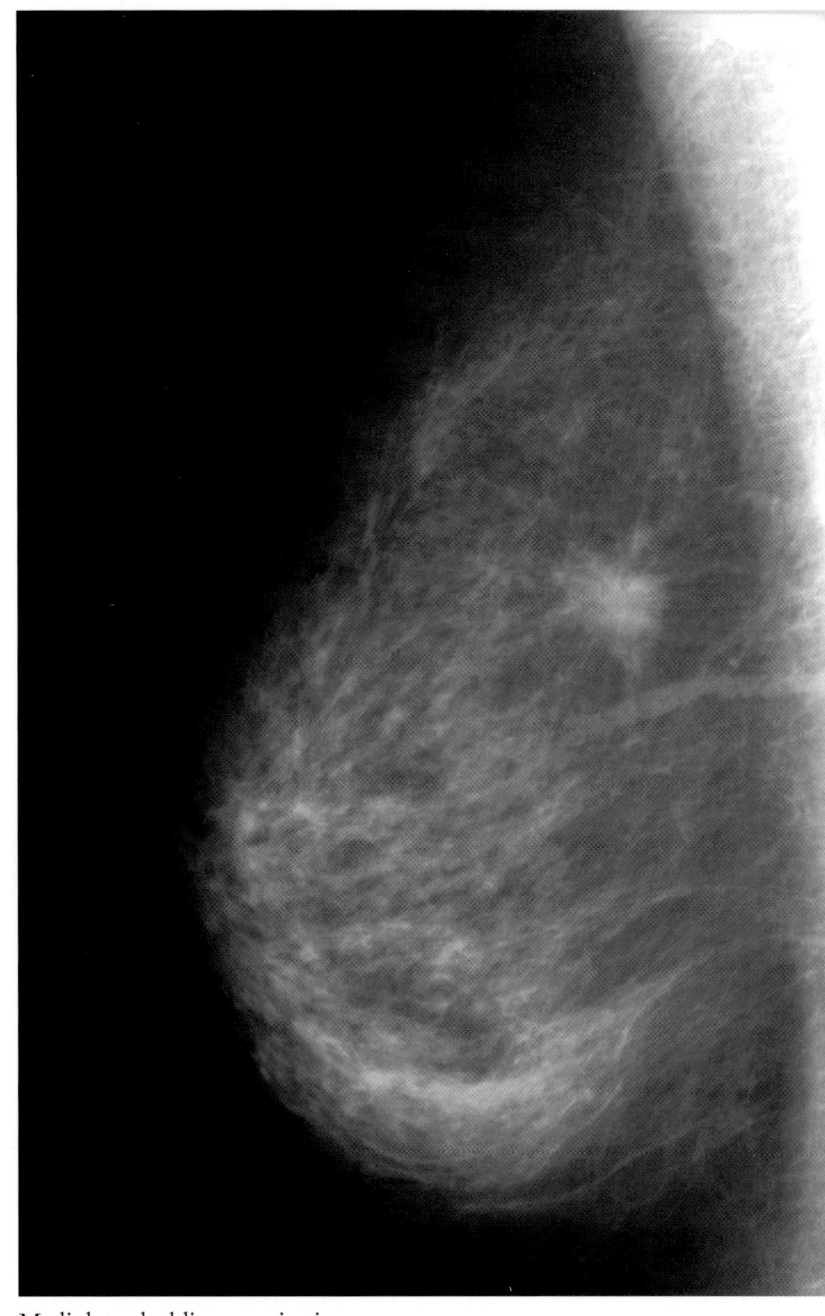

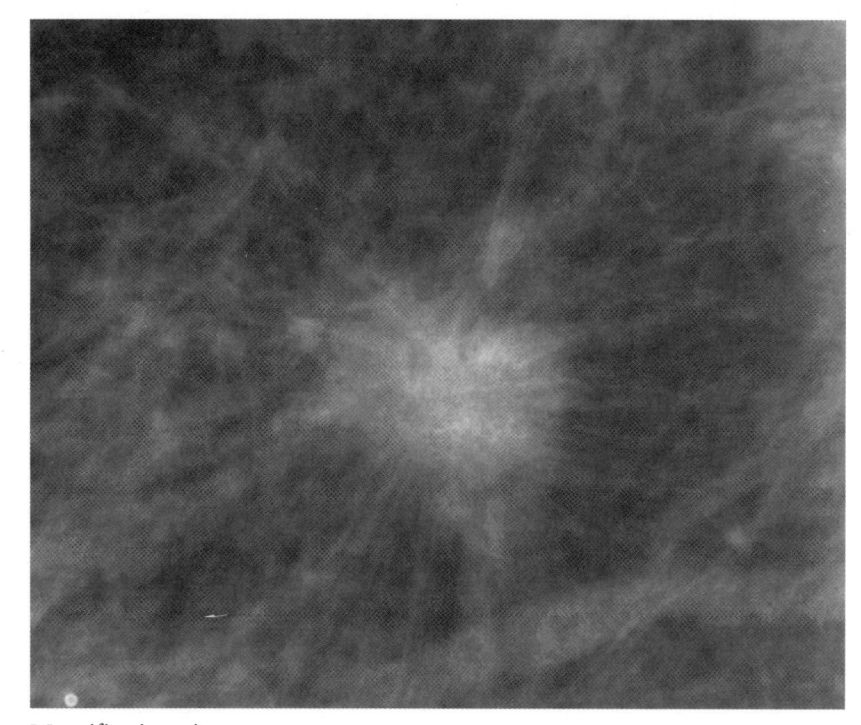

Magnification view

Mediolateral oblique projection

STELLATE OPACITY

A hyperlucent, stellate opacity is visible, its spicules running out into the surrounding tissue and towards the areolar skin, which appears thickened and retracted. The spot compression view, in the tangential craniocaudal projection, shows the thickened skin better. The tumour centre is well defined, with stubby, homogeneous spicules proportionate in length to the size of the nucleus.

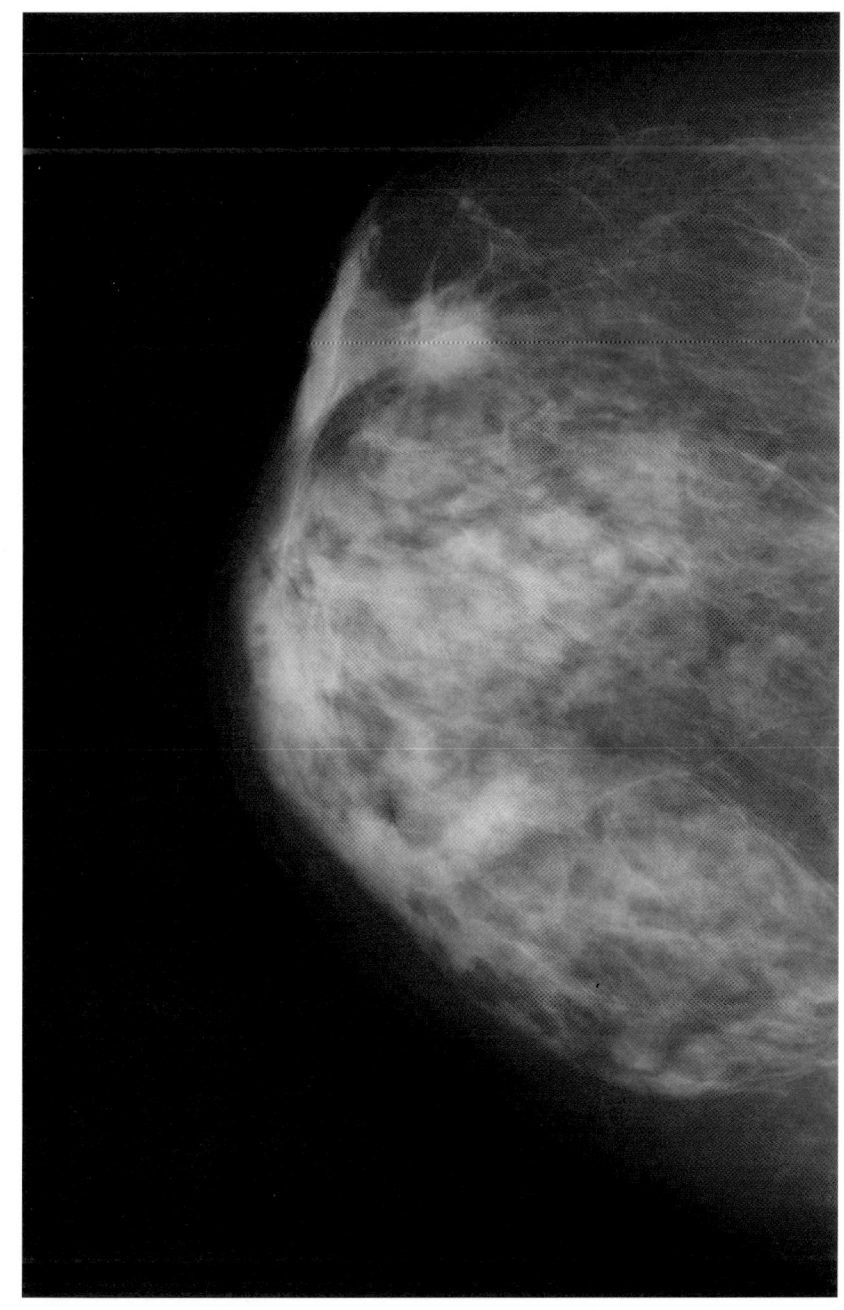

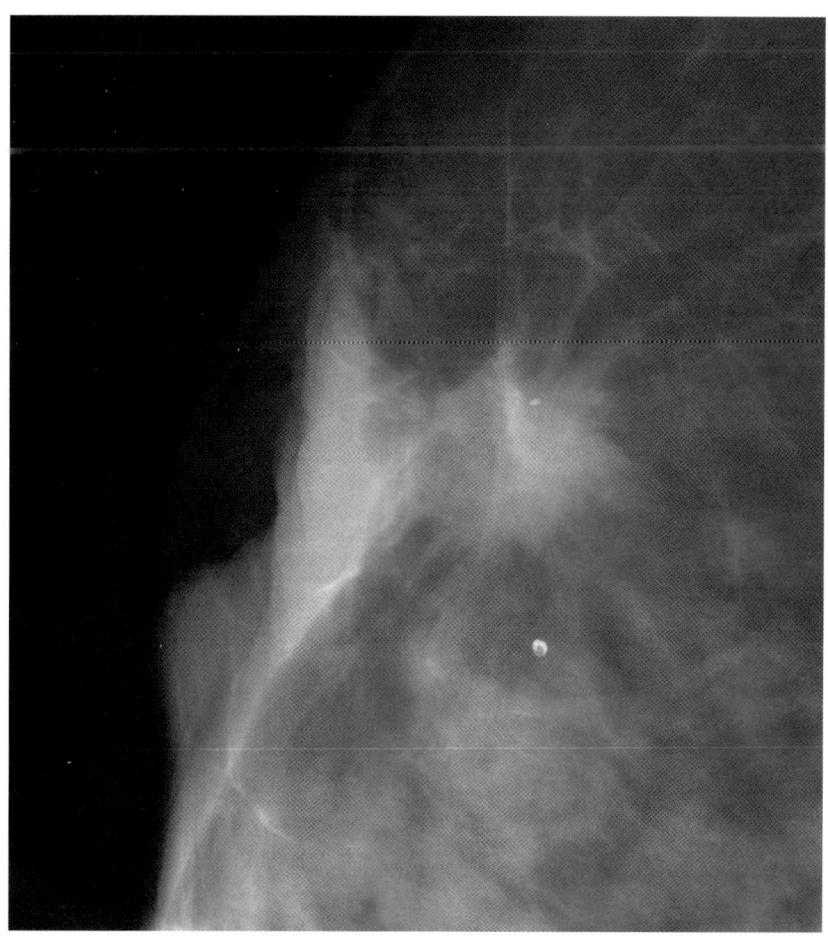

Detail of the craniocaudal projection

Craniocaudal projection

STELLATE OPACITY

Behind the areola, a non-homogeneous stellate opacity is visible with spicules running into the surrounding parenchyma and towards the areolar skin, which appears thickened and retracted.

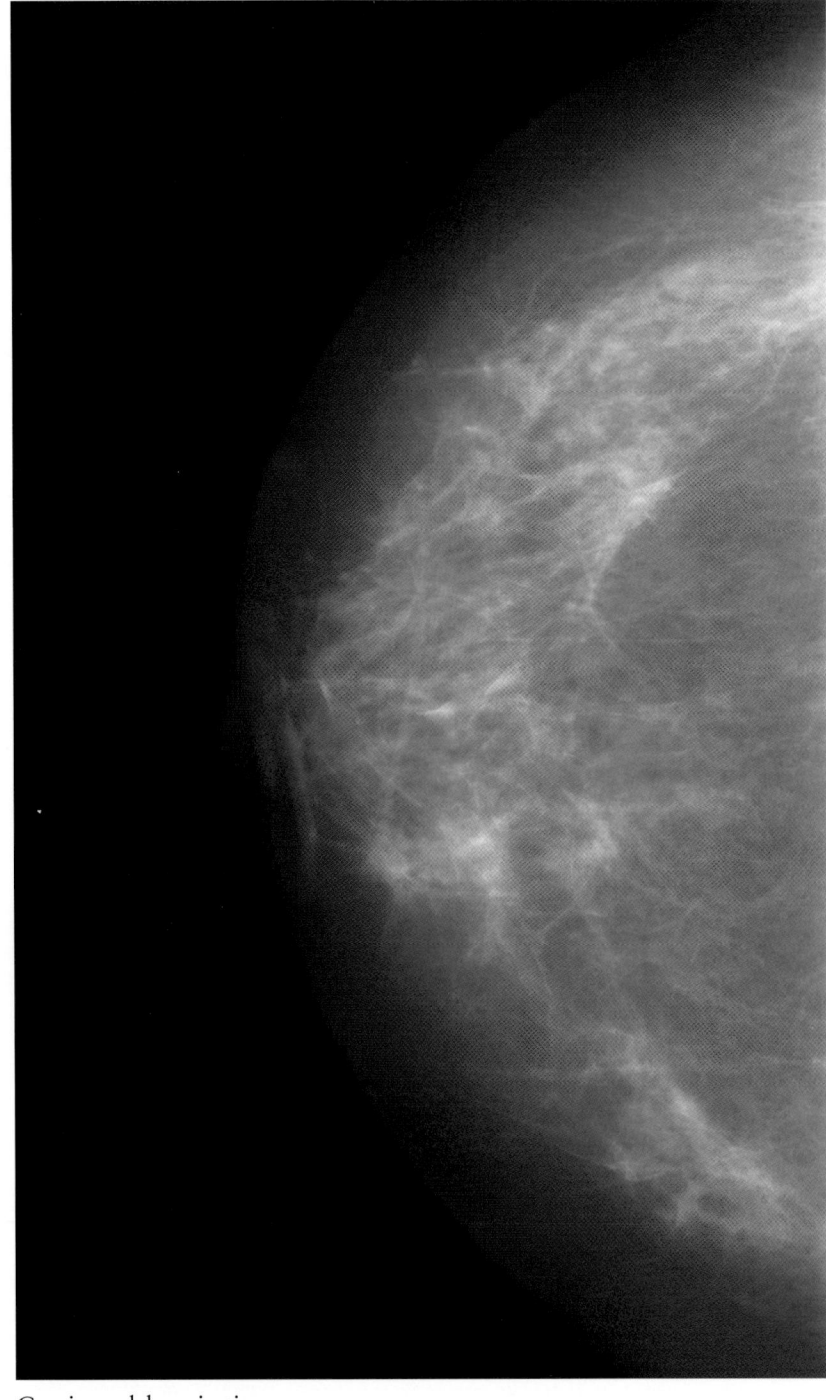

Craniocaudal projection

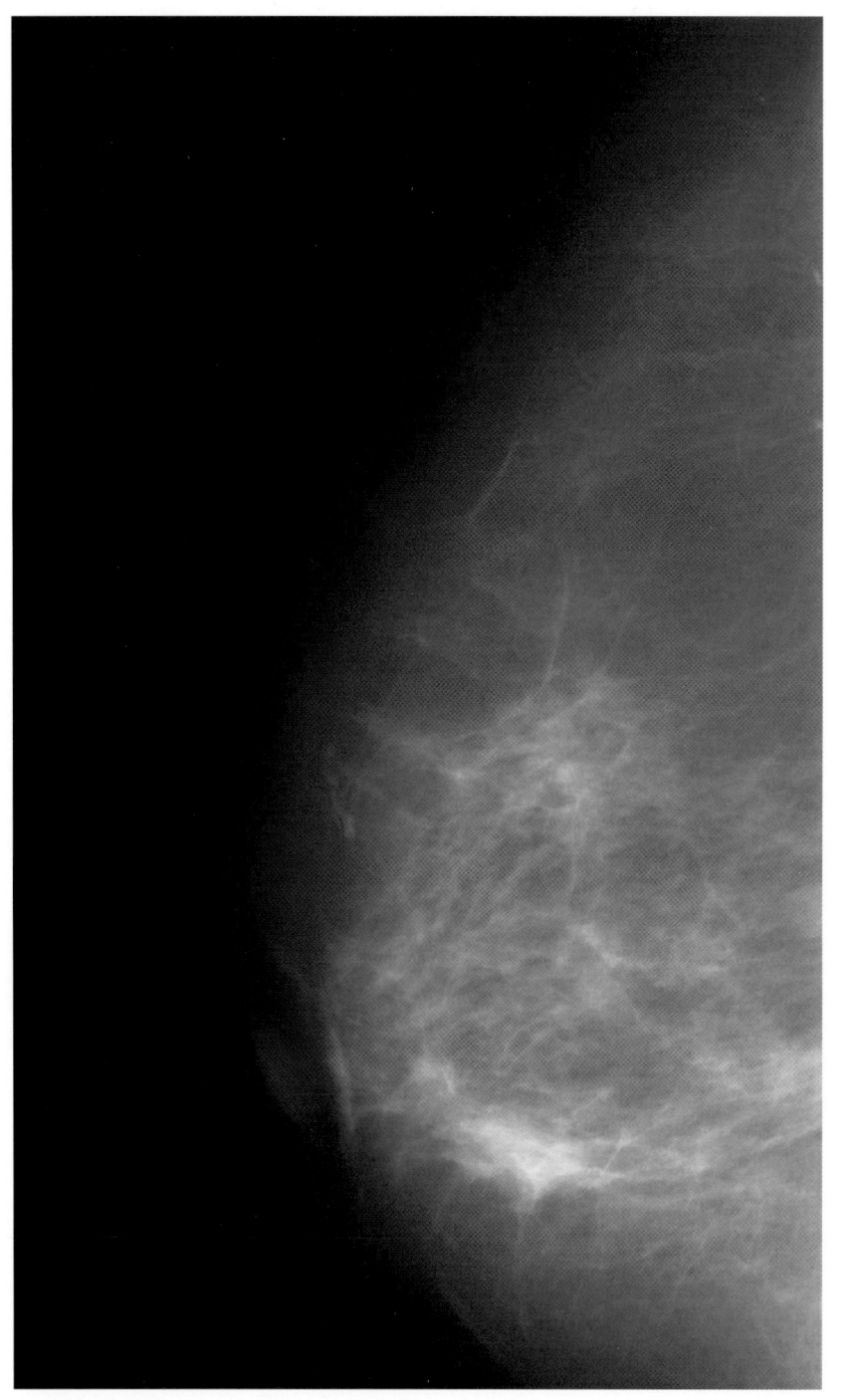

Lateral projection

Behind the areola, a non-homogeneous stellate opacity is visible with spicules running into the surrounding parenchyma and towards the areolar skin, which appears thickened and retracted. The spot compression view, in the tangential craniocaudal projection, shows the thickened skin better. A tangential projection is often decisive for defining lesions in the retroareolar region.

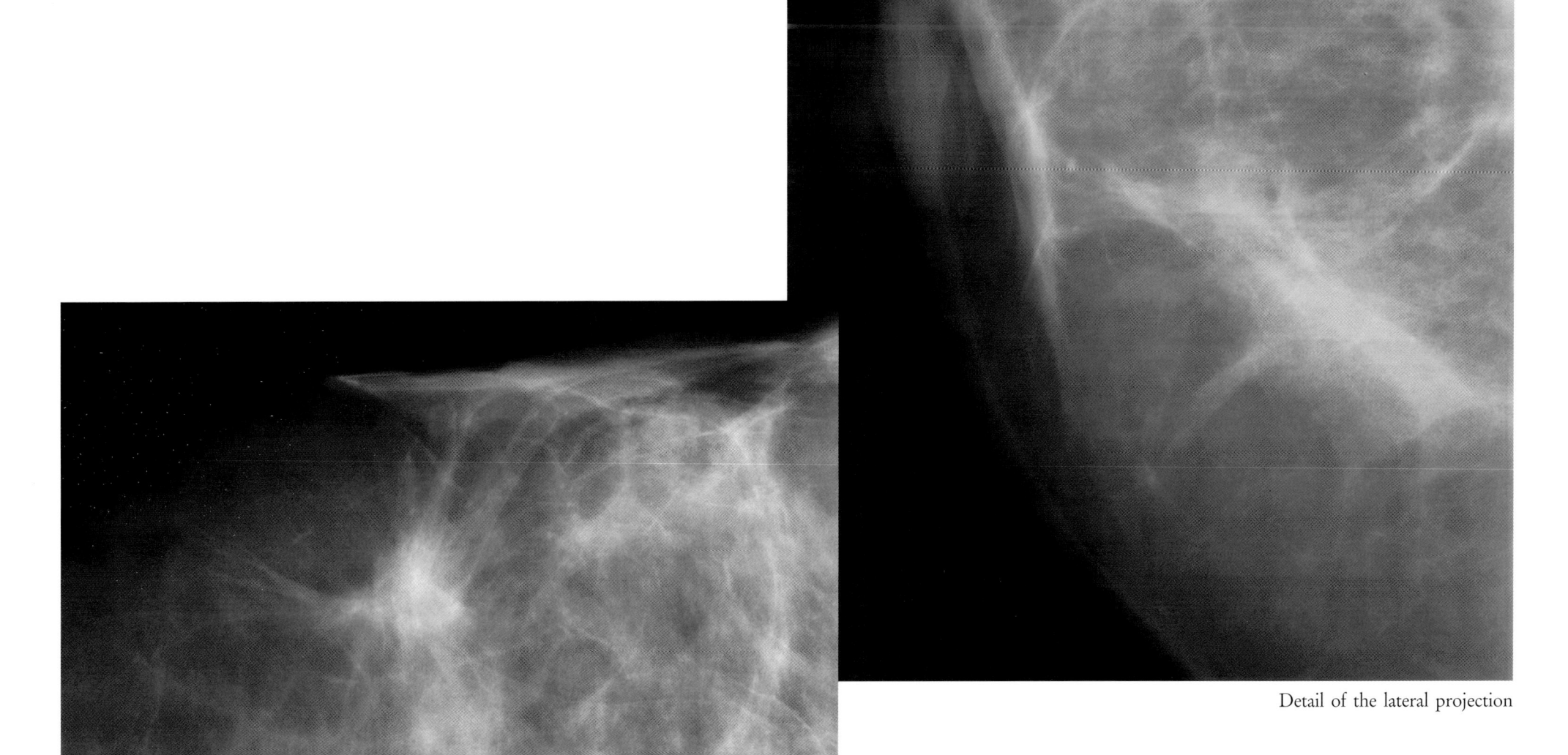

Detail of the lateral projection

Detail of the craniocaudal projection

STELLATE OPACITY

A stellate opacity is visible in an outer anterior location; it is denser than the surrounding parenchyma and has homogeneous spicules proportionate in length to the size of the tumour centre. Posteriorly, the mass appears to be joined to another smaller opacity with poorly defined margins (A). In an upper anterior location there is a stellate opacity with a dense tumour centre and radiating spicules that are mostly homogeneous, except for some elongated, asymmetrical dendritic spicules (B).

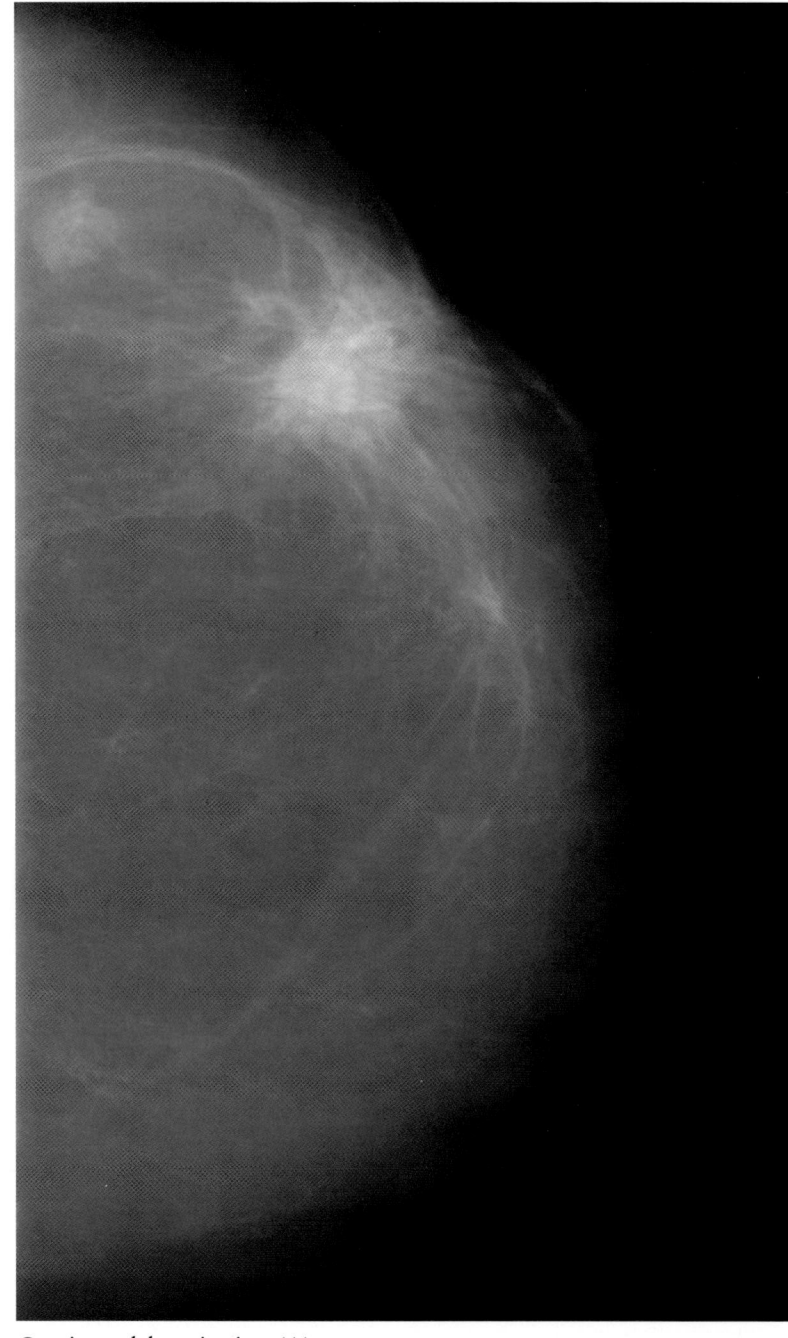

Craniocaudal projection (A)

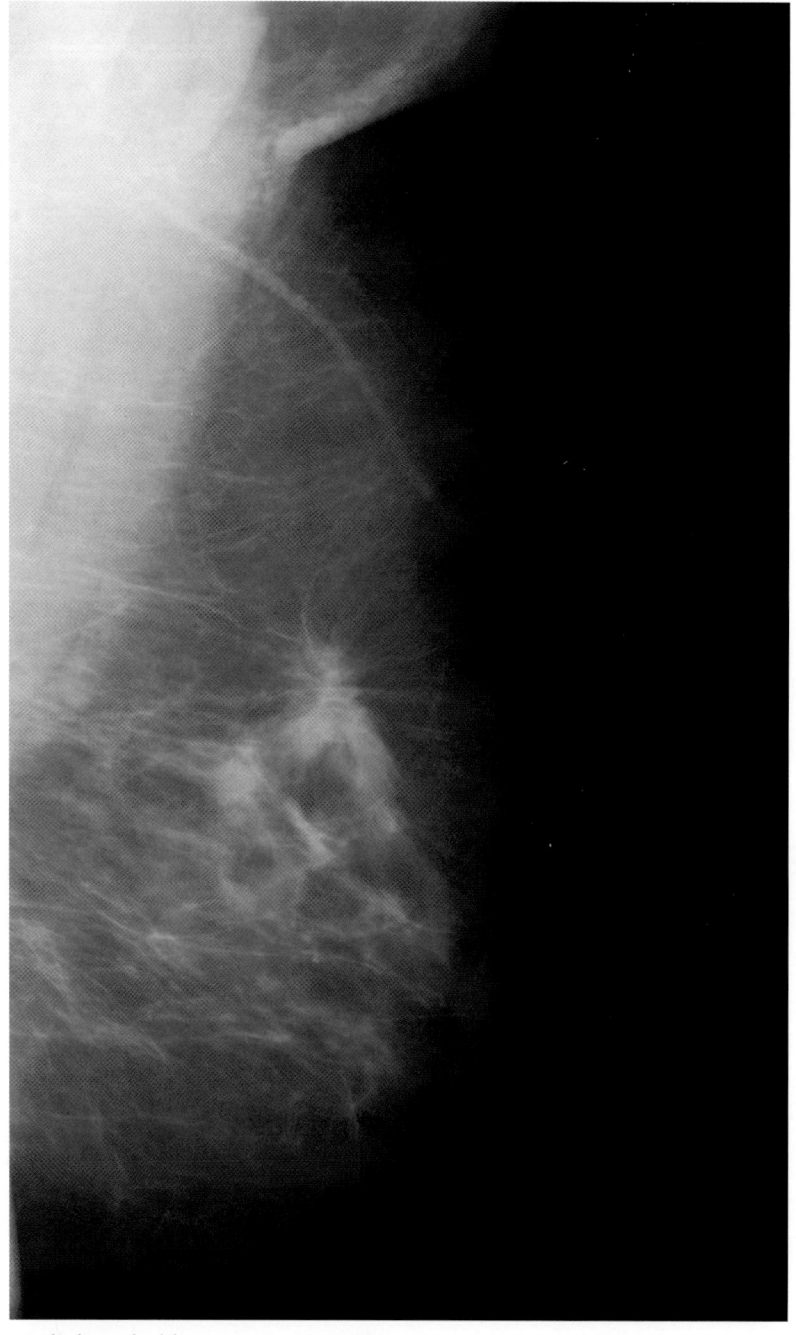

Mediolateral oblique projection (B)

STELLATE OPACITY

A stellate opacity is visible in an outer anterior location; it is denser than the surrounding parenchyma and has homogeneous spicules proportionate in length to the size of the tumour centre. Posteriorly, the mass appears to be joined to another smaller opacity with poorly defined margins (A). In an upper anterior location there is a stellate opacity with a dense tumour centre and radiating spicules that are mostly homogeneous, except for some elongated, asymmetrical dendritic spicules (B).

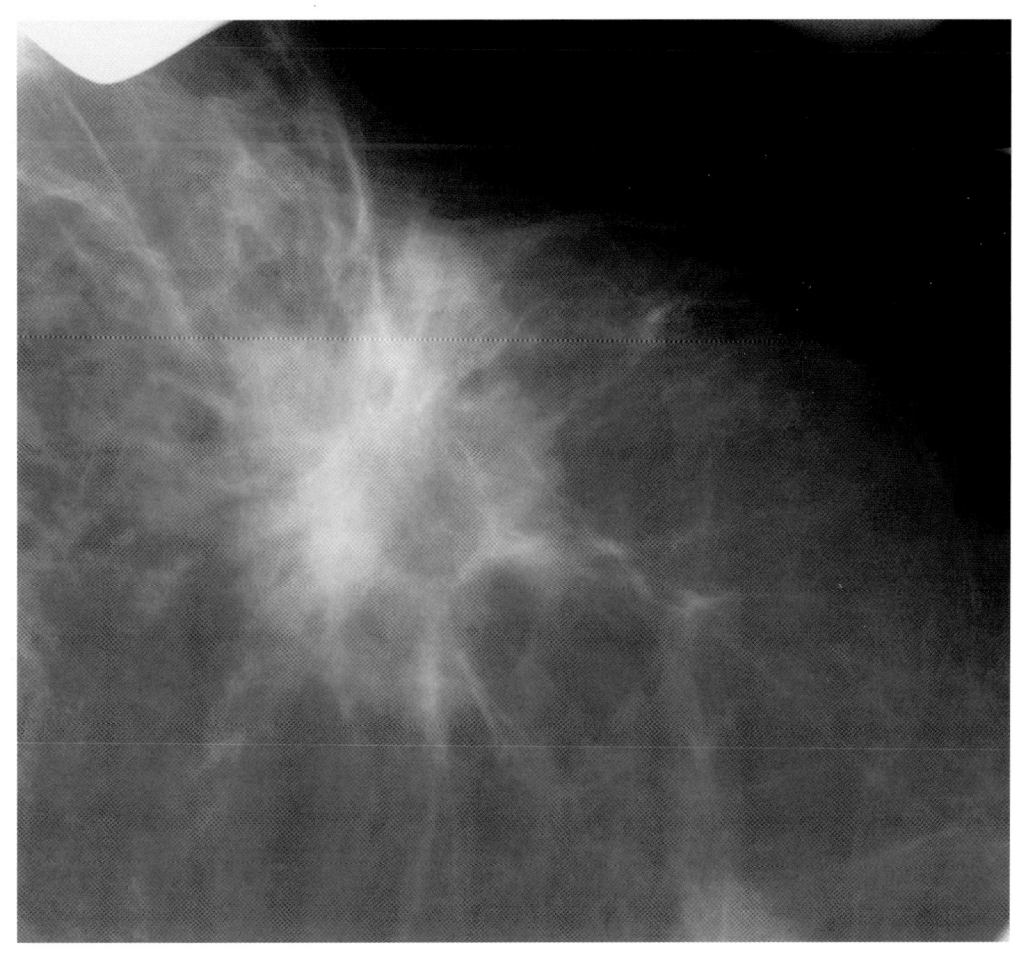

Detail of the craniocaudal projection (A)

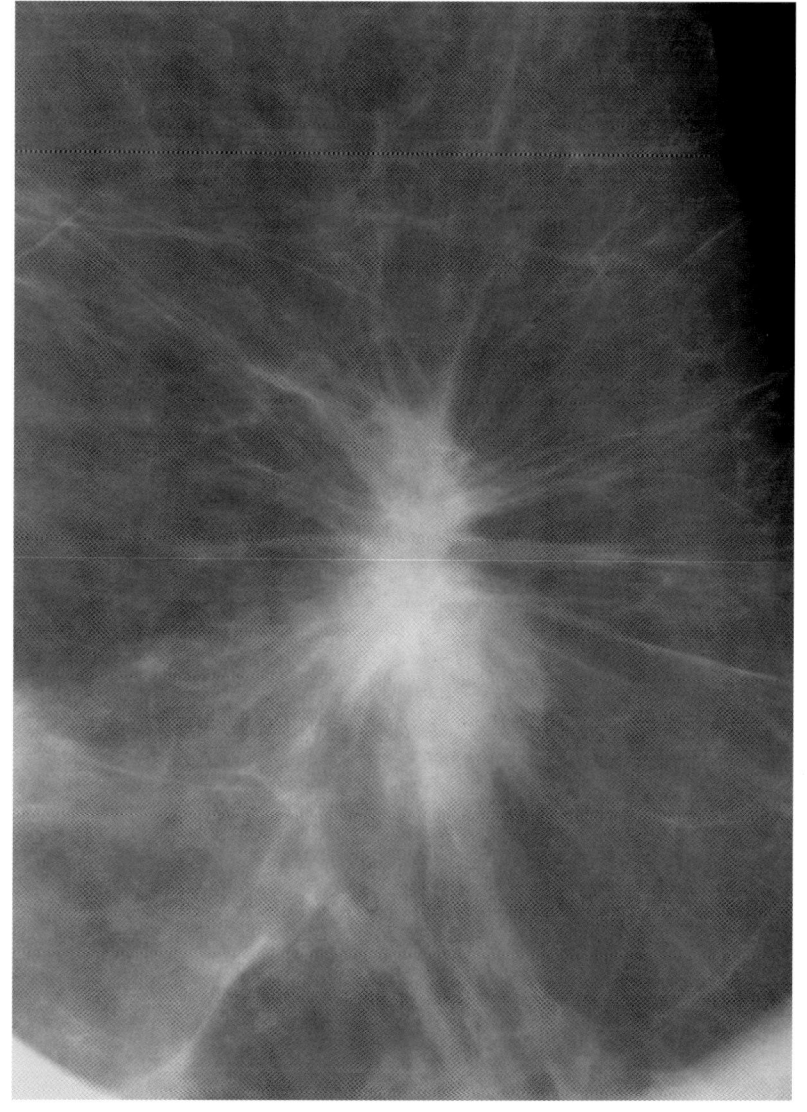

Detail of the oblique projection (B)

STELLATE OPACITY

In the retroareolar space a stellate hyperlucent opacity is visible. It is adjacent to the areolar skin, which appears markedly thickened and retracted, with the nipple stretched over and adhering to the opacity (A). In the upper anterior area there is a low-density stellate opacity with homogeneous radiating spicules proportionate in length to the size of the tumour centre (B).

Note the different density of the two stellate masses, the more lucent one (A) caused by an infiltrating ductal carcinoma and the other (B) by an infiltrating tubular carcinoma.

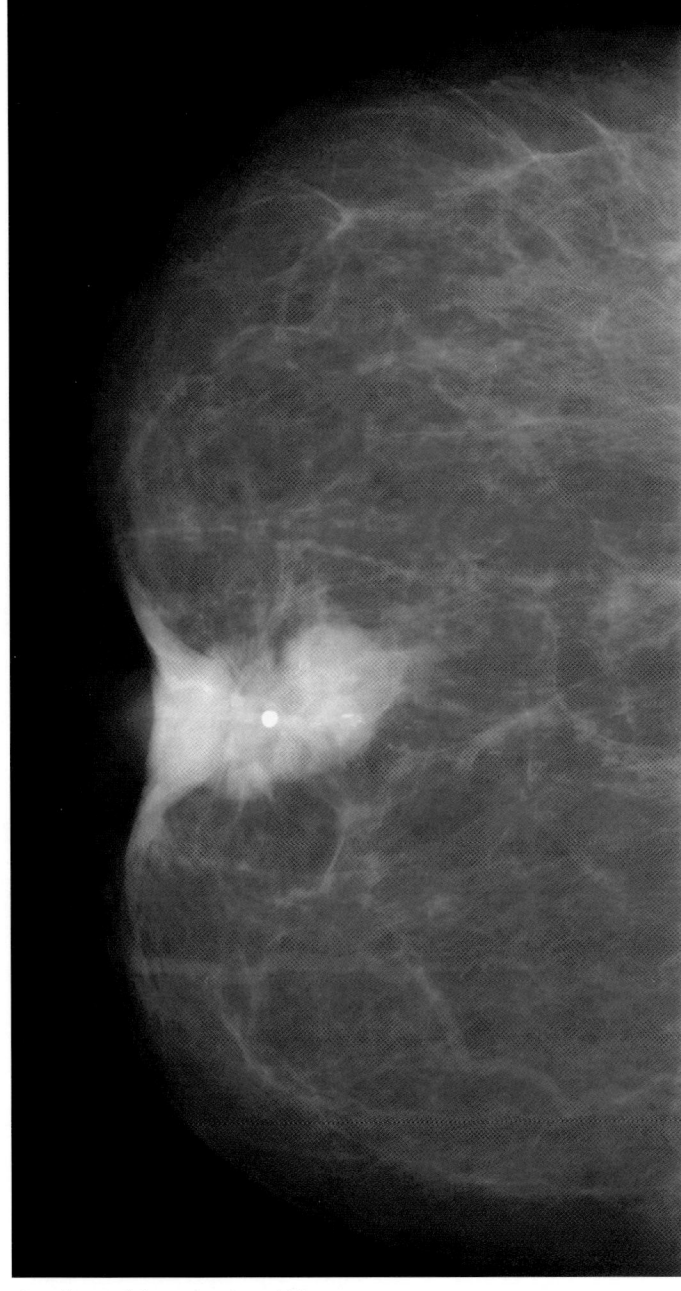

Craniocaudal projection (A)

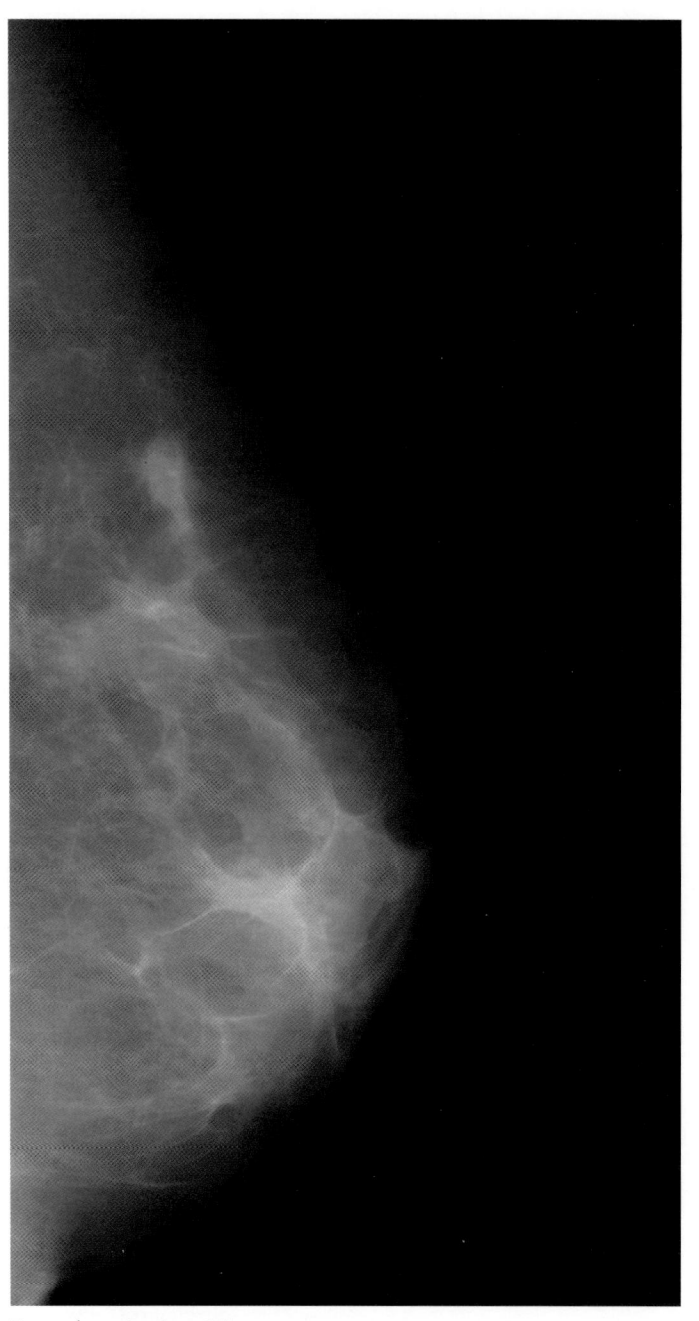

Lateral projection (B)

STELLATE OPACITY

In the retroareolar space a high-density stellate opacity is visible. It is adjacent to the areolar skin, which appears markedly thickened and retracted, with the nipple stretched over and adhering to the opacity (A). In an upper anterior location there is a low-density stellate opacity with homogeneous short radiating spicules proportionate in length to the size of the tumour centre (B).

Note the different density of the two stellate masses, the denser one (A) caused by an infiltrating ductal carcinoma and the other (B) by an infiltrating tubular carcinoma.

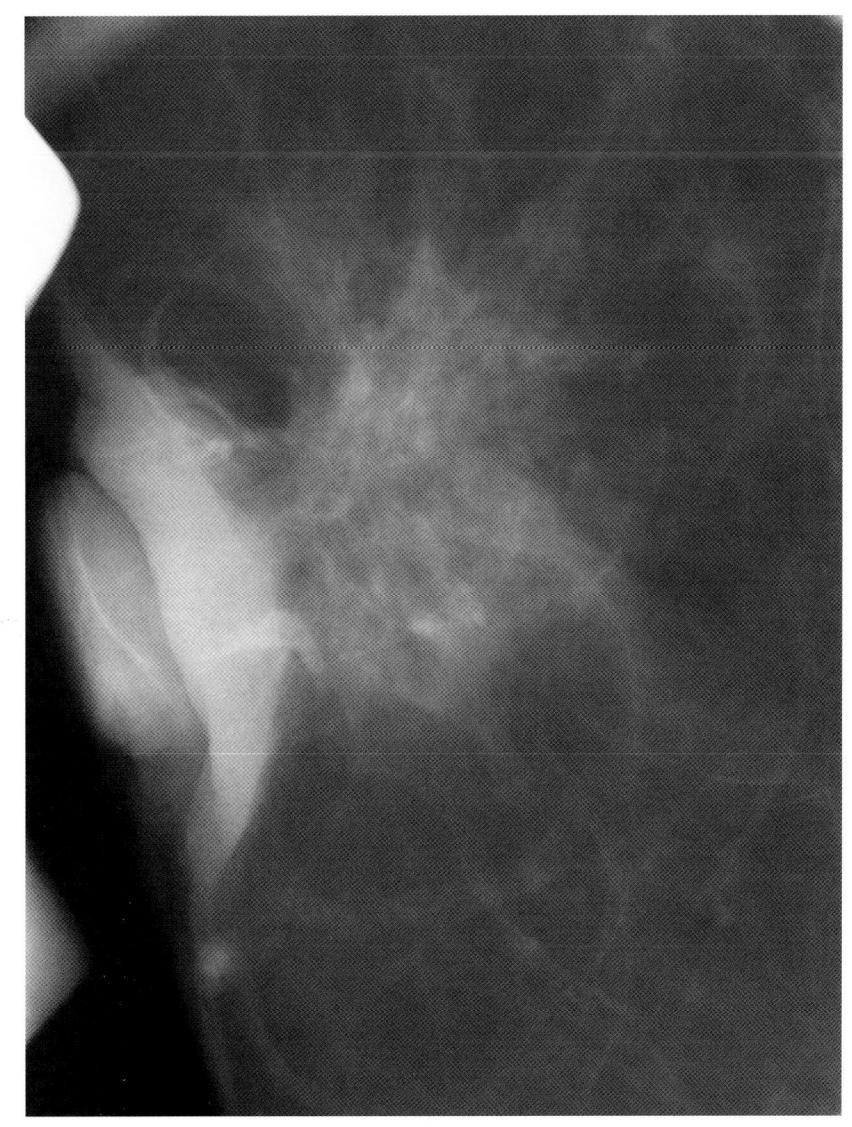

Detail of the craniocaudal projection (A)

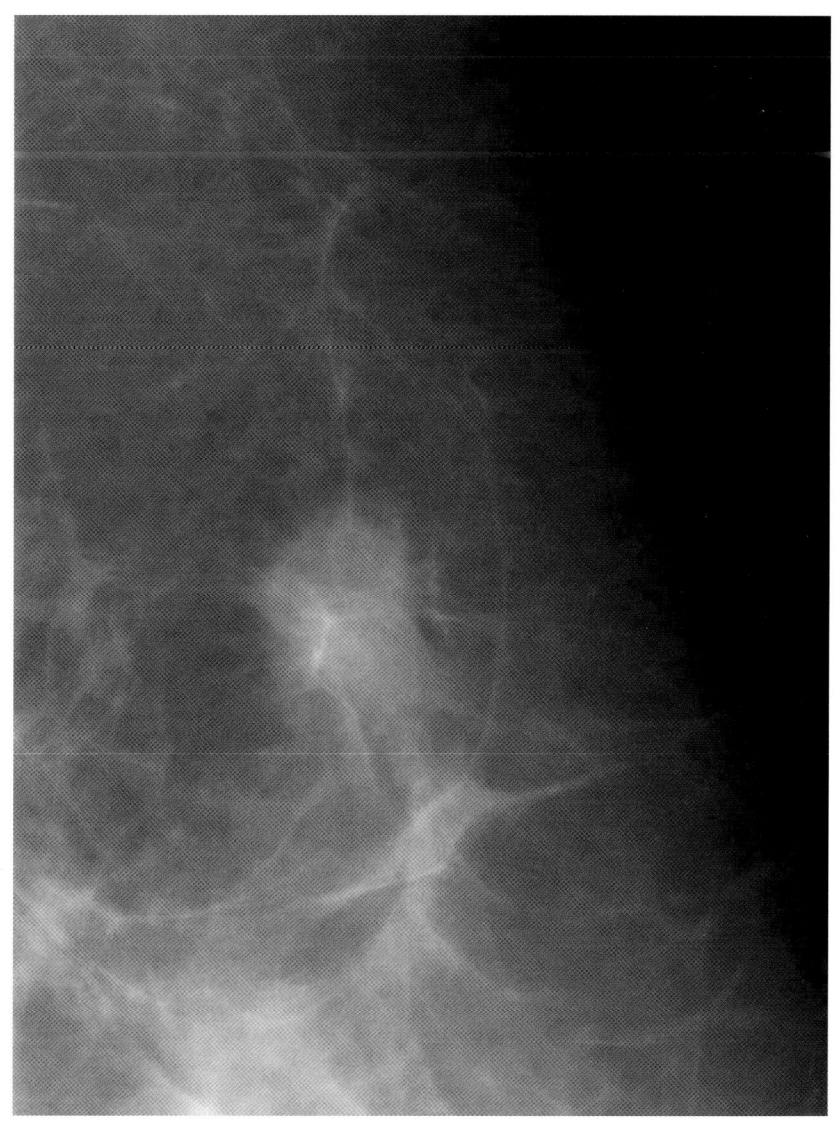

Detail of the lateral projection (B)

STELLATE OPACITY

In the upper outer quadrant and in a central location, there is a stellate opacity of the same density as the surrounding tissue, with non-homogeneous spicules at its margins and a moderately dense tumour centre, which can be identified only in the craniocaudal projection.

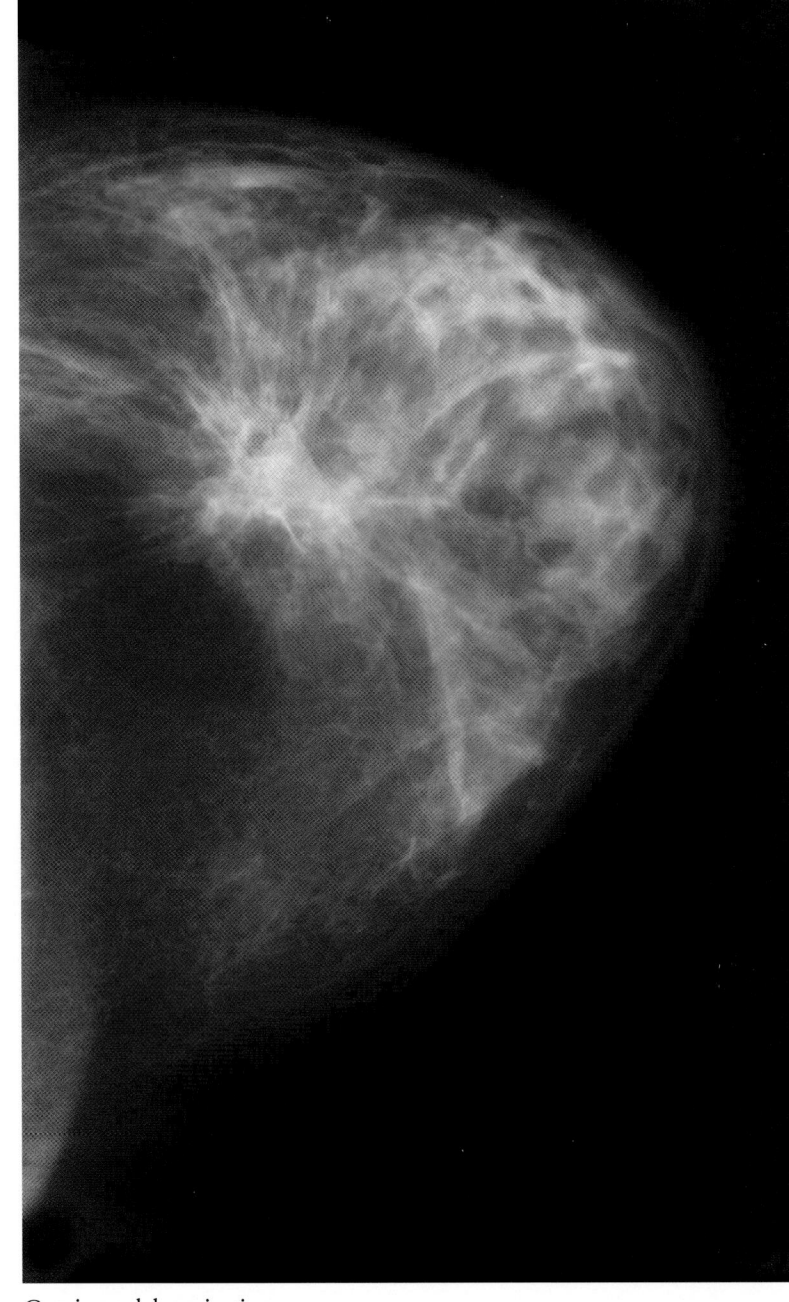

Craniocaudal projection

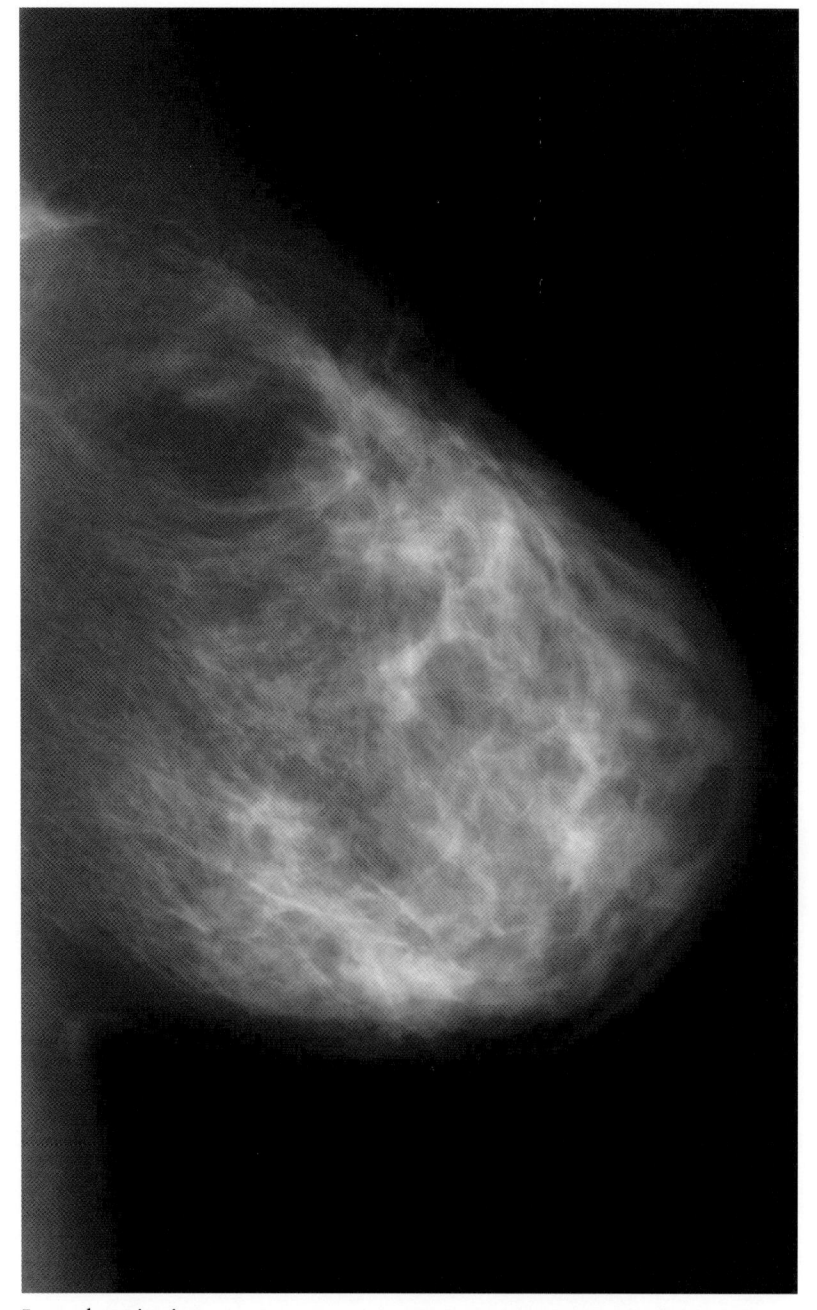

Lateral projection

STELLATE OPACITY

The spot compression view shows a stellate opacity of comparable density to the surrounding parenchyma, with non-homogeneous spicules at its margins and an irregular shape in the lateral projection. Here the radiating pattern is no longer recognizable, but multiple, confluent, radiolucent vacuoles are visible (post-quadrantectomy scarring with foci of fat necrosis).

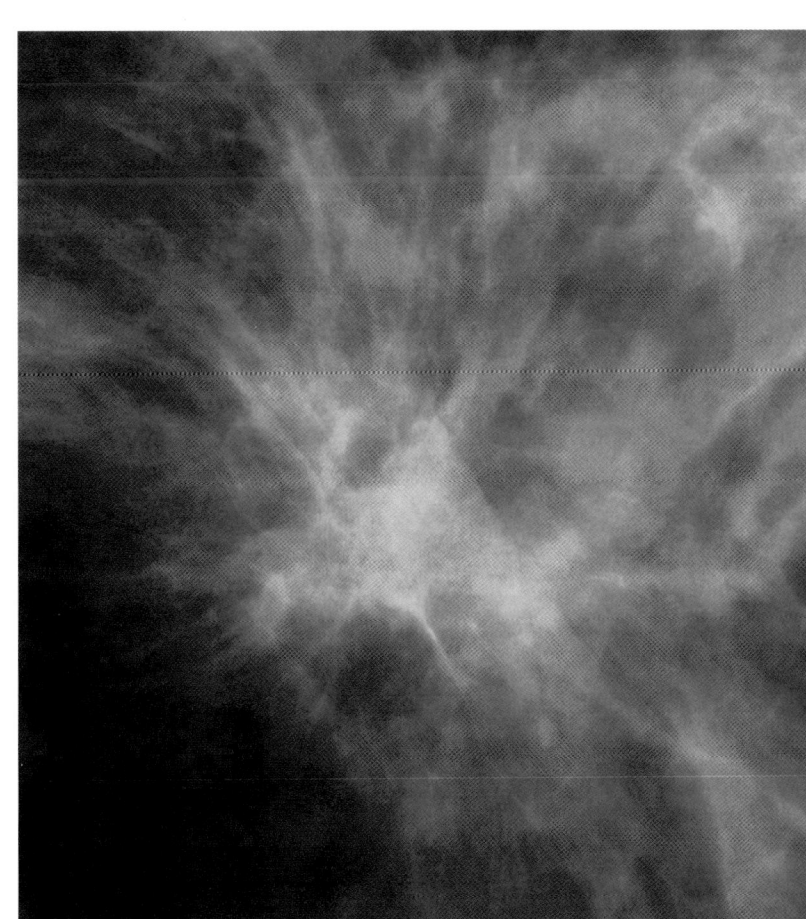

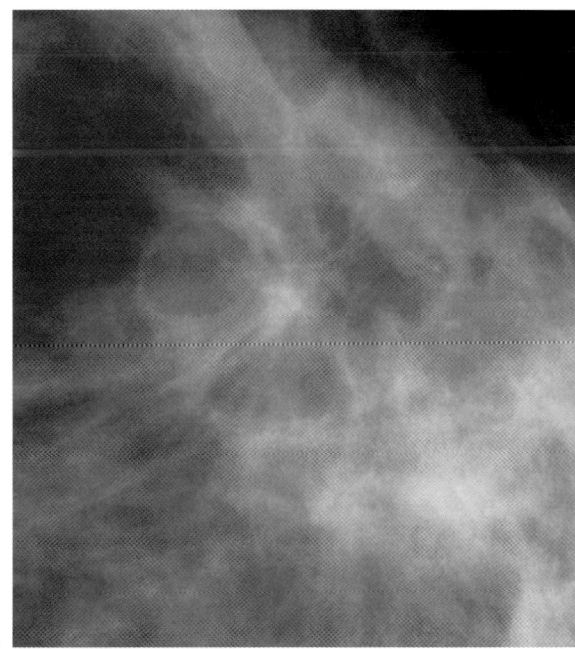

Detail of the lateral projection

Detail of the craniocaudal projection

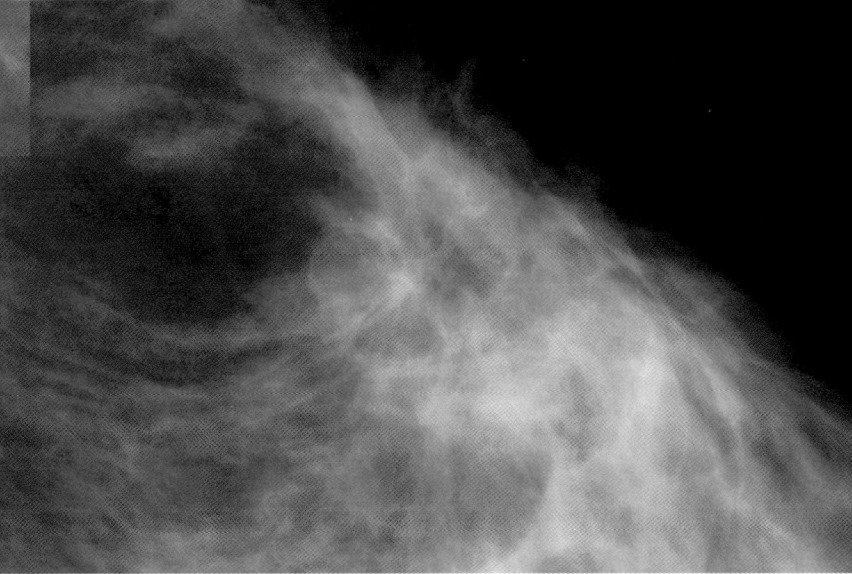

STELLATE OPACITY

A stellate lesion is visible in an outer central location, of similar low density to the surrounding tissues. There is no clearly visible high-density tumour centre, and the two orthogonal projections do not give the same morphological patterns. The lateral projection shows the thin non-homogeneous spicules of variable length better, which seem to converge on a central area with no sign of a nucleus. The parenchyma appears wrinkled and irregular, forming a rosette-like pattern. These features are consistent with a benign proliferative lesion, but make it difficult to distinguish a stellate lesion from an architectural distortion.

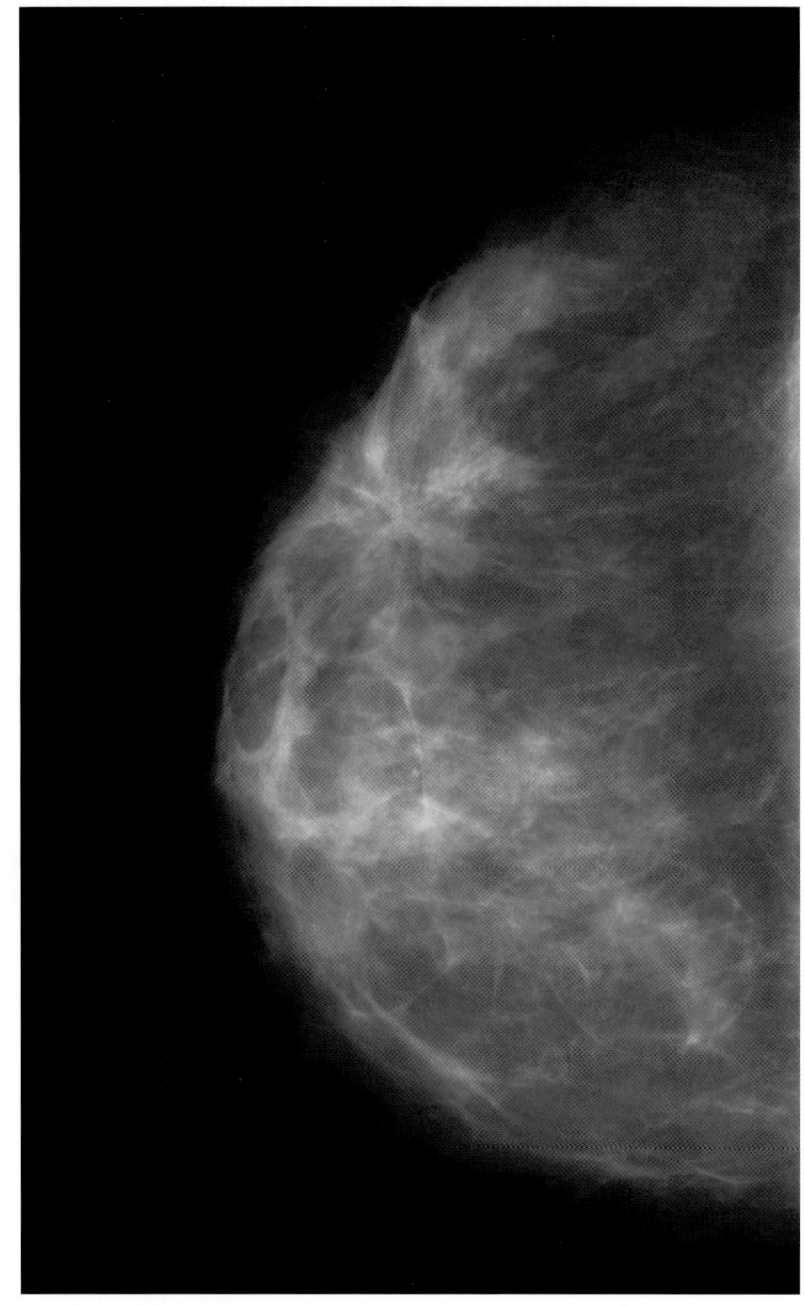

Craniocaudal projection

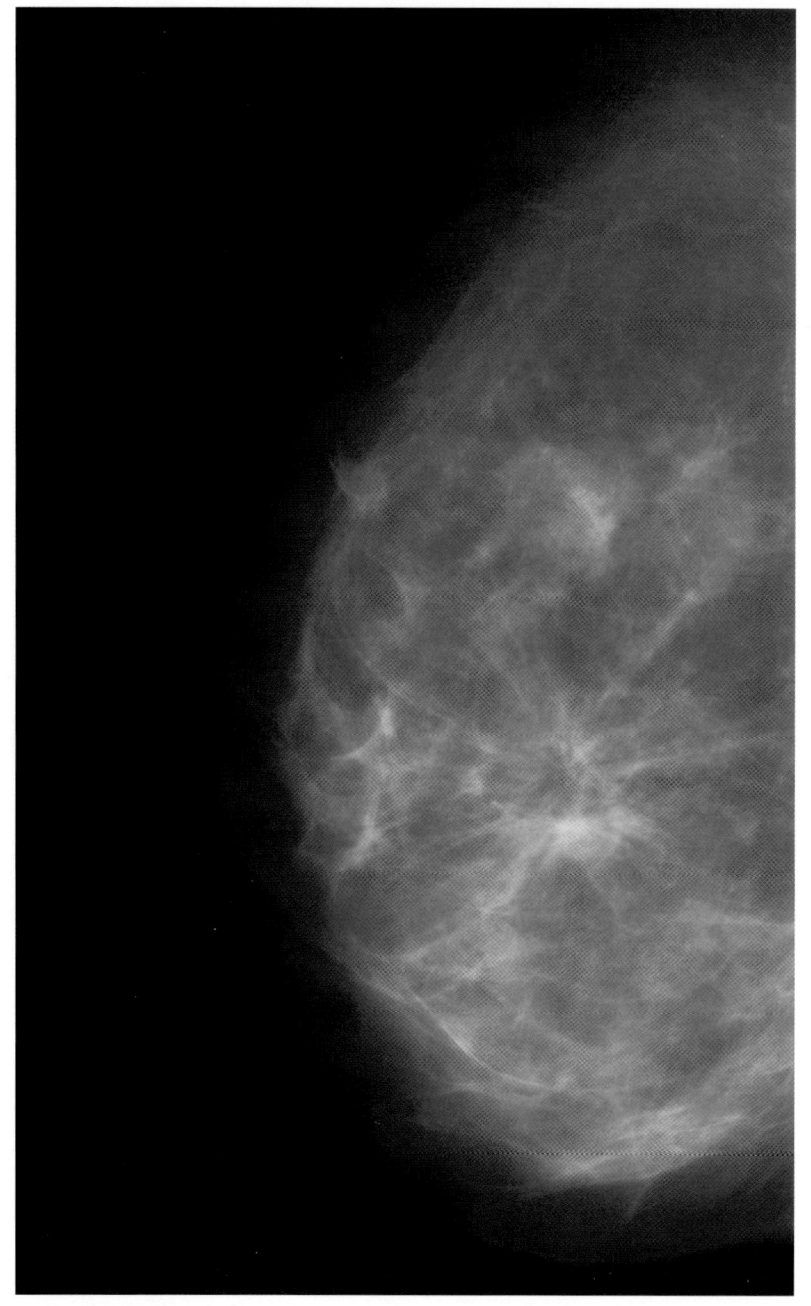

Lateral projection

STELLATE OPACITY

A stellate lesion is visible in an outer central location, of similar low density to the surrounding tissues. There is no clearly visible dense tumour centre, and the two orthogonal projections do not give the same morphological patterns. The lateral projection shows the thin non-homogeneous spicules of variable length better, which seem to converge on a central area with no sign of a dense nucleus. The parenchyma appears wrinkled and irregular, forming a rosette-like pattern. These features are consistent with a benign proliferative lesion, but make it difficult to distinguish a stellate lesion from an architectural distortion.

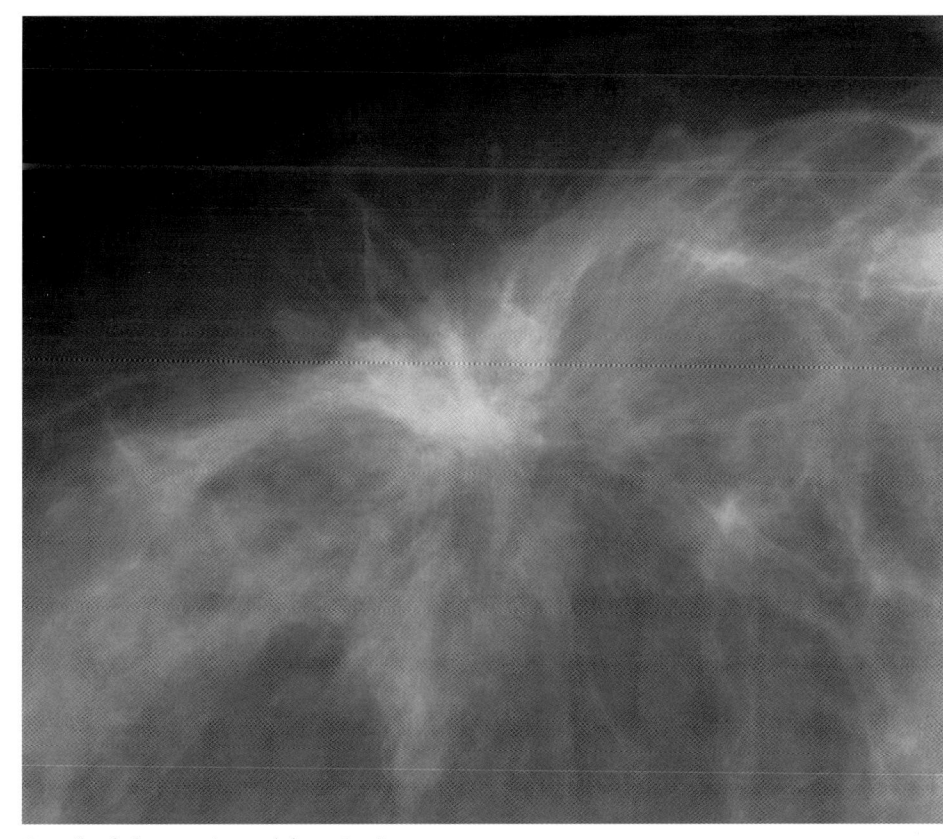

Detail of the craniocaudal projection

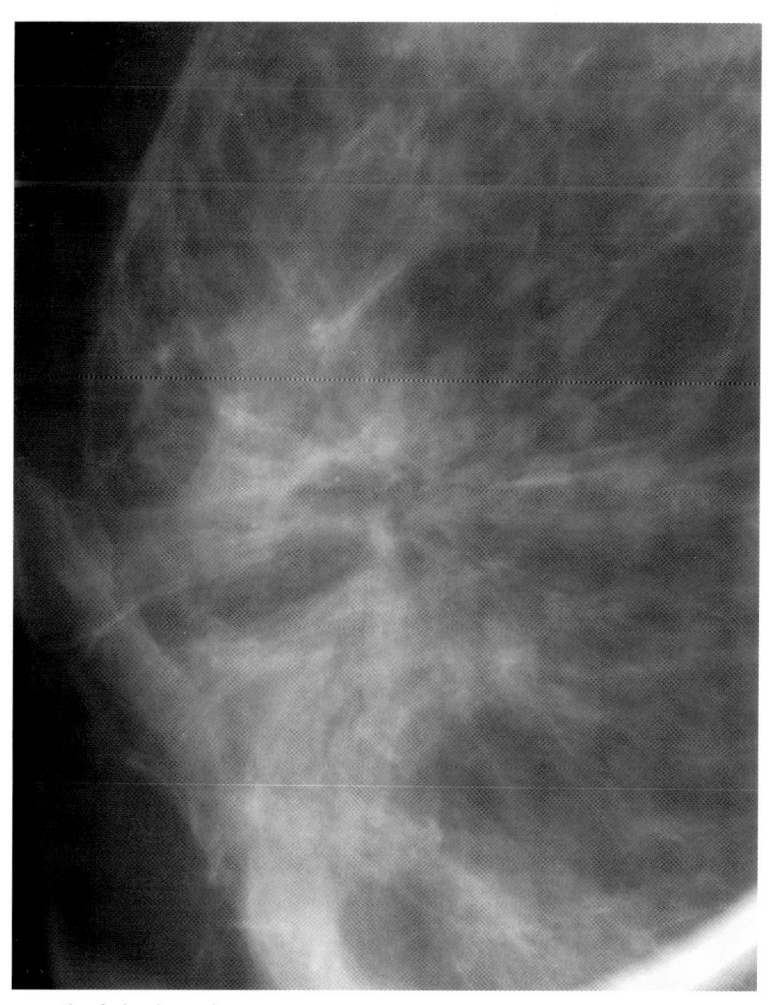

Detail of the lateral projection

Histological finding: atypical lobular hyperplasia

STELLATE OPACITY

In a central posterior location there is a small, low-density stellate opacity with fine, short, homogeneous, radiating spicules proportionate in length to the size of the nucleus.

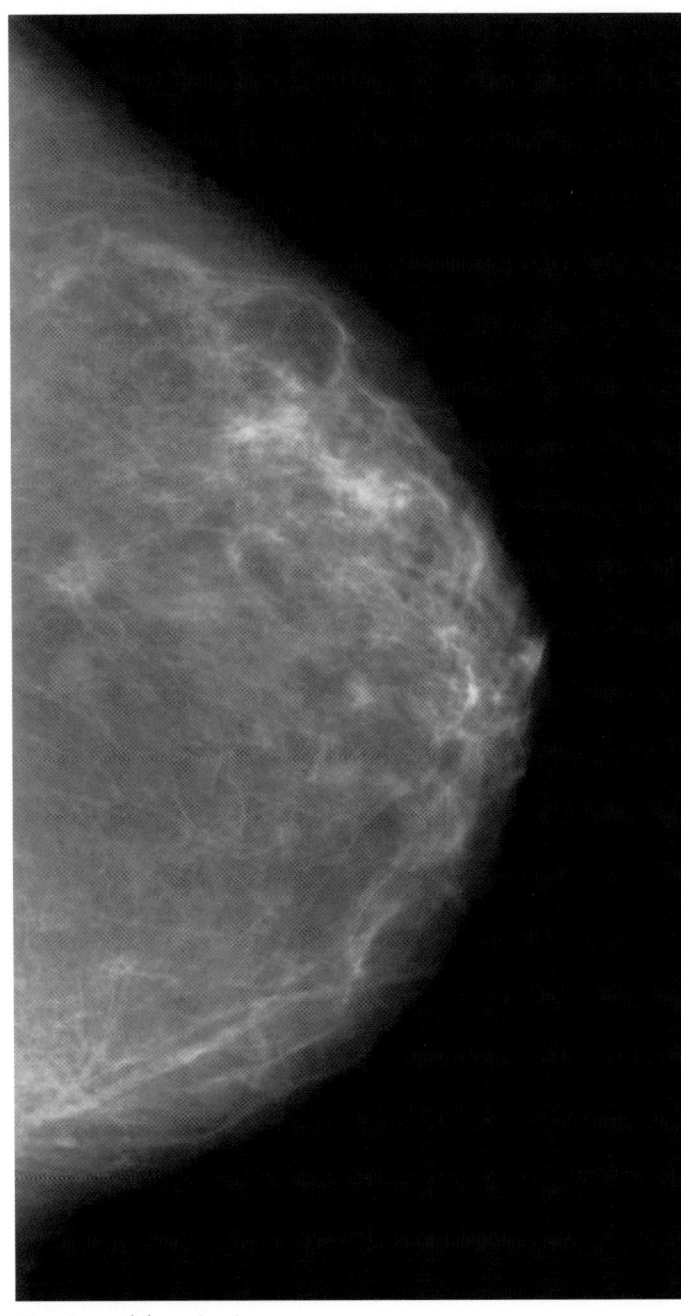

Magnification view

Craniocaudal projection

Histological finding: infiltrating ductal carcinoma

STELLATE OPACITY

In a middle and central location there is a low-density stellate opacity with non-homogeneous spicules radiating into the surrounding tissues. In the magnification view the tumour centre appears clearer, with multiple small radiolucent areas and one single coarse calcification inside it. The spicules are asymmetric, some proportionate to the tumour centre, others thin and alternating with elongated and radiolucent ones.

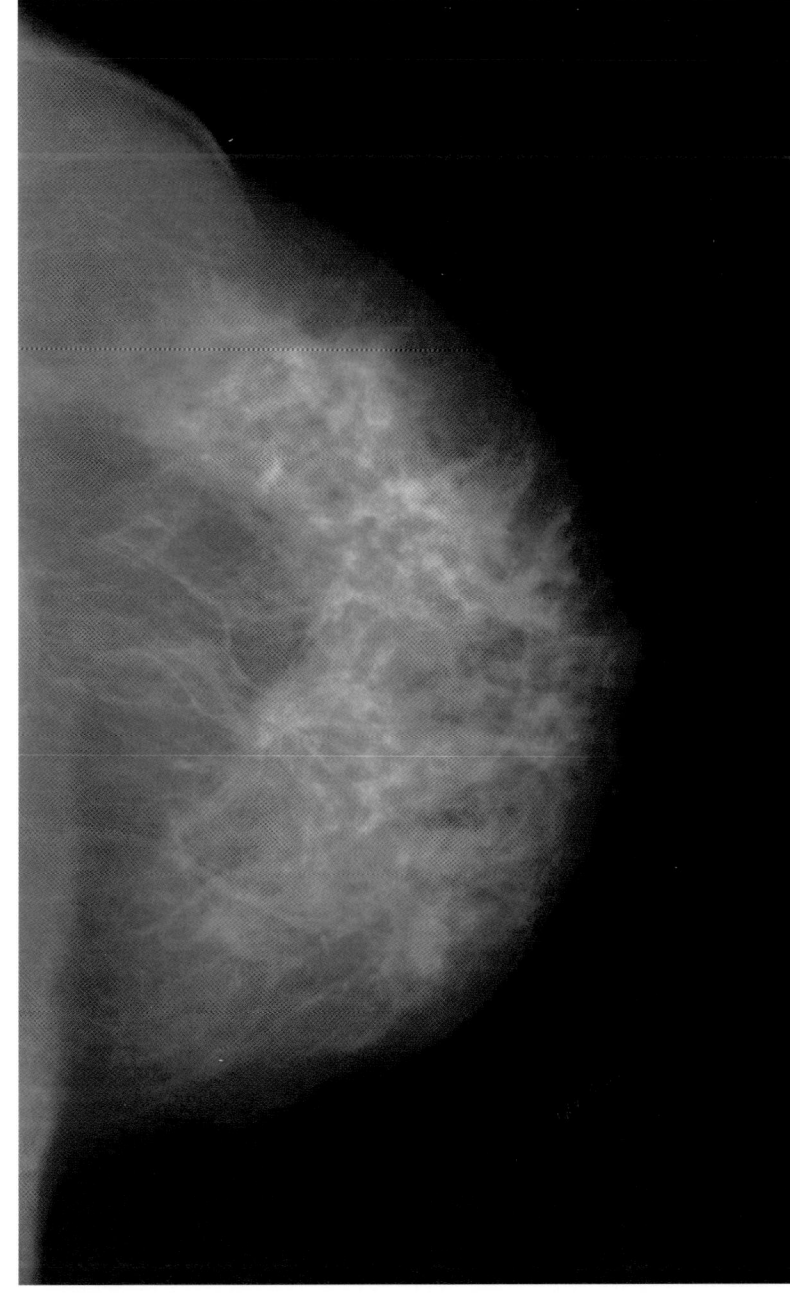

Craniocaudal projection

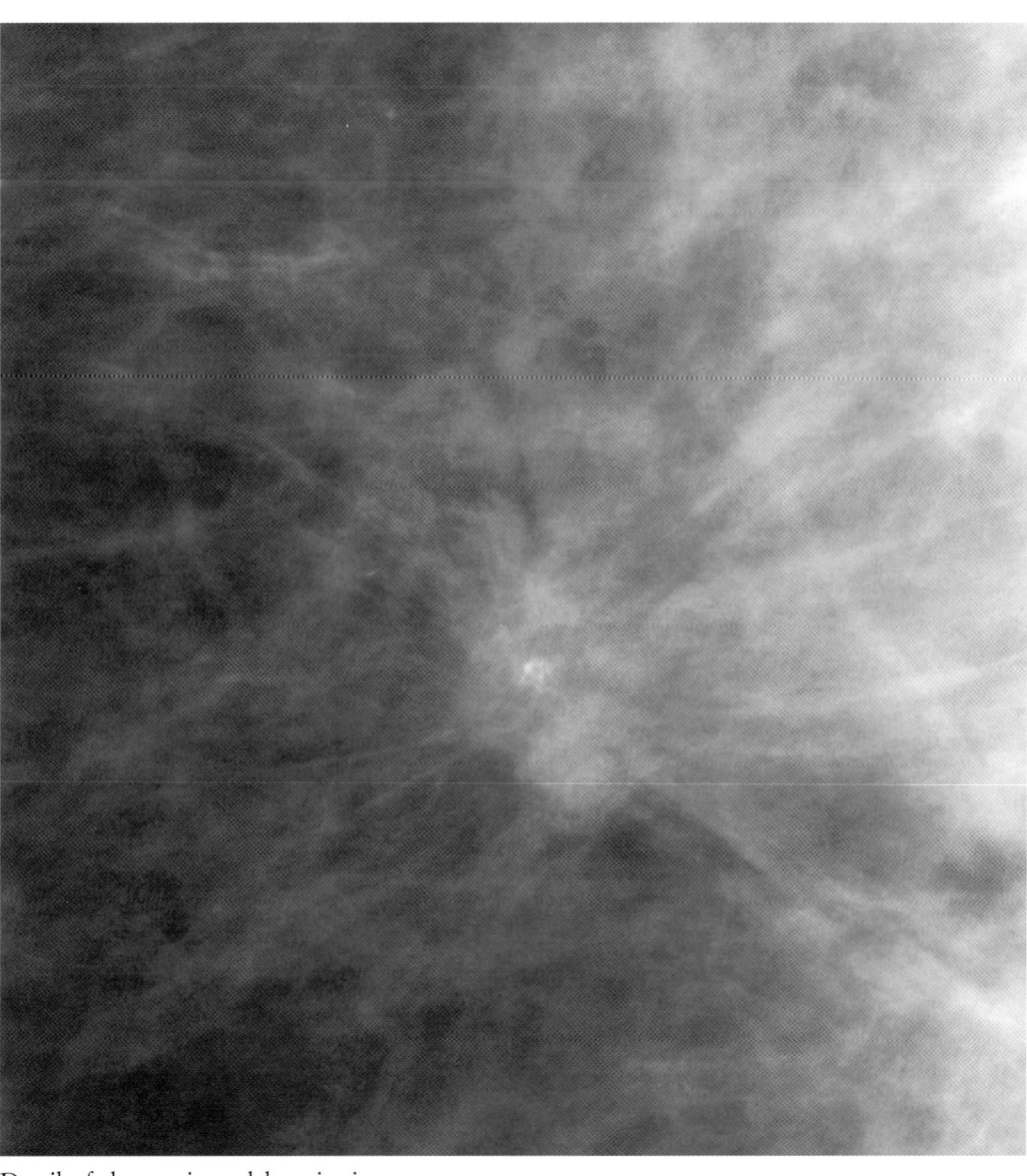

Detail of the craniocaudal projection

Histological finding: atypical lobular hyperplasia

STELLATE OPACITY

Small stellate opacities of varying density which on closer examination present scalloped or spiculated margins. The real length of the spicules can be grasped more easily in the magnification view of the specimen.

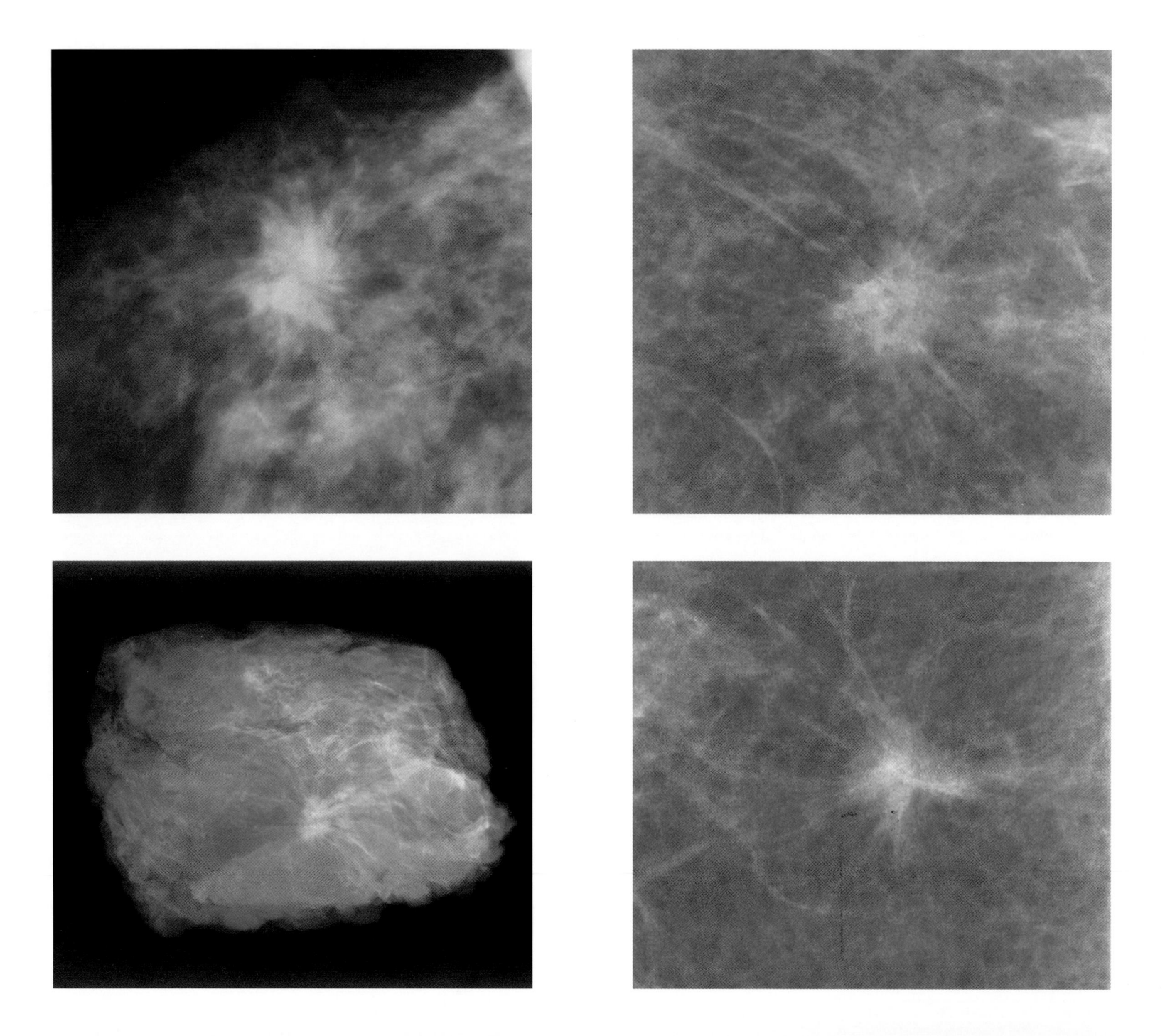

Stellate opacity:
differential diagnosis of benign proliferative lesion and carcinoma

Benign proliferative lesion

- The morphology of the opacity may vary in different projections
- No palpable mass and/or skin retraction, even when the lesion is bulky or superficial
- Few, coarse calcifications
- No central dense, solid tumour centre
- Radiolucent central vacuoles
- Non-homogeneous, long, thin spicules, not proportionate to the size of the nucleus, bunched together like "sheaves of wheat"

Carcinoma

- Dense solid tumour centre
- Dense, well-defined radiating spicules, proportionate in length to the size of the tumour centre
- Small carcinomas may have serrated or scalloped margins
- There may be skin retraction
- The lesions may contain casting-like or granular calcifications

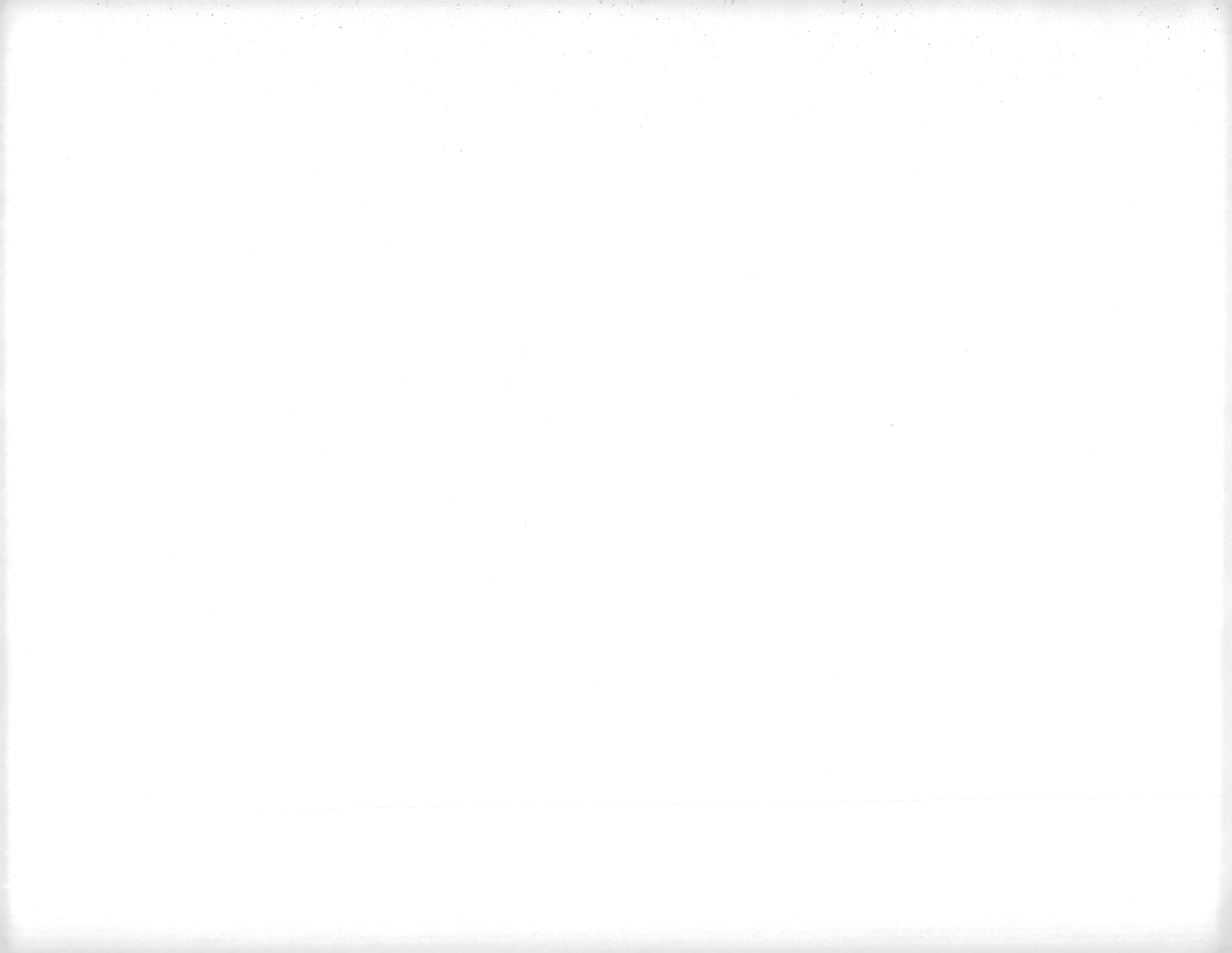

Diffuse opacity

Definition
Morphologically poorly defined or circumscribed opacity, occupying more or less extensive parts of the fibro-glandular architecture. It may be objectively difficult to distinguish diffuse opacity from focal asymmetry or density due to diffuse edema. Focal asymmetry may merely indicate a diversity of anatomical structure, but diffuse opacities are almost always associated with disease. Unlike oedematous thickening, diffuse opacities are not accompanied by obvious signs of inflammation.

Margins
Poorly defined.

Density
Density is generally higher than the surrounding parenchyma, and relatively homogeneous.

DIFFUSE OPACITY

On the left, behind the areola, there is diffuse low-density opacity with poorly defined margins fading gradually into the surrounding fatty tissue. No evident signs of inflammation.

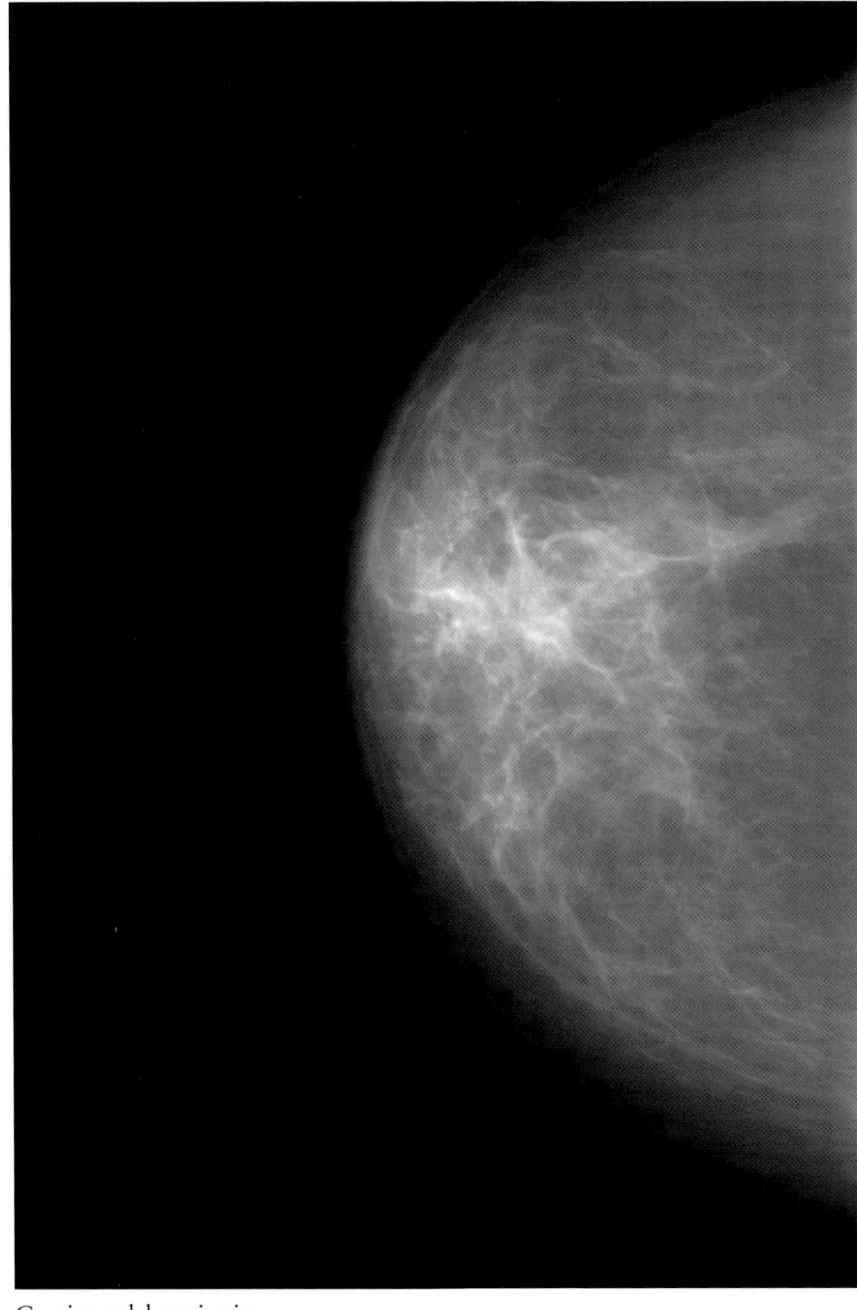

Craniocaudal projection

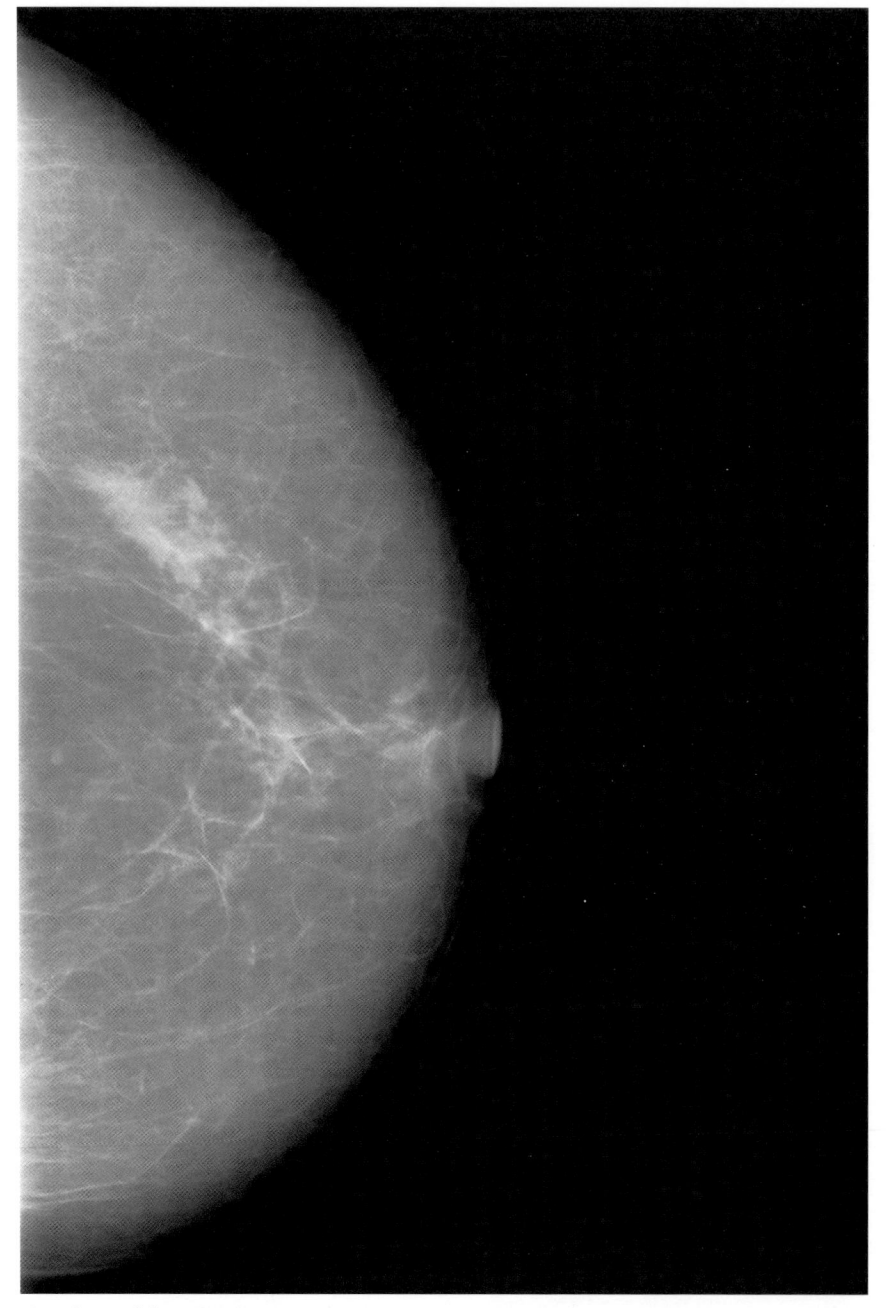

Craniocaudal projection

DIFFUSE OPACITY

On the left, behind the areola, there is diffuse low-density opacity with poorly defined margins fading gradually into the surrounding fatty tissue. No evident signs of inflammation.

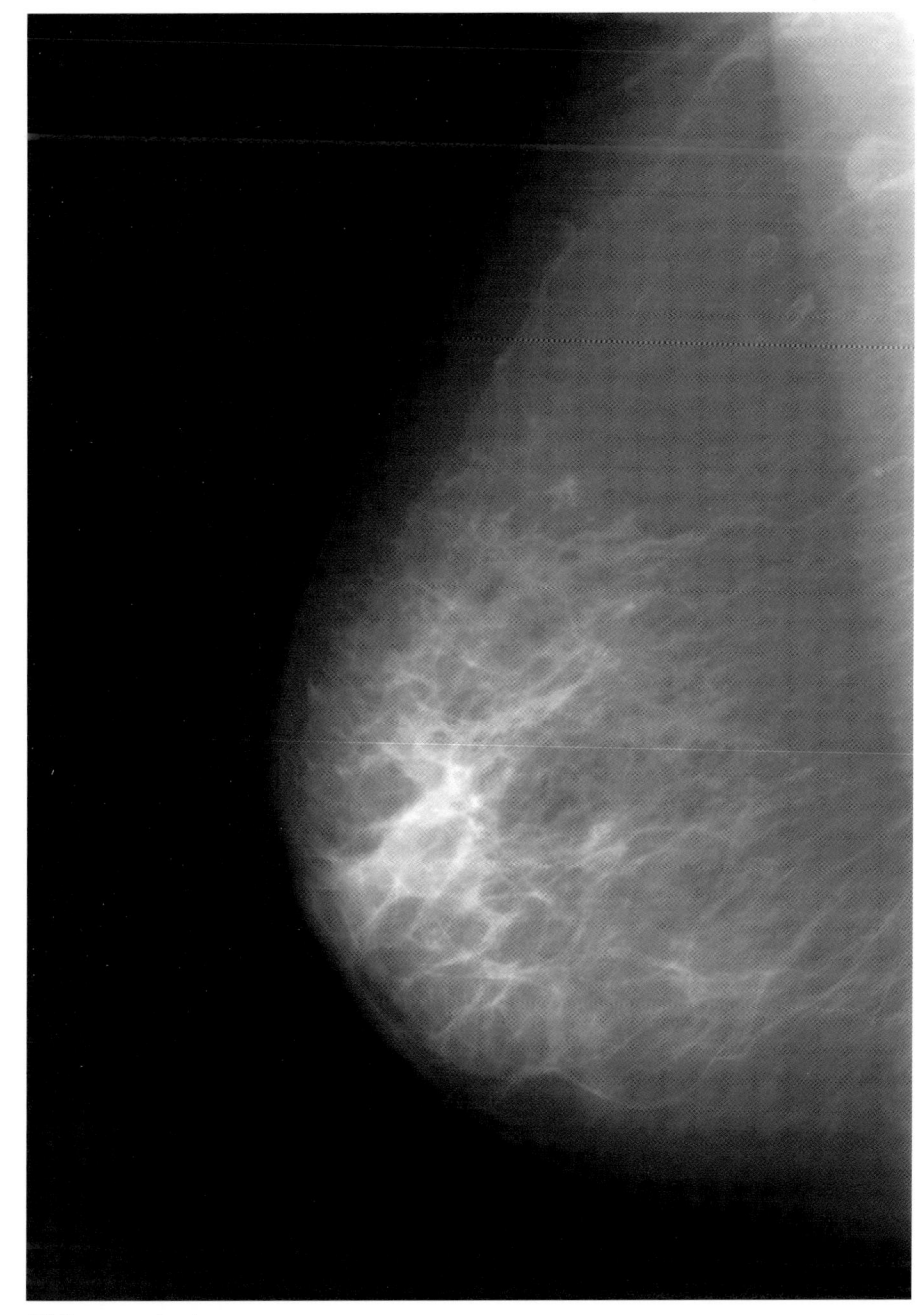

Oblique projection

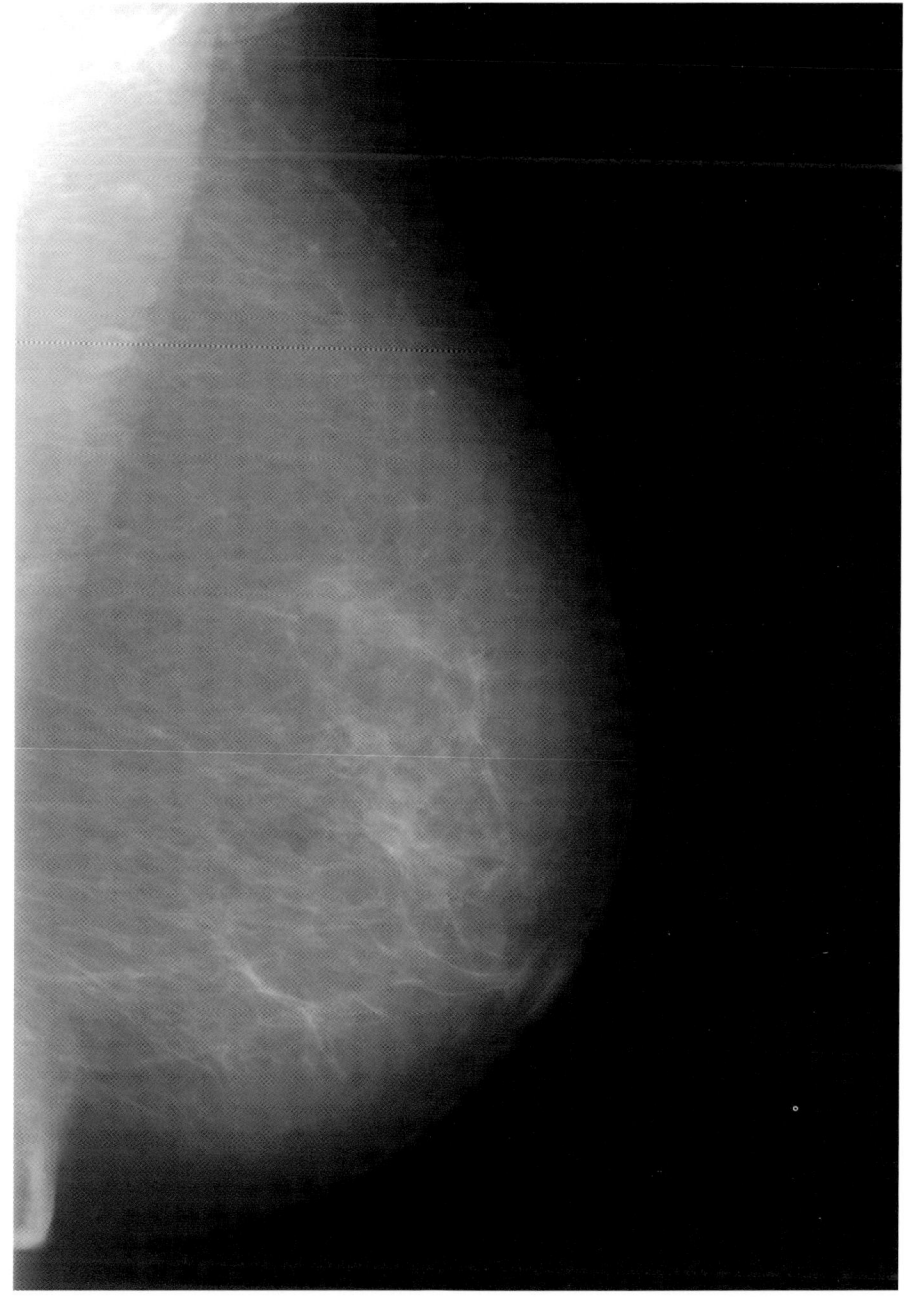

Mediolateral oblique projection

DIFFUSE OPACITY

On the right, in the upper central area behind the areola, there is diffuse opacity with poorly defined margins, clearly denser than the surrounding parenchyma. No evident signs of inflammation.

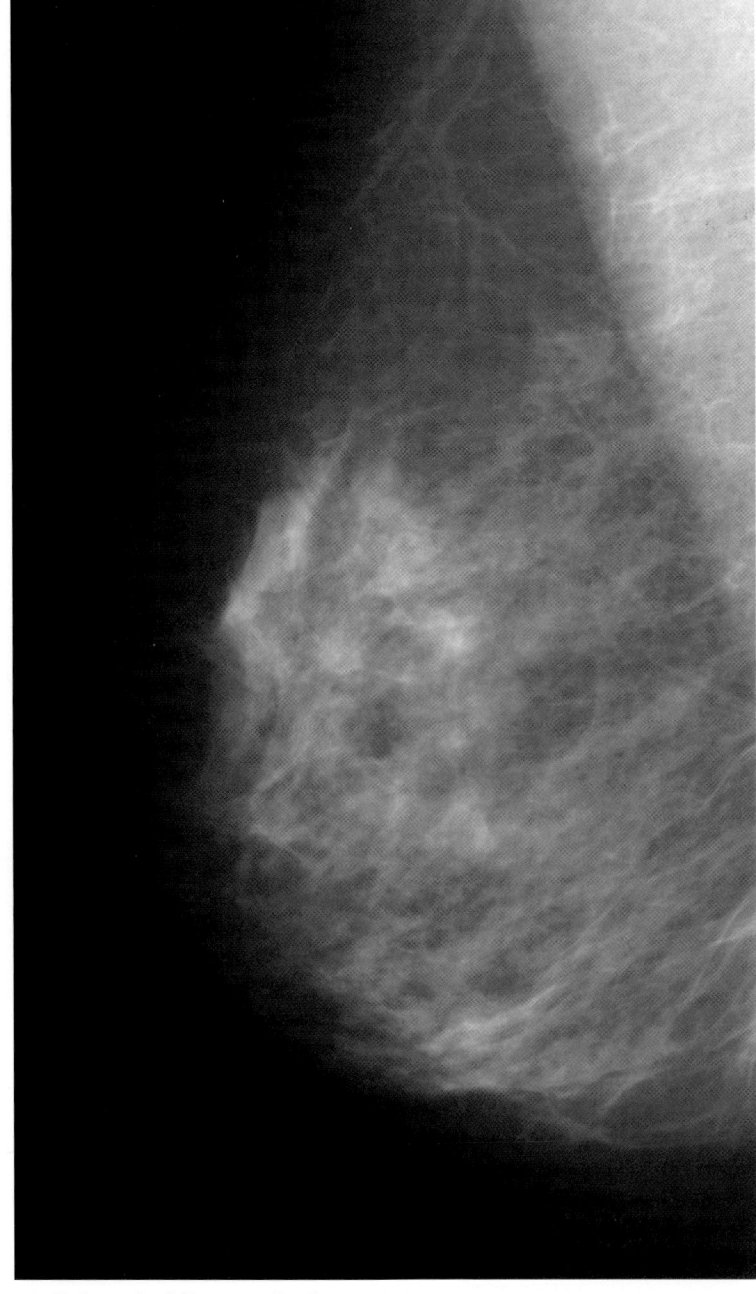

Mediolateral oblique projection

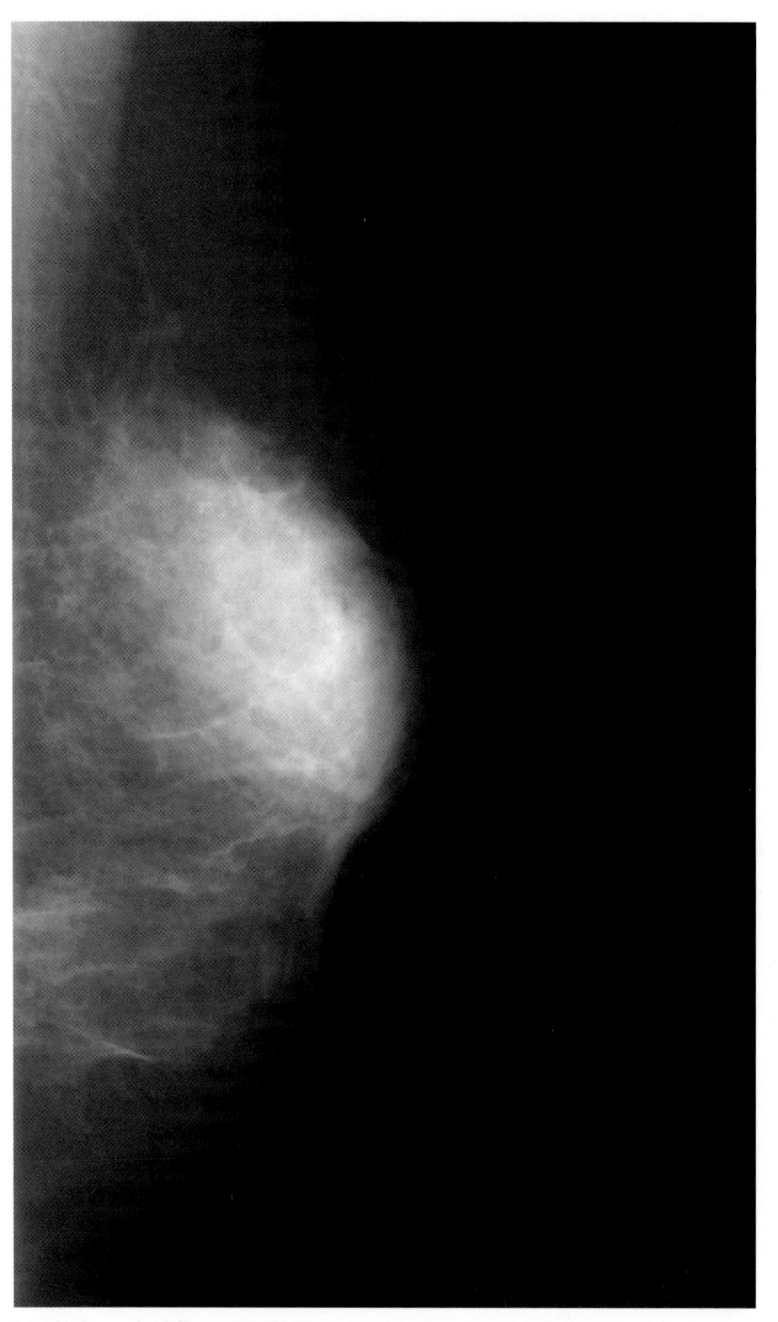

Mediolateral oblique projection

DIFFUSE OPACITY

In the upper medial area behind the areola, there is a palpable parenchymatous thickening, giving diffuse opacity with poorly defined margins, denser than the surrounding parenchyma. No evident signs of inflammation.

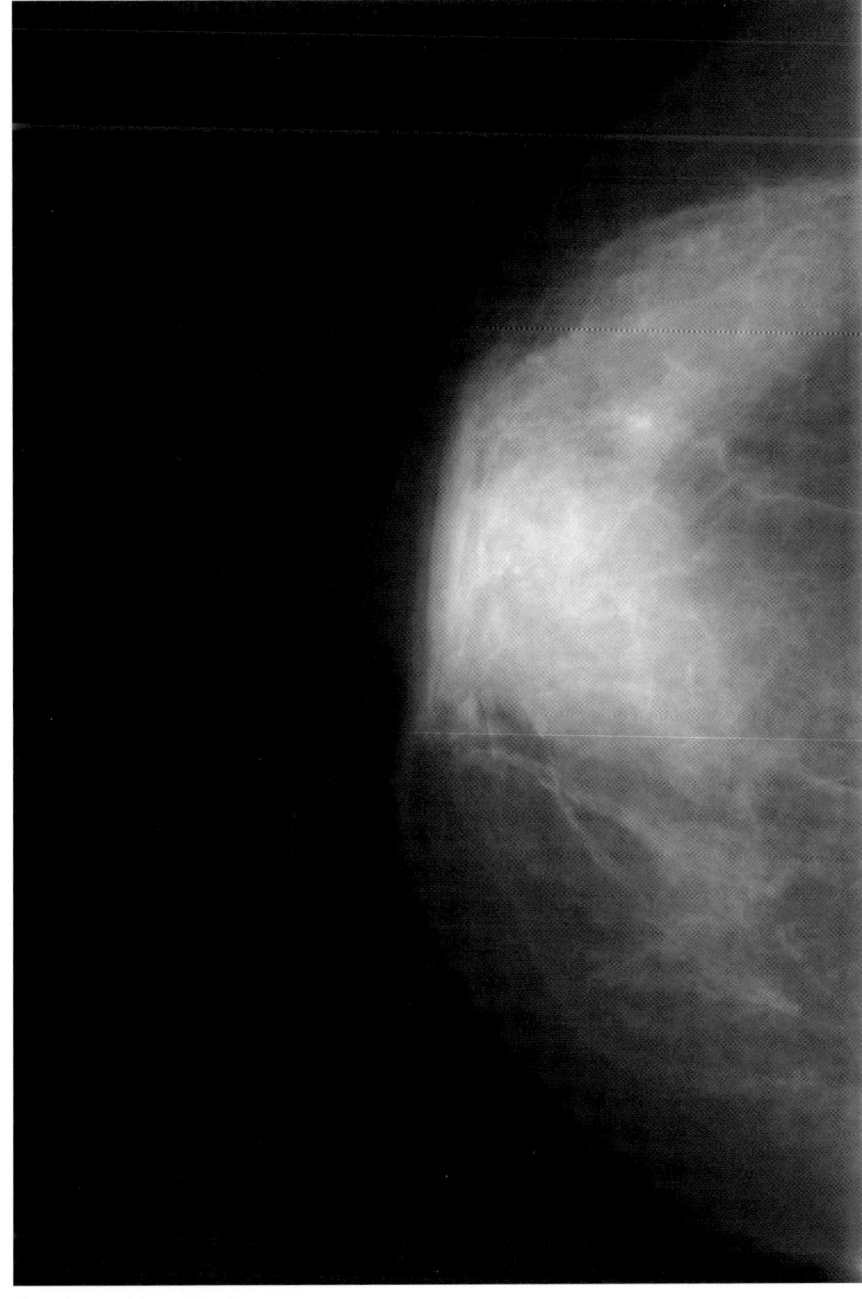

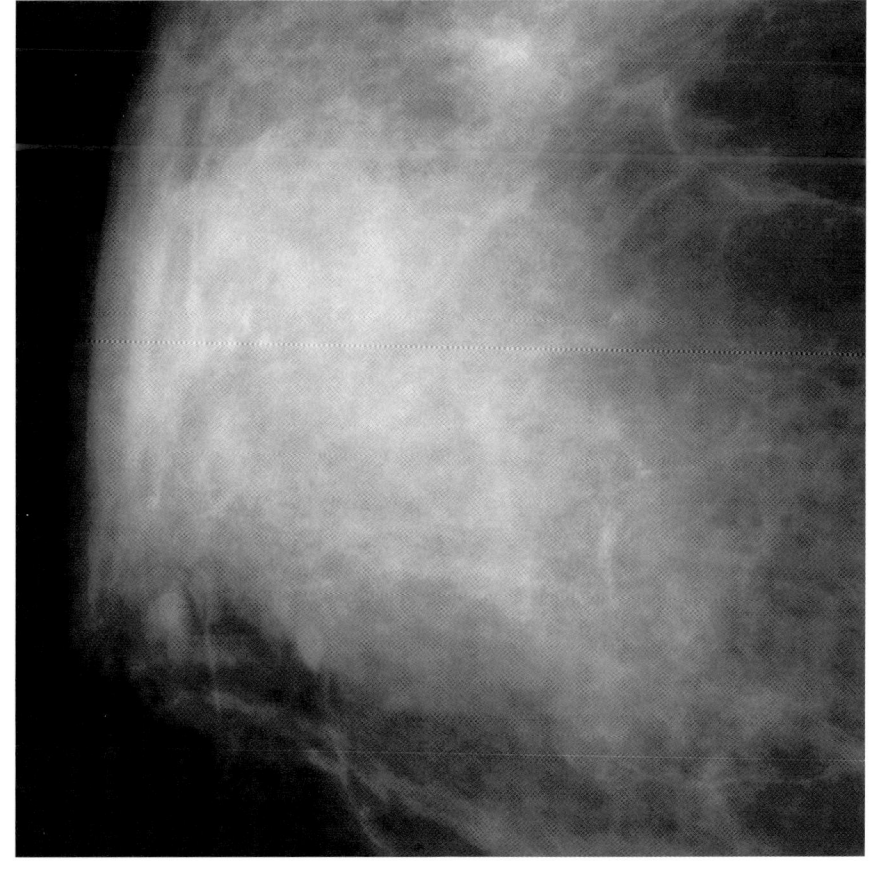

Craniocaudal projection

Craniocaudal projection

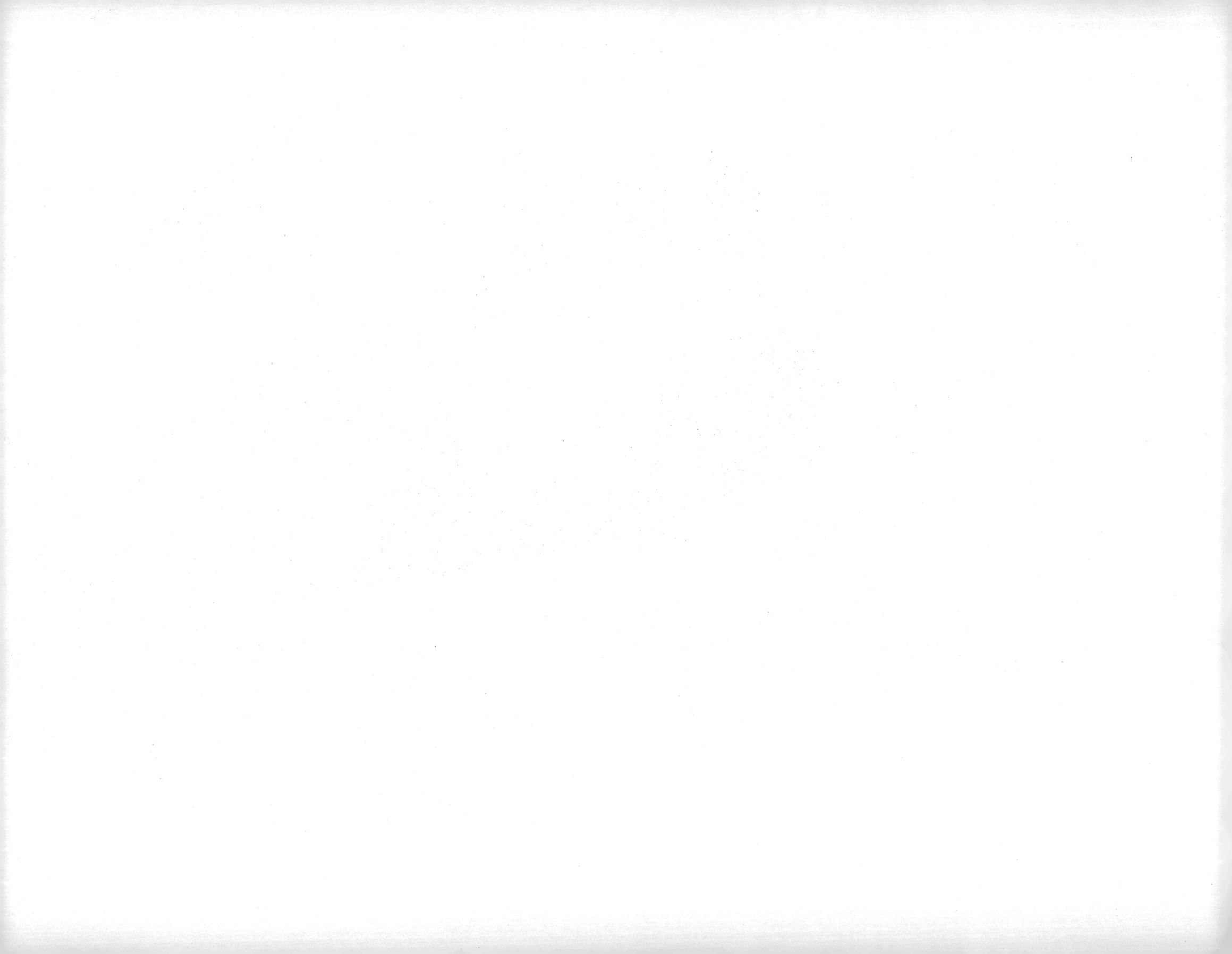

ARCHITECTURAL DISTORTION

Definition
An alteration in the normal direction of an area of the breast structure towards the nipple. The density of the alteration is generally low and its appearance may change to some extent in different projections. Its anterior and posterior profile may look abnormally straight, pulled in or wavy and bumpy, with no visible mass. This is the main characteristic of architectural distortion. When the central or internal parts of the breast are involved, the parenchyma appears wrinkled, folded or disorderly, with multiple contiguous radiopaque strands. This may give a rosette-like or "scalloped" pattern, depending on whether the alteration is circular or arc-shaped.

Classification
Depending on the location of the architectural distortion, i.e. at the anterior or posterior margins of the breast, or within it, it is termed either marginal or intra-parenchymal distortion.

Evaluation
In breasts with parenchymal distortion, it is essential to take a thorough history to establish whether the onset was subsequent to trauma, and identify any morphological changes noticed since it appeared. Any association with clinical and/or ultrasound-detected irregularities must also be evaluated.

ARCHITECTURAL DISTORTION

Intra-parenchymal distortion
Extensive low-density architectural distortion is visible, with a radiating pattern, somewhat stellate, centrally in the upper outer quadrant, especially in the lateral projection. No radiopaque tumour centre.

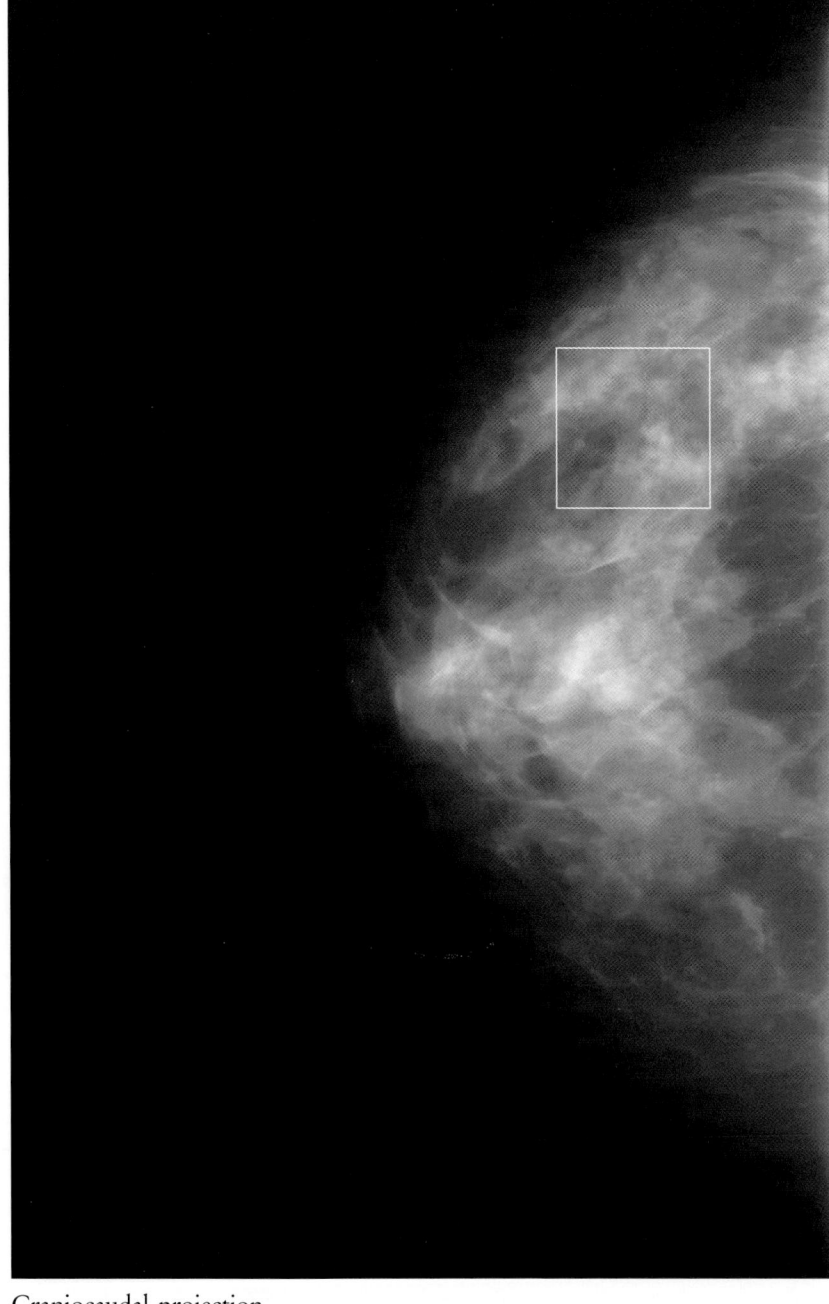

Craniocaudal projection

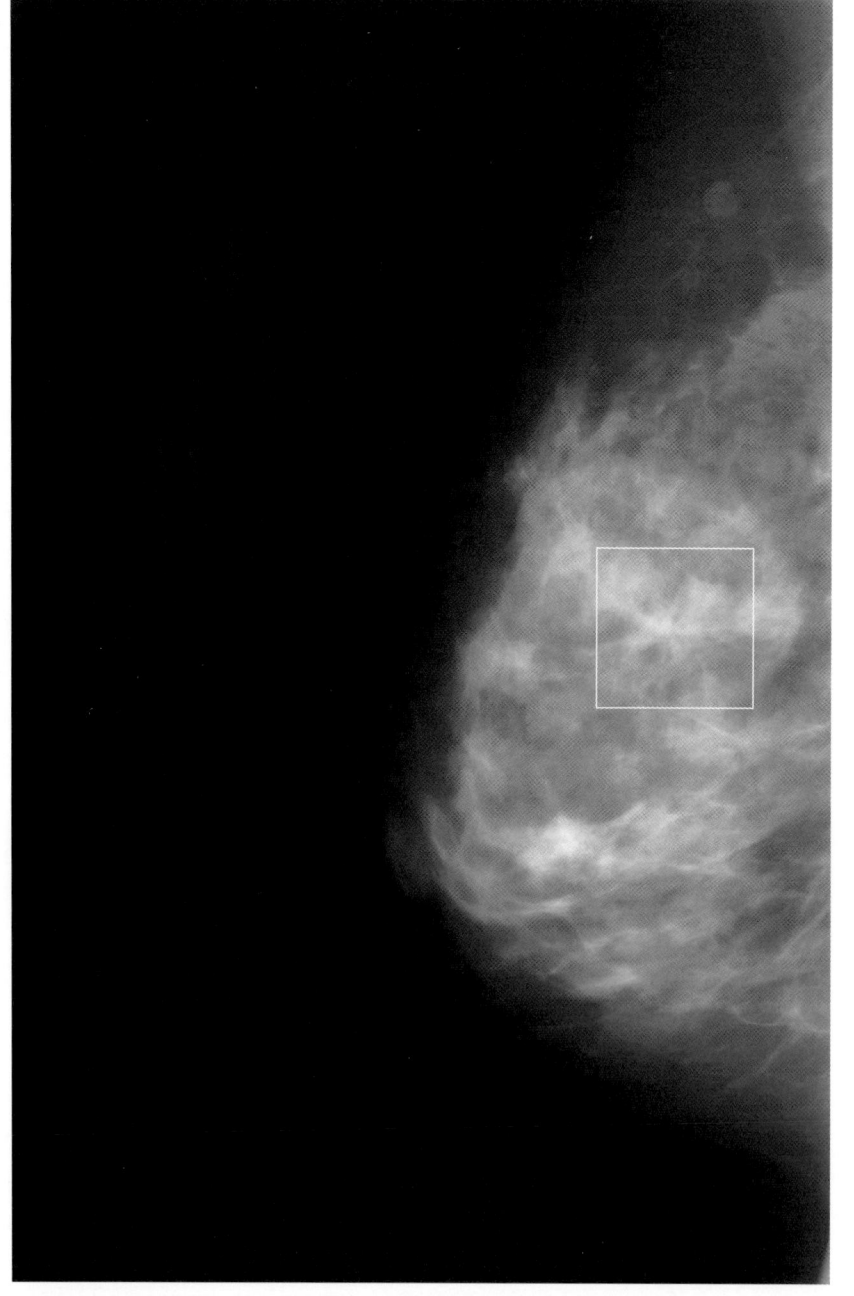

Lateral projection

Intra-parenchymal distortion

These magnification views show more clearly intra-parenchymal distortion that is difficult to detect owing to its lowdensity. The parenchyma appears wrinkled and has a rosette-like appearance.

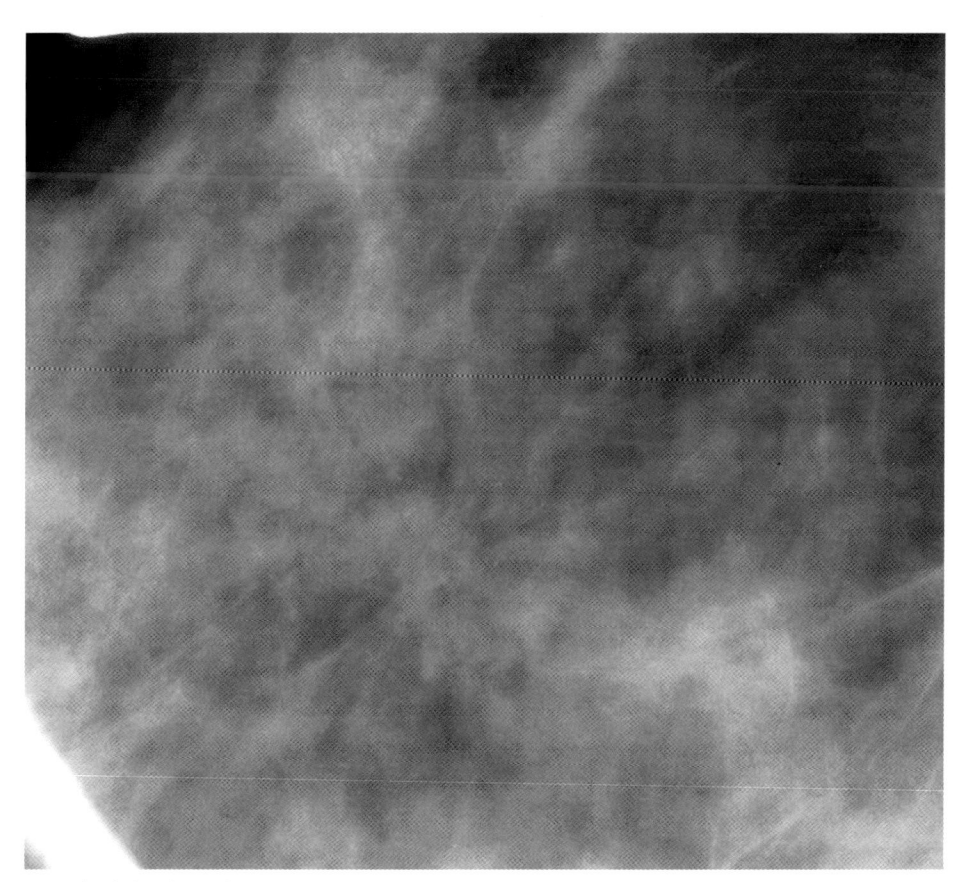

Detail of the lateral projection

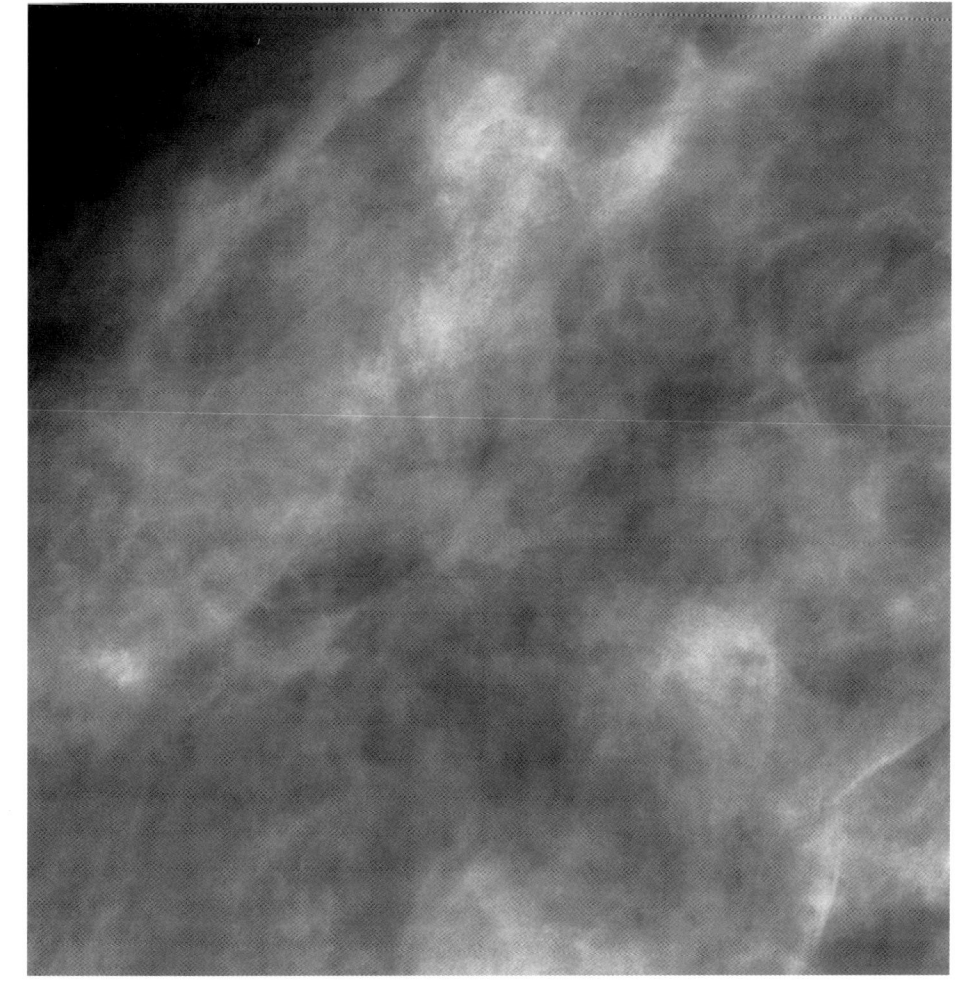

Detail of the craniocaudal projection

Histological finding: infiltrating ductal carcinoma

ARCHITECTURAL DISTORTION

Intra-parenchymal distortion

Low-density intra-parenchymal distortion is visible, with a radiating pattern, centrally in the upper medial quadrant. There is no tumour centre. The magnification view clearly shows mixed hyperlucent and radiopaque strands, and several central hyperlucent vacuoles. The round lucent-centred calcification is dysplastic.

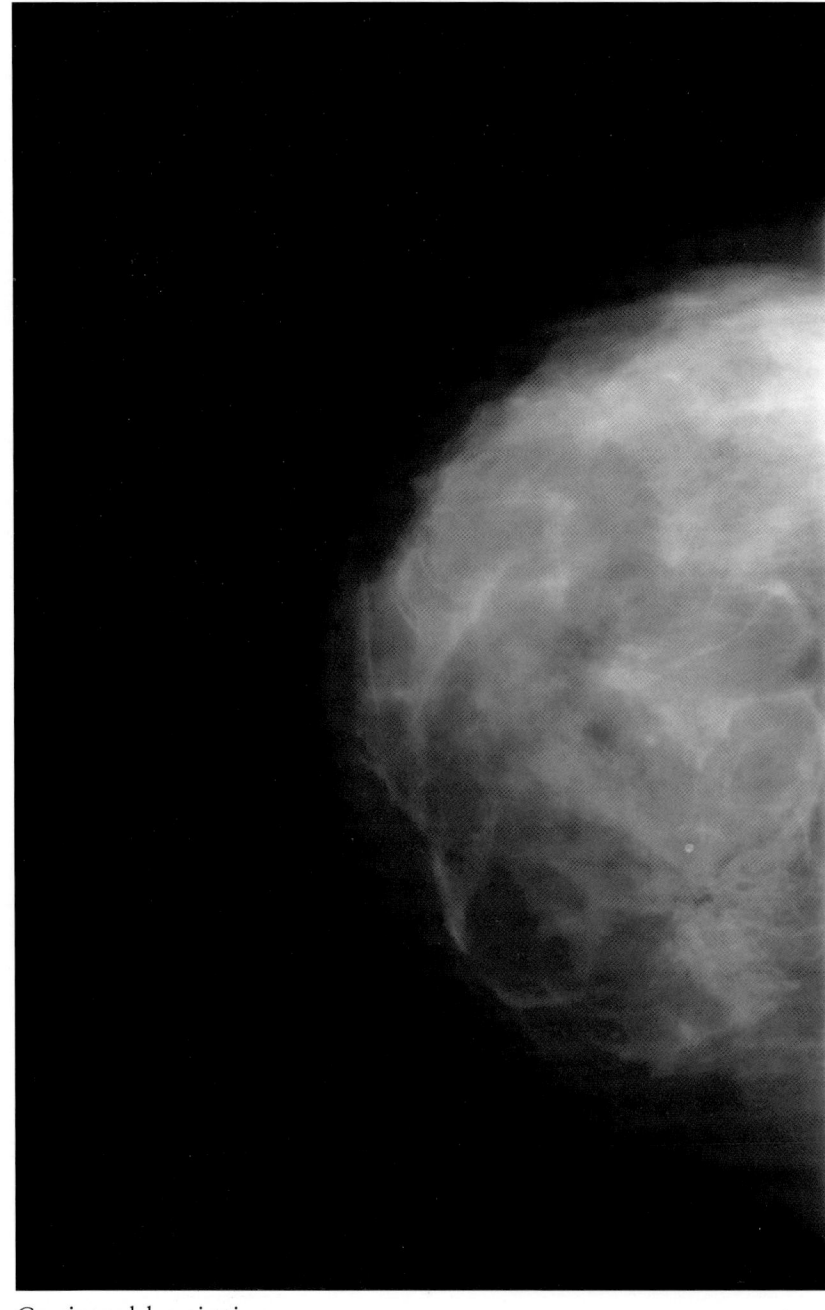

Craniocaudal projection

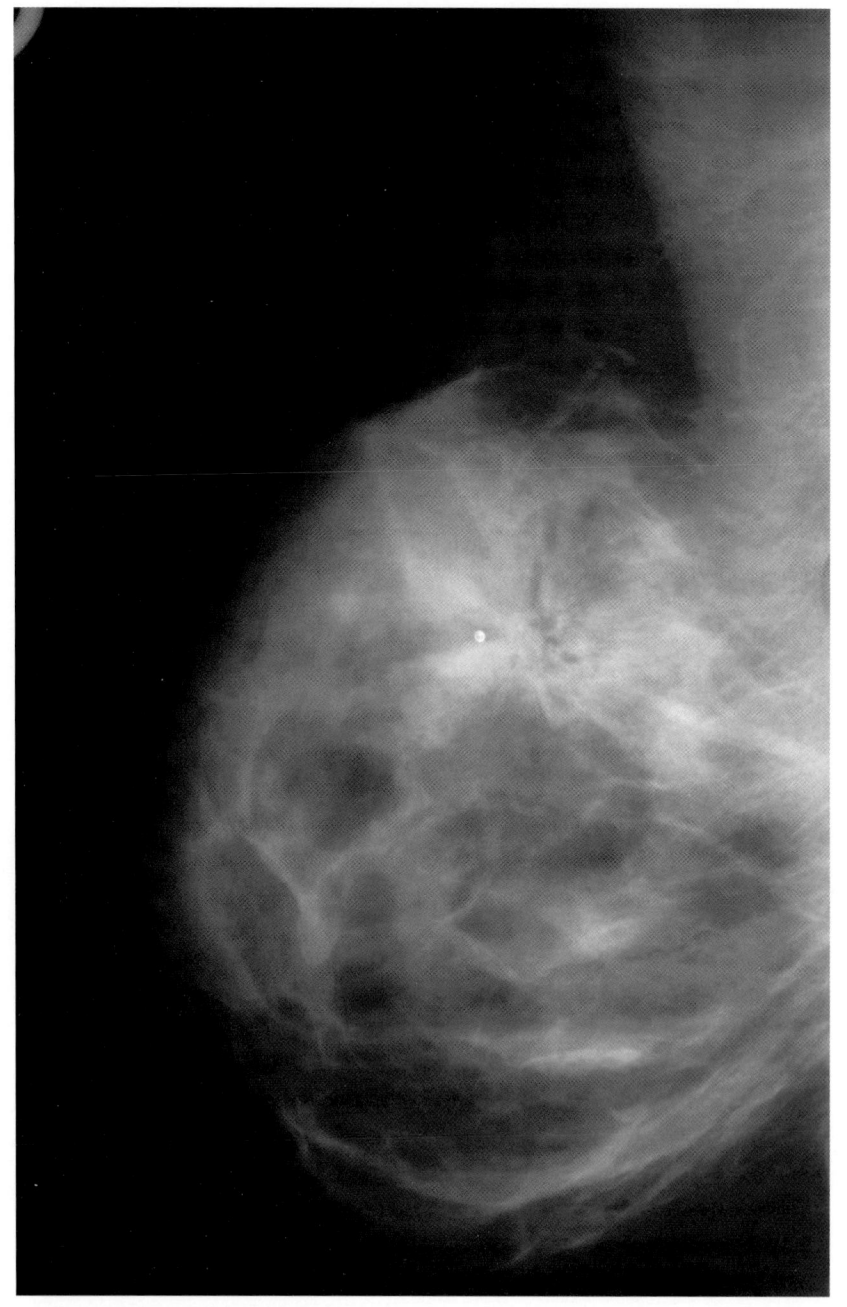

Mediolateral oblique projection

Intra-parenchymal distortion

In the inner upper quadrant, in a posterior location, there is low-density intra-parechymal distortion with a radiating pattern and no tumour. The magnification view shows alternating radiolucent and radiopaque strands and several mixed central radiolucent vacuoles. The round lucent-centred calcification is clearly dysplastic.

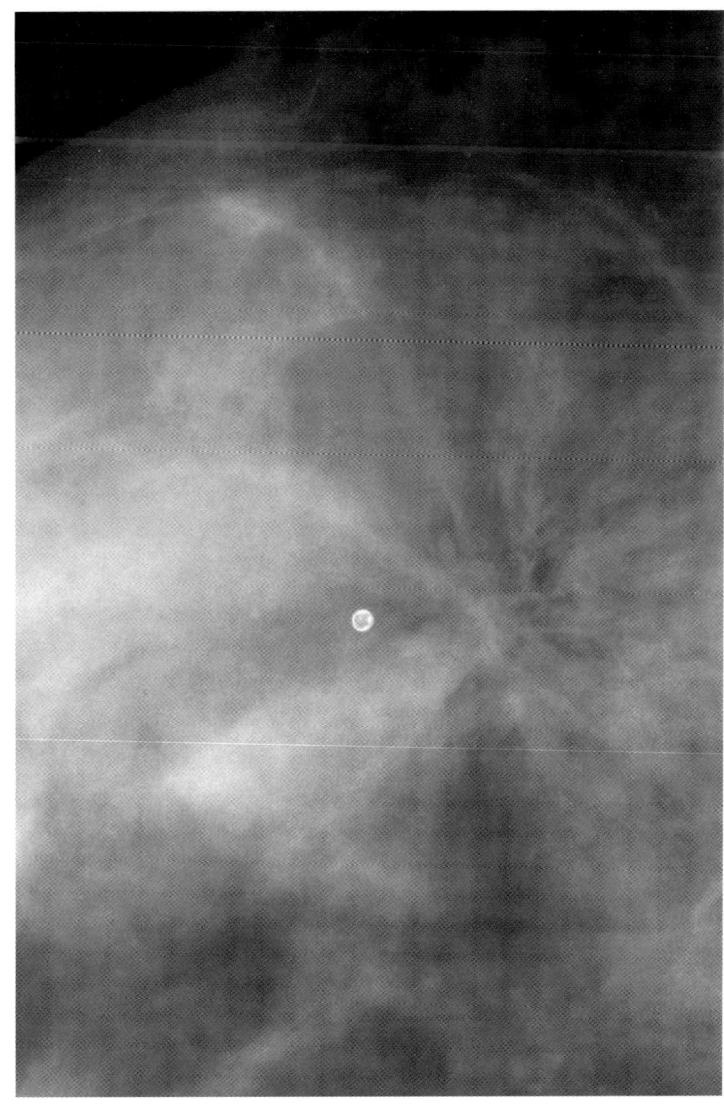

Detail of the craniocaudal projection

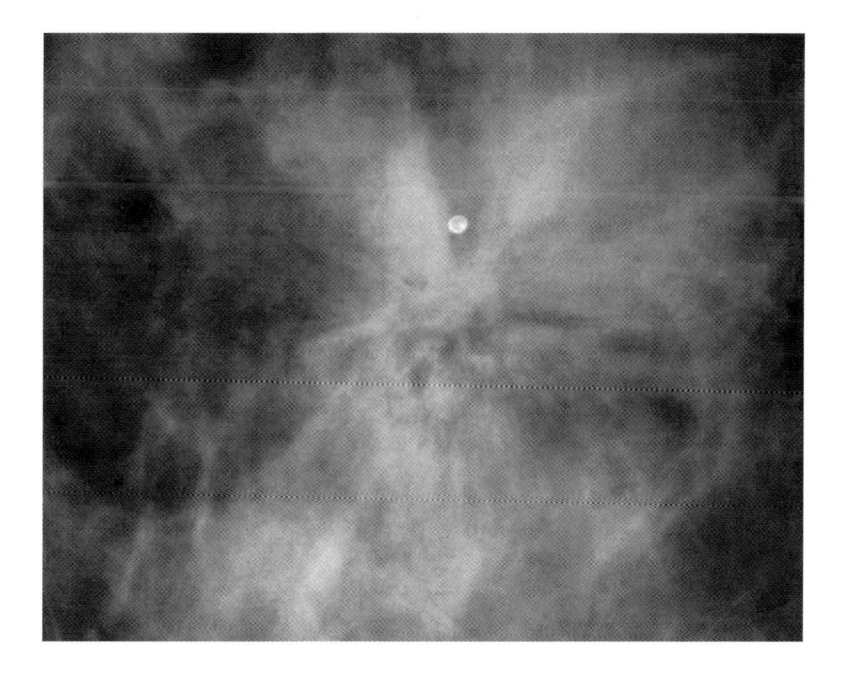

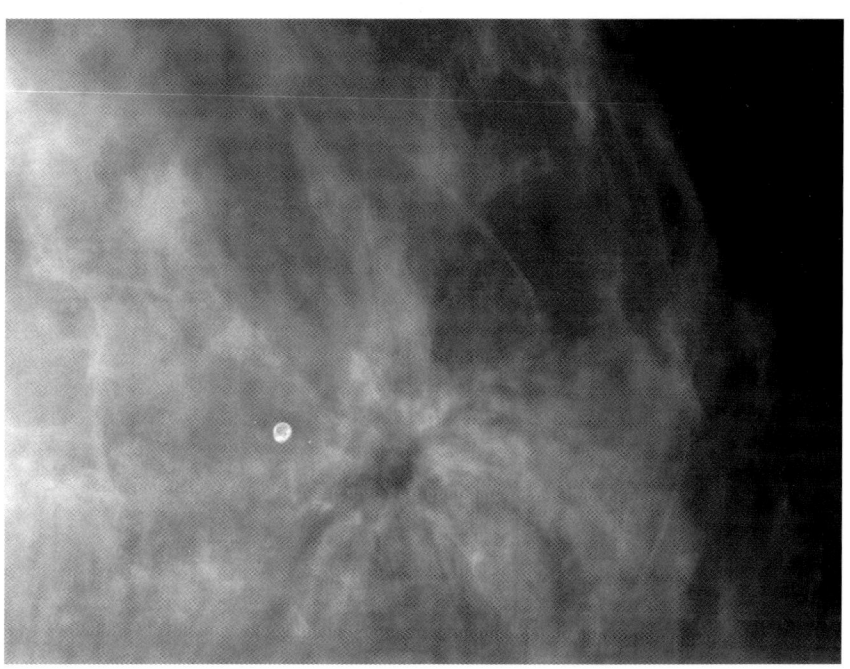

Histological finding: sclerosing adenosis

ARCHITECTURAL DISTORTION

Intra-parenchymal distortion

In the upper outer quadrant the parenchimal-stromal architecture is abnormally oriented and looks disorderly or wrinkled. There is a low-density rosette image, whose appearance changes depending on the orthogonal projections.

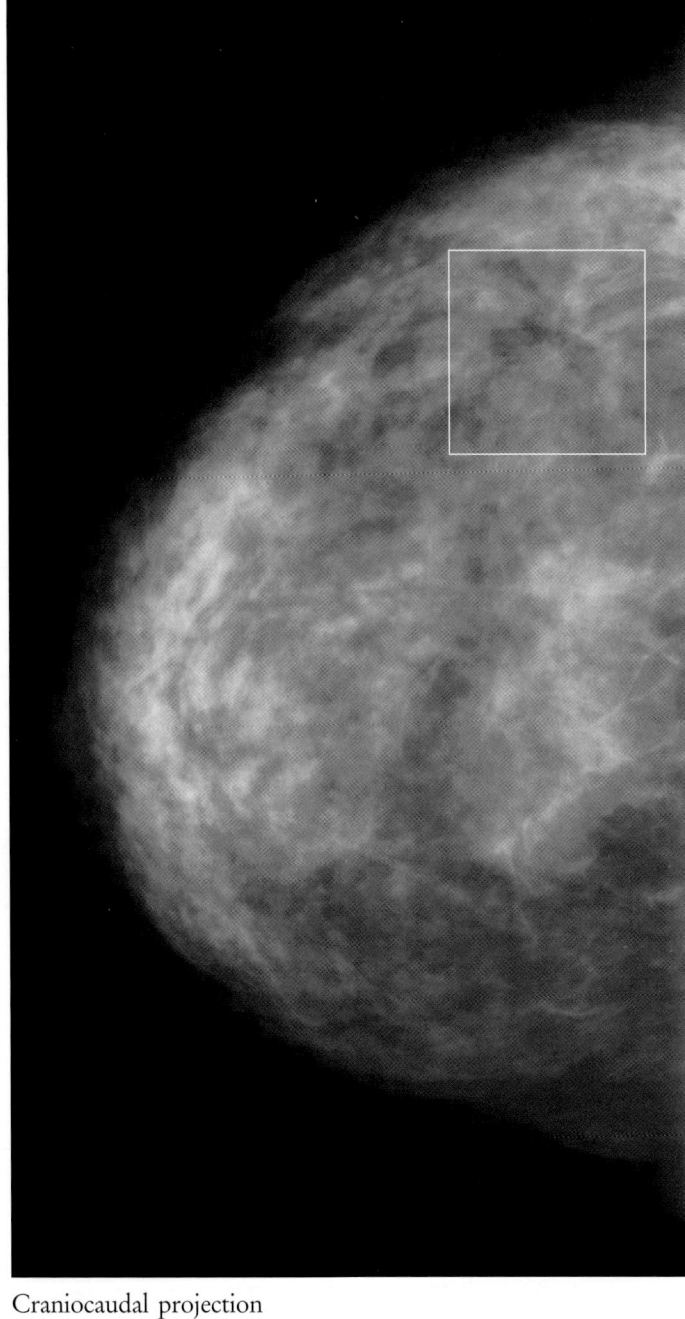

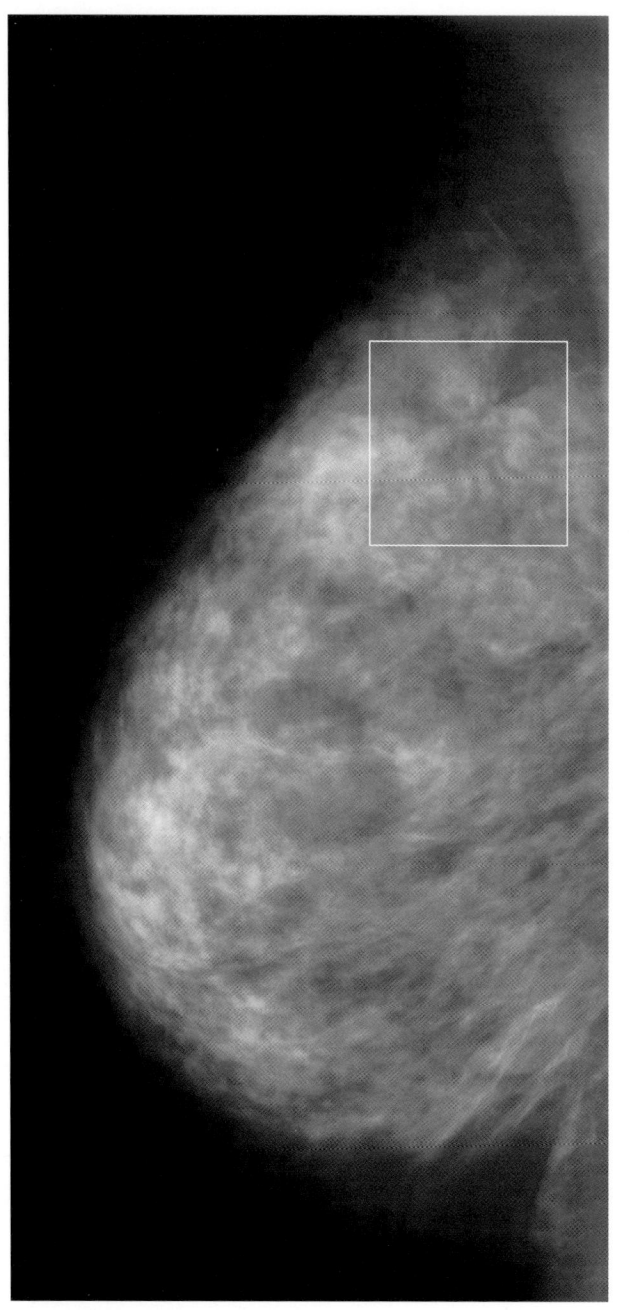

Craniocaudal projection

Lateral projection

Intra-parenchymal distortion

The upper outer quadrant displays an abnormal parenchymal-stromal architecture: it looks disorderly or wrinkled. The image shows a low-density rosette, whose appearance changes depending on the orthogonal projections.

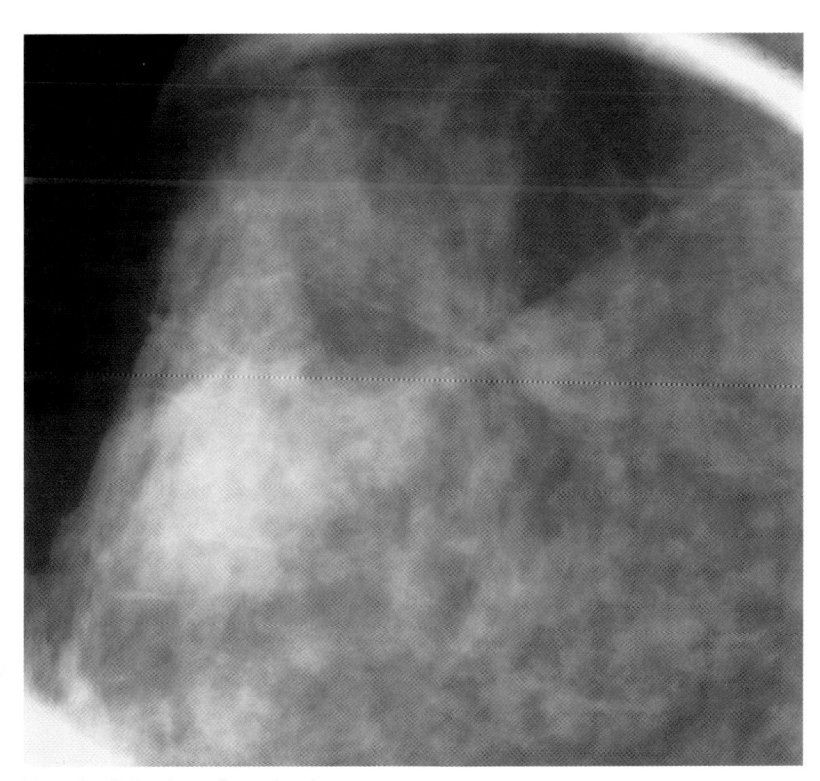

Detail of the lateral projection

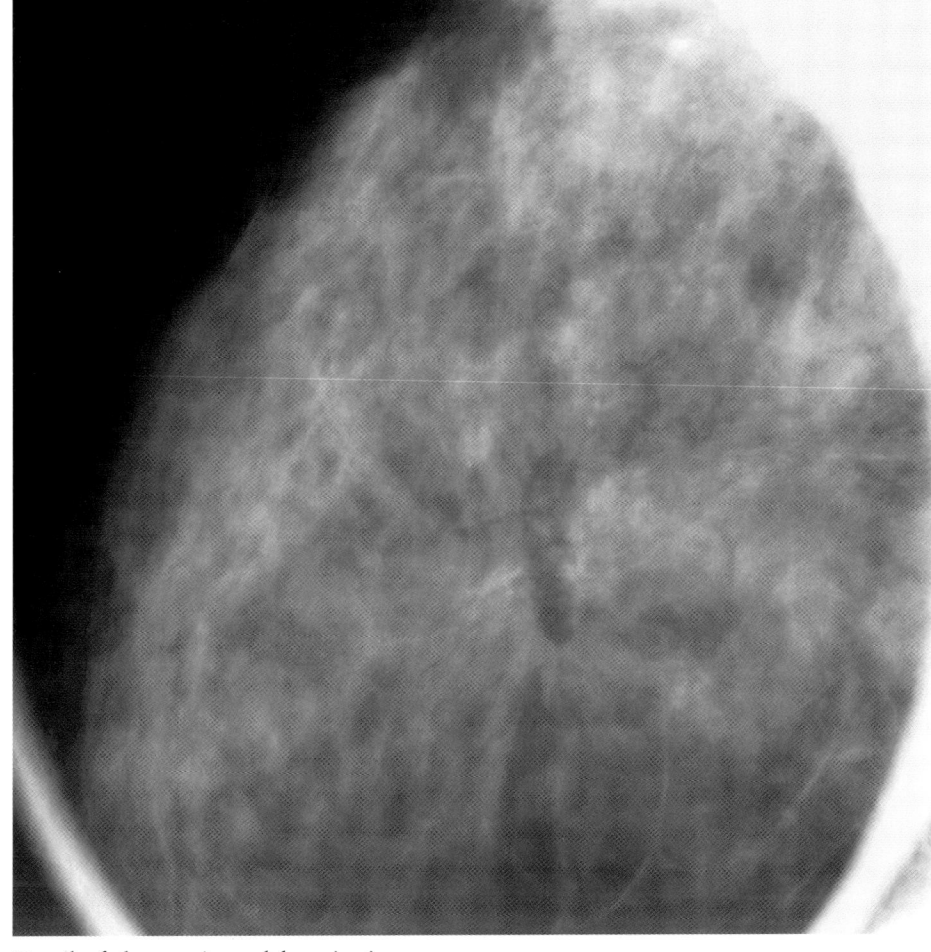

Detail of the craniocaudal projection

Histological finding: infiltrating tubular carcinoma

ARCHITECTURAL DISTORTION

Intra-parenchymal distortion

Low-density architectural distortion in central lower location, resulting from multiple converging ribbon-like opacities. In the craniocaudal projection, the distortion seems to radiate outwards, almost in a star pattern, while in the lateral projection the morphology is more irregular.

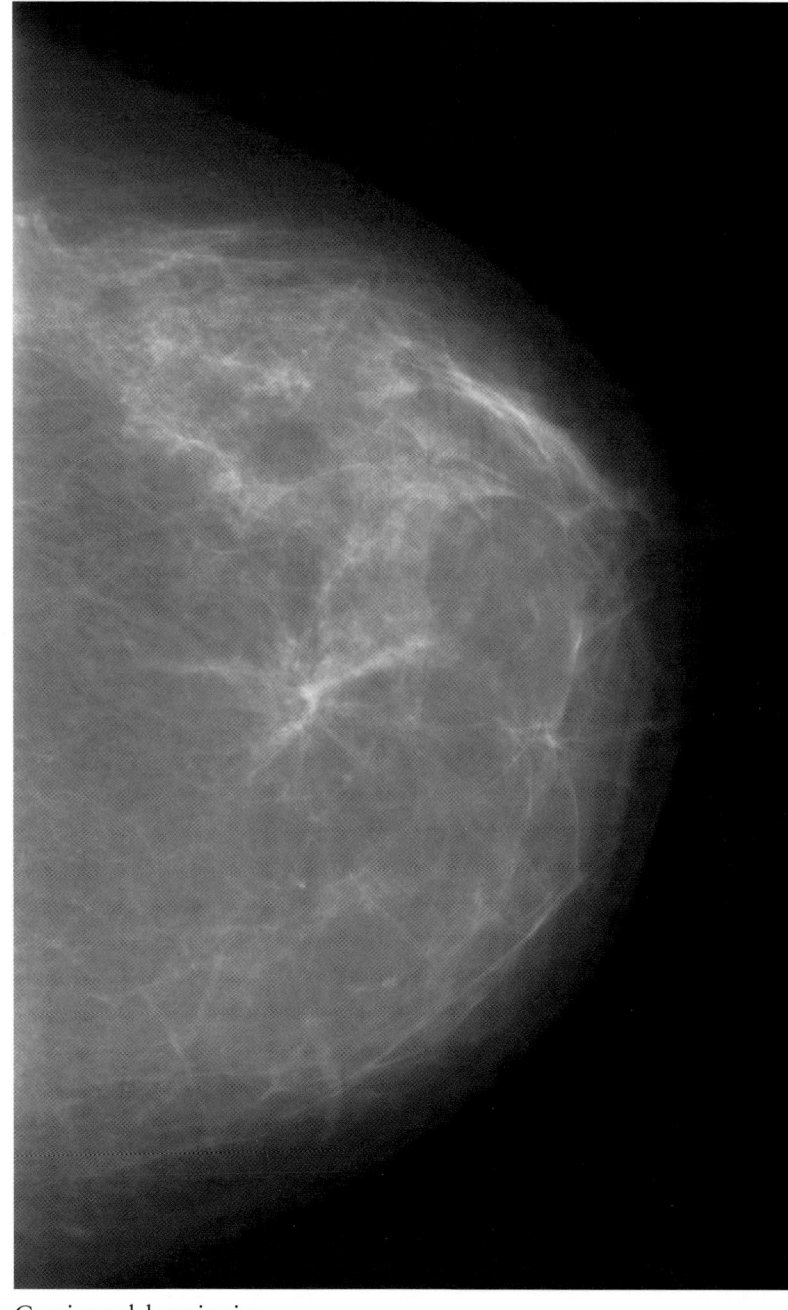

Craniocaudal projection

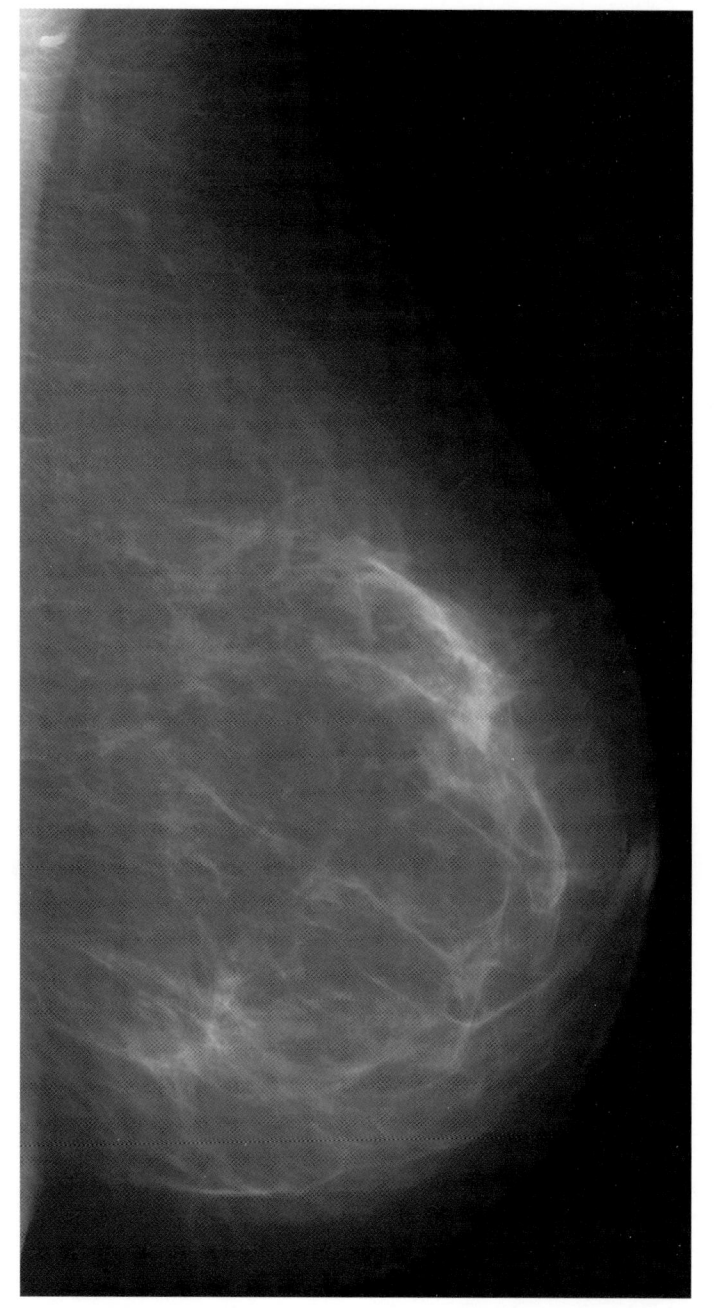

Lateral projection

Intra-parenchymal distortion

Low-density architectural distortion in central lower location, radiating outwards, almost in a star pattern. Note how the image changes in the two projections. No radiopaque tumour centre.

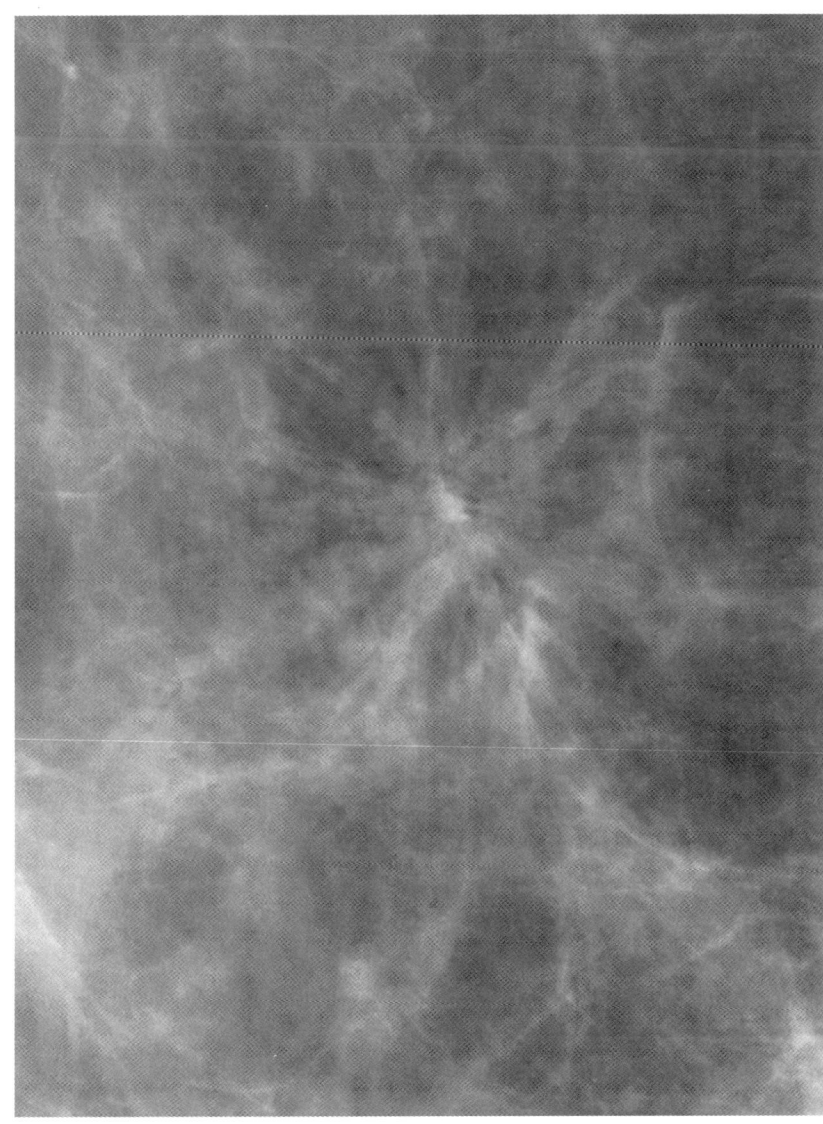

Detail of the craniocaudal projection

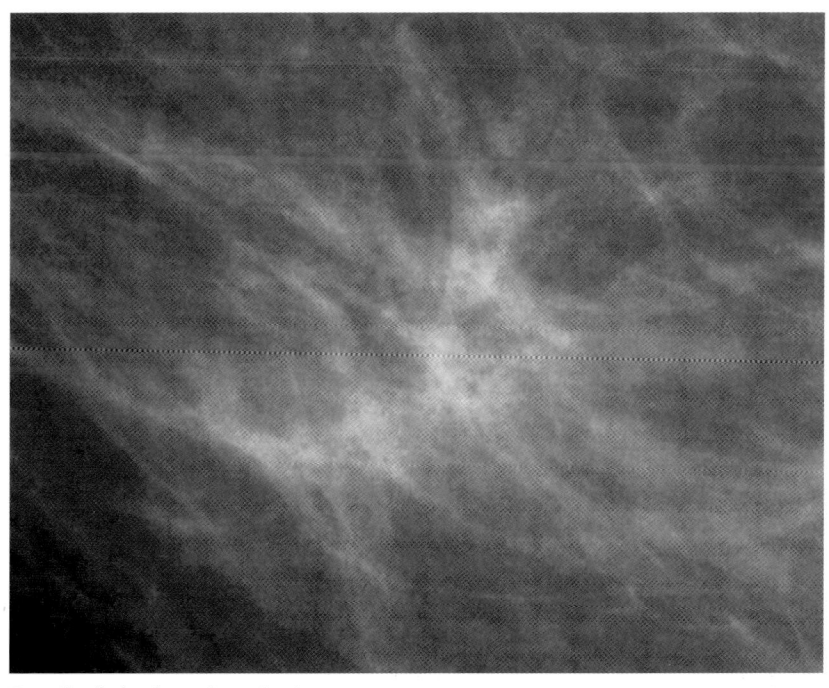

Detail of the lateral projection

Histological finding: atypical ductal hyperplasia

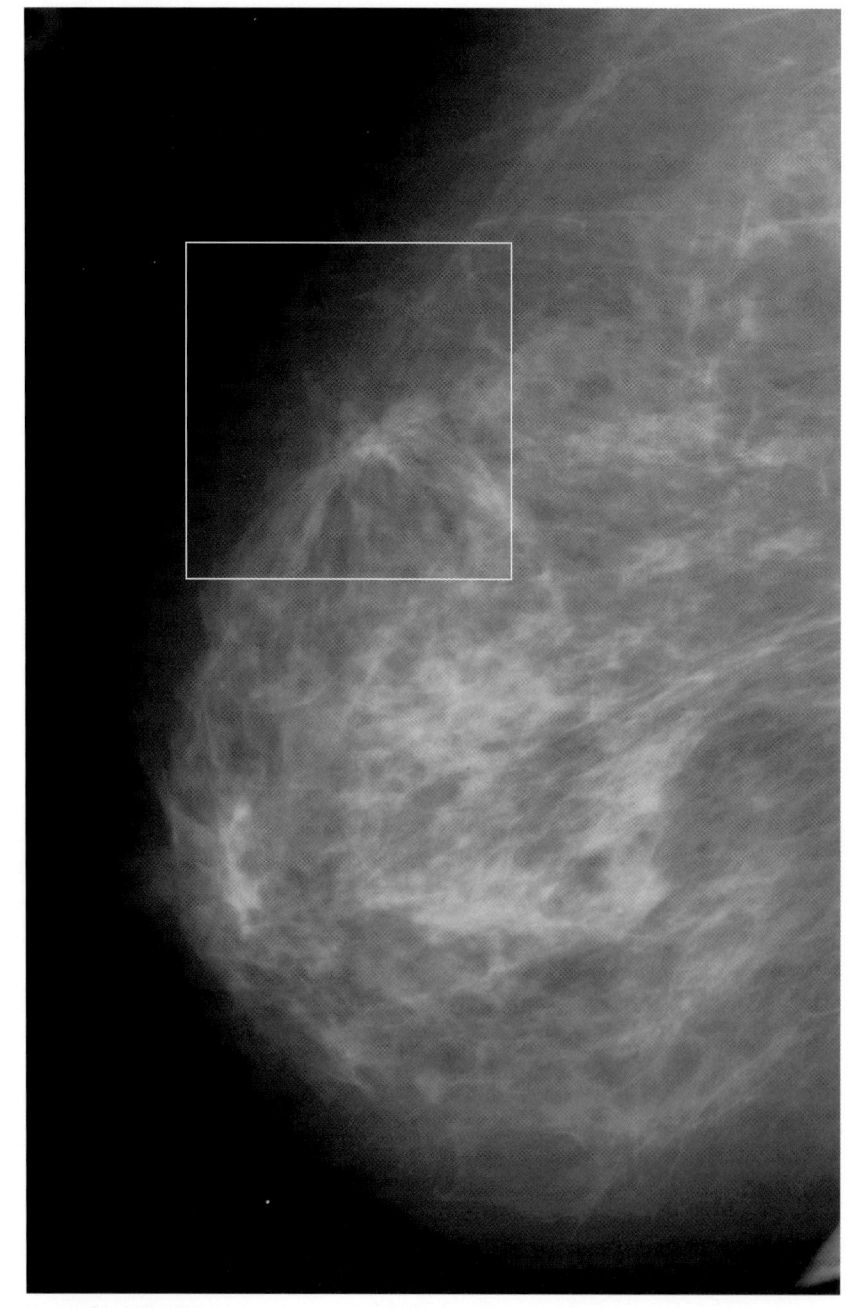

ARCHITECTURAL DISTORTION

Intra-parenchymal distortion

Low-density architectural distortion in the lower inner quadrant, radiating outwards, in a star-like pattern, especially in the craniocaudal projection. In the lateral projection the image is quite different, with radiopaque strands bunched together, like a "sheaf of wheat". No clinical or ultrasound findings are associated.

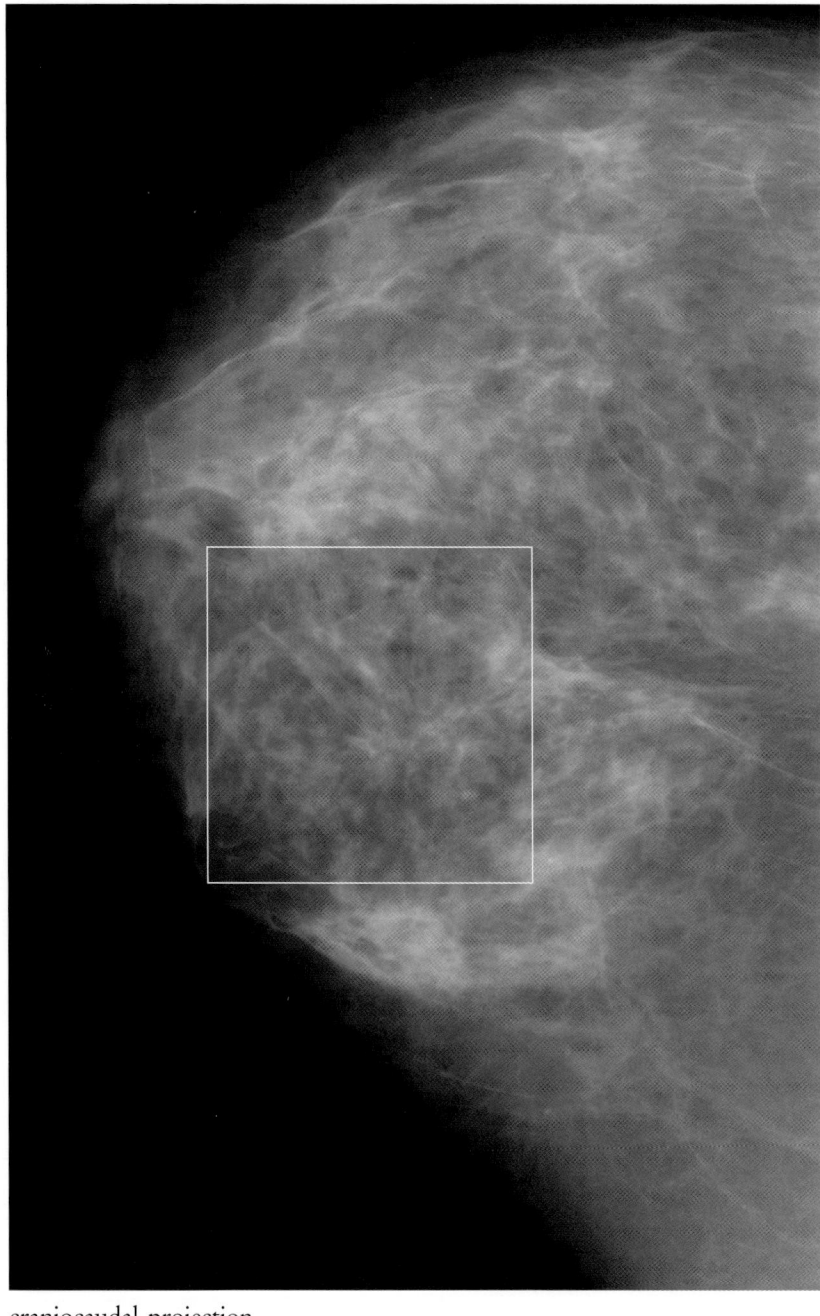

craniocaudal projection

Lateral projection

Intra-parenchymal distortion

Low-density architectural distortion in the upper inner quadrant, radiating outwards, in a star-like pattern, especially in the craniocaudal projection. Note how the image changes in the two projections. No radiopaque tumour centre.

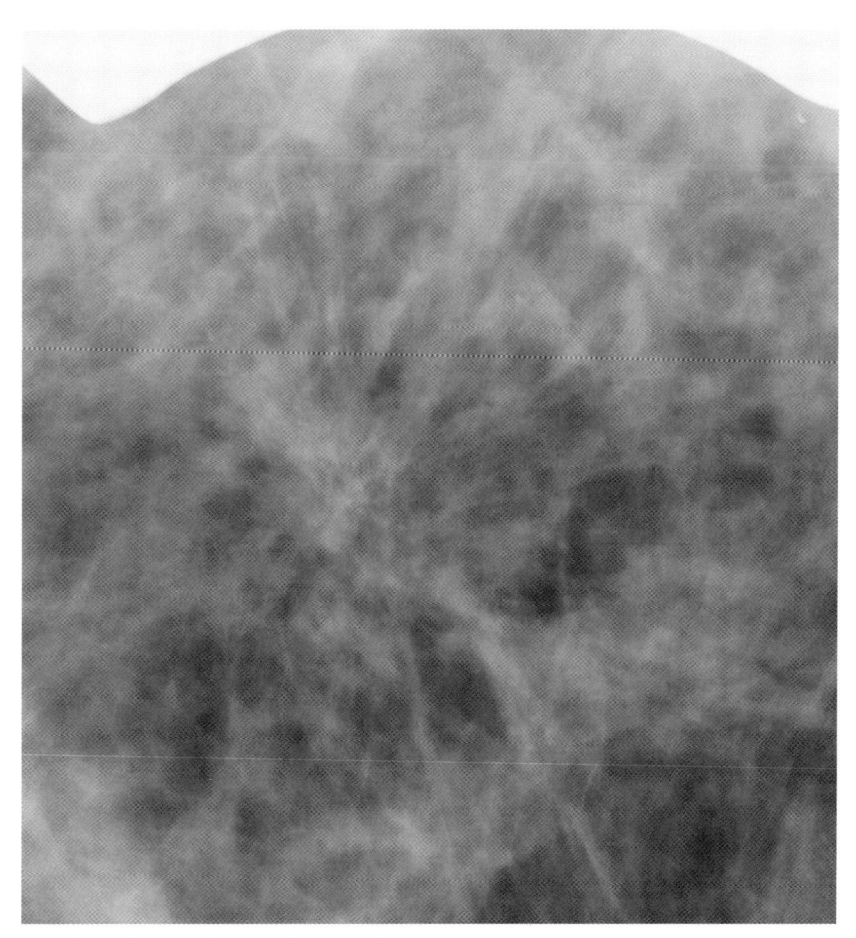

Detail of the craniocaudal projection

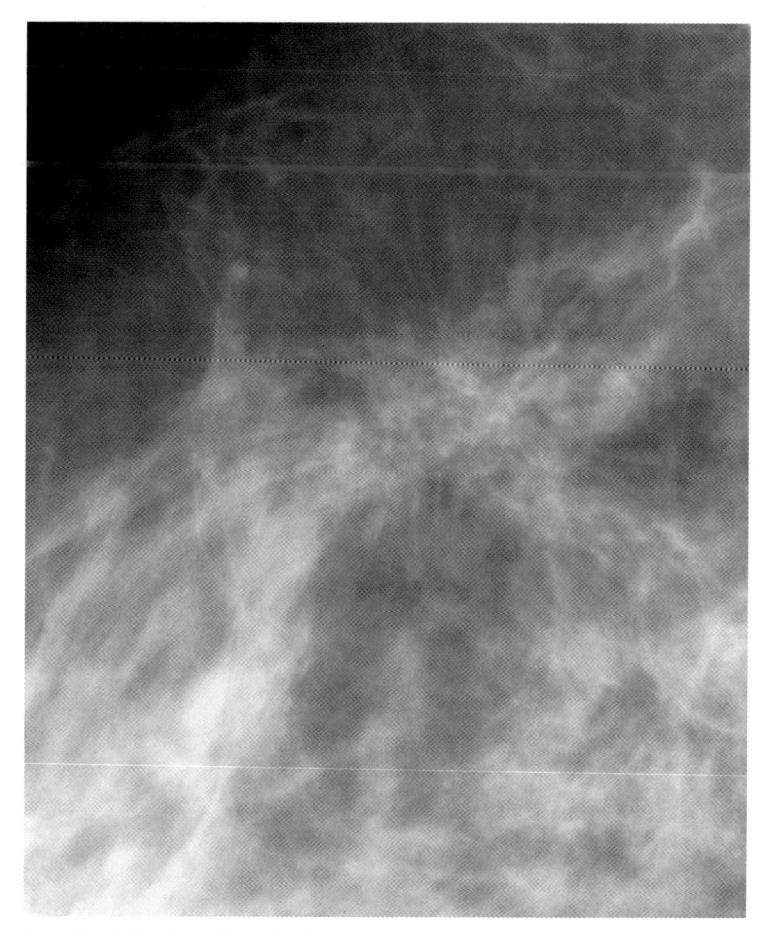

Detail of the lateral projection

Histological finding: adenosis and epitheliosis

ARCHITECTURAL DISTORTION

Anterior marginal distortion

The left outer quadrant shows an abnormal anterior profile of the breast, with a serrated, spiculated contour. No space-occupying mass is detectable.

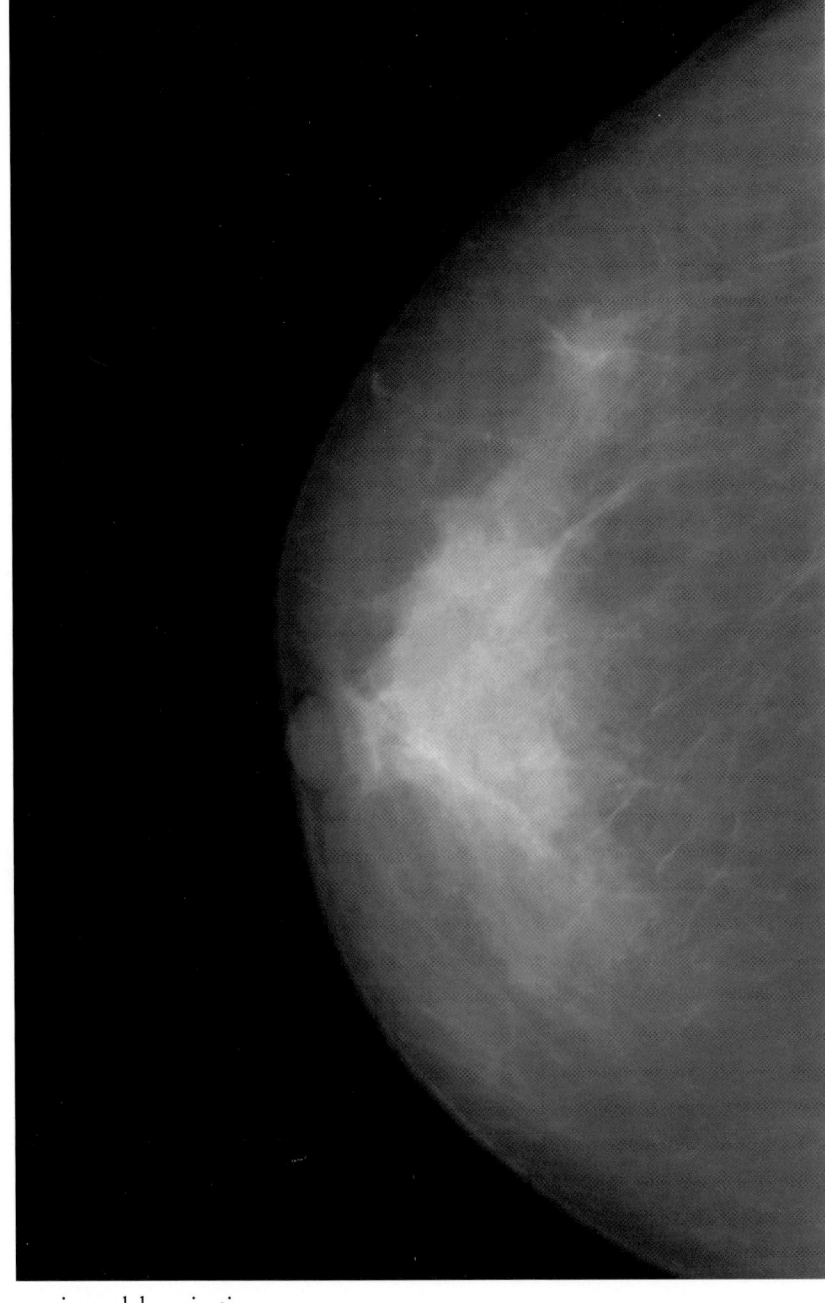

craniocaudal projection

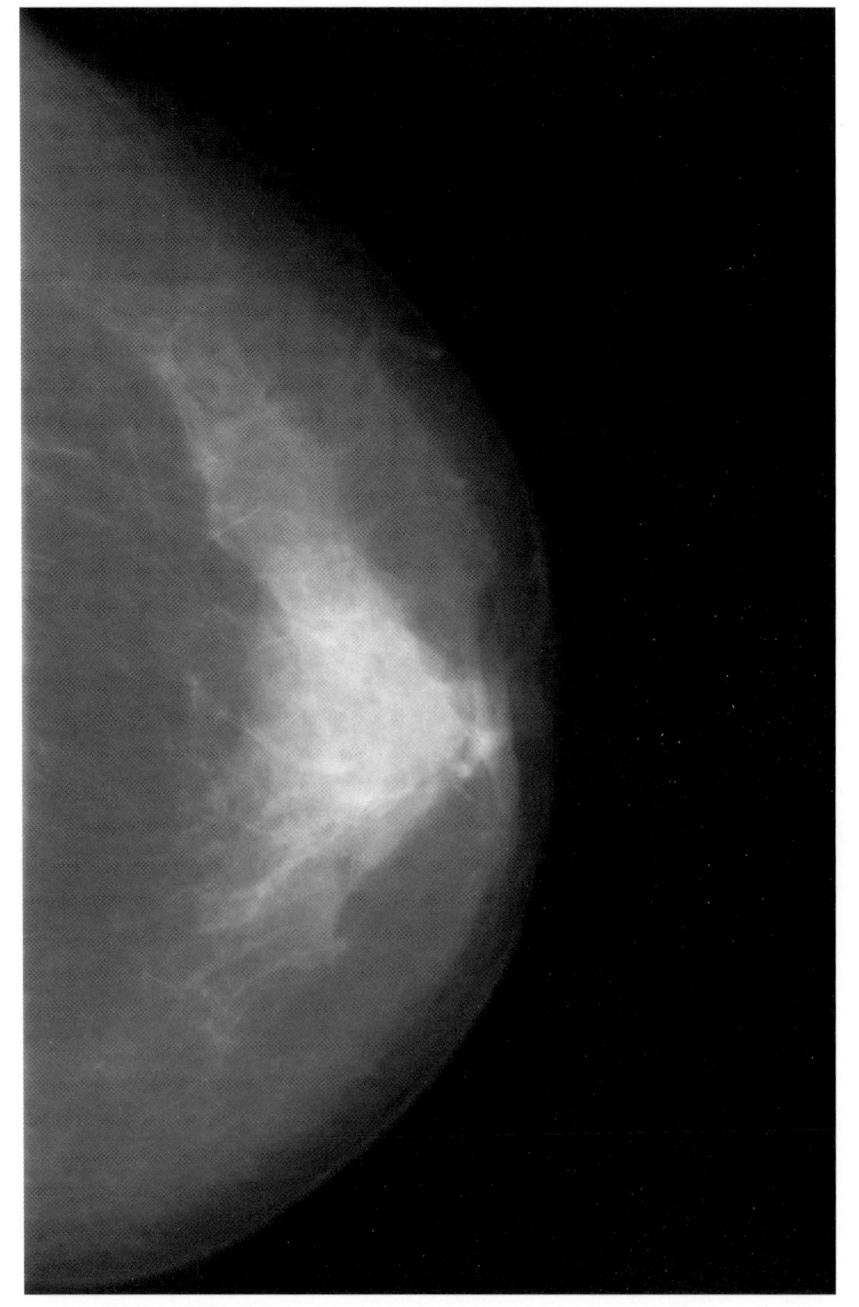

craniocaudal projection

Anterior marginal distortion
The spot compression views show more clearly the irregularly shaped opacity with spicules at the margins.

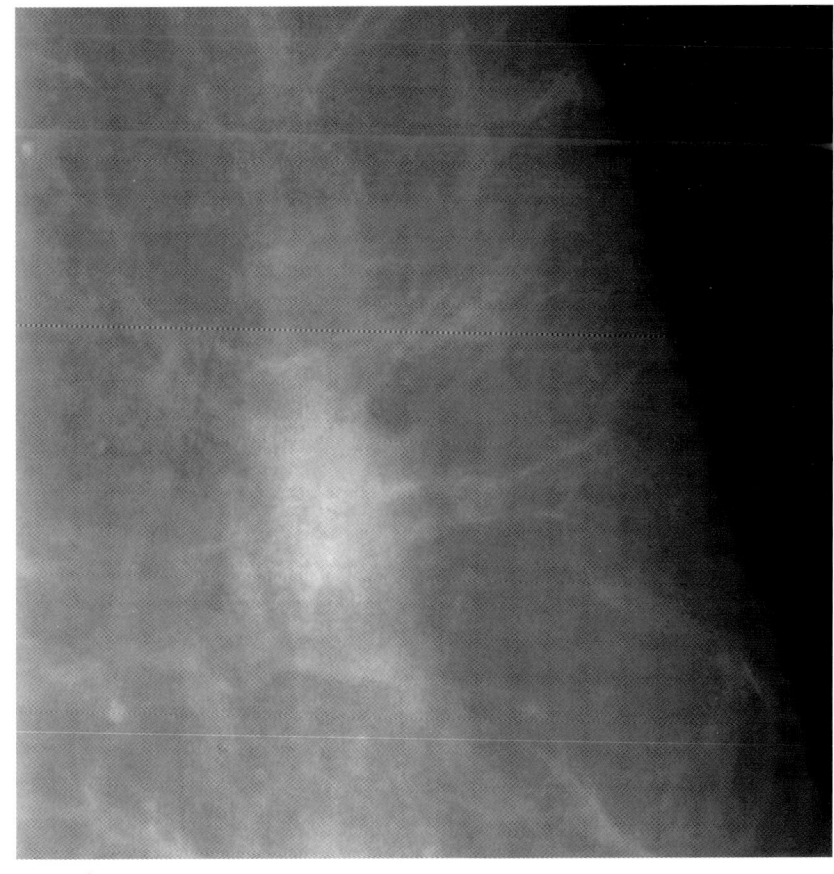

Magnification view

Magnification view

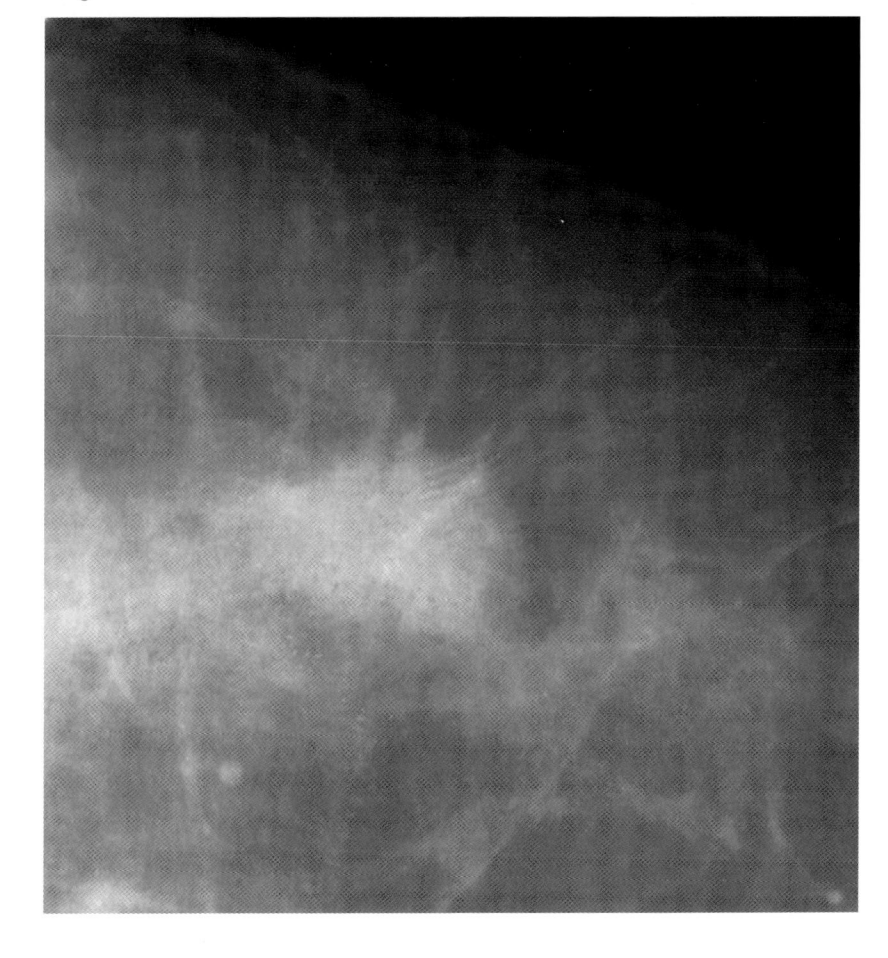

Histological finding: infiltrating ductal carcinoma

ARCHITECTURAL DISTORTION

Posterior marginal distortion

In the right upper outer quadrant, in a posterior location, the body of the mammary gland is markedly abnormal, with a disorderly rosette-like appearance. The distortion gives a low-density image, changing partially according to the projection.

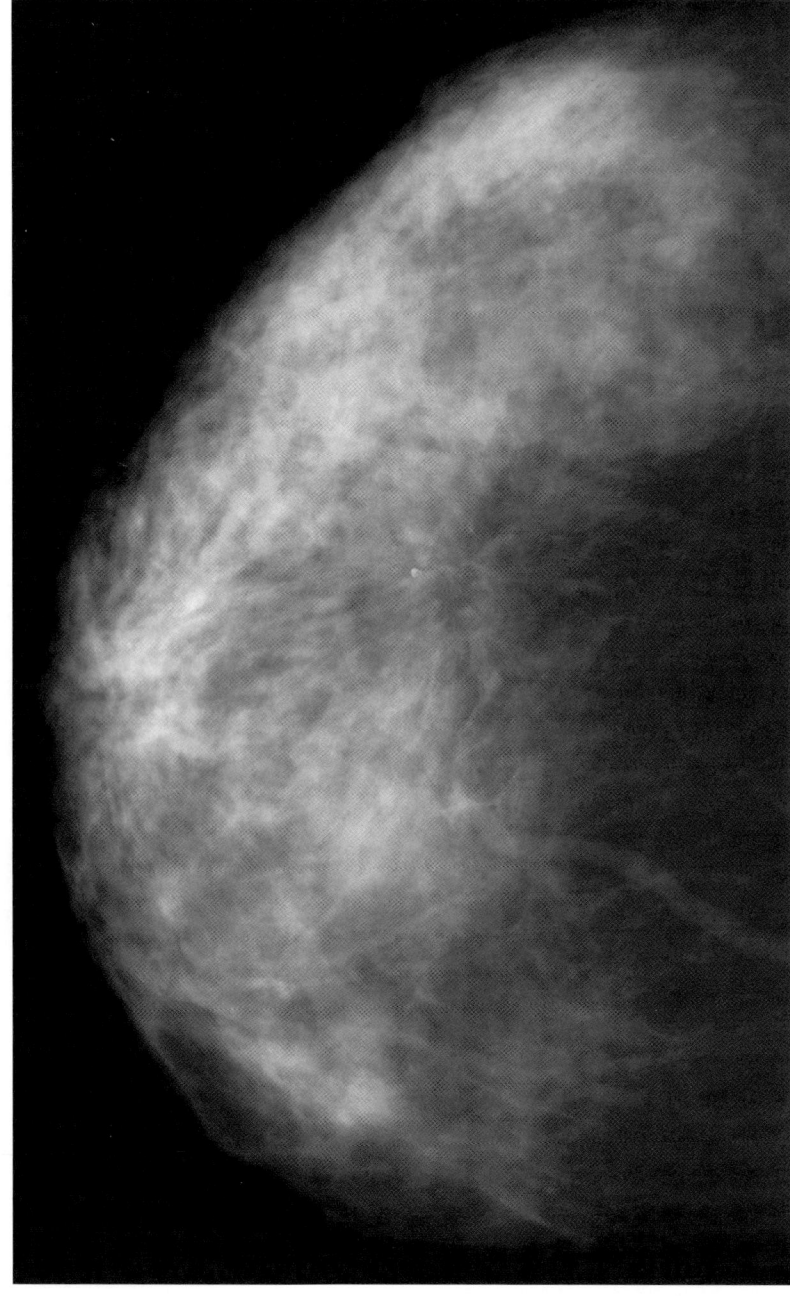

Craniocaudal projection

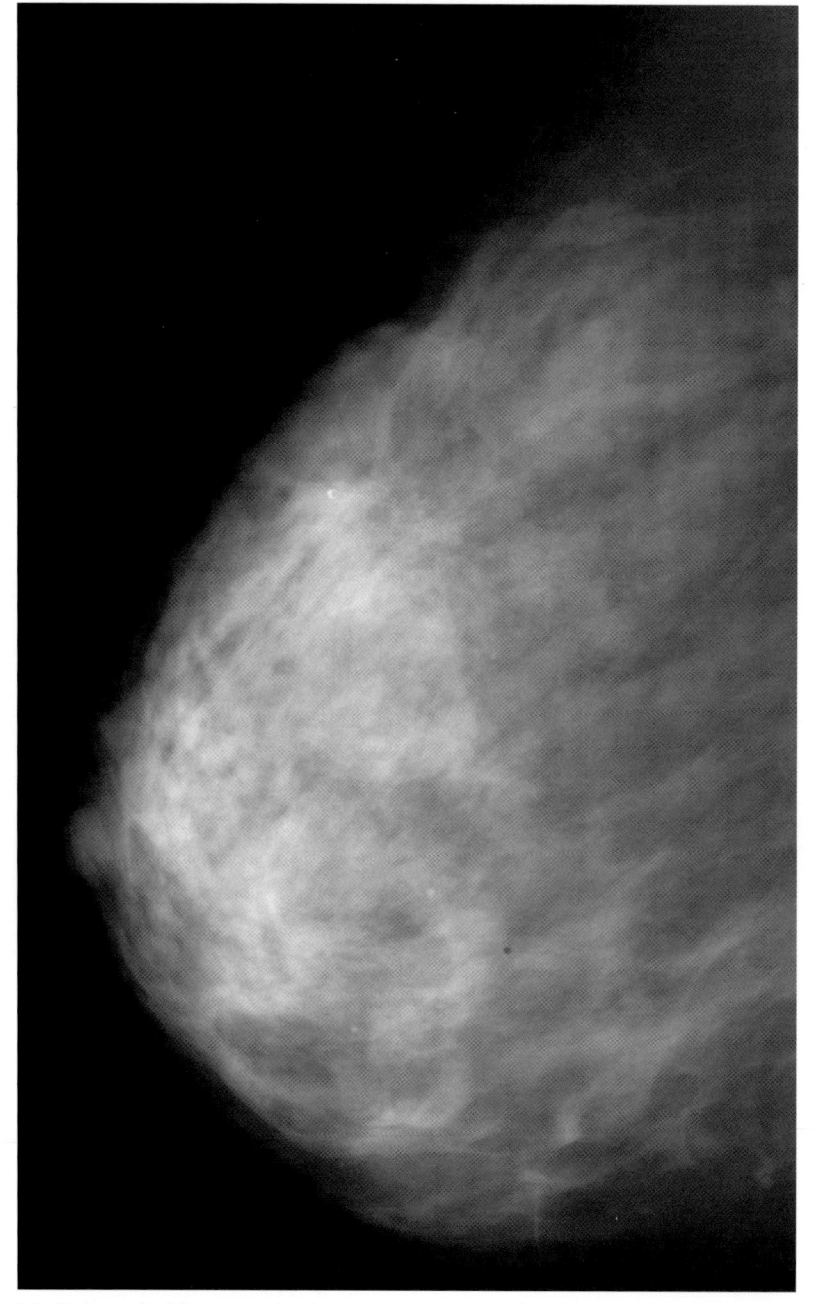

Mediolateral oblique projection

Posterior marginal distortion

In the right upper outer quadrant, in a posterior location, the body of the mammary gland is markedly abnormal, with a disorderly rosette-like appearance. The distortion gives a low-density image, changing partially according to the projection.

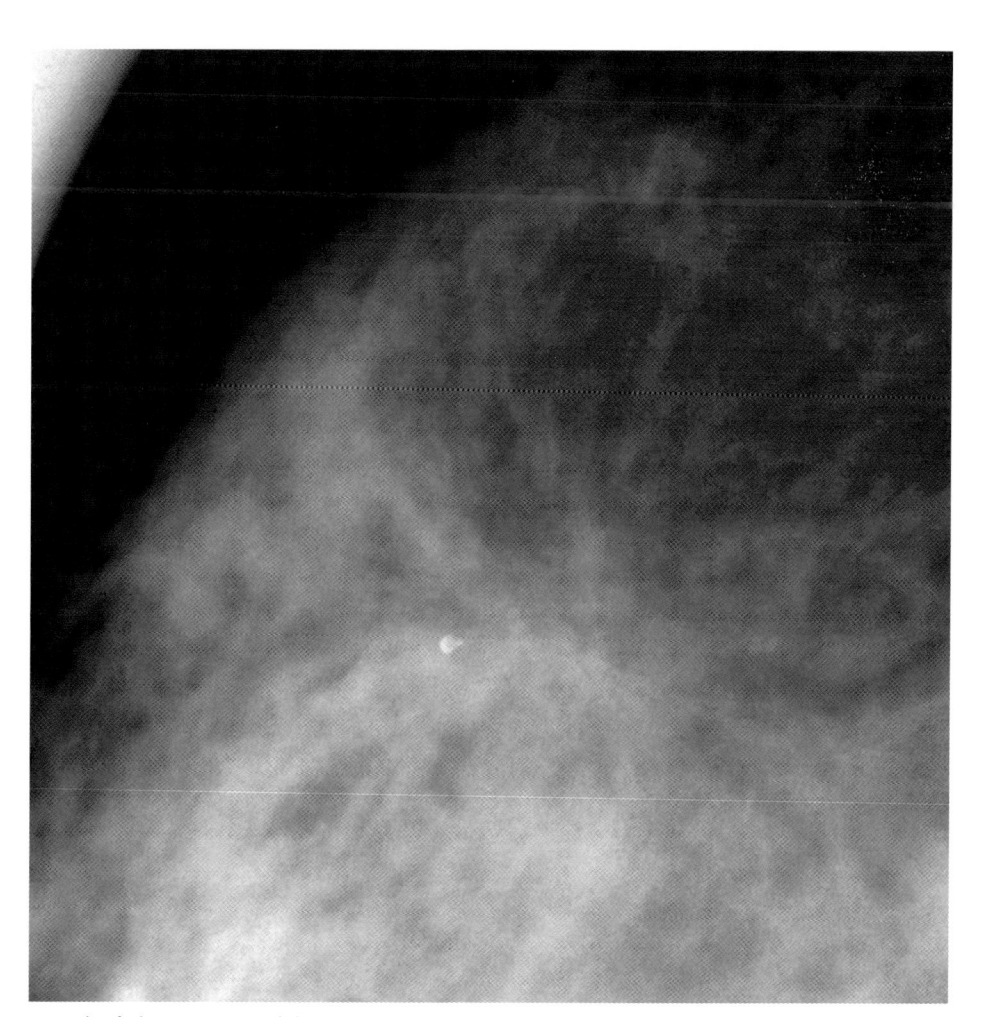

Detail of the craniocaudal projection

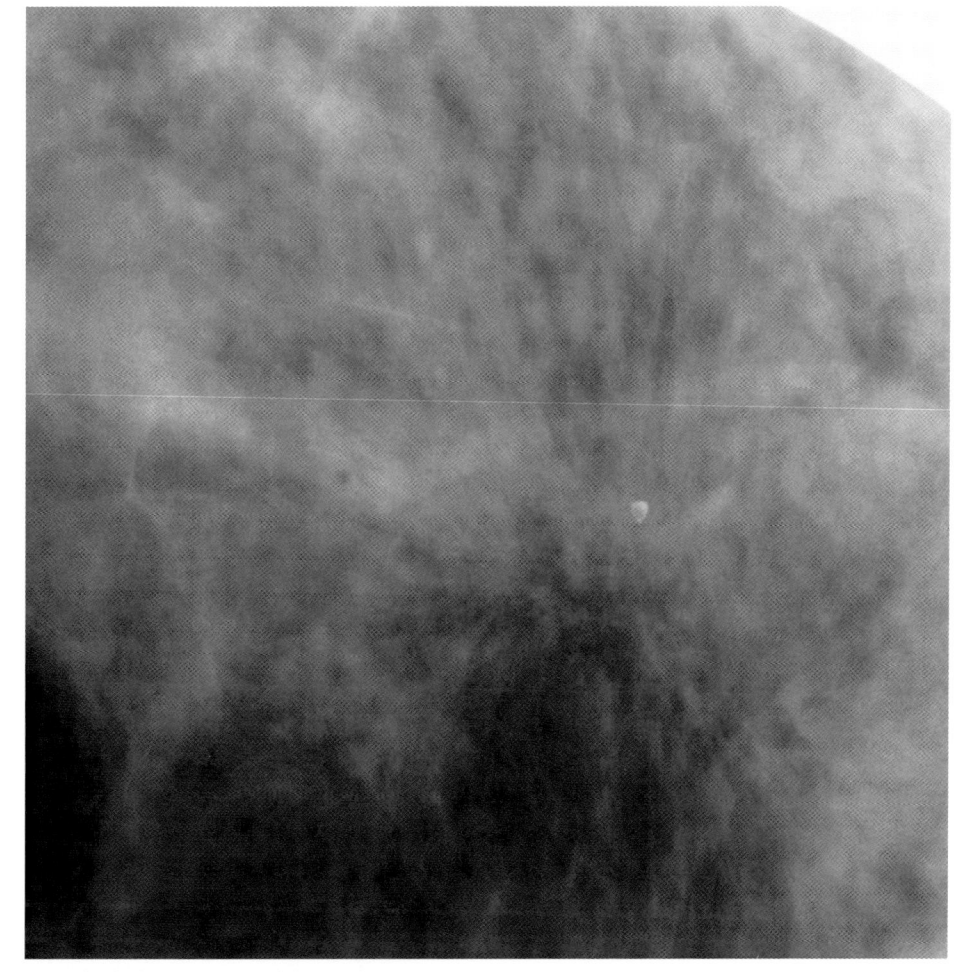

Detail of the craniocaudal projection

Histological finding: benign proliferative hyperplasia

ARCHITECTURAL DISTORTION

Anterior marginal distortion

Externally, the normal orientation of the body of the breast is altered. The anterior profile shows a long spiculated groove interrupting the normal convex shape, but in the standard craniocaudal projection no real mass is visible. In the magnification view, the distortion looks somewhat stellate, with a non-homogeneous central portion containing multiple radiolucent vacuoles and a coarse calcification.

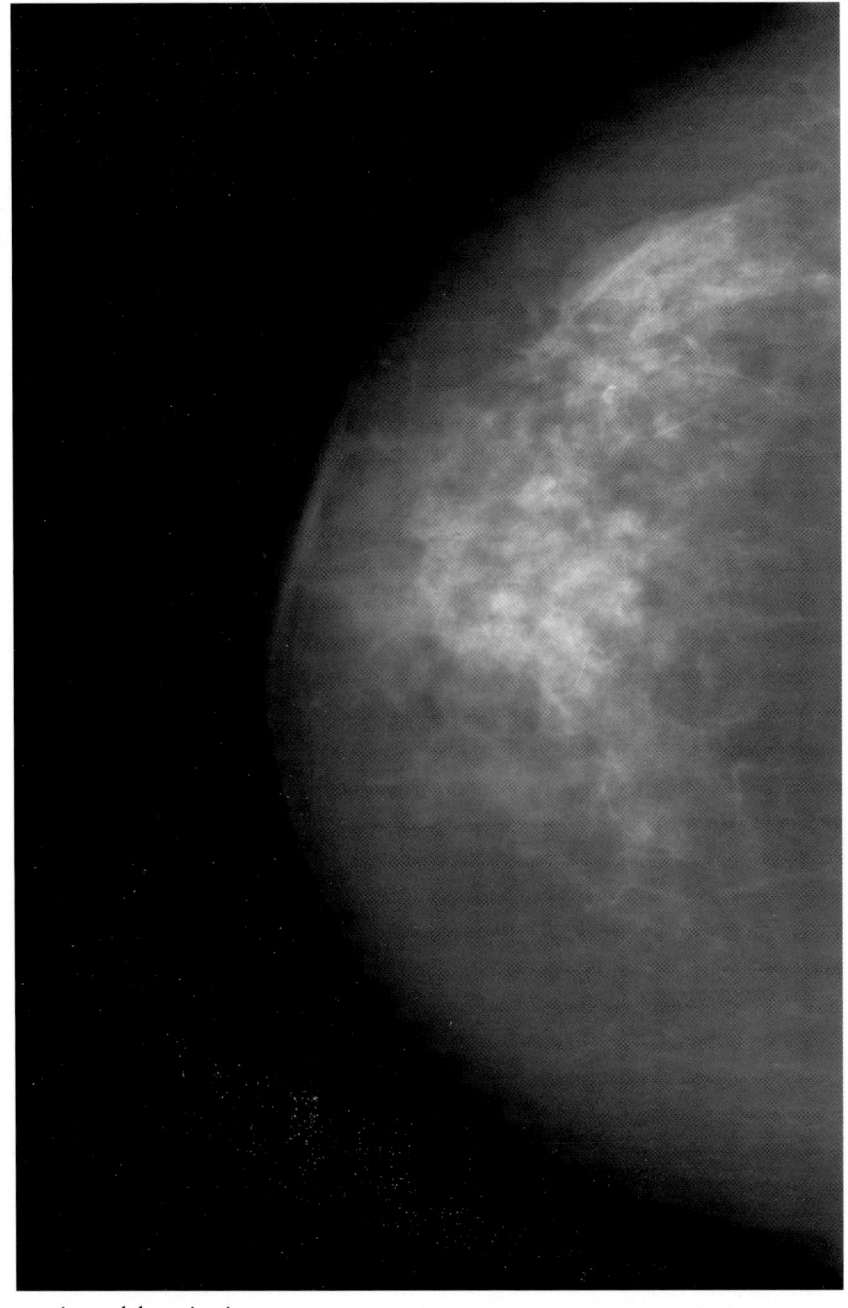

craniocaudal projection

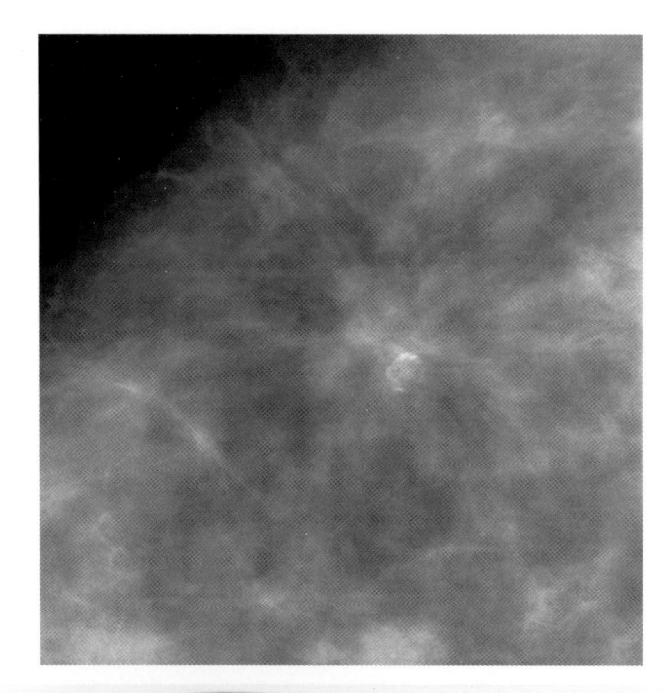

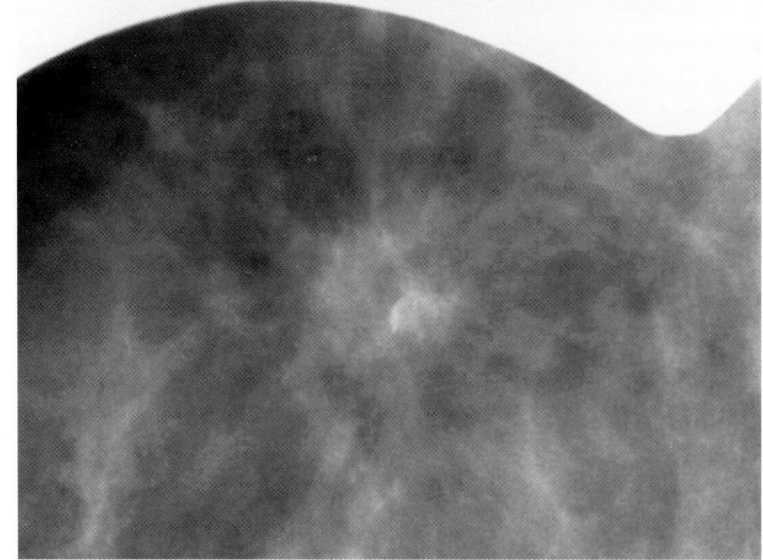

Magnification view of the craniocaudal projection

Histological finding: infiltrating ductal carcinoma

CALCIFICATIONS

Definition
Calcifications are amorphous, radiopaque, acellular entities produced by calcium deposits. They vary widely in density, shape and size, reflecting the secretory or degenerative processes of the breast. Malignant calcifications may be caused either by cellular secretion or by calcification of necrotic cancer cells.
The detection of calcium deposits in a suspicious opacity, or more often, isolated calcified clusters, is only possible with mammography, and has made it possible to recognize many cancers at a very early stage, permitting conservative surgery and reducing the mortality rate for breast cancer. Calcifications are among the most frequent mammographic signs and can also be amongst the most difficult to define and interpret. It is useful to distinguish between calcifications in the proper sense or microcalcifications and coarse calcifications. Calcifications can be solitary or associated with opacities.

Classification
In relation to their site of origin, calcifications are classified as ductal, when they originate in ducts or ductules, or lobular, when they come from dilated lobules or pseudocysts.

Evaluation
Several features must be evaluated in order to establish the nature of calcifications:
- Shape
- Distribution
- Site
- Size
- Number

CLASSIFICATION

Ductal calcifications
- granular type
- "casting type"
- mixed
- rod-shaped, tubular

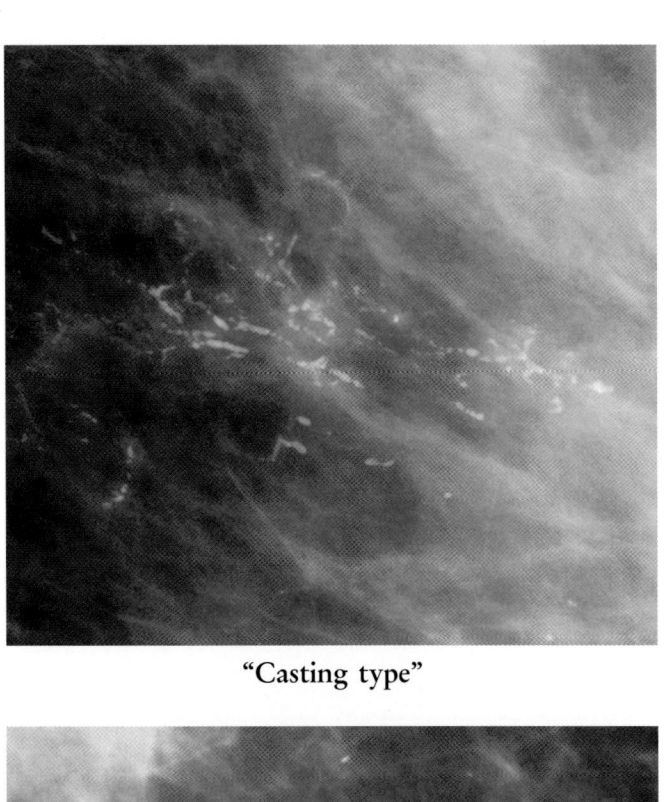

"Casting type"

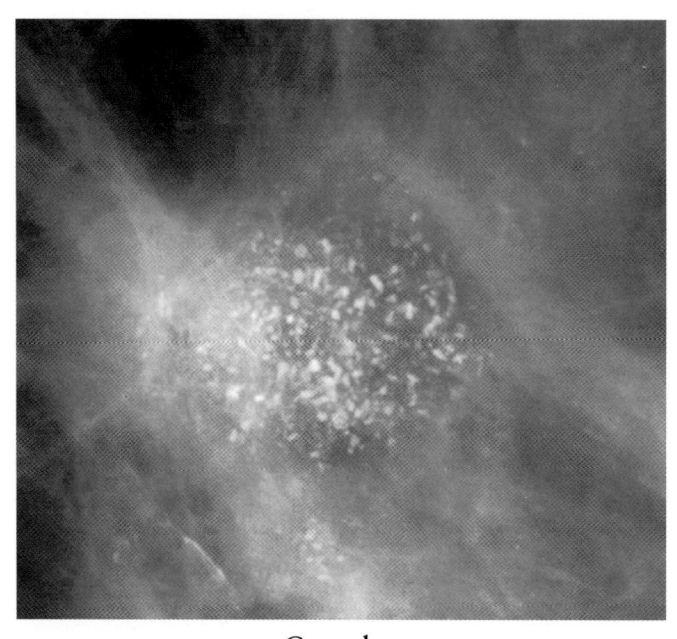

Granular

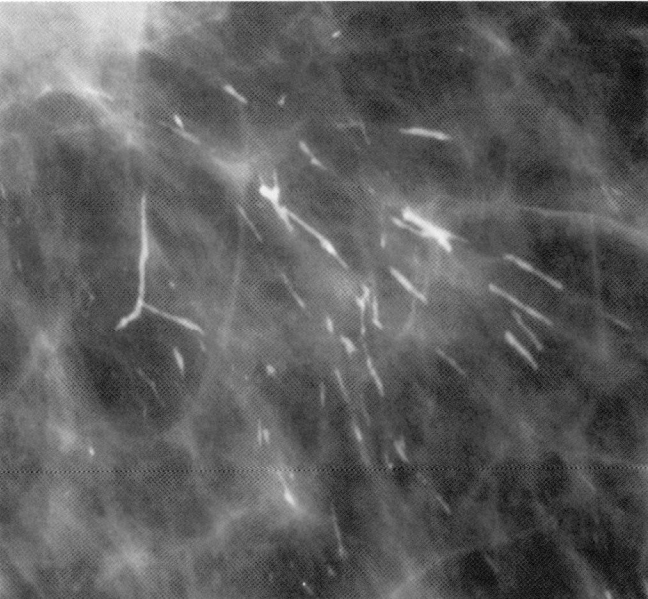

Rod-shaped

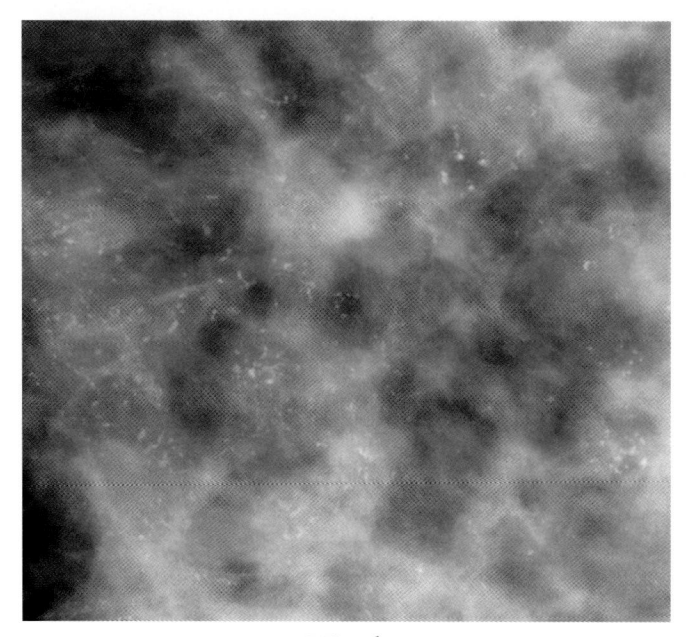

Mixed

Lobular calcifications
- rounded or bead-like (punctate, powdery)
- "milk-of-calcium" ("tea-cup", "meniscus-like")
- spherical with lucent centre
- "egg-shell"

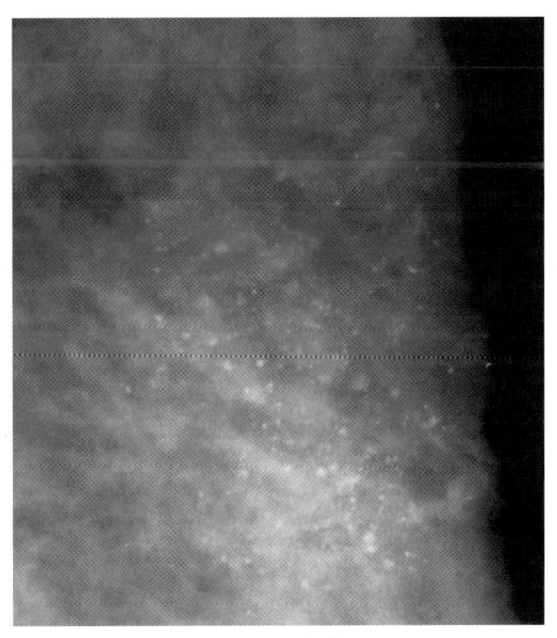

Rounded

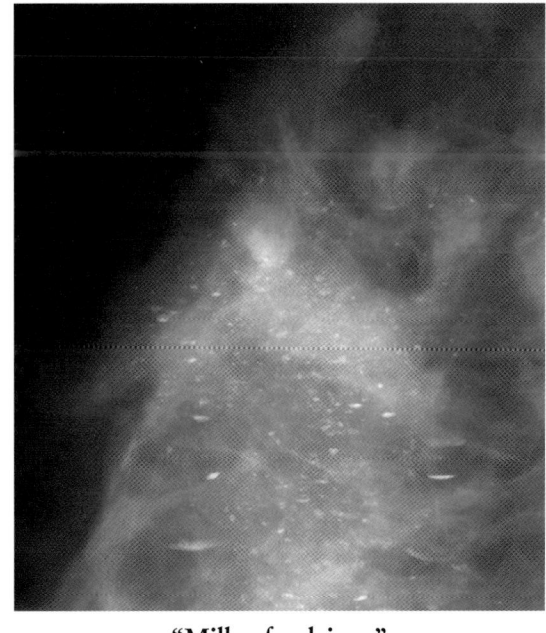

"Milk-of-calcium"

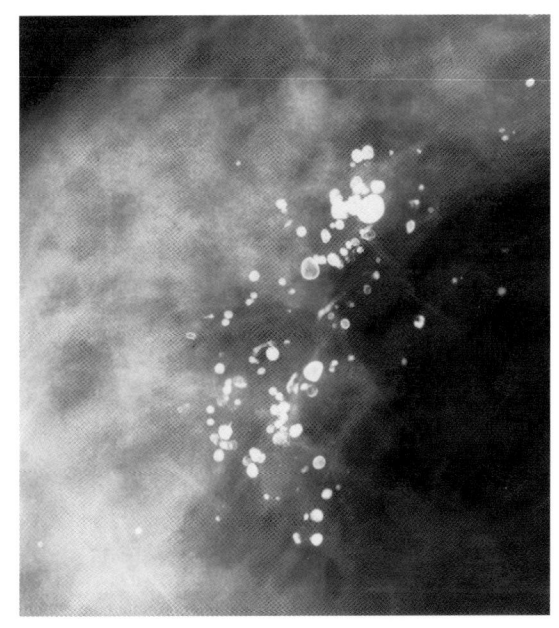

Spherical with lucent centre

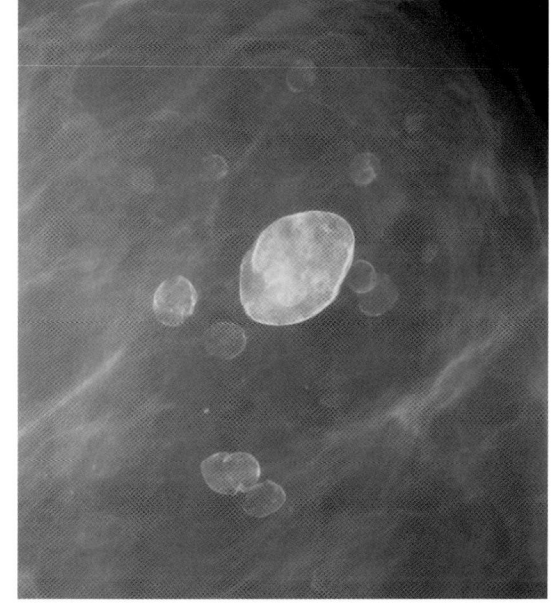

"Egg-shell"

CLASSIFICATION

Coarse calcifications
- patches ("popcorn", "candle-wax")
- vascular
- dystrophic
- skin calcifacations
- foreign body-induced
- pseudocalcifications

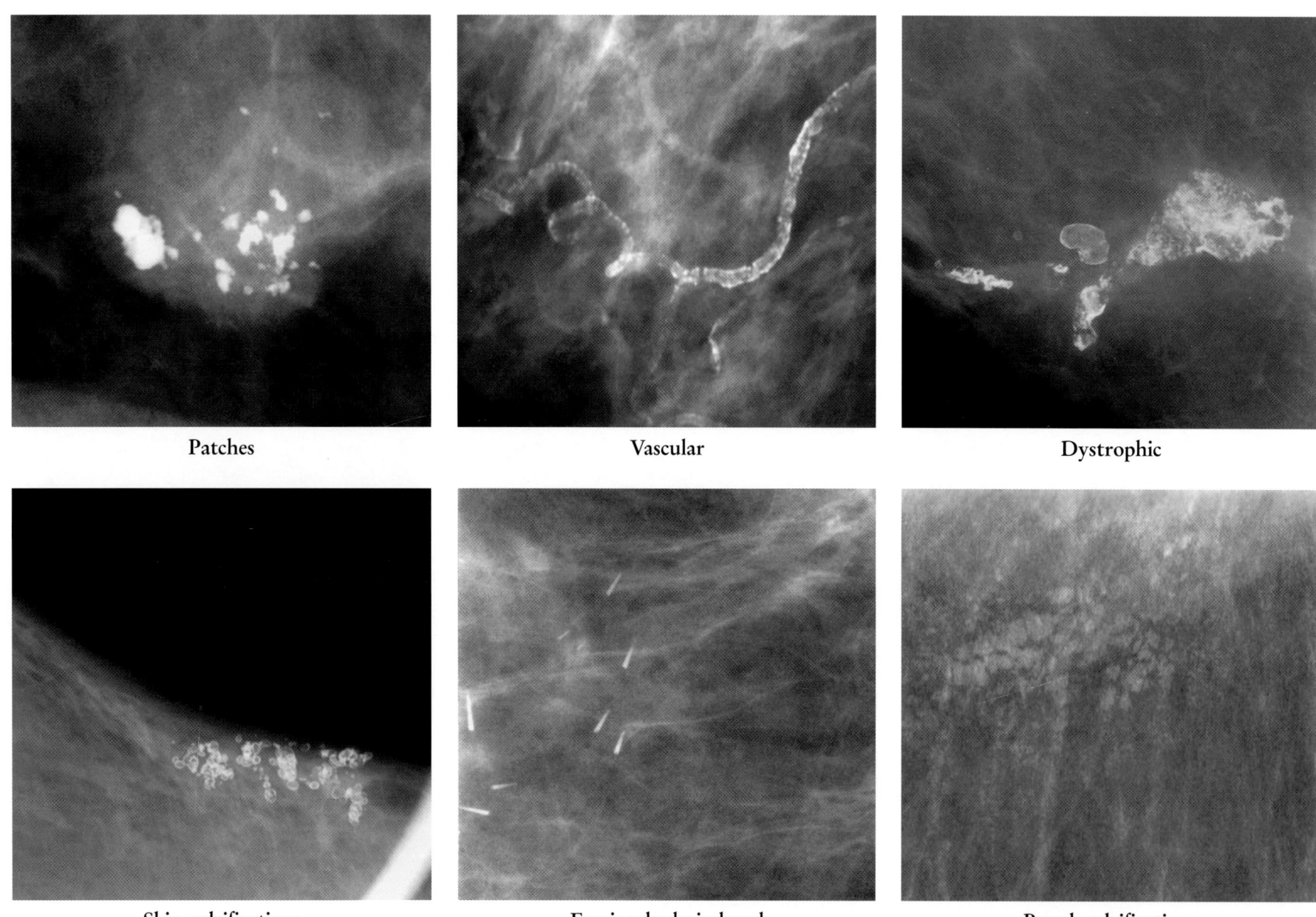

| Patches | Vascular | Dystrophic |

| Skin calcifications | Foreign body-induced | Pseudocalcifications |

Morphology: Morphology is the most important feature, with density, in the analysis of calcifications, either isolated or clustered. The shape often helps establish how they were formed. A cluster of calcifications with heterogeneous morphology and density should always arouse concern.

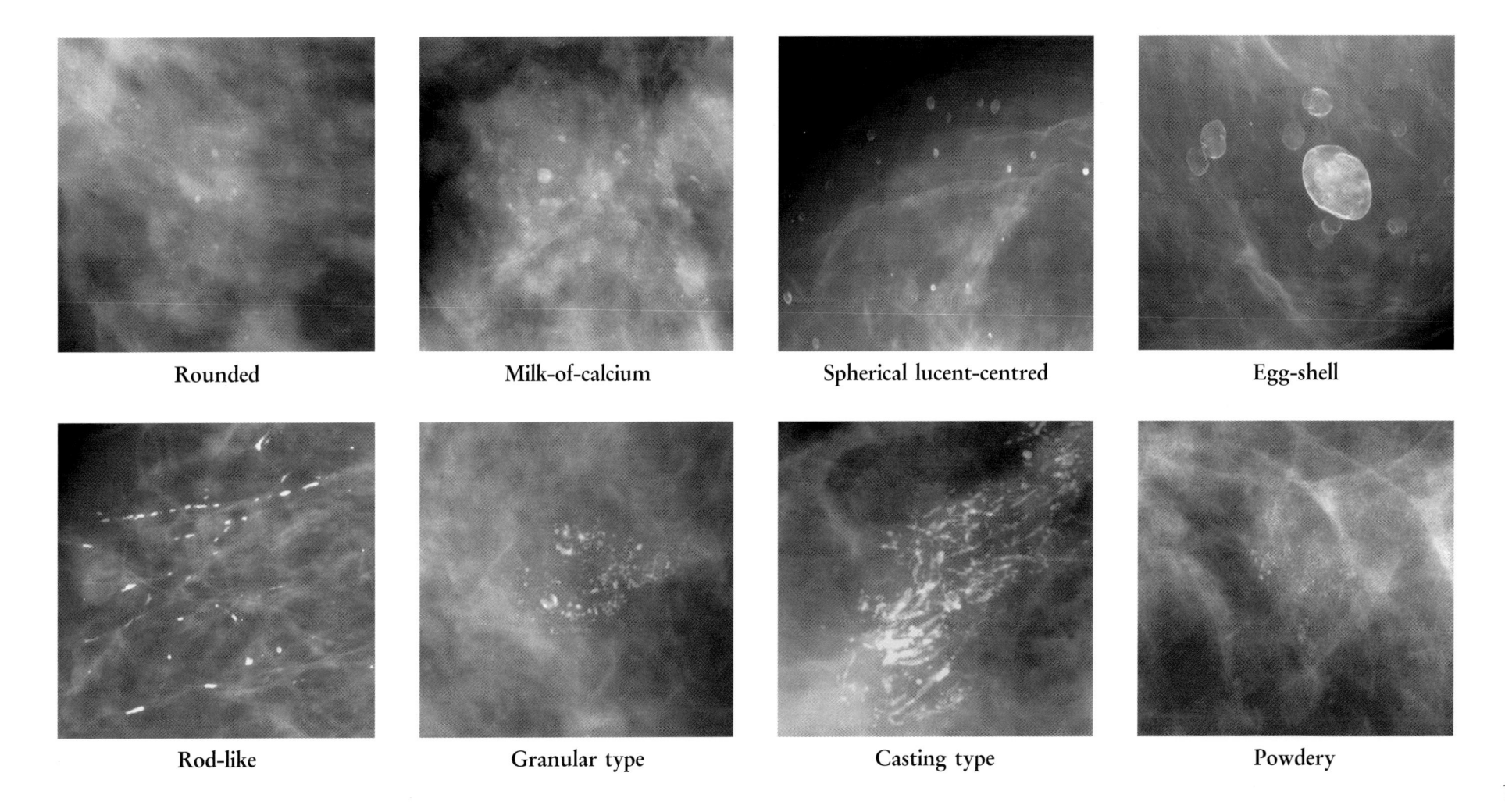

Rounded | Milk-of-calcium | Spherical lucent-centred | Egg-shell

Rod-like | Granular type | Casting type | Powdery

EVALUATION

Distribution: This is the second most important feature. Though calcifications often have no particular pattern of distribution, it is sometimes possible to establish the intraductal or lobular origin and progression of their growth in the parenchymal-stromal tissue, and this may help identify the underlying pathology. Linear and clustered distribution patterns mainly suggest intraductal carcinomas, as do segmental or lobar patterns. The distribution is more likely to be regional or diffuse in degenerative processes. The morphology and density of calcifications must always be assessed together with their distribution.

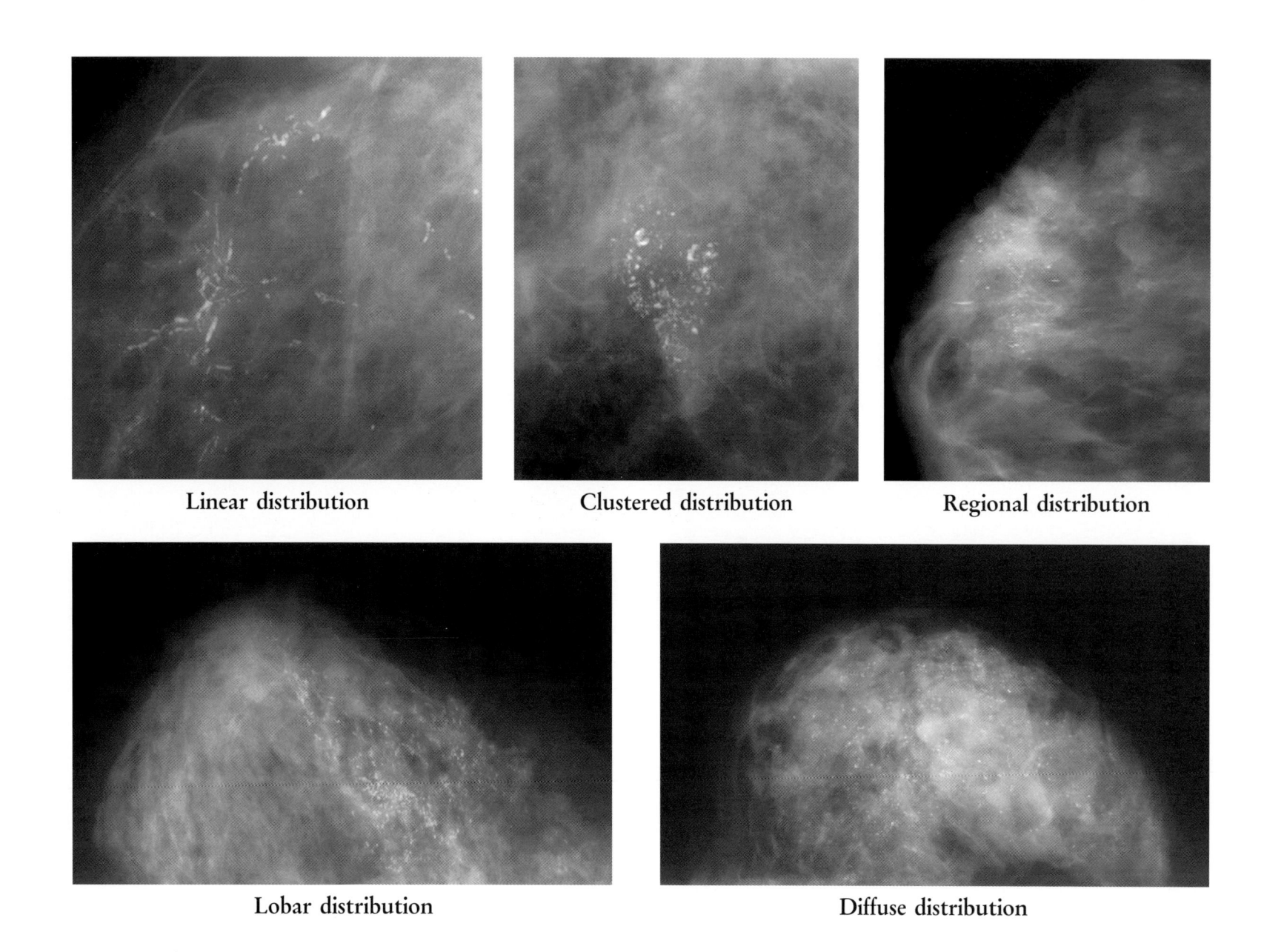

Linear distribution

Clustered distribution

Regional distribution

Lobar distribution

Diffuse distribution

Site: Before starting to analyse calcifications, it is advisable to ascertain that calcifications are truly intra-mammary, to rule out skin or pseudo-calcifications due to artefacts.

Size: Many different dimensions are reported, but calcifications associated with malignancies are generally between 0.5 and 2 mm, though often even smaller.

Number: There is no consensus on the smallest number of calcifications beyond which it is likely that a lesion is malignant. Some authors maintain that more than five calcifications in an area of 0.5/1 cm x 0.5/1 cm is suggestive of a neoplastic focus. Obviously the number of calcifications must be evaluated together with their morphology and distribution.

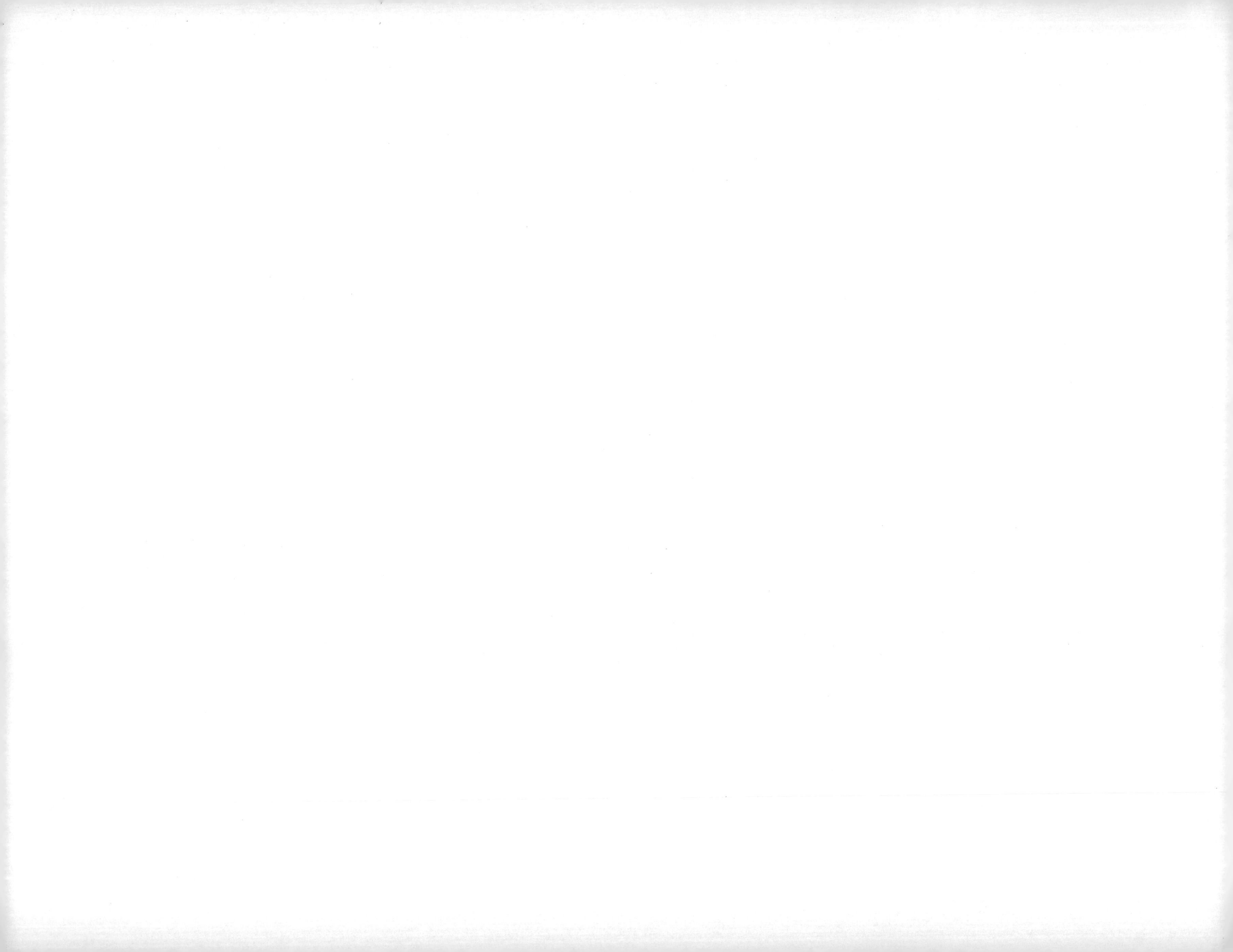

Distribution

The most frequent and easily recognized distribution patterns are:
- *linear*
- *clustered*
- *lobar or segmental*
- *regional*
- *diffusely scattered*

Linear distribution

This pattern alone suggests an intraductal process; if the calcifications are linear, elongated and irregular with a tendency to branch out, they are generally consistent with carcinoma in situ, but if the morphology is more regular, the density fairly homogeneous, and above all if the distribution is radial, starting from the nipple, these calcifications are often early signs of plasma cell mastitis.

DISTRIBUTION

Linear distribution
A stellate opacity with intralesional calcifications is visible in the median aspect. Posteriorly, and stretching linearly and posteriorly, some linear "casting type" are also visible.

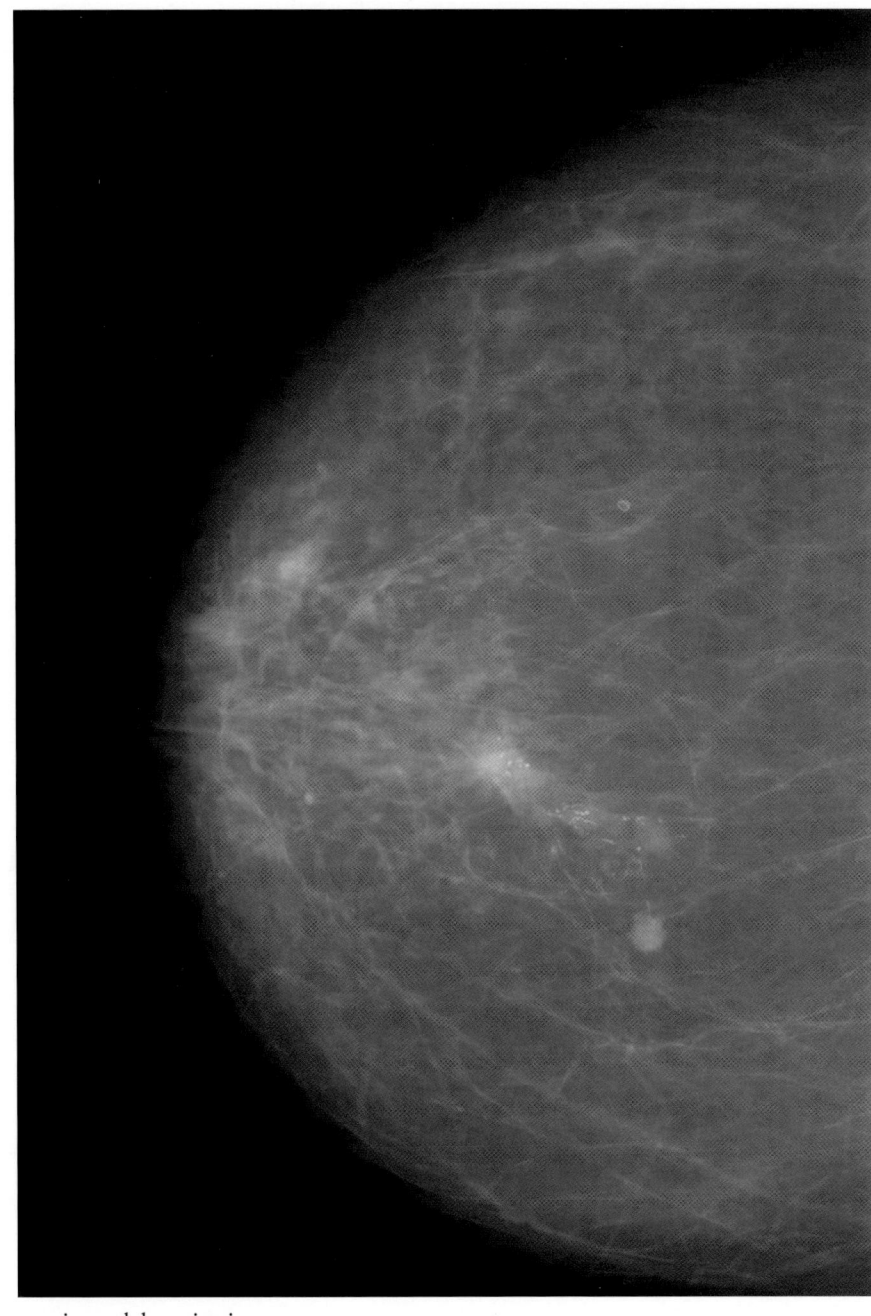

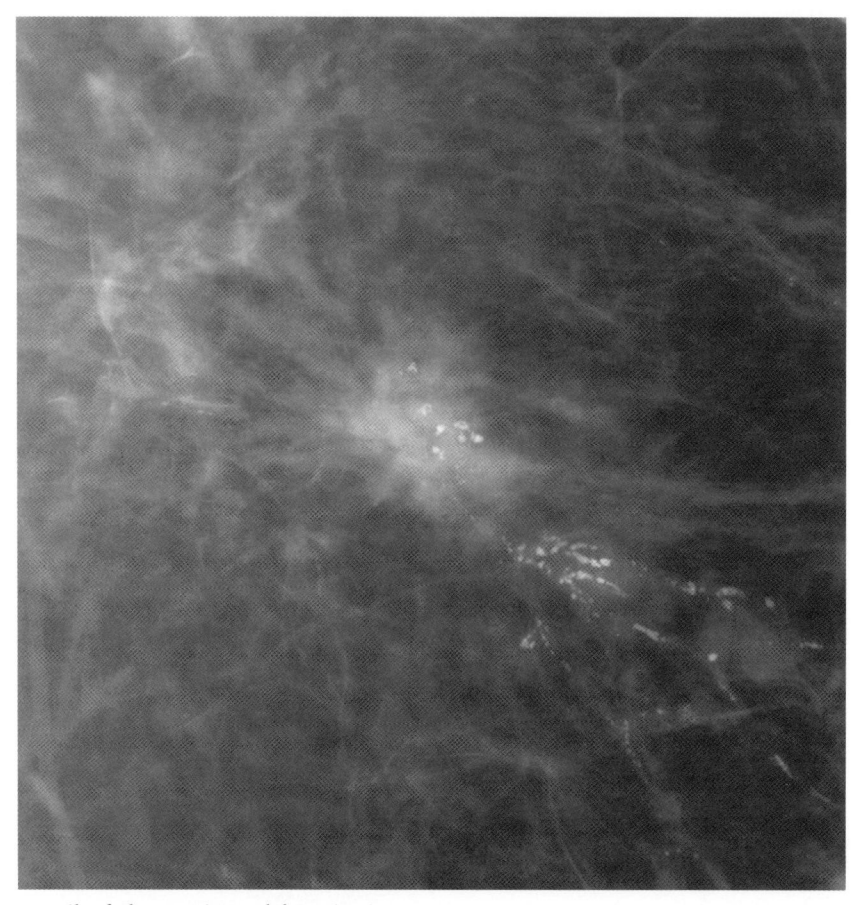

Detail of the craniocaudal projection

craniocaudal projection

Linear distribution

The image shows "casting type" microcalcifications behind the areola, tightly packed in a first-order duct, reproducing the morphology of its lumen precisely. The distribution is linear in the underlying parenchyma (A). Linear distribution in a retroareolar duct, with a hint of first and second-order branching (B).

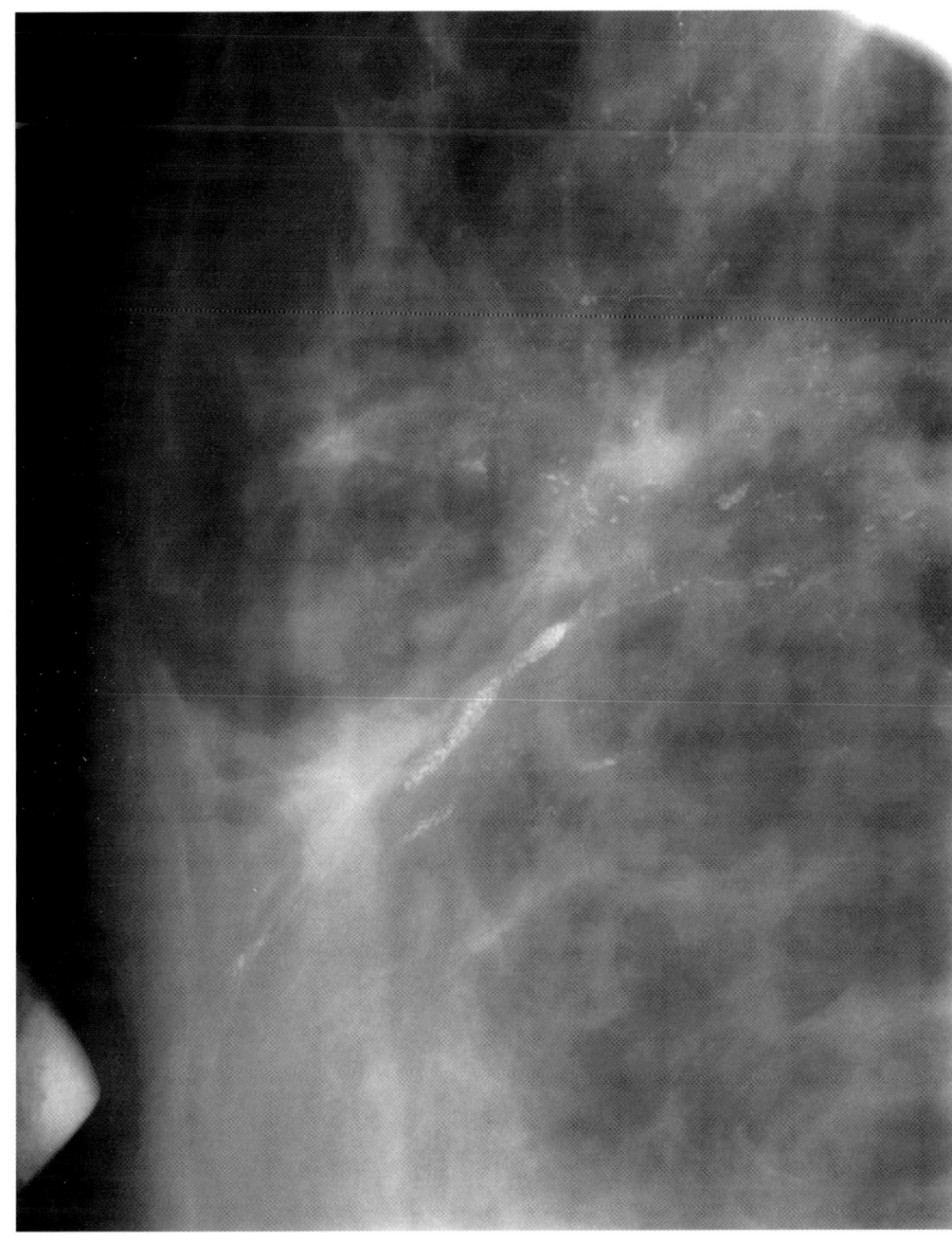

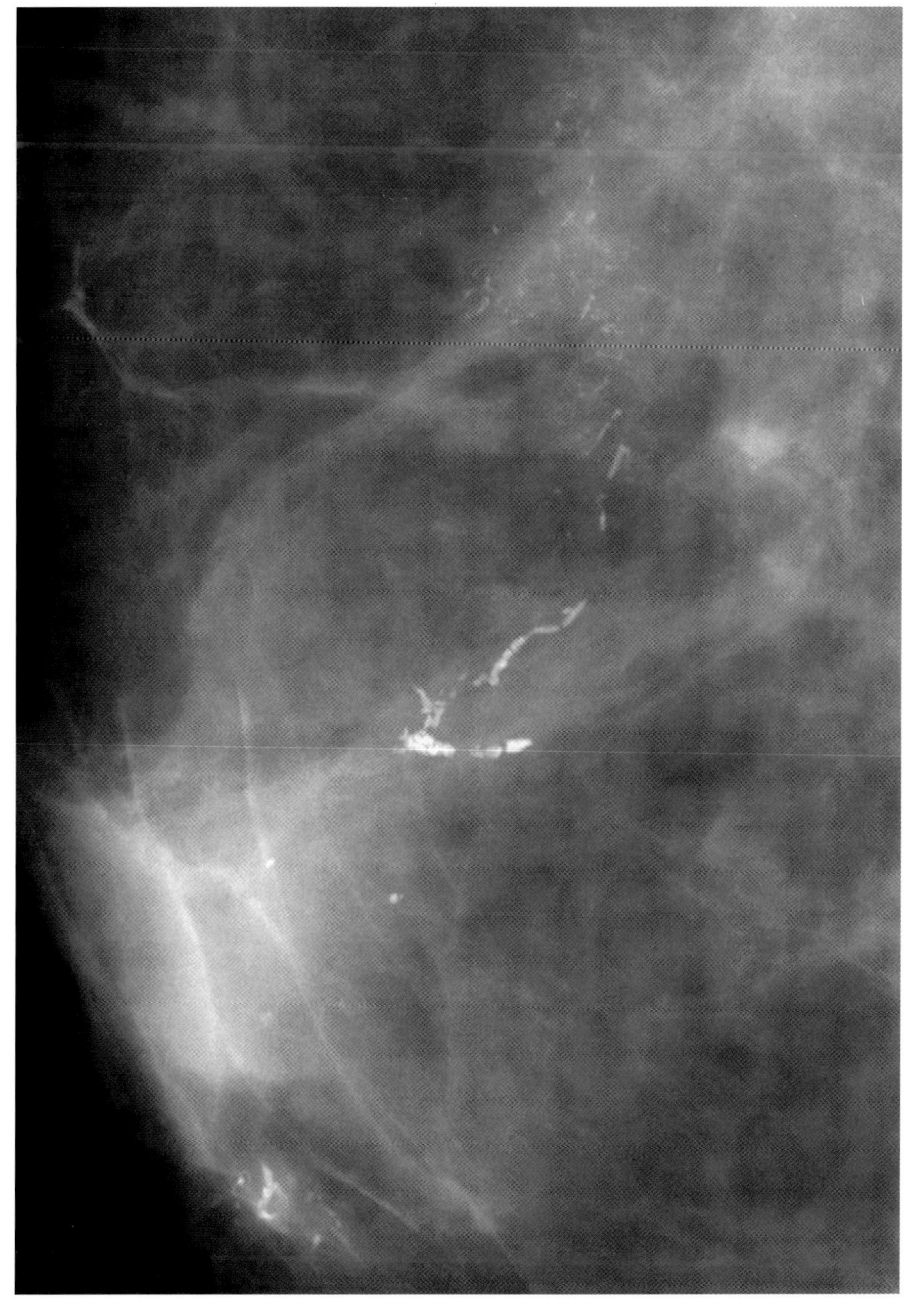

Lateral projection (A)

Lateral projection (B)

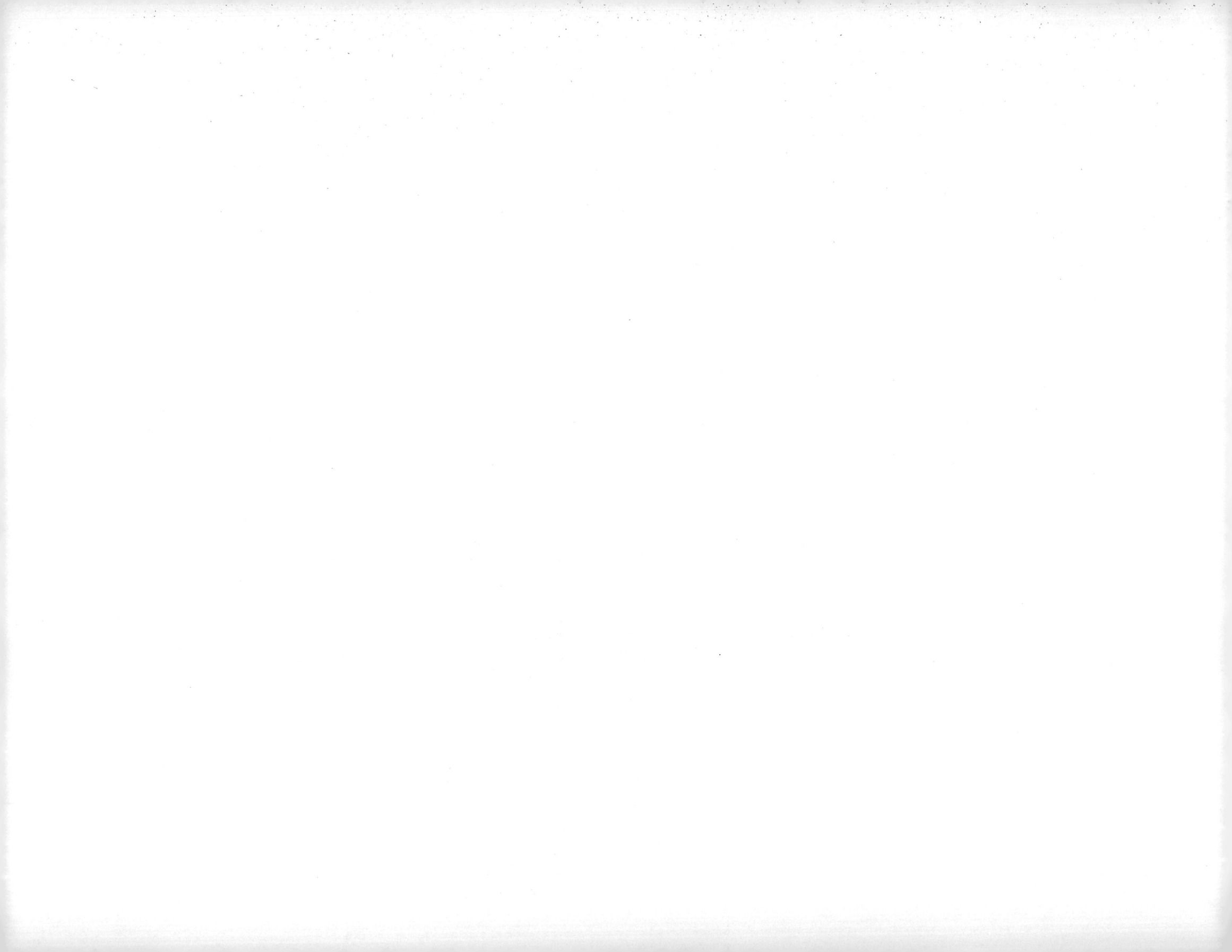

Clustered distribution

This term is used to indicate calcifications clustered in a small area, no bigger than 1-2 cm. Calcifications that are granular type, uneven in size and density strongly suggest a and predominantly intraductal carcinoma, while rounded or punctate ones with a regular outline may be benign proliferative lesions of the lobular acini, such as areas of adenosis or atypical hyperplasia. In the latter case, there are usually multiple foci, spread over a large area, often bilaterally.

DISTRIBUTION

Clustered distribution

A cluster of granular type calcifications is visible in the upper central region, irregular in density and morphology (A), approximately 5 mm in diameter. In a posterior inferior location there is a cluster of rounded calcifications, approximately 1 cm in diameter, homogeneous in density (B).

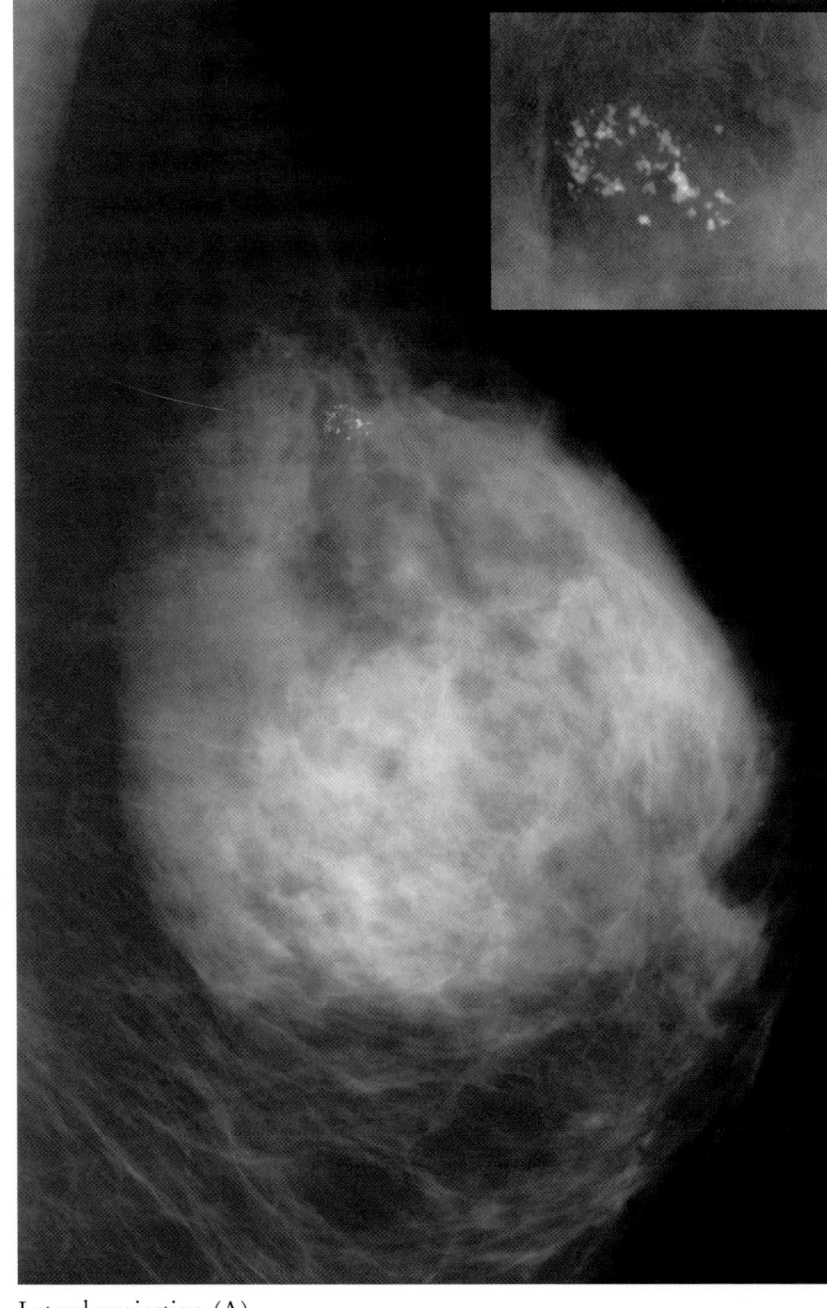

Lateral projection (A)

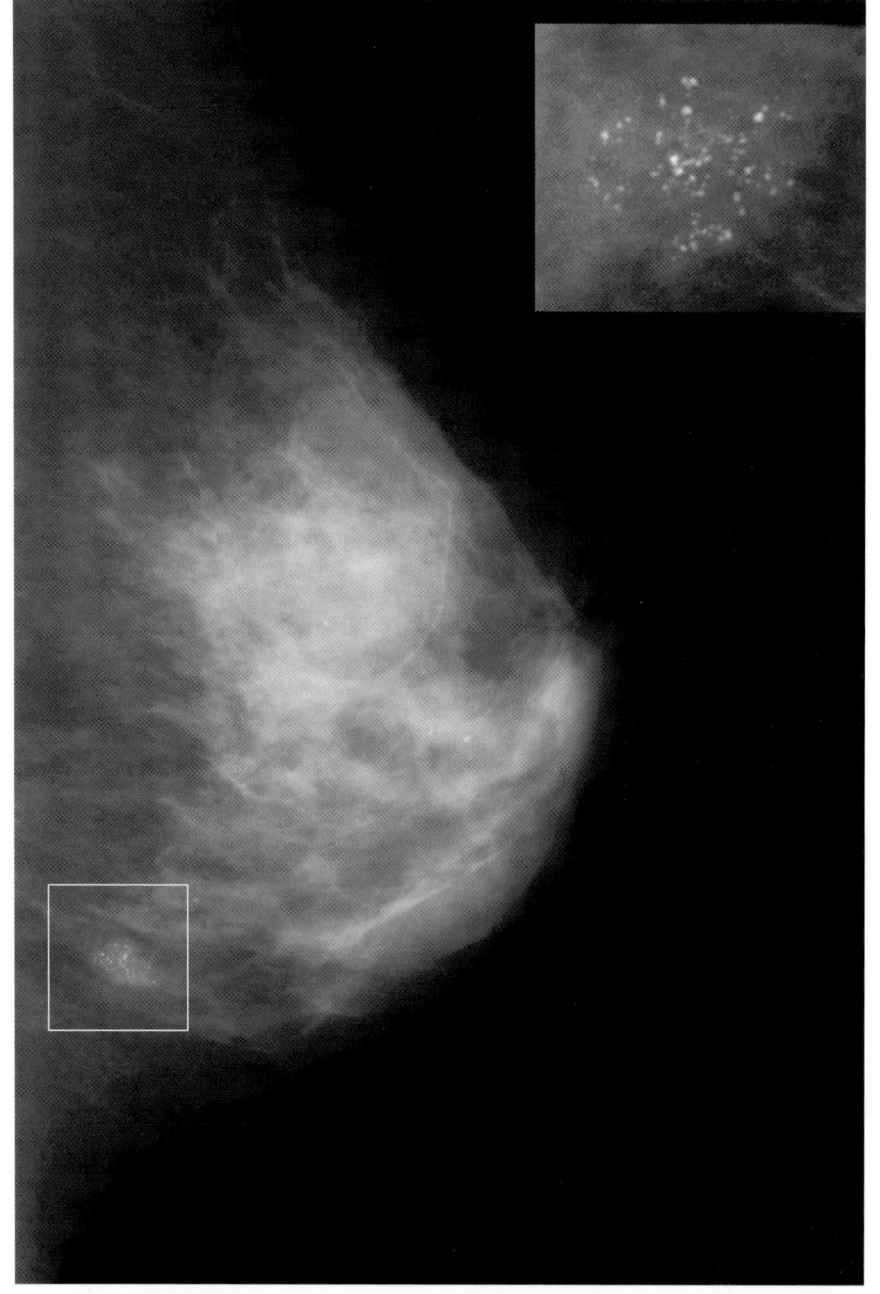

Lateral projection (B)

Multiclustered distribution

Behind the areola there are clusters of granular type calcifications, irregular in density and morphology. Their linear distribution faithfully follows a lactiferous duct (A). In the upper retroareolar space there are multiple clusters of granular type calcifications with irregular density and morphology, some isolated and others tending to converge, within a lobe (B).

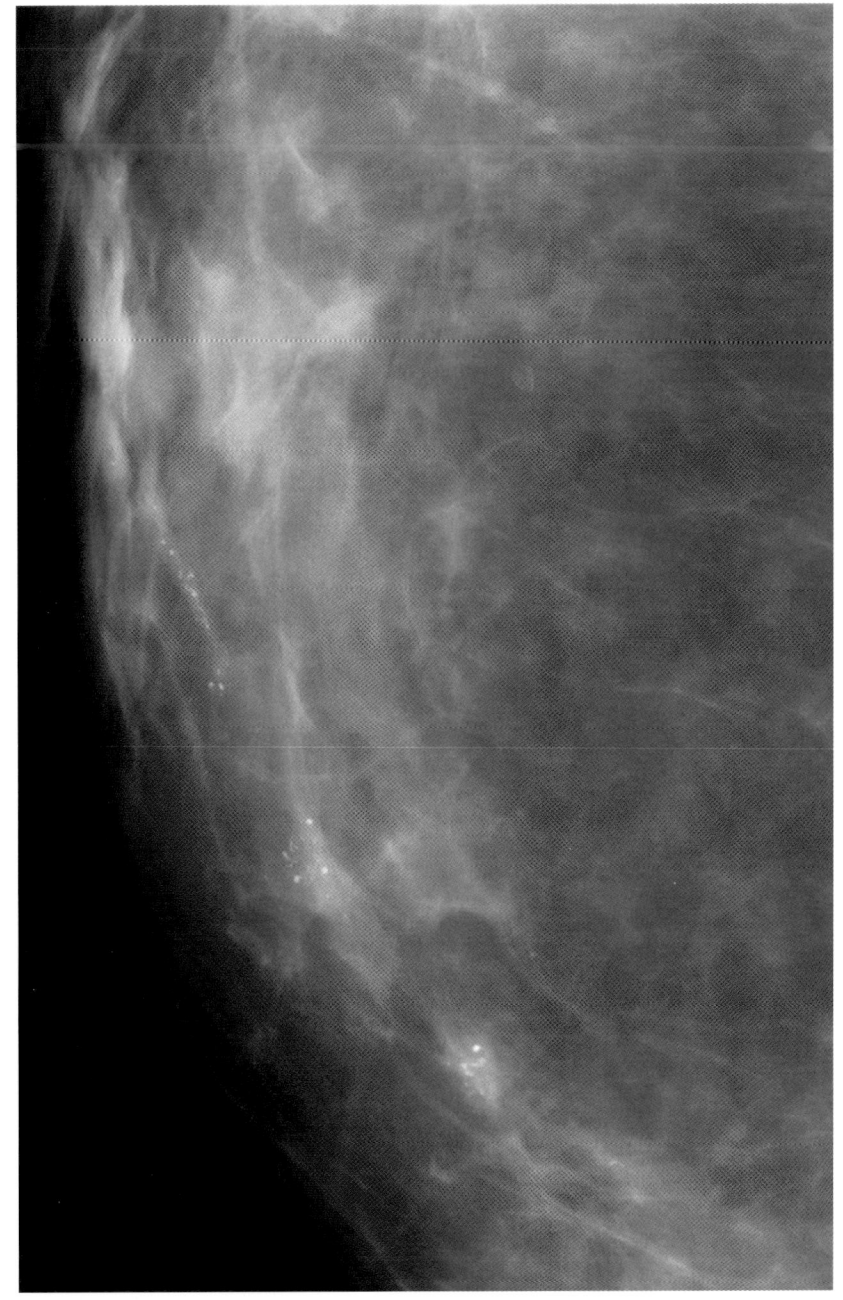

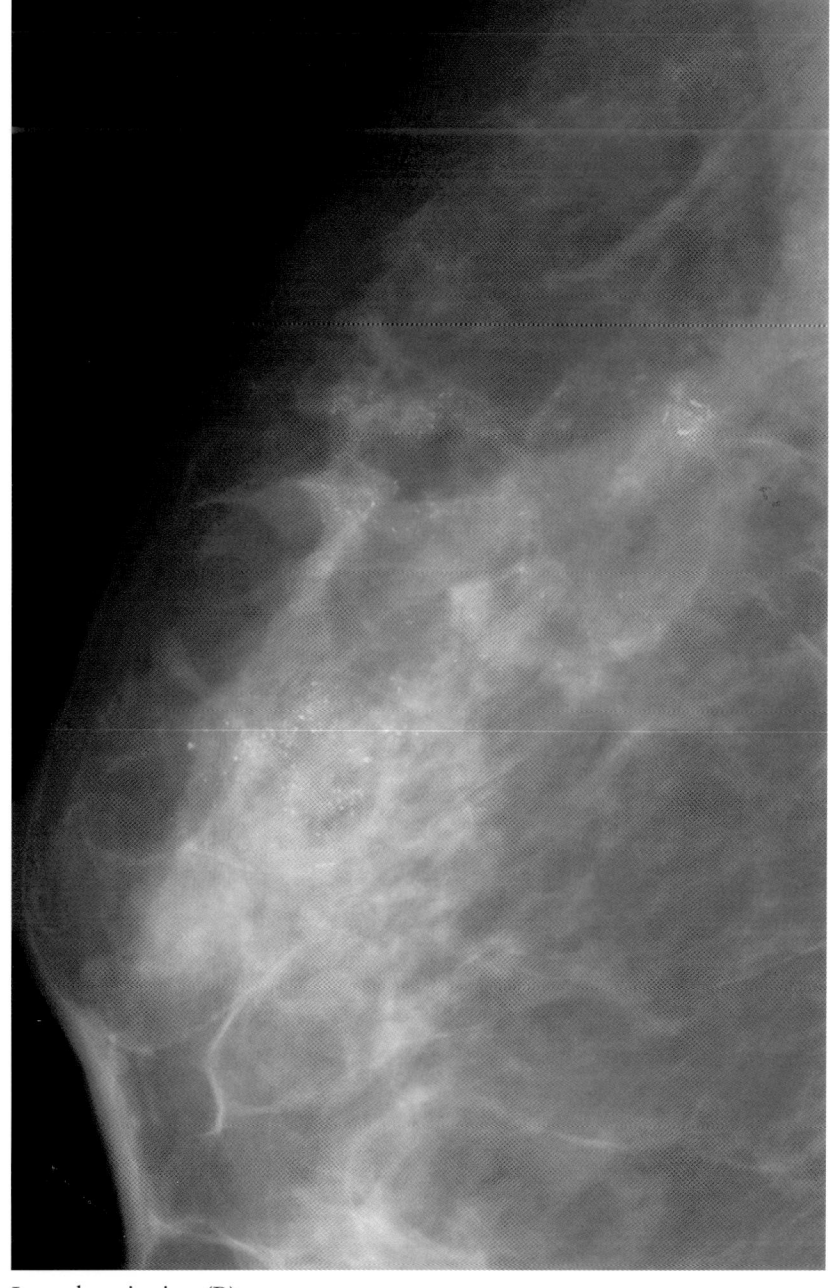

Lateral projection (A)

Lateral projection (B)

Lobar (or segmental) distribution

The ductal network of a whole mammary lobe or segment is involved, from the first-order retroareolar duct to the outermost ramifications. The ductal network may be only partially involved, or several ducts may be involved, suggesting multifocal or multicentric malignancy. This pattern is seldom seen in benign processes such as secretory disease or, later, plasma cell mastitis, in which the morphology of the individual calcifications is benign and the distribution is typically radial, in parallel planes.

DISTRIBUTION

Lobar (or segmental) distribution

Numerous "casting type" calcifications are visible, following the shape of the duct where they arise, in the outer portion of the lobe (A). In the middle retroarcolar region, there is another cluster of "casting type" calcifications in a segmental pattern, again closely reproducing the lobar anatomy. Note the thickened tissue in which the microcalcifications are visible (B).

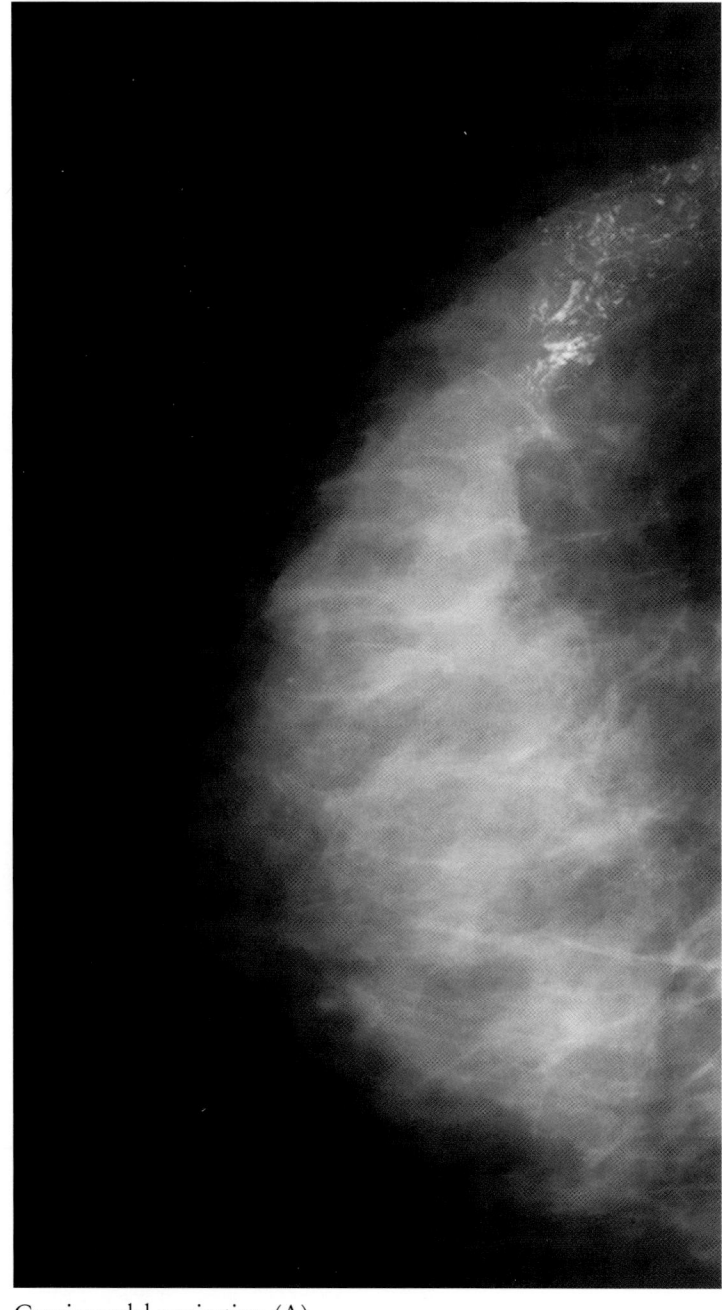

Craniocaudal projection (A)

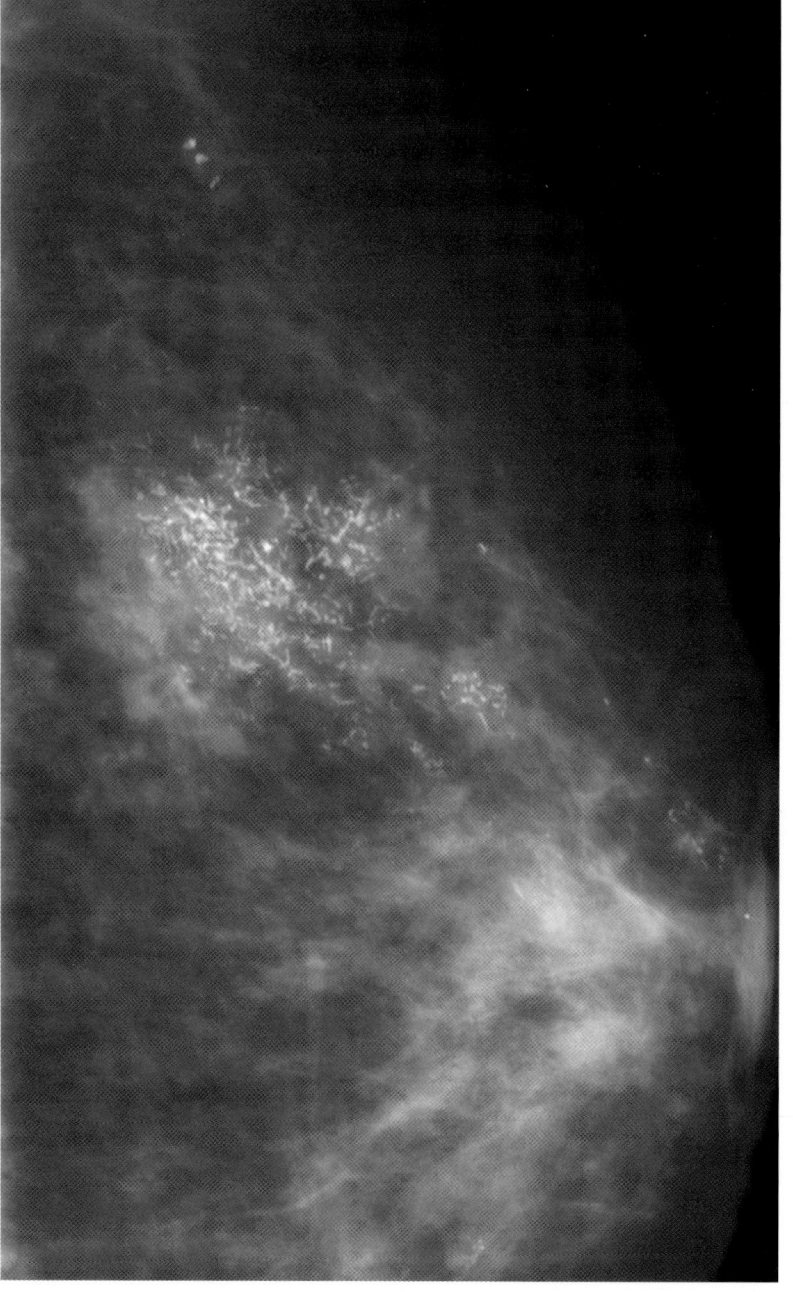

Lateral projection (B)

Lobar (or segmental) distribution

In a upper retroareolar location there are numerous mixed calcifications, "casting" and granular type, following the ductal lumen which is their site of origin, and involving the whole lobe as far as the axillary tail. Lobar distribution is frequently associated with multifocal or multicentric malignancies, especially if the morphology of the individual calcifications is irregular. Sometimes, however, secretory disease can give a segmental pattern.

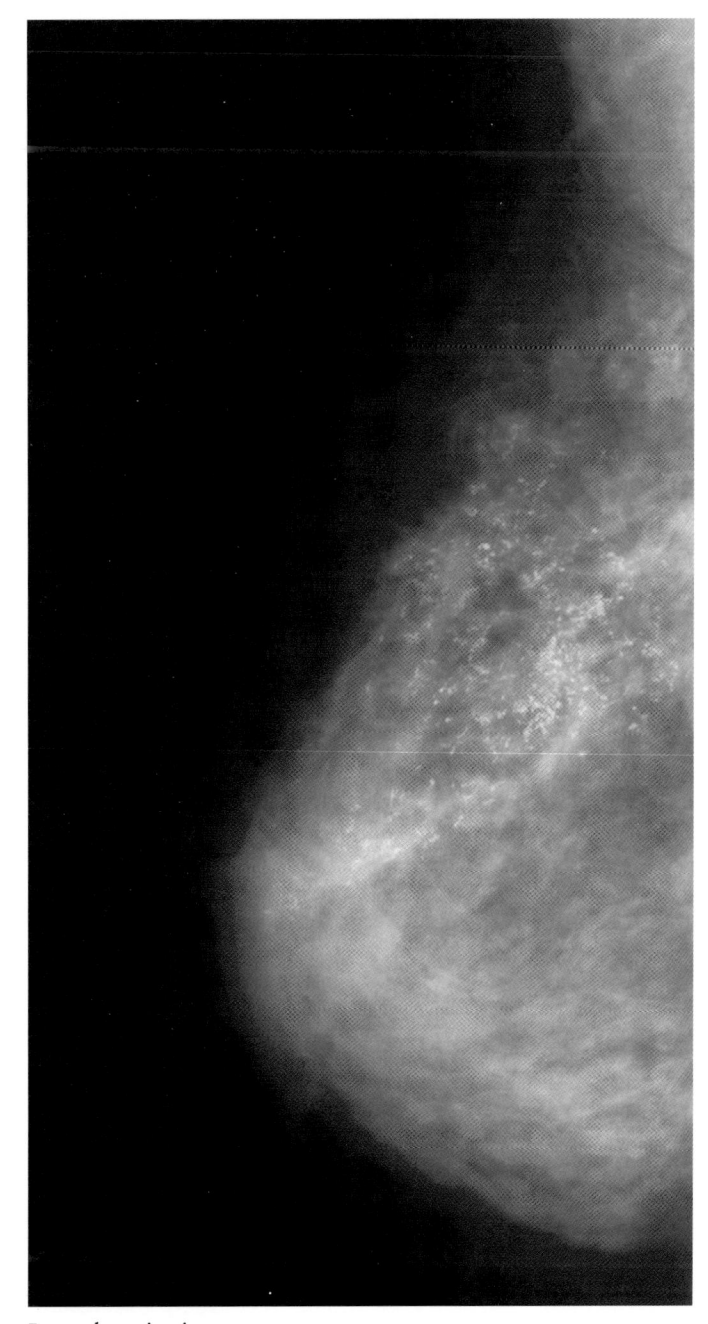

Lateral projection

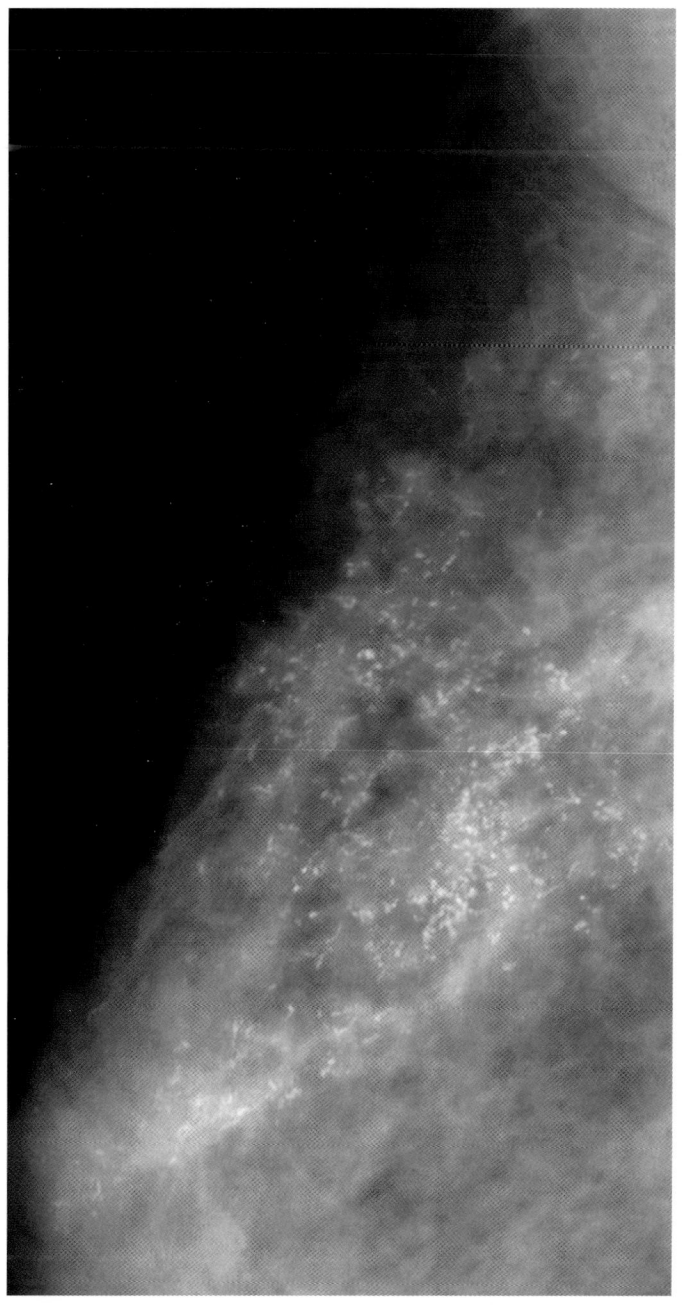

Detail of the lateral projection

DISTRIBUTION

Lobar (or segmental) distribution

In the upper outer quadrant numerous mixed calcifications follow the pattern of their origin in the ductal lumen, involving several adjacent lobes. Anteriorly, some clusters of calcifications seem to reproduce the shape of individual ducts, whilst posteriorly the deposits are tightly packed almost throughout the parenchyma.

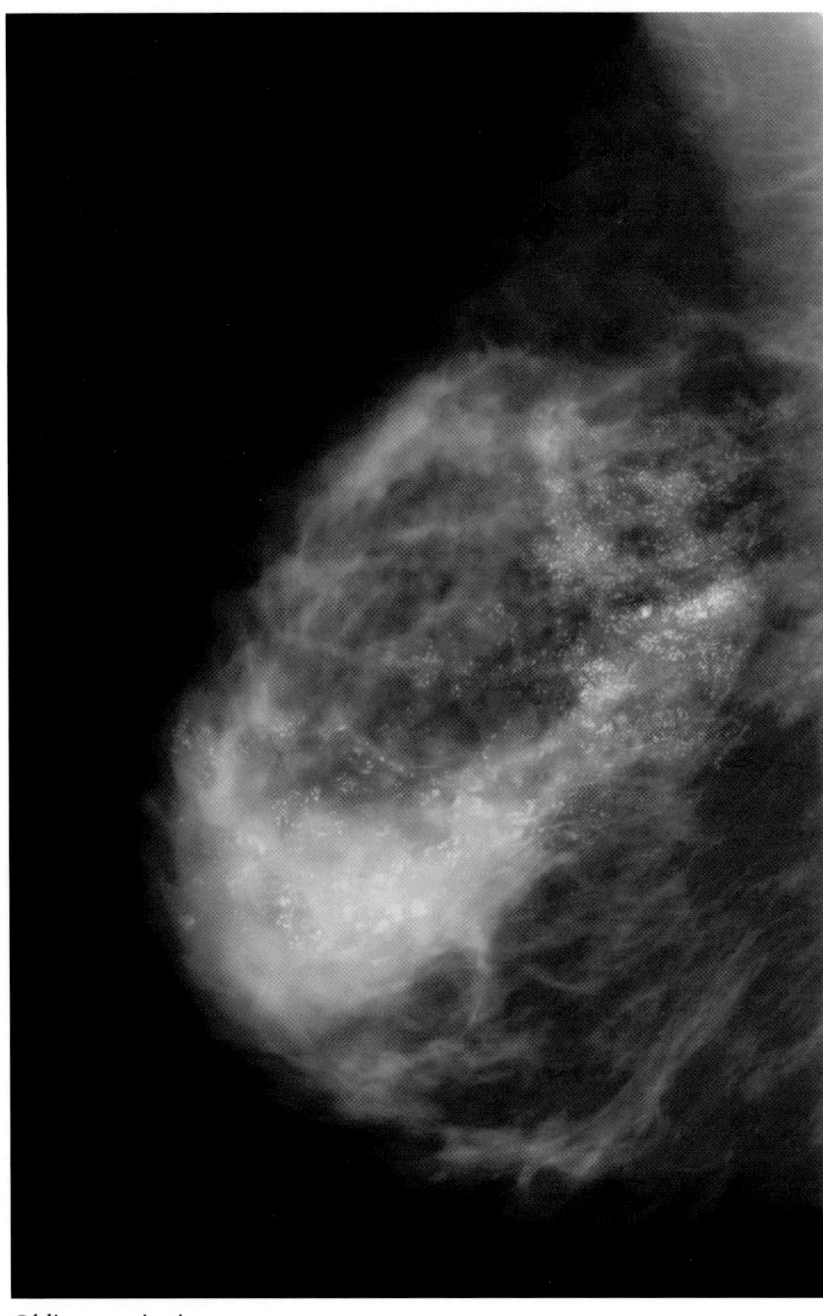

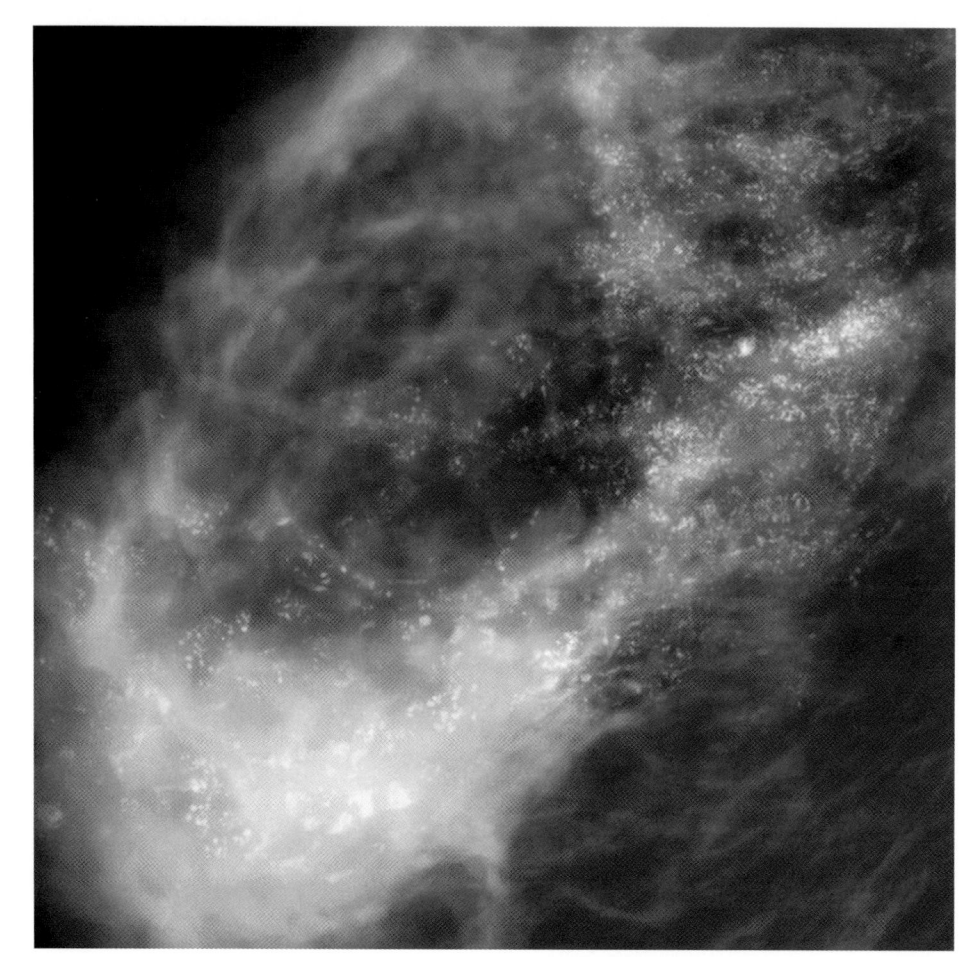

Detail of the oblique projection

Oblique projection

Regional distribution

The calcifications are scattered widely through the breast tissue, not necessarily suggesting a ductal distribution. A regressive process of microcystic dilatation of lobular acini, such as "milk-of-calcium" deposits, may also be regionally distributed.

DISTRIBUTION

Regional distribution

Multiple rounded calcifications are visible in the upper and central areas; they are scattered unevenly, in clusters or singly, throughout a fairly large part of the breast tissue. Note the circumscribed round opacity with sharp anterior and blurred posterior margins, of the same density as the surrounding parenchyma (A). In the upper area the calcifications are rounded and "milky", and lie within a limited area of the breast which is dense, but not suggestive of a ductal pattern distribution (B).

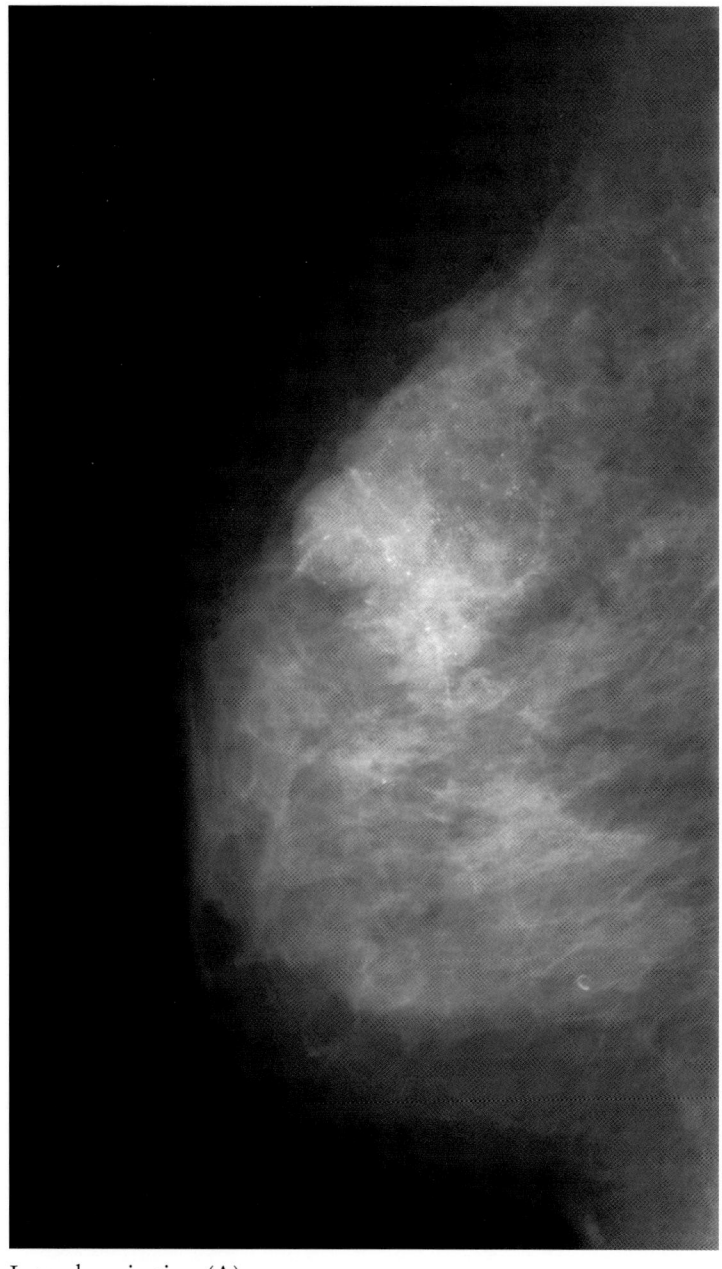

Lateral projection (A)

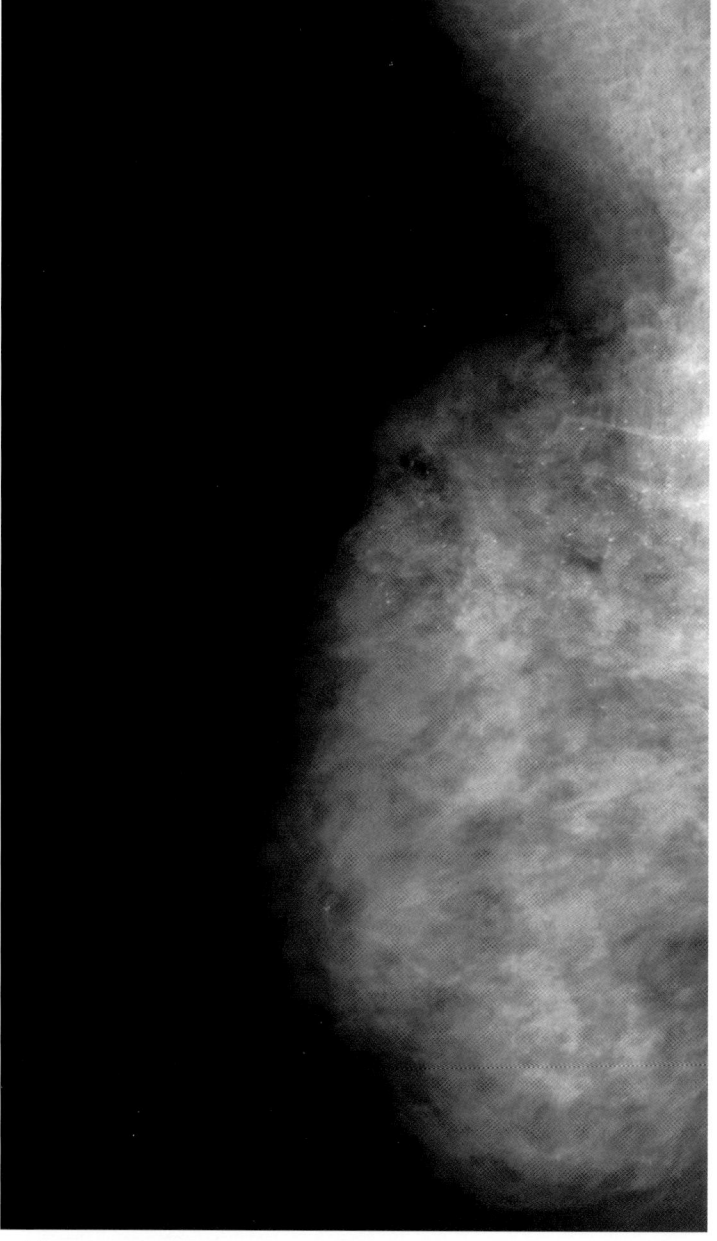

Oblique projection (B)

Regional distribution

The magnification view shows the morphology and regional distribution of the calcifications more clearly.

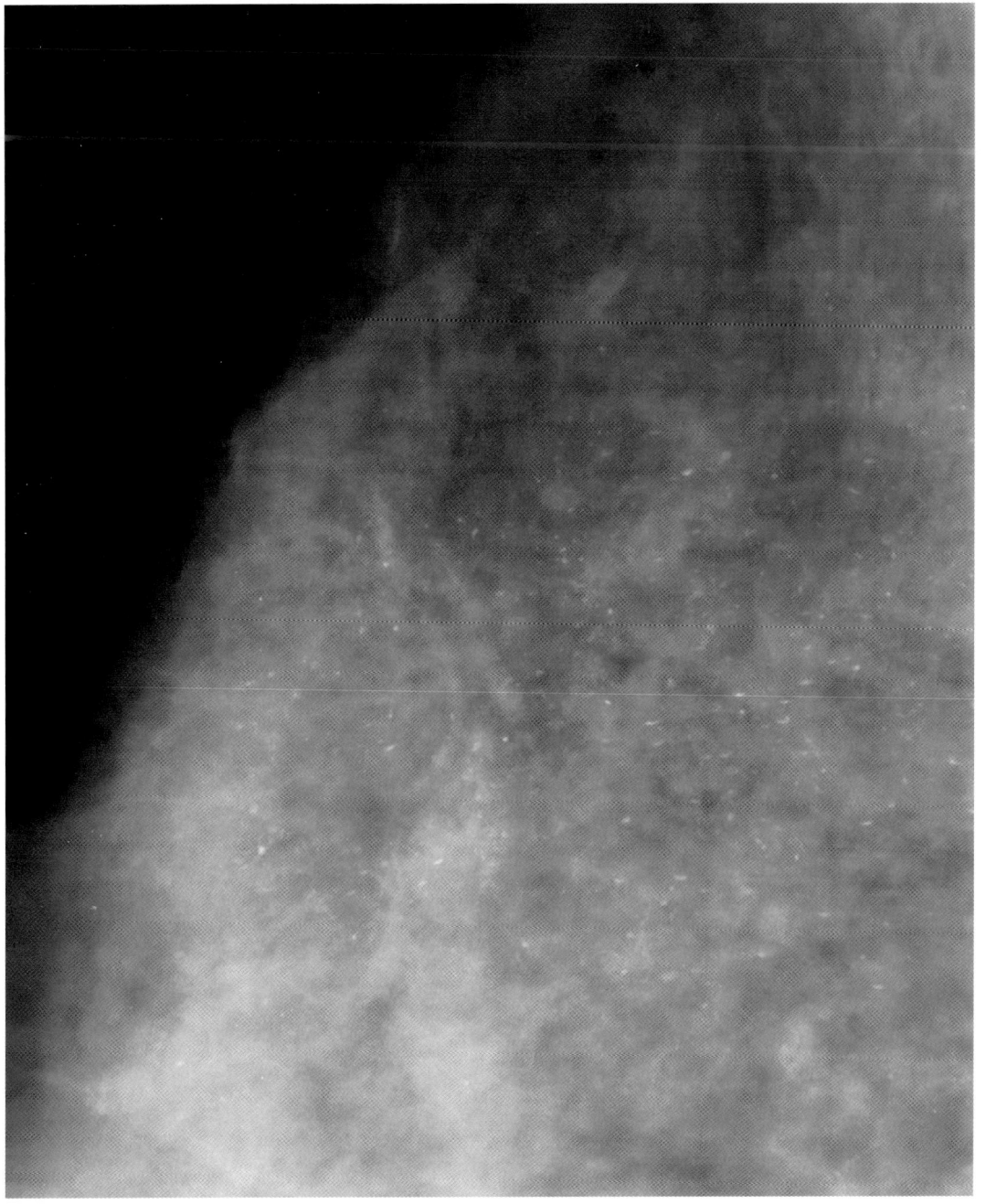

Magnification view

Diffusely scattered distribution

These calcifications are scattered at random, with no real pattern, throughout the whole breast. Generally benign, they are only very occasionally due to diffuse in situ malignancies. The presence of a large number of calcifications of varying size and density may impede the detection and analysis of a suspicious clustered lesion, or mask the diffuse or generalized distribution of a process, making it difficult to clarify its true extent.

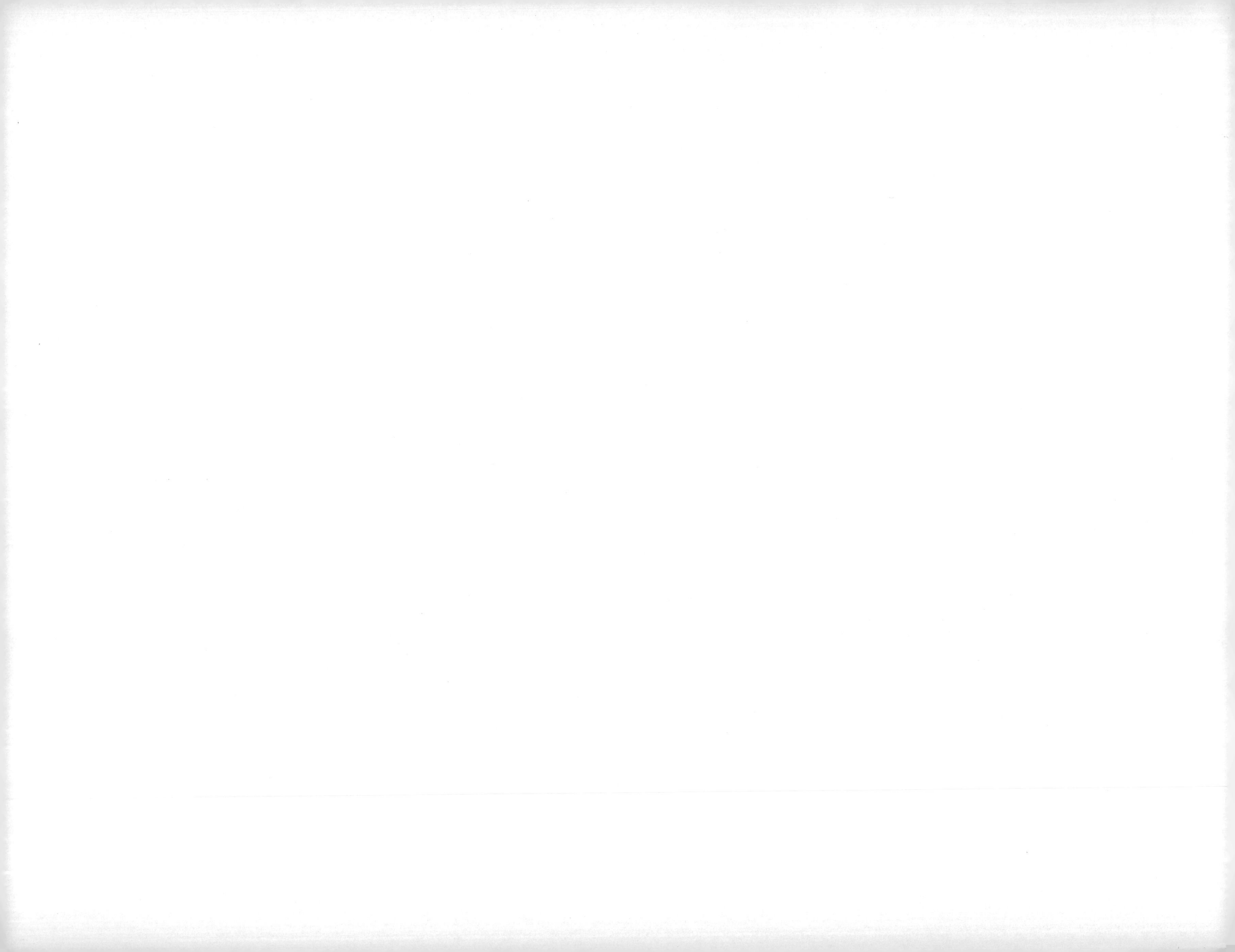

Diffusely scattered distribution

Calcifications with mixed morphology (rounded and "milk-of-calcium") appear randomly distributed, with no regular pattern, throughout the breast.

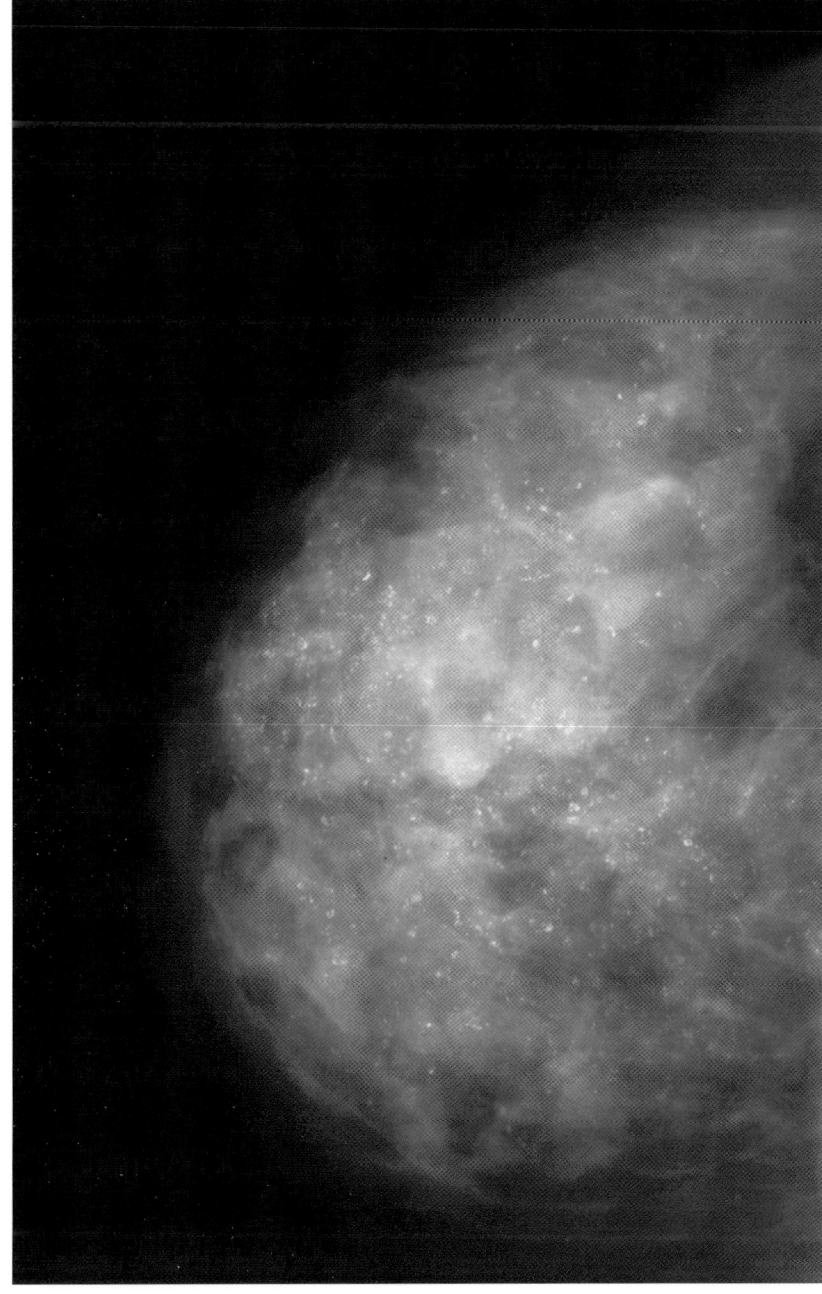

craniocaudal projection

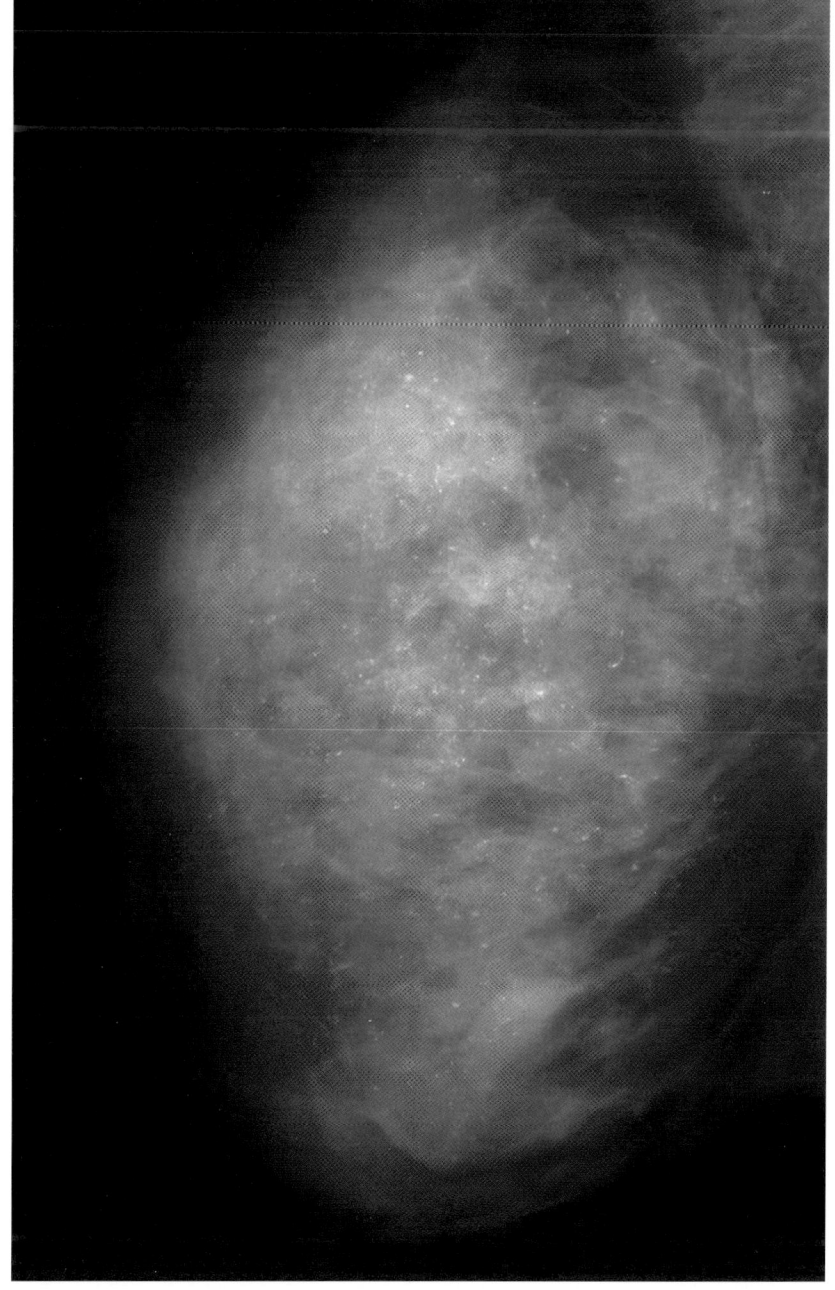

Mediolateral oblique projection

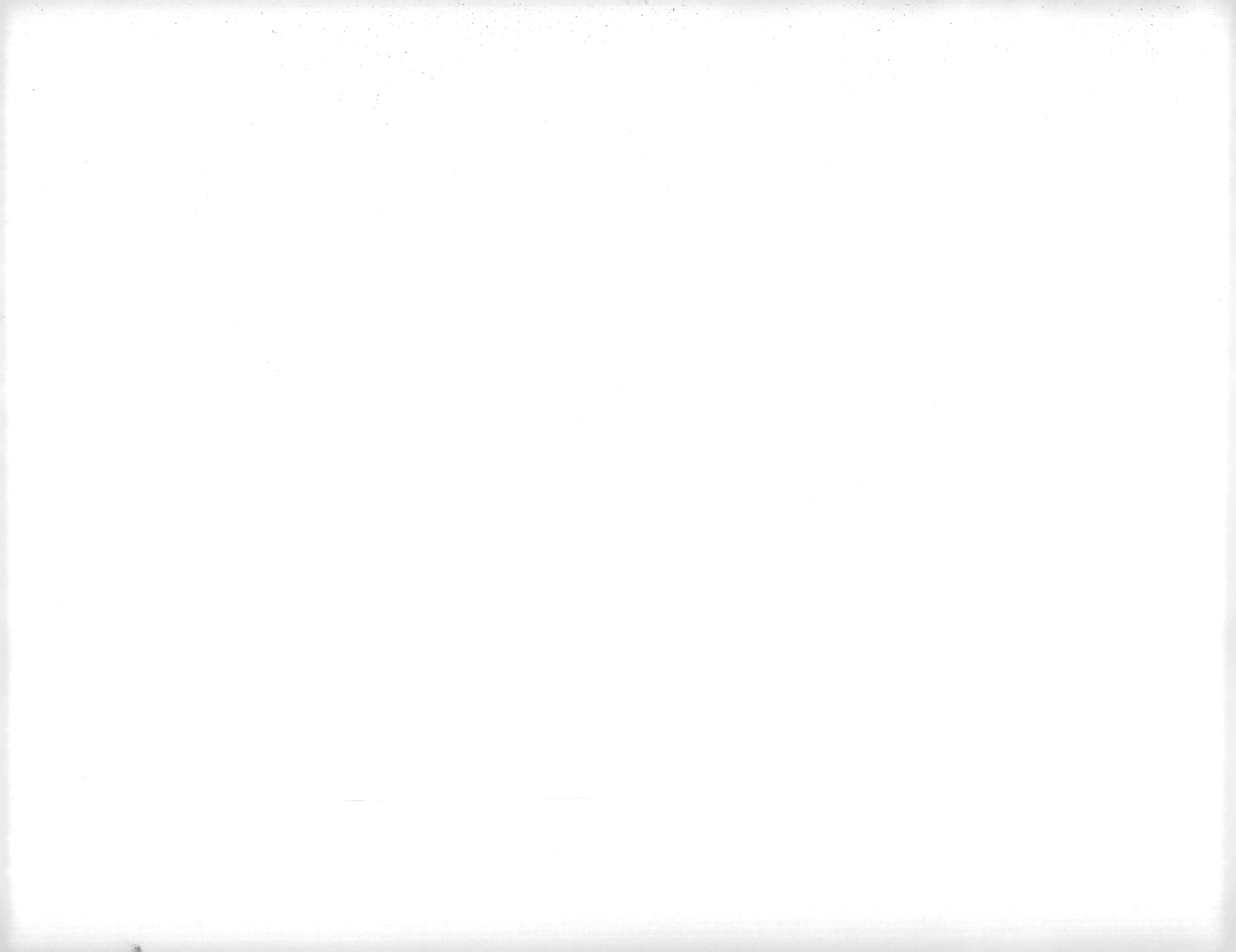

Morphology

Morphology can help establish the predictive value of calcifications, which may be classified as probably benign, doubtful or indeterminate and probably malignant.

Probably benign

- *round (or bead-like)*
- *"milk-of-calcium"*
- *round lucent-centred*
- *"egg-shell"*
- *rod-shaped or tubular*
- *coarse ("popcorn", "candle-wax")*
- *vascular*
- *dystrophic*
- *skin calcifications*
- *foreign body-induced*
- *pseudocalcifications*

Doubtful or indeterminate

- *powdery*
- *rounded*
- *granular type*

Probably malignant

- *casting type*
- *granular type*
- *mixed*

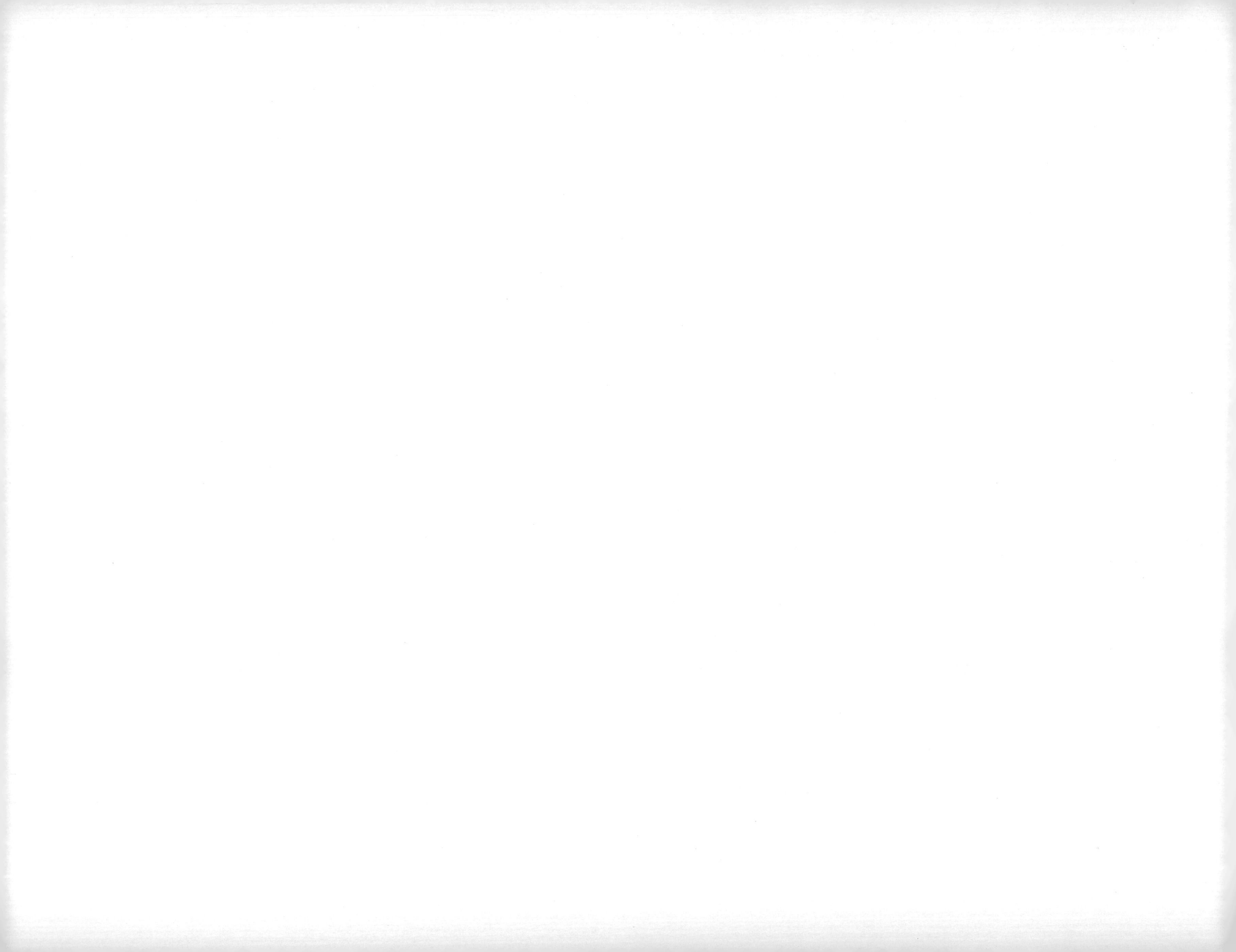

Probably benign calcifications

- *round (or bead-like)*
- *"milk-of-calcium"*
- *round lucent-centred*
- *"egg-shell"*
- *rod-shaped or tubular*
- *coarse ("popcorn", candle-wax")*
- *vascular*
- *dystrophic*
- *skin calcifications*
- *foreign body-induced*
- *pseudocalcifications*

Round calcifications

Round calcifications come in different sizes, sometimes with perfectly smooth, bead-like surfaces; they form clusters in the acini of lobules. When they are smaller than 0.5 mm they should be defined as "punctate" or "powdery".

PROBABLY BENIGN CALCIFICATIONS

Round calcifications

In the upper middle location there are multiple round calcifications distributed unevenly; a few are solitary but the majority are clustered together in a large part of the breast. There is a circumscribed round opacity with sharp anterior margins and unclear posterior margins, of the same density as the surrounding parenchyma (A). A cluster of regularly shaped round calcifications with uniformly higher density is visible in the lower periareolar region, within a circumscribed opacity with blurred margins (B).

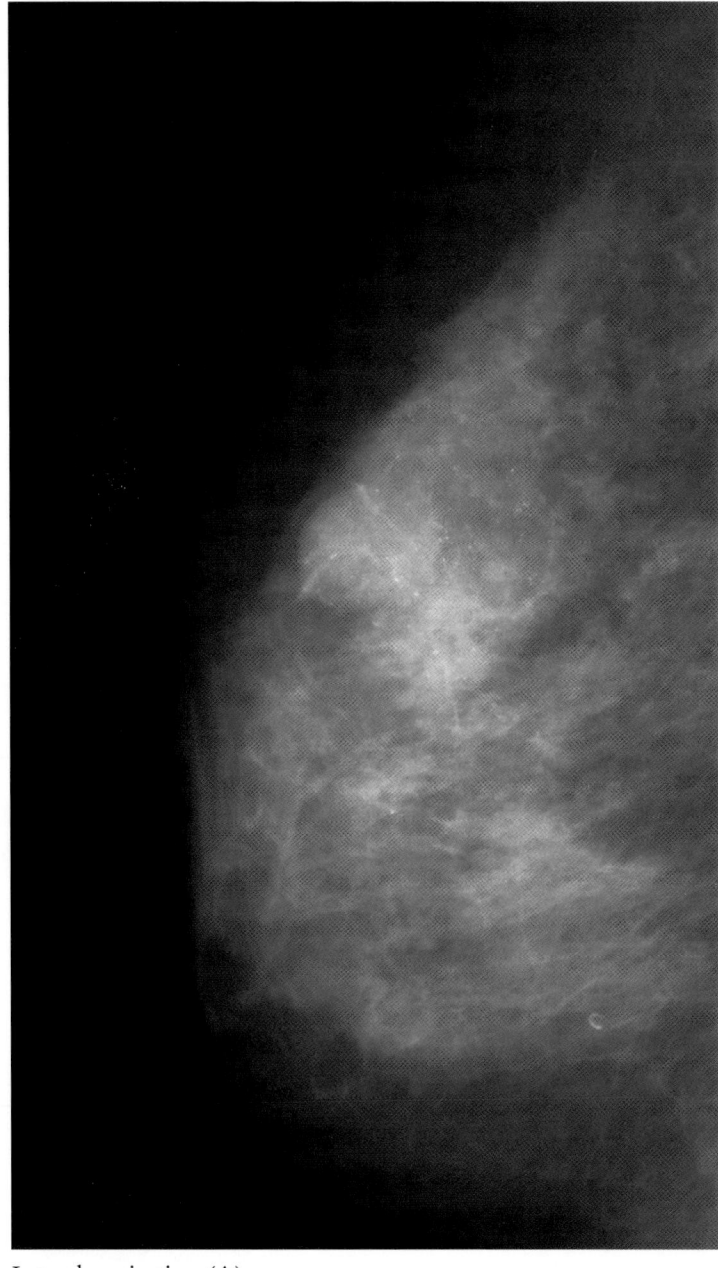

Lateral projection (A)

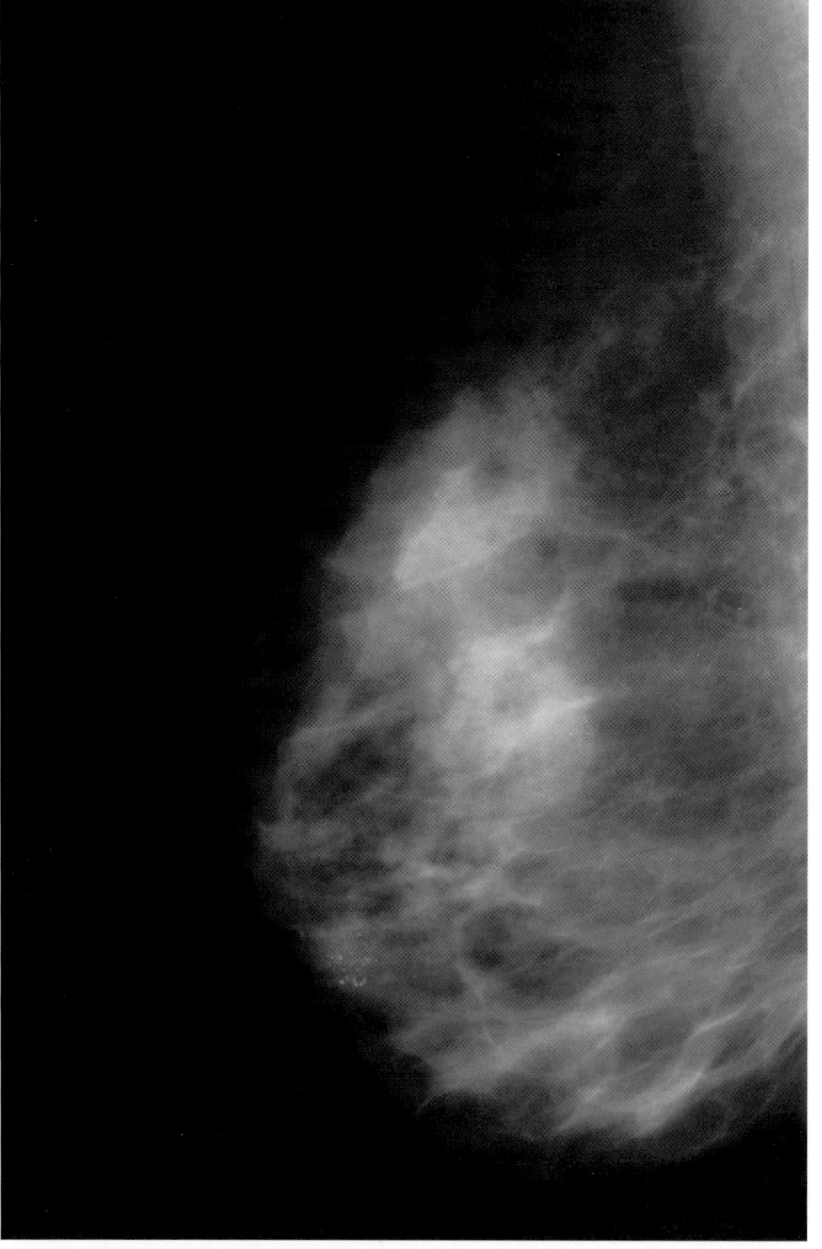

Mediolateral oblique projection (B)

Round calcifications

Multiple round calcifications distributed unevenly; a few are solitary but the majority are clustered together in a large part of the breast. There is a circumscribed round opacity with sharp anterior margins and blurred posterior margins, of the same density as the surrounding parenchyma (A). A cluster of regularly shaped round calcifications with uniformly higher density is visible within a circumscribed opacity with blurred margins (B).

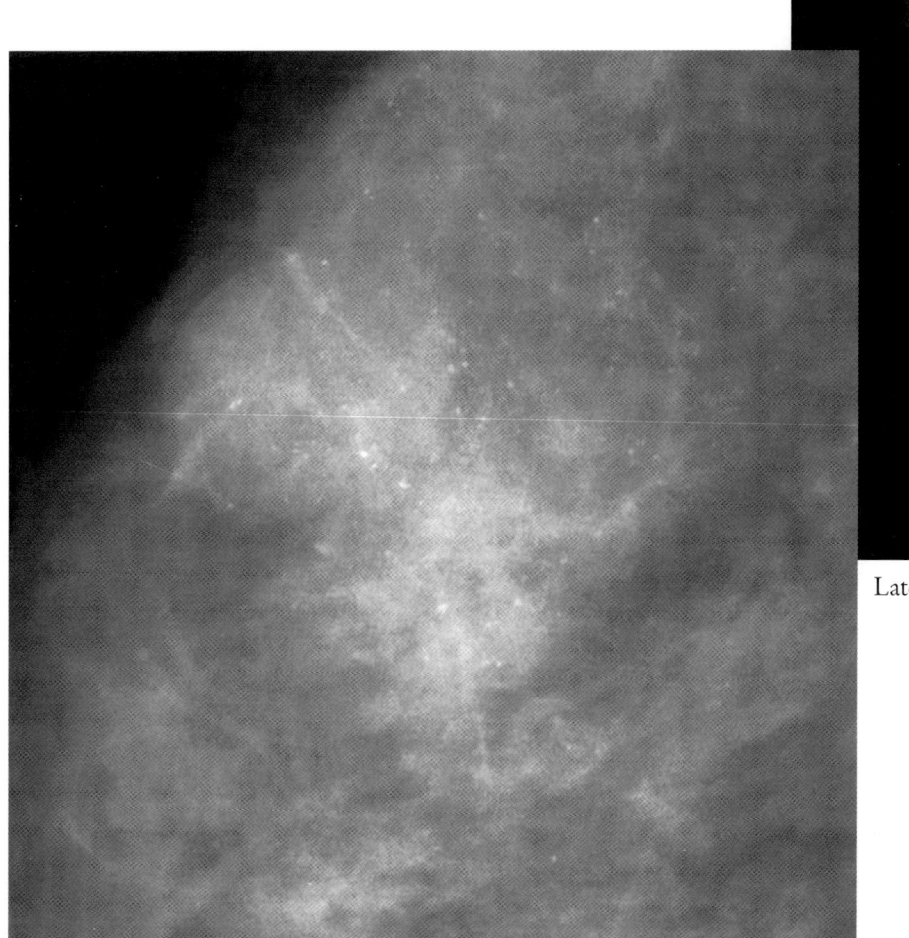

Lateral magnification view

Lateral magnification view

Histological finding: intracanalicular fibroadenoma

PROBABLY BENIGN CALCIFICATIONS

Round calcifications
Numerous round calcifications are distributed unevenly on both sides, throughout the breast; some are solitary and coarse and others are finer and more numerous.

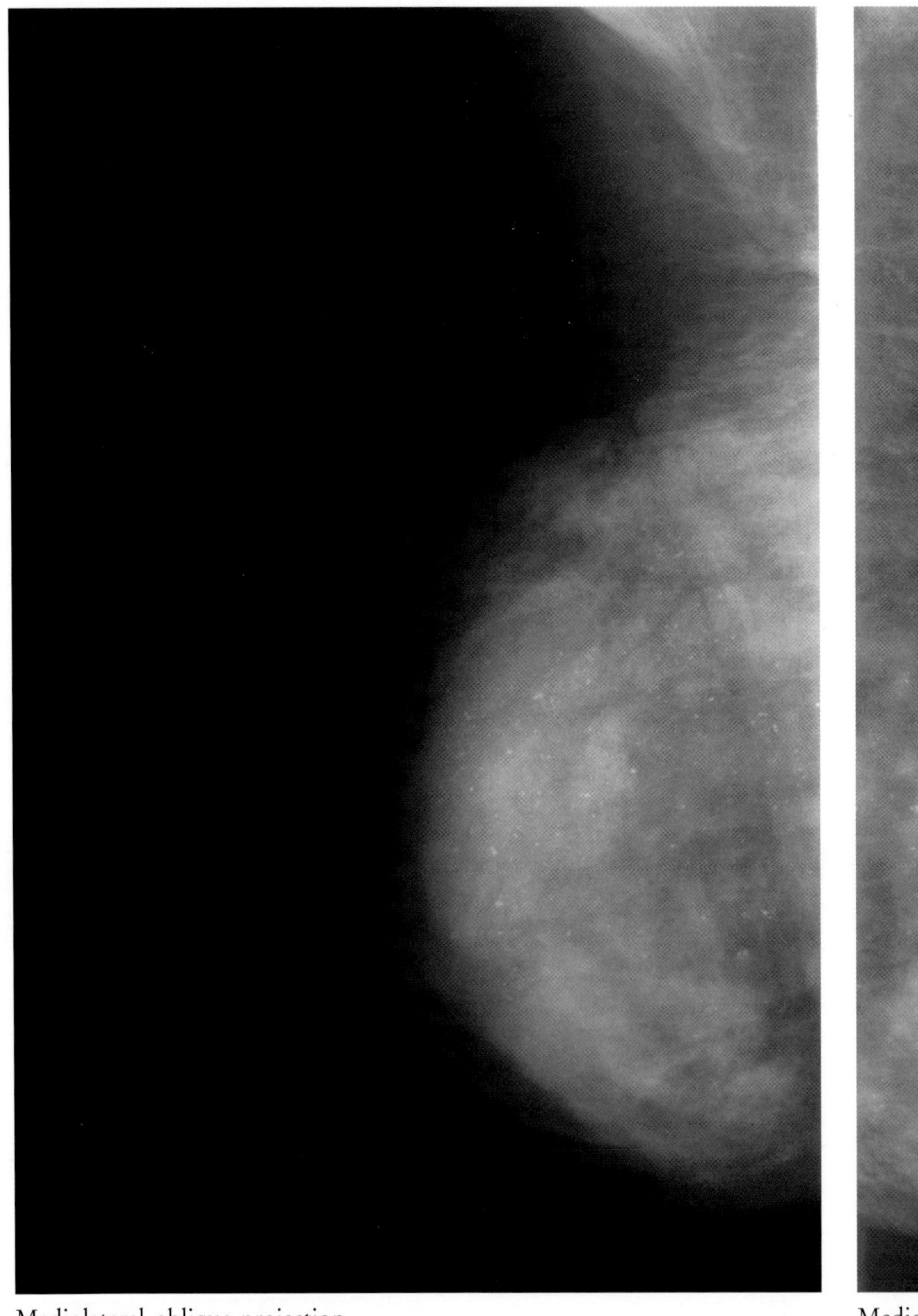

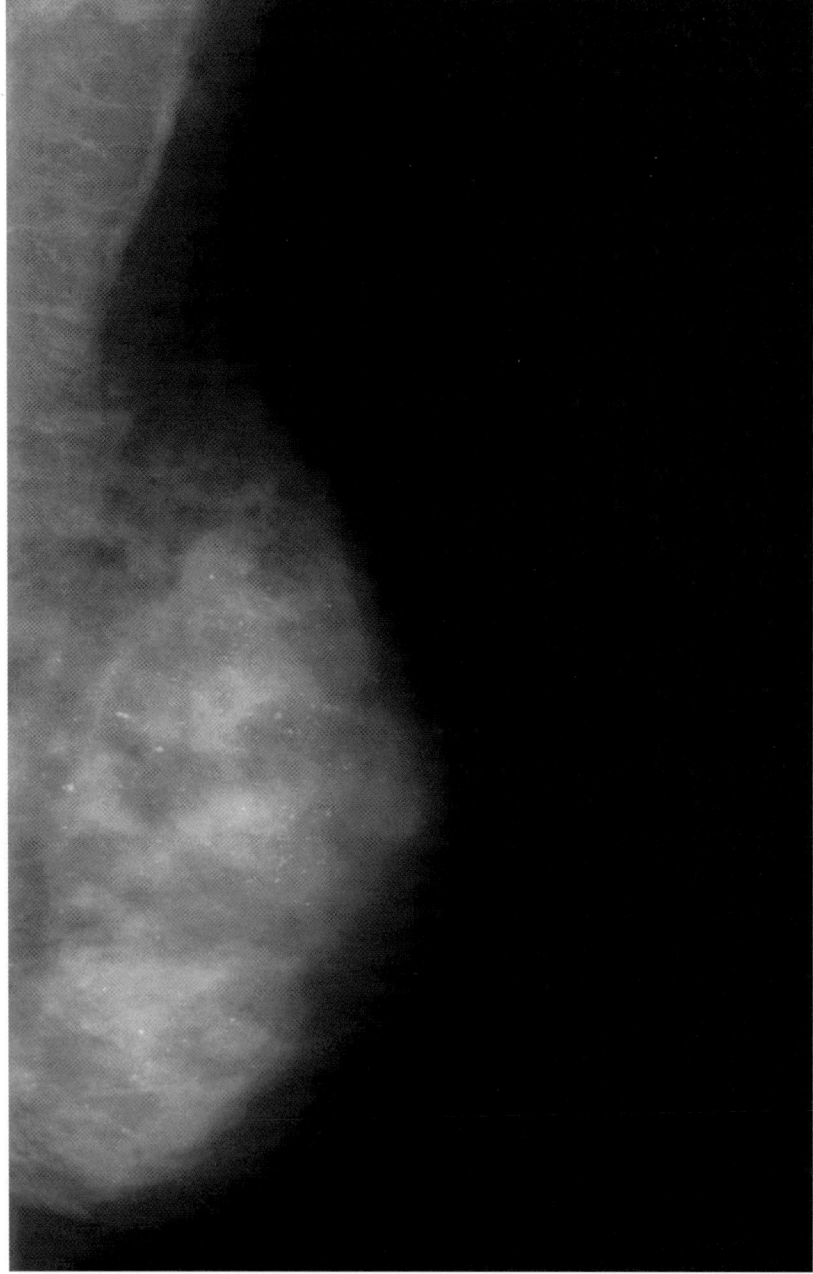

Mediolateral oblique projection

Mediolateral oblique projection

Round calcifications

Numerous round calcifications are distributed unevenly on both sides, throughout the breast; some are solitary and coarse and others are finer and more numerous.

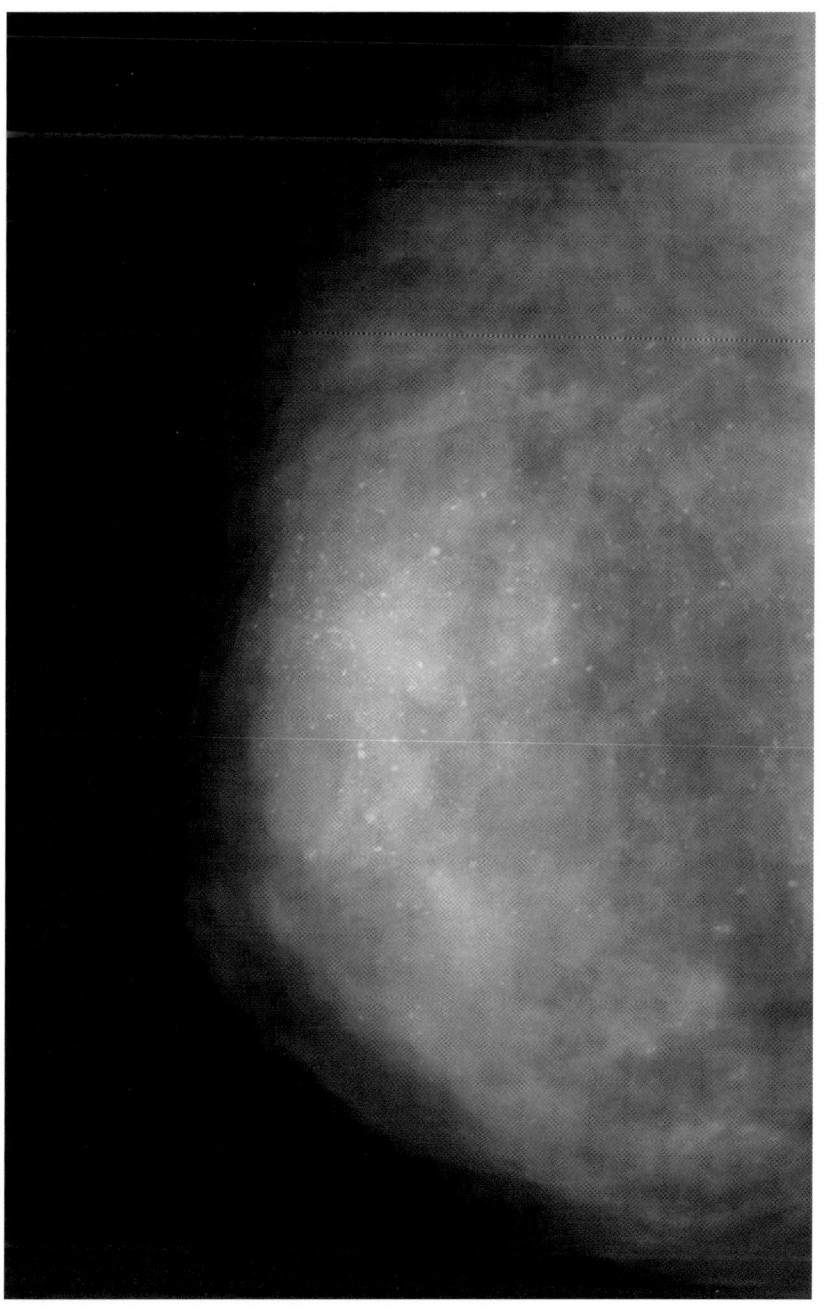

Close-up of the mediolateral oblique projection

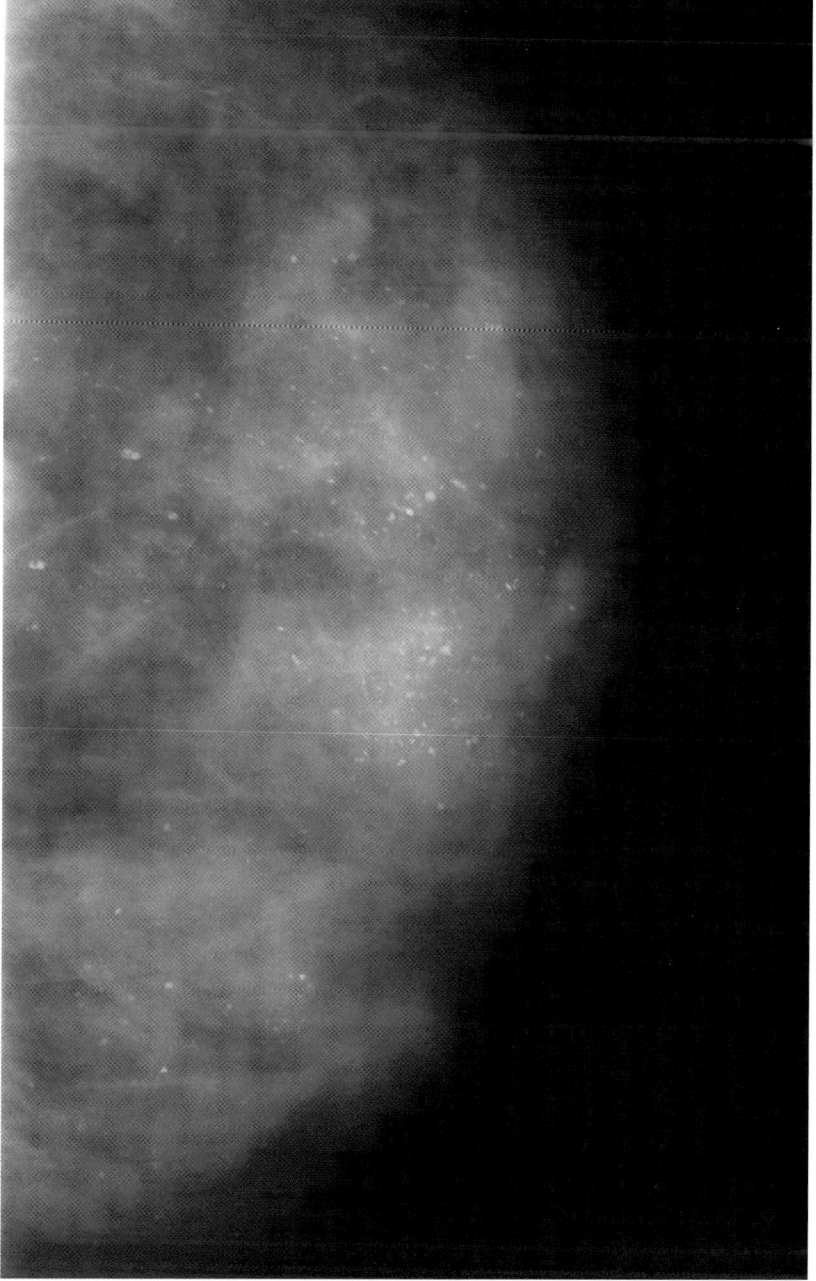

Close-up of the mediolateral oblique projection

PROBABLY BENIGN CALCIFICATIONS

Round calcifications
Multiple round calcifications, varying in diameter and density, distributed in a circumscribed area, with no segmental pattern.

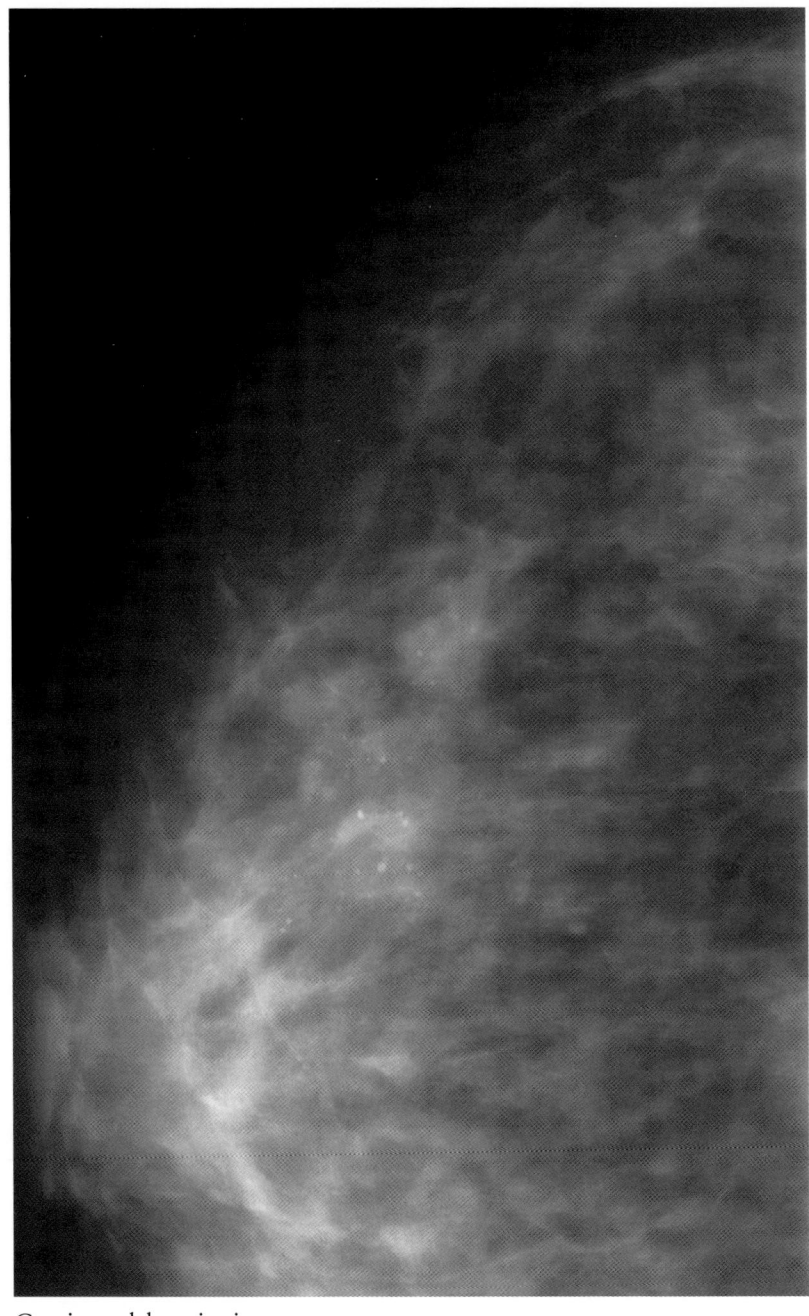

Craniocaudal projection

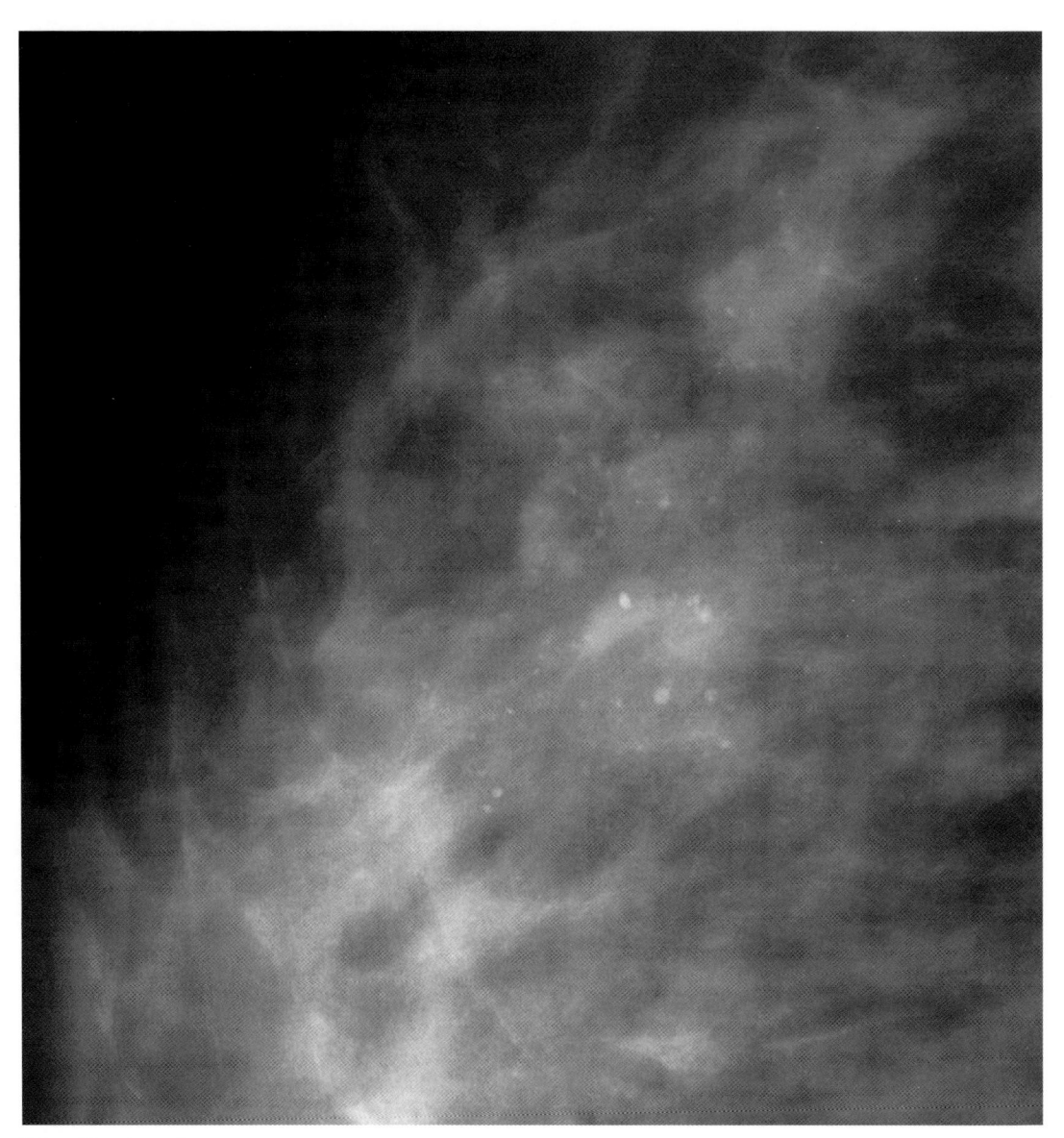

Magnification view

"Milk-of-calcium" calcifications

These calcifications are crescent or "teacup" shaped when observed in the oblique projection, while in the craniocaudal projection they look round, faint, amorphous, sometimes like small, fuzzy, non-homogeneous patches. The fact that the calcifications look different in the two projections is pathognomonic, but when there are only a few with an elongated shape or they occupy only a small area, they may be more difficult to interpret. "Milk-of-calcium" calcifications are produced by calcium secretions from microcysts that form as a delayed epiphenomenon of adenosis (microcystic adenosis)

"Milk-of-calcium" calcifications

These calcifications are crescent or "teacup" shaped when observed in the oblique projection, while in the craniocaudal projection they look round, faint, amorphous, sometimes like small, fuzzy, non-homogeneous patches. The fact that the calcifications look different in the two projections is pathognomonic, but when there are only a few with an elongated shape or they occupy only a small area, they may be more difficult to interpret. "Milk-of-calcium" calcifications are produced by calcium secretions from microcysts that form as a delayed epiphenomenon of adenosis (microcystic adenosis).

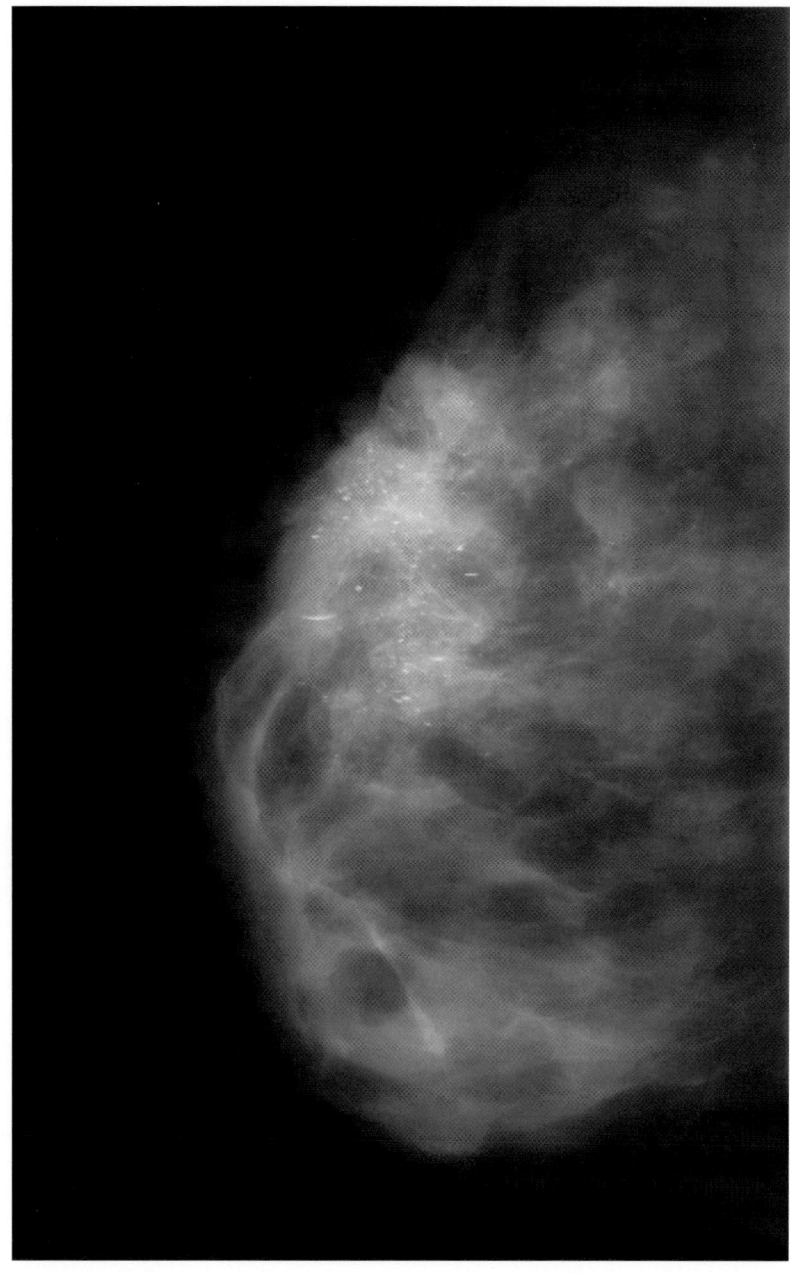

Lateral projection

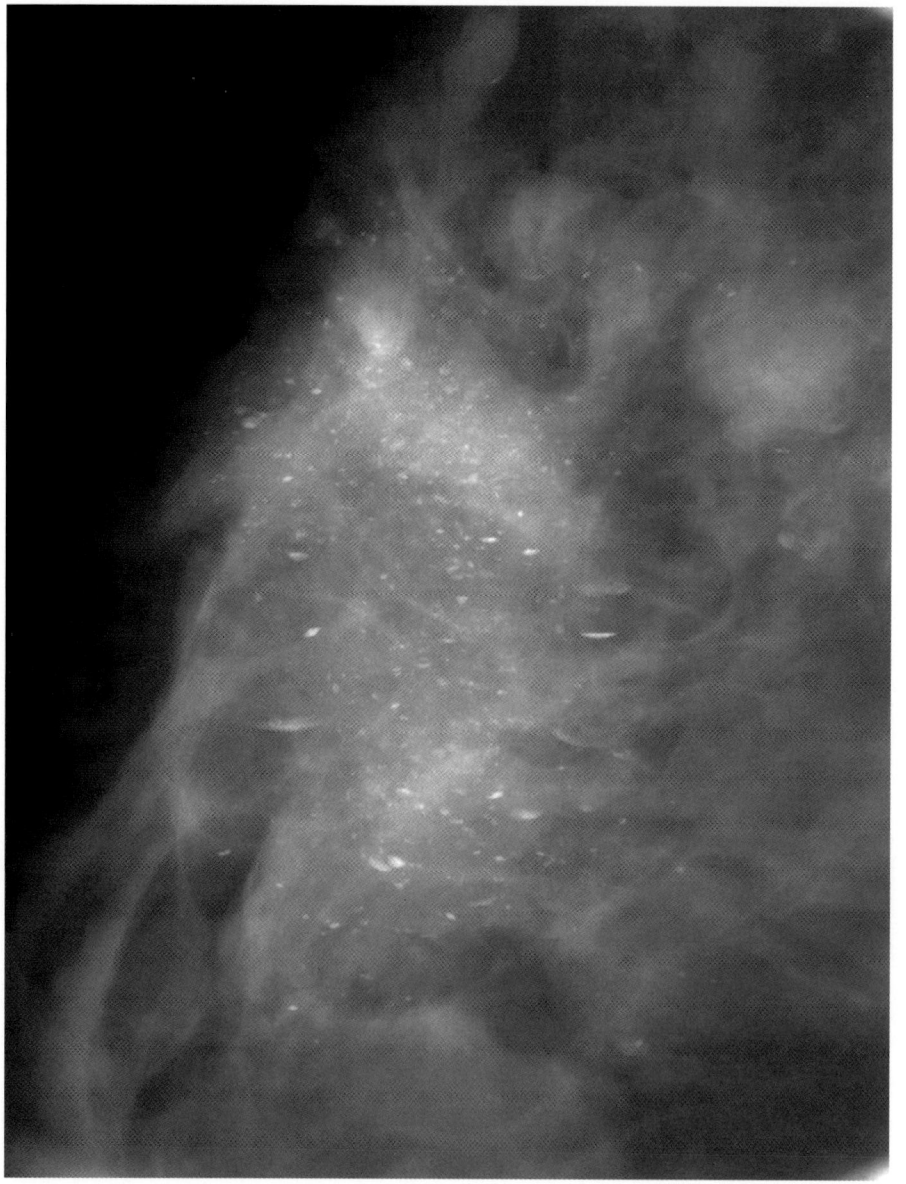

Magnification view

"Milk-of-calcium" calcifications

The magnification views better show these calcifications: some are neatly round, others are less distinct, sometimes looking like small, fuzzy, non-homogeneous patches in the craniocaudal projection; in the lateral or oblique projection, they are crescent shaped, due to the calcium deposits settling on the concave floor of the microcysts. The fact that the calcifications look different in the two projections is pathognomonic, but when there are only a few or they occupy only a small area, they may be more difficult to interpret. "Milk-of-calcium" calcifications are produced by calcium secretions from microcysts that form as a delayed epiphenomenon of adenosis.

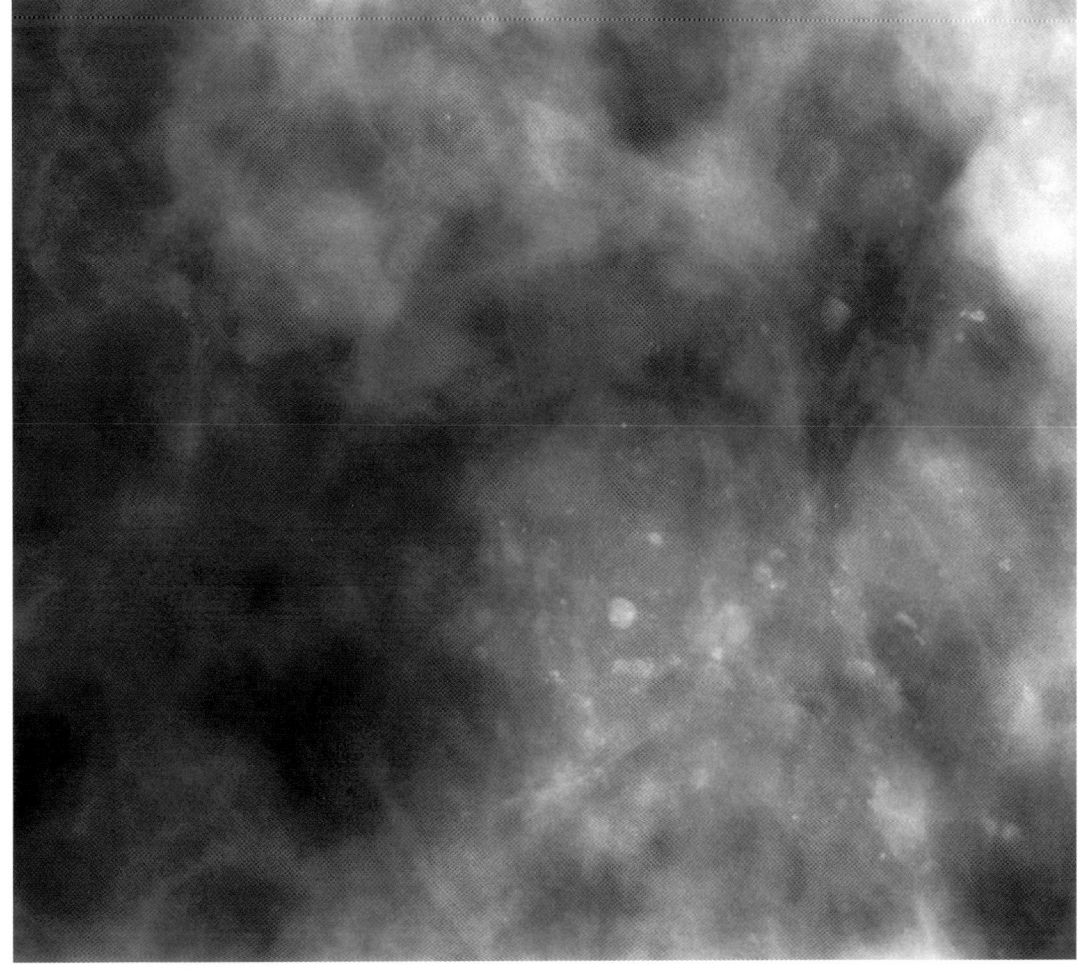

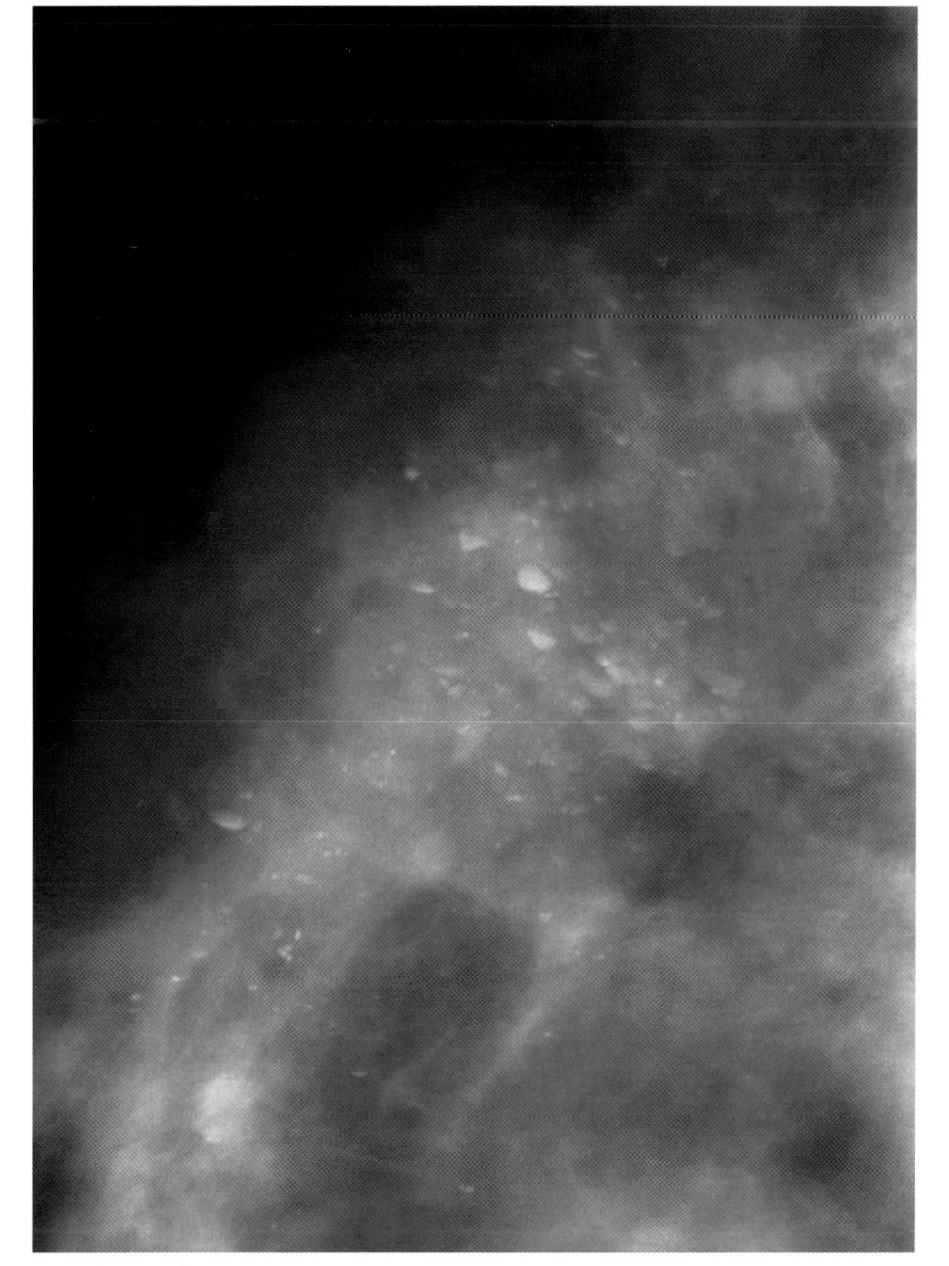

Craniocaudal magnification view

Lateral magnification view

PROBABLY BENIGN CALCIFICATIONS

"Milk-of-calcium" calcifications

These calcifications are polymorphous: some are neatly round, others are less distinct, sometimes looking like small, fuzzy, non-homogeneous patches in the craniocaudal projection; in the lateral or oblique projection, they are crescent shaped, due to the calcium deposits settling on the concave floor of the microcysts. "Milk-of-calcium" calcifications are produced by calcium secretions from microcysts that form as a delayed epiphenomenon of adenosis.

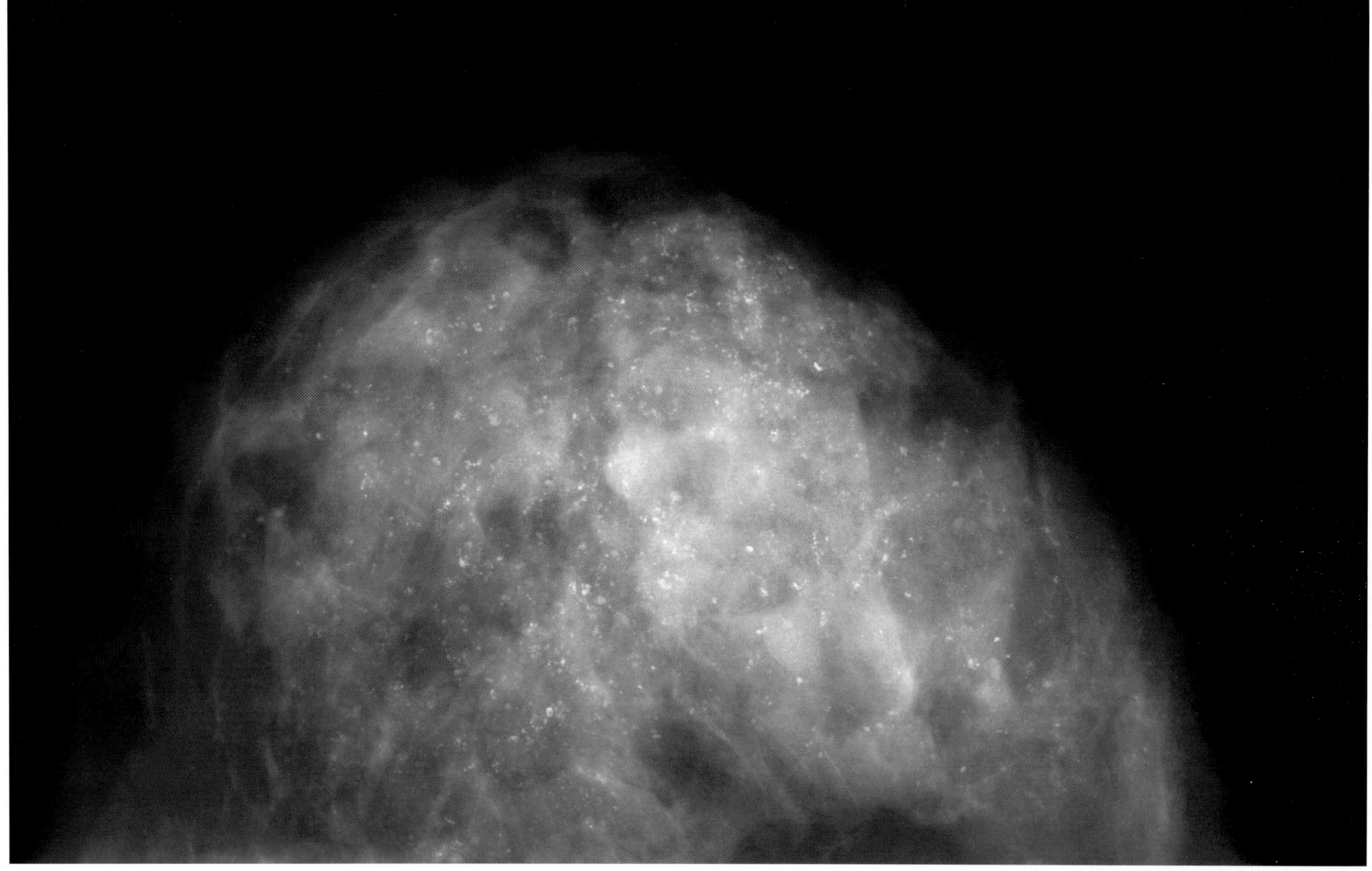

Craniocaudal projection

"Milk-of-calcium" calcifications

The magnification views show the steps in the formation of milk of calcium. There are some lower-density round spots, which are the start of the calcification, with solitary or coalescing formations, and some round and ring-like lucent-centred calcifications.

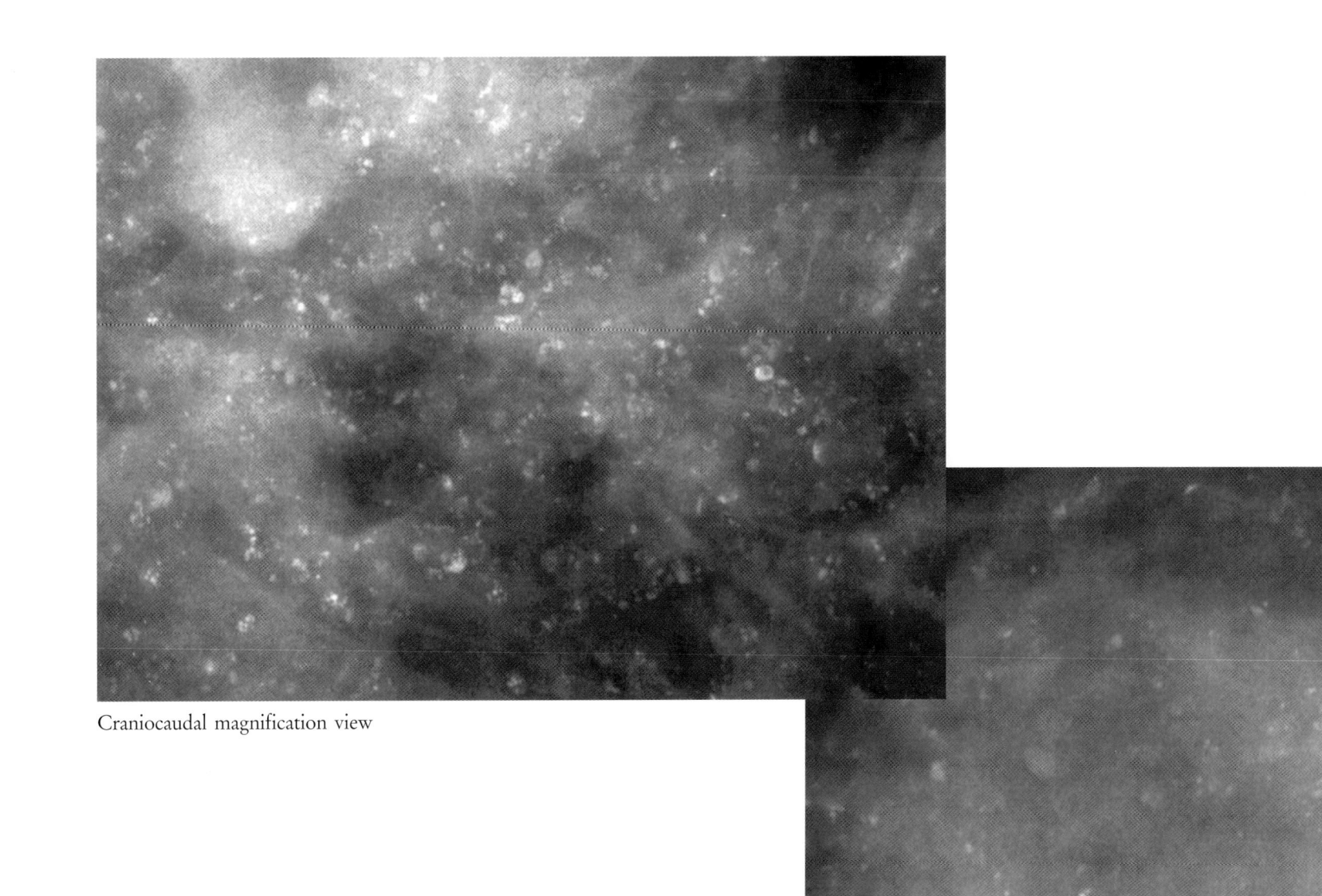

Craniocaudal magnification view

Craniocaudal magnification view

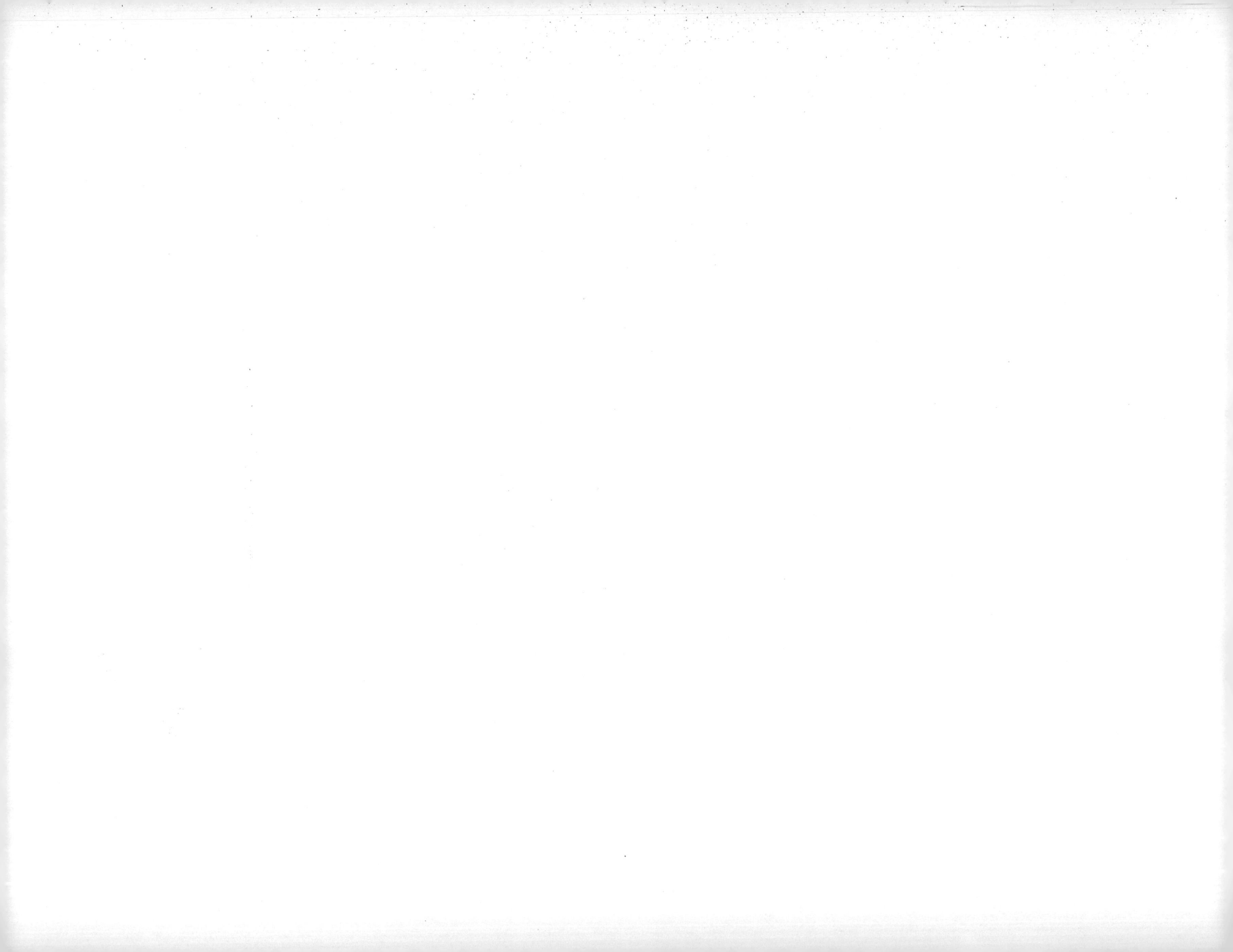

Round lucent-centred calcifications

These are radiolucent round entities with a sharp, regular calcified rim, measuring approximately 1 mm. They occur in small cysts or fat necrosis foci. Lucent-centred calcifications may be totally calcified or at various stages of calcification.

PROBABLY BENIGN CALCIFICATIONS

Round lucent-centred calcifications
Round masses of mixed appearance, 1-3 mm in diameter, are visible in the middleposterior region; most are confluent. Some are totally and homogeneously radiopaque, while others have a ring-like rim capsule (A). Ring-like lucent-centred calcifications are disseminated throughout the breast (B).

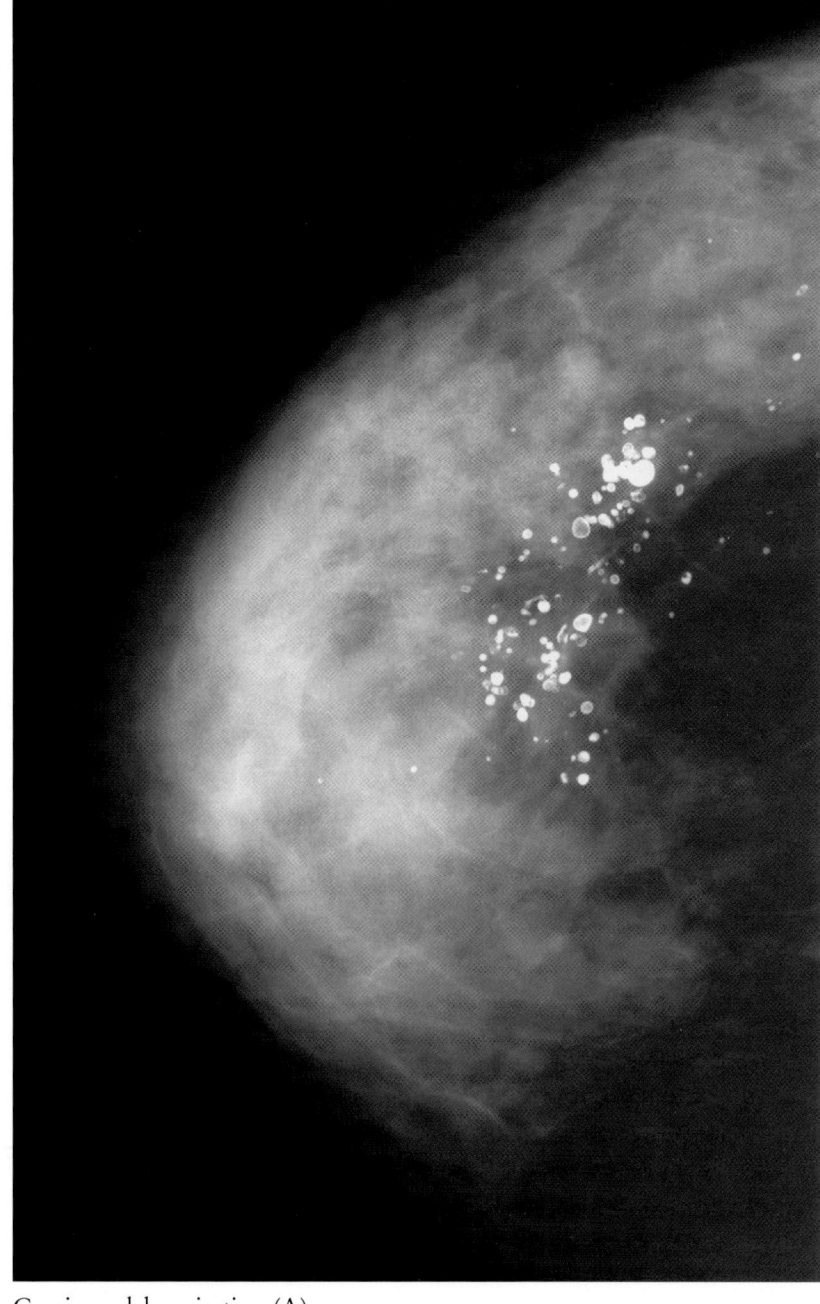

Craniocaudal projection (A)

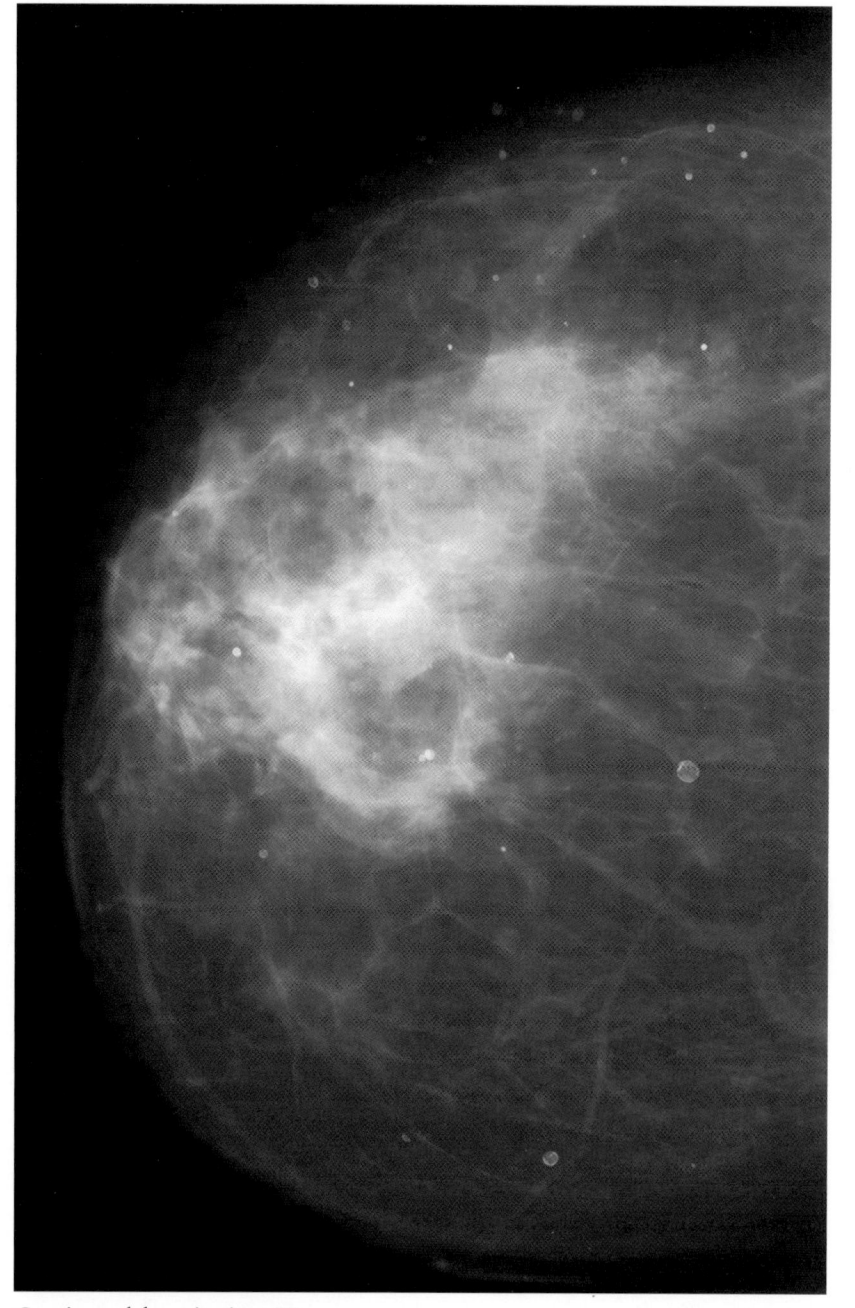

Craniocaudal projection (B)

Round lucent-centred calcifications

Round masses of mixed appearance, 1-3 mm in diameter, mostly confluent. Some are totally and homogeneously radiopaque, while others have a ring-like rim (A). Ring-like lucent-centred calcifications are disseminated throughout the breast (B).

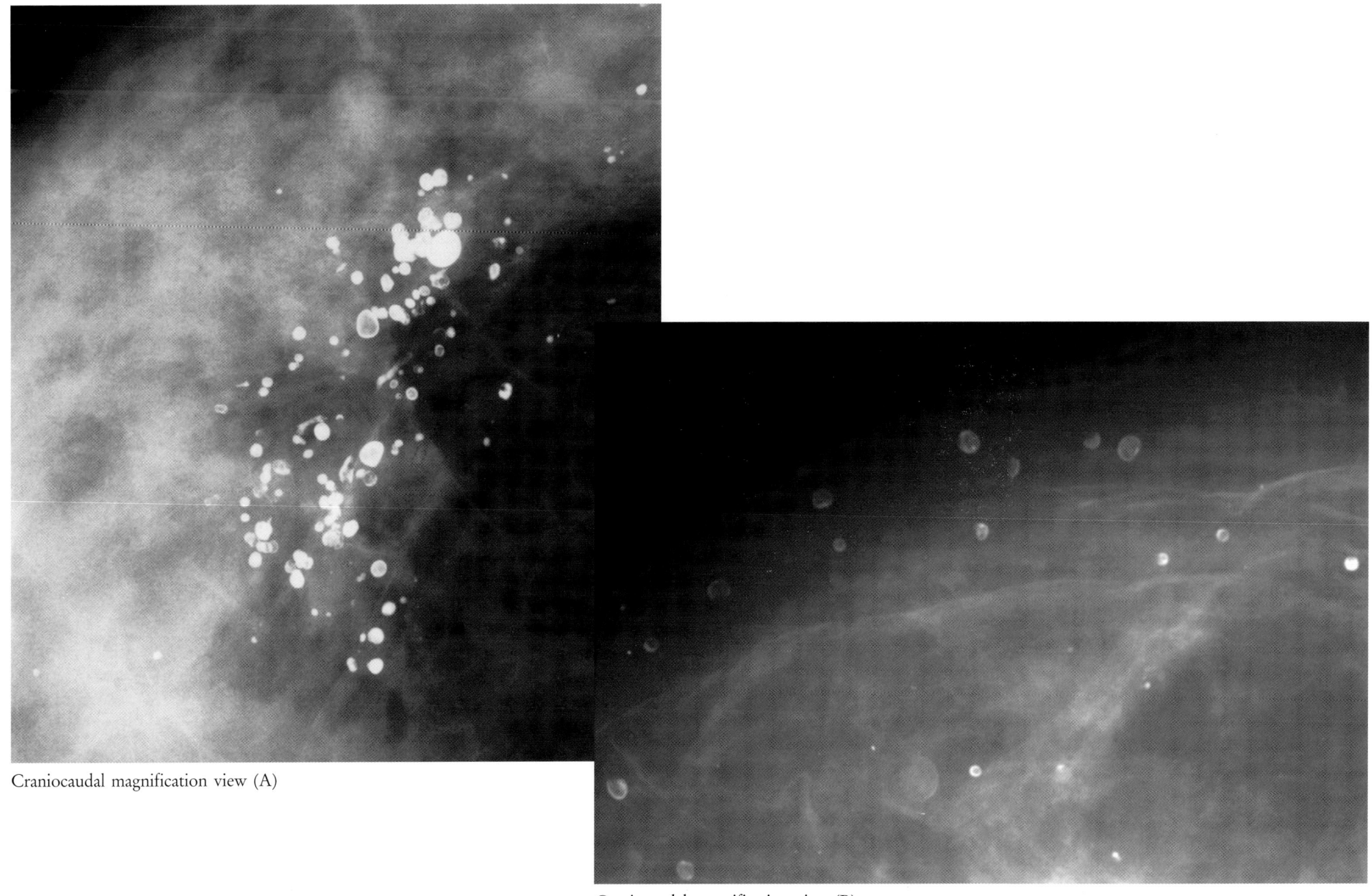

Craniocaudal magnification view (A)

Craniocaudal magnification view (B)

"Egg-shell" calcifications

These are generally ring-like calcifications approximately 1 cm in diameter, with a thicker calcified rim, looking like calcified spheres. They may be subsequent to traumatic fat necrosis, surgical excision, radiotherapy or ductal ectasia.

PROBABLY BENIGN CALCIFICATIONS

"Egg-shell" calcifications

In the upper aspect there is an oval radiolucent image almost entirely surrounded by an intensely calcified radiopaque rim and containing areas in the early stages of calcification (A). The calcified spheres are occasionally poorly lucent, with a "blown glass" or "milky" appearance (B).

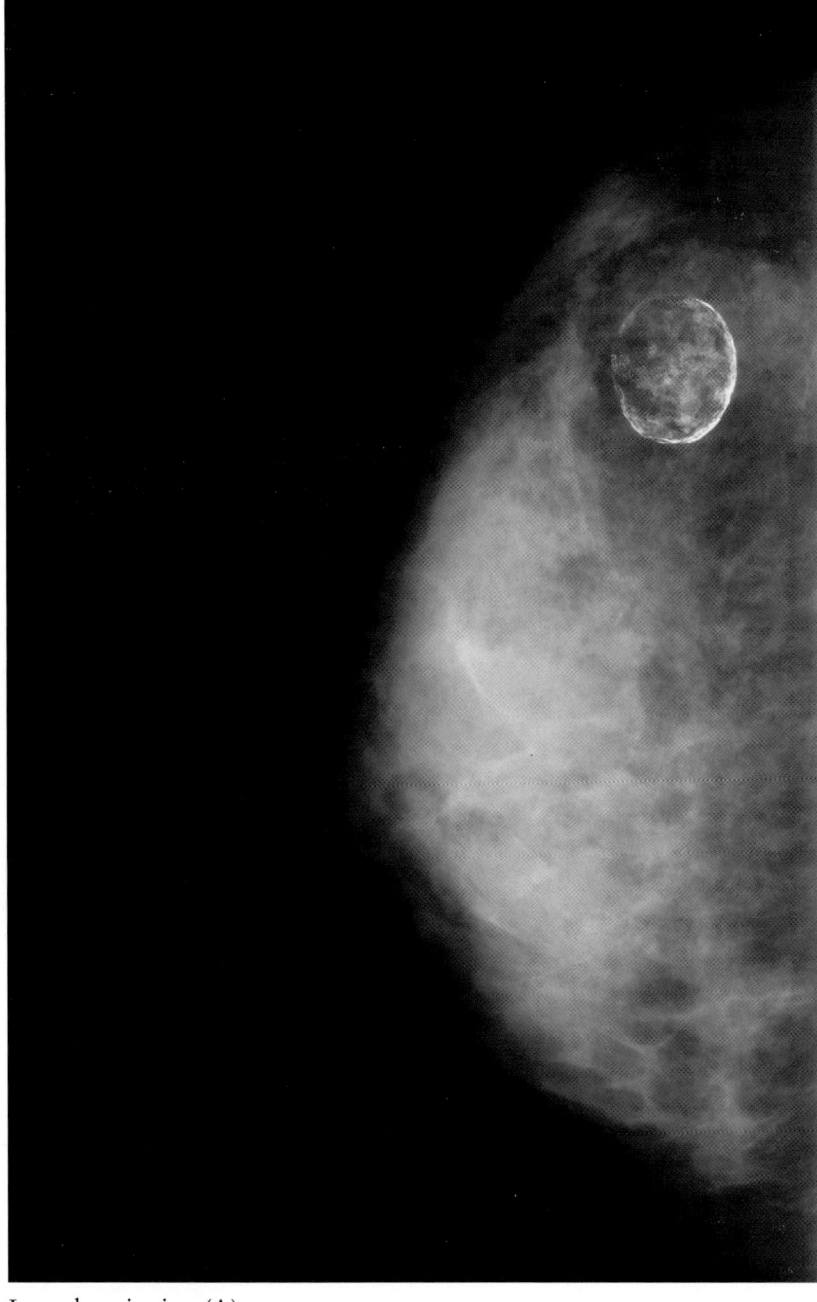

Lateral projection (A)

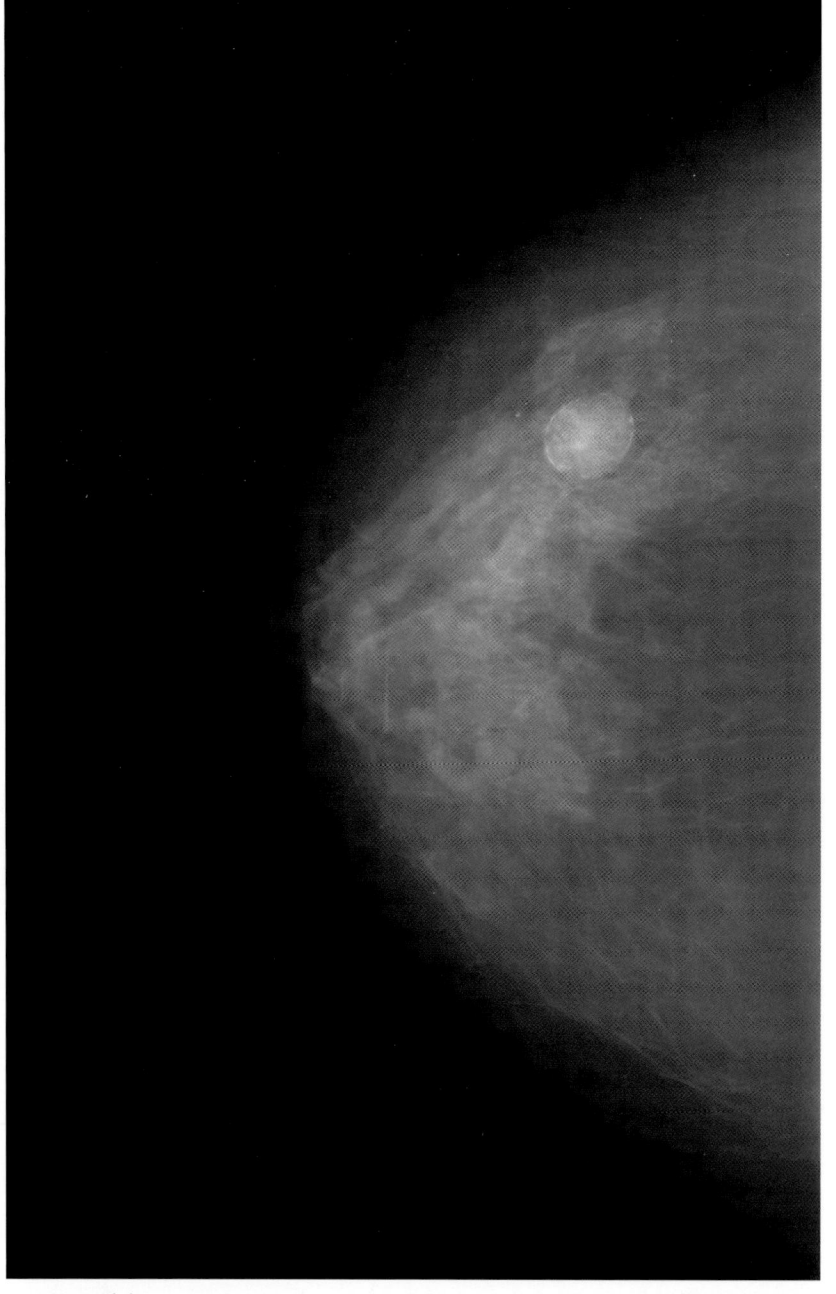

craniocaudal projection (B)

"Egg-shell" calcifications

This oval radiolucent mass is almost entirely surrounded by an intensely calcified radiopaque rim and contains areas in the early stages of calcification (A). The calcified sphere is poorly lucent, with a "blown glass" or "milky" appearance (B).

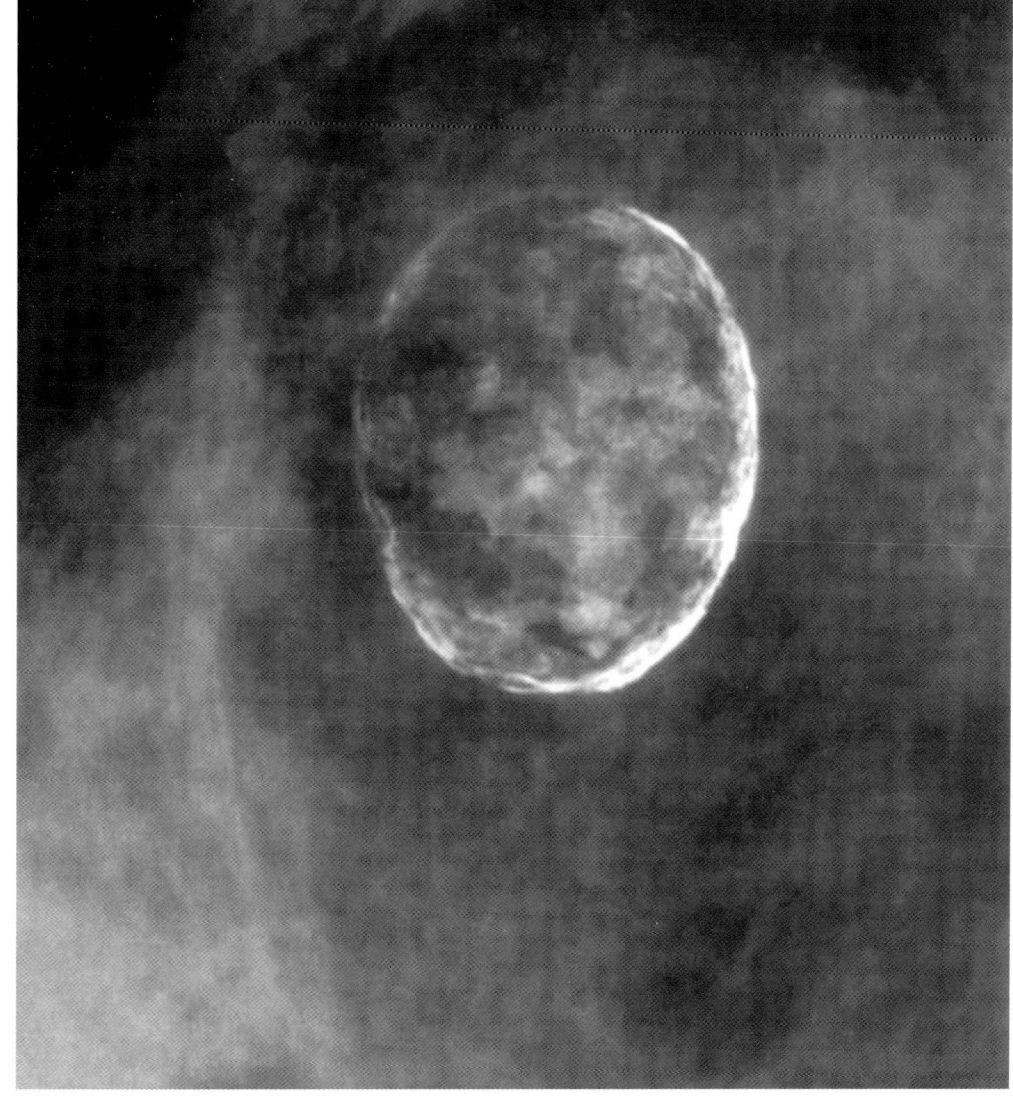

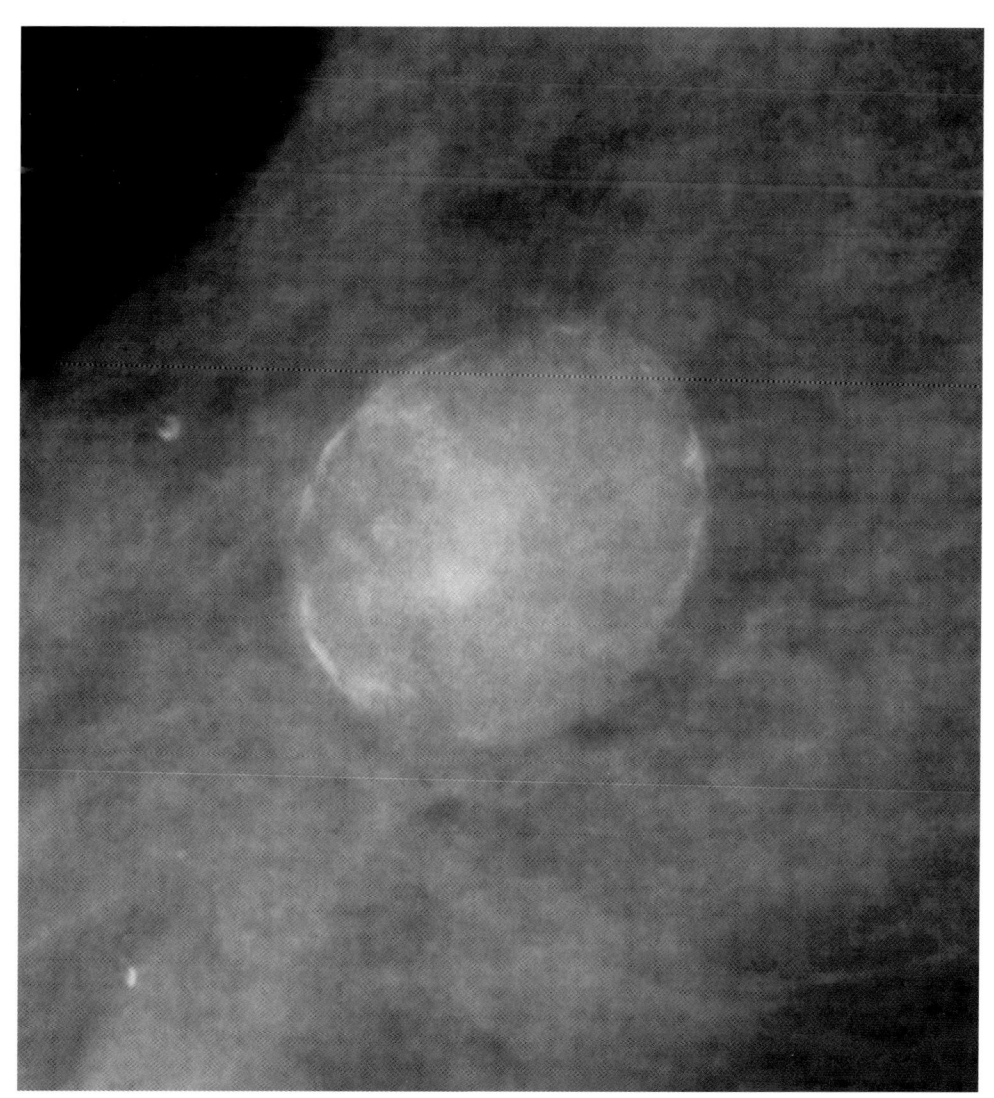

Lateral magnification view (A)

Craniocaudal magnification view (B)

PROBABLY BENIGN CALCIFICATIONS

"Egg-shell" calcifications
Multiple radiolucent images with clear-cut margins and a sometimes incompletly calcified rim. Generally the calcified spheres are poorly lucent, with a "blown glass" or "milky" appearance.

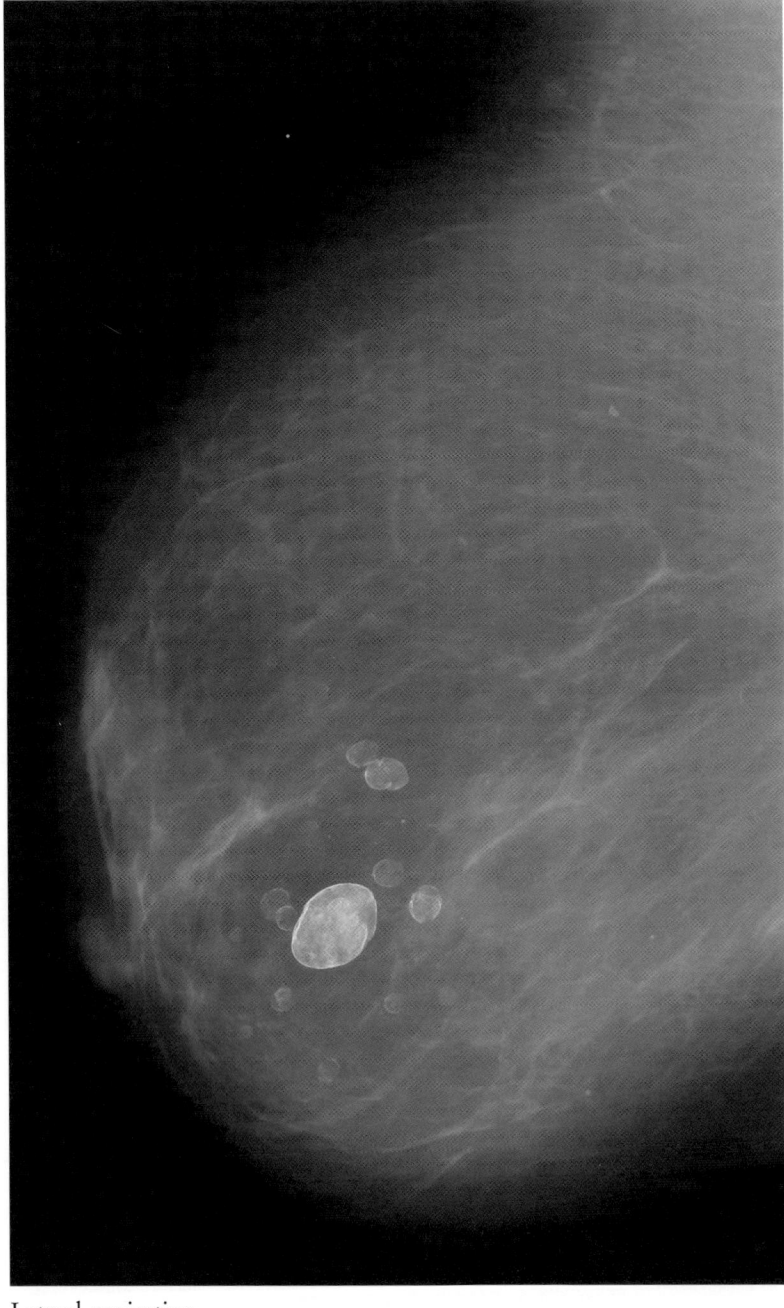

Lateral projection

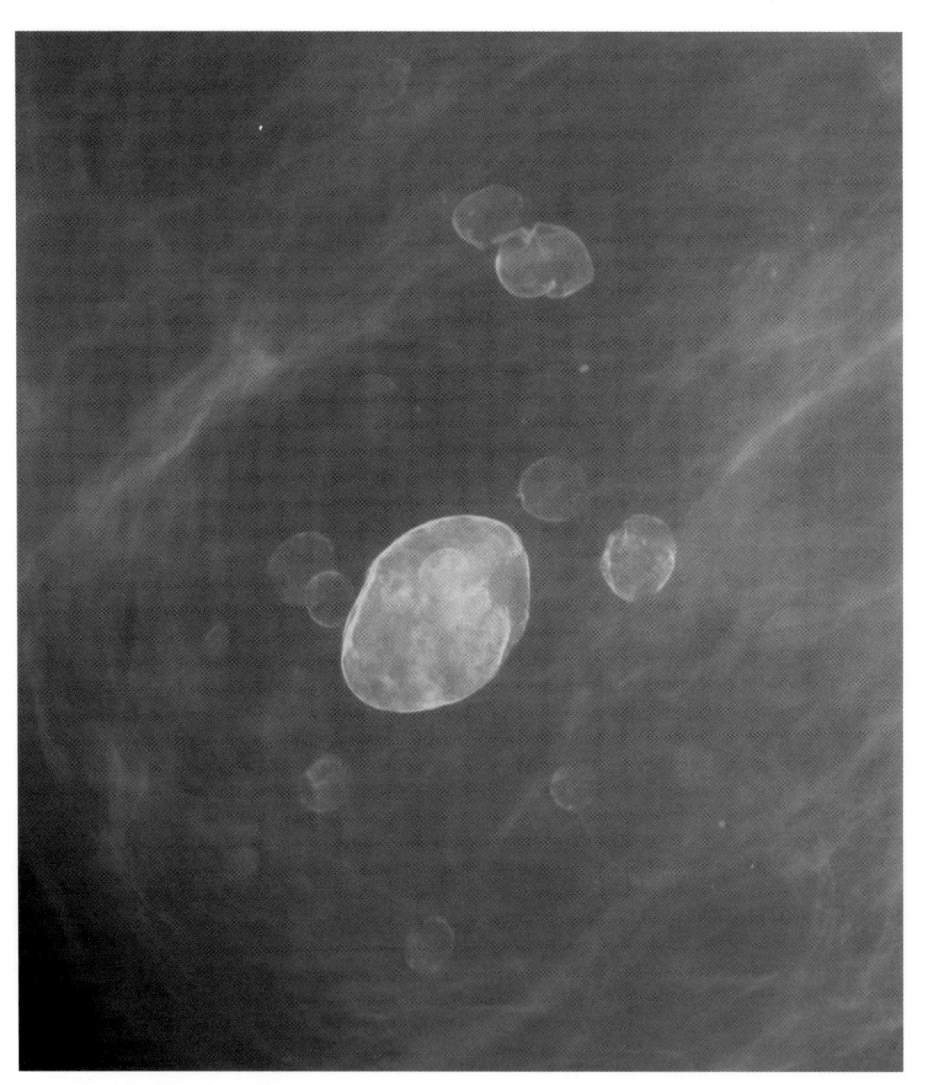

Lateral magnification view

Rod-shaped or tubular calcifications

Rod-shaped calcifications are straight, bright and relatively regular. Rod-shaped and tubular calcifications may fill or surround dilated ducts; they consist of solid "cores" with blunt, smooth edges when they fill the ductal lumen and look like hollow cylinders when they are in the walls. These calcifications form a radiating pattern from the areola, following the ducts and their ramifications. They are caused by secretory disease, ductal ectasia and plasma cell mastitis, and result from the extravasation of irritants into the mammary parenchyma through the dilated duct walls.

PROBABLY BENIGN CALCIFICATIONS

Rod-shaped or tubular calcifications

Rod-shaped calcifications are intensely radiopaque, linear, and regular shaped, following the ductal lumen from which they originate. Generally they radiate out evenly from the areola, in the pattern of the ducts and their ramifications (A) (B). These calcifications are frequently associated with ductal ectasia or plasma cell mastitis.

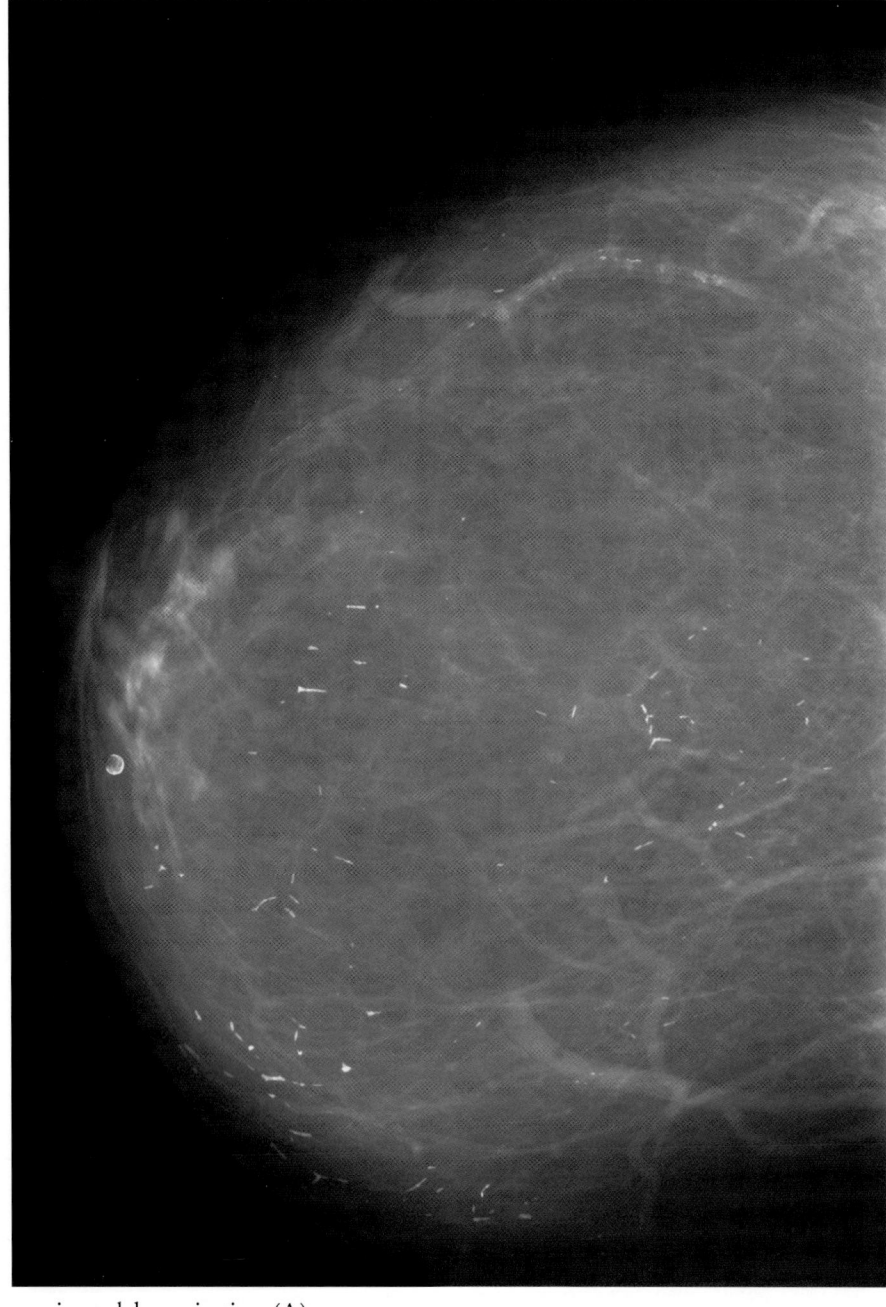

craniocaudal projection (A)

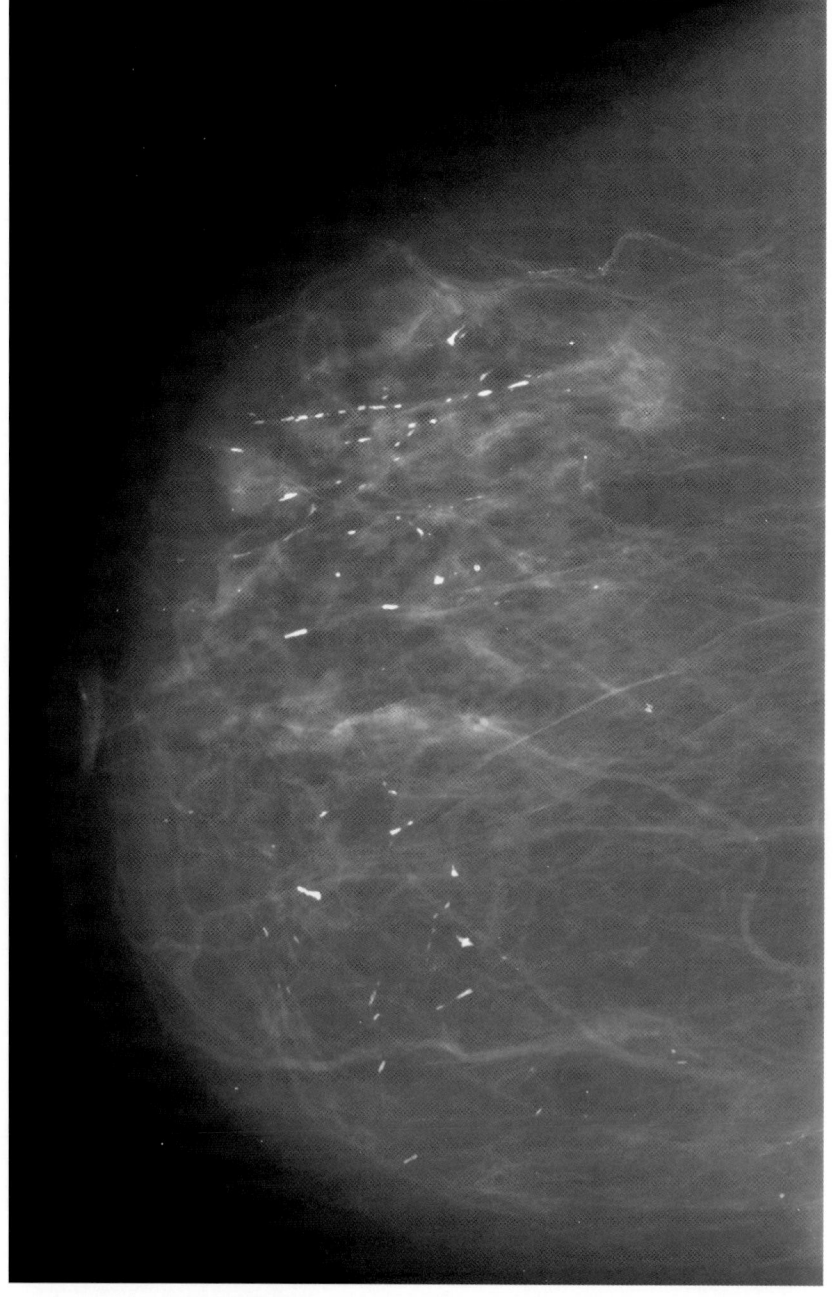

craniocaudal projection (B)

Rod-shaped calcifications

Intensely radiopaque linear calcifications, reproducing the ductal lumen from which they originate. Generally they radiate out evenly from the areola, following the pattern of the ducts and their ramifications (A) (B). These calcifications are frequently associated with ductal ectasia or plasma cell mastitis.

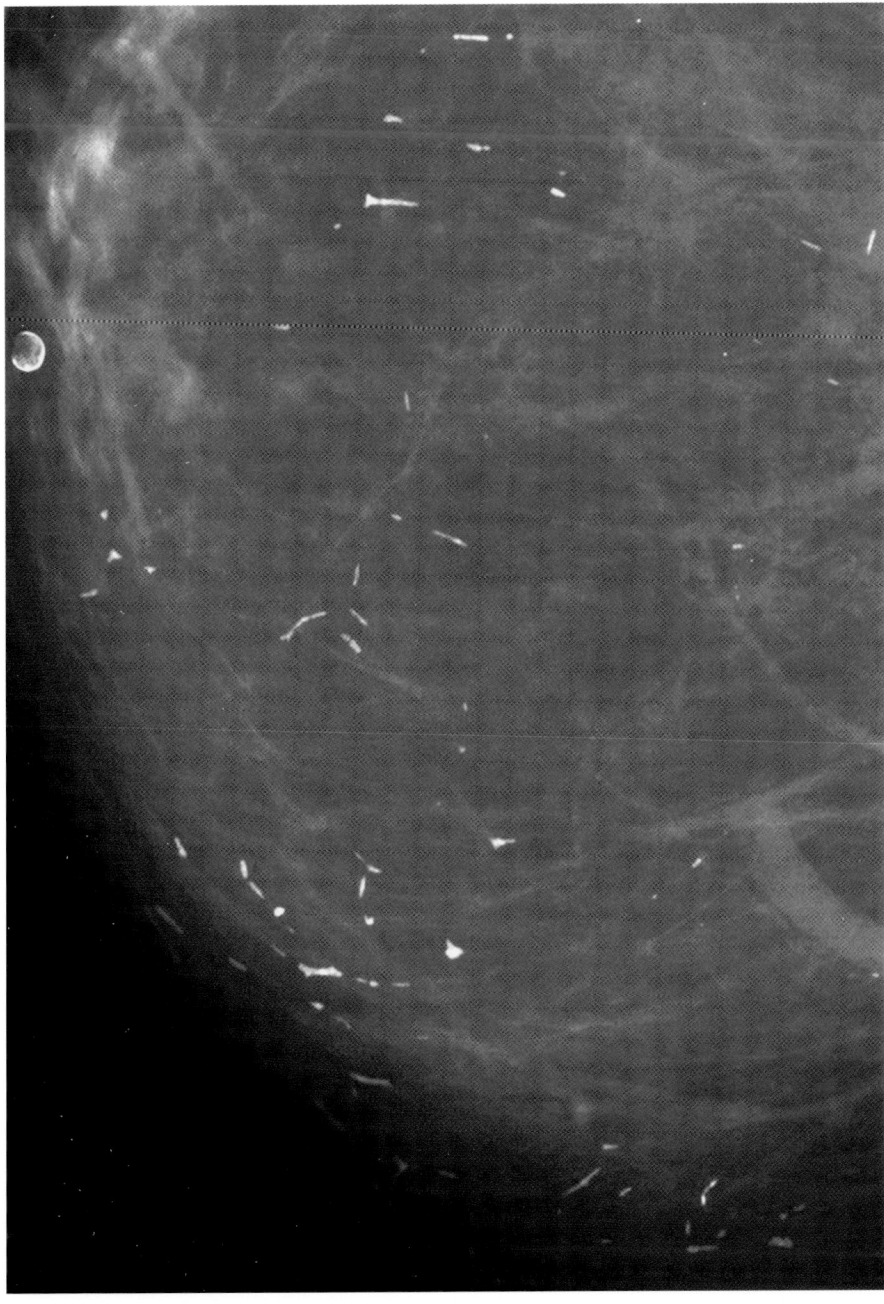

Craniocaudal magnification view (B)

Craniocaudal magnification view (A)

PROBABLY BENIGN CALCIFICATIONS

Rod-shaped calcifications

Intensely radiopaque linear calcifications, reproducing the ductal lumen from which they originate. Generally they radiate out evenly from the areola, following the pattern of the ducts and their ramifications (A) (B). A mass is visible behind the areola, with thickening of the overlying skin. These elongated calcifications, the way they radiate out following the ductal architecture, and the presence of retroareolar thickening are all strongly predictive of ductal ectasia and plasma cell mastitis (A) (B).

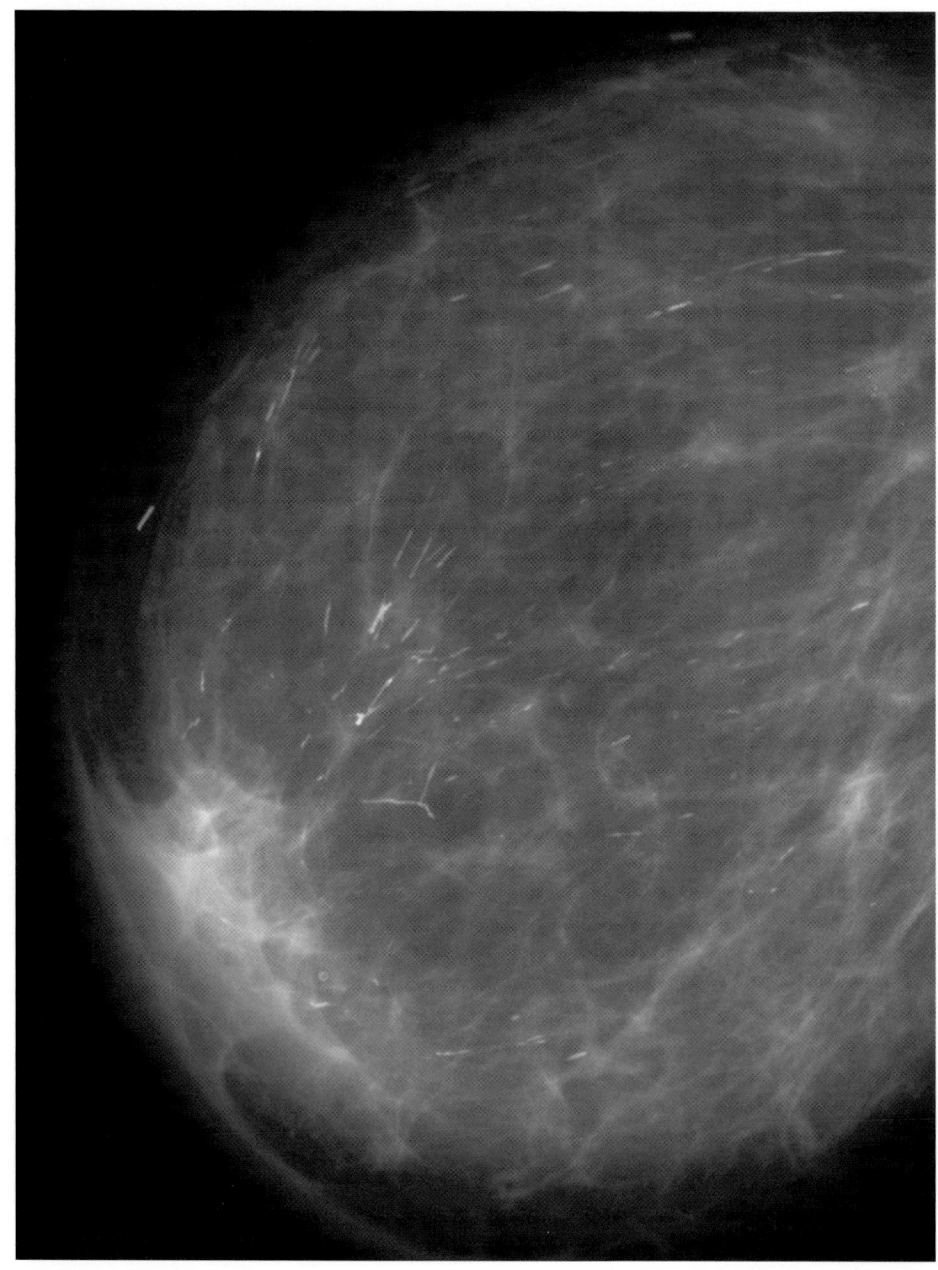

Lateral projection (A)

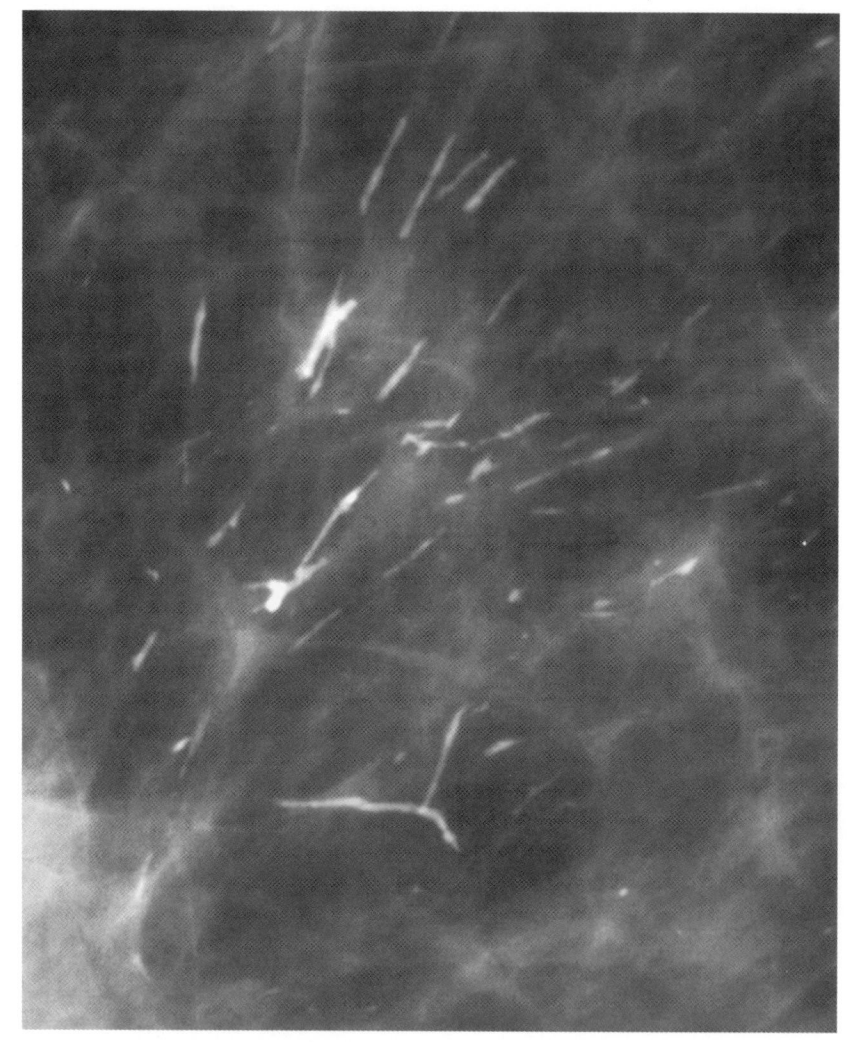

Lateral magnification view (B)

Tubular or rod-shaped calcifications

Calcifications of various types are seen scattered throughout the breast, some rod-shaped, or solid "cores" with blunt, smooth margins following the pattern of the ducts, others like sleeves or tubes, surrounding enlarged ducts. In the deeper tissues, there are two round "egg-shell" calcifications, probably due to sacciform ductal ectasia.

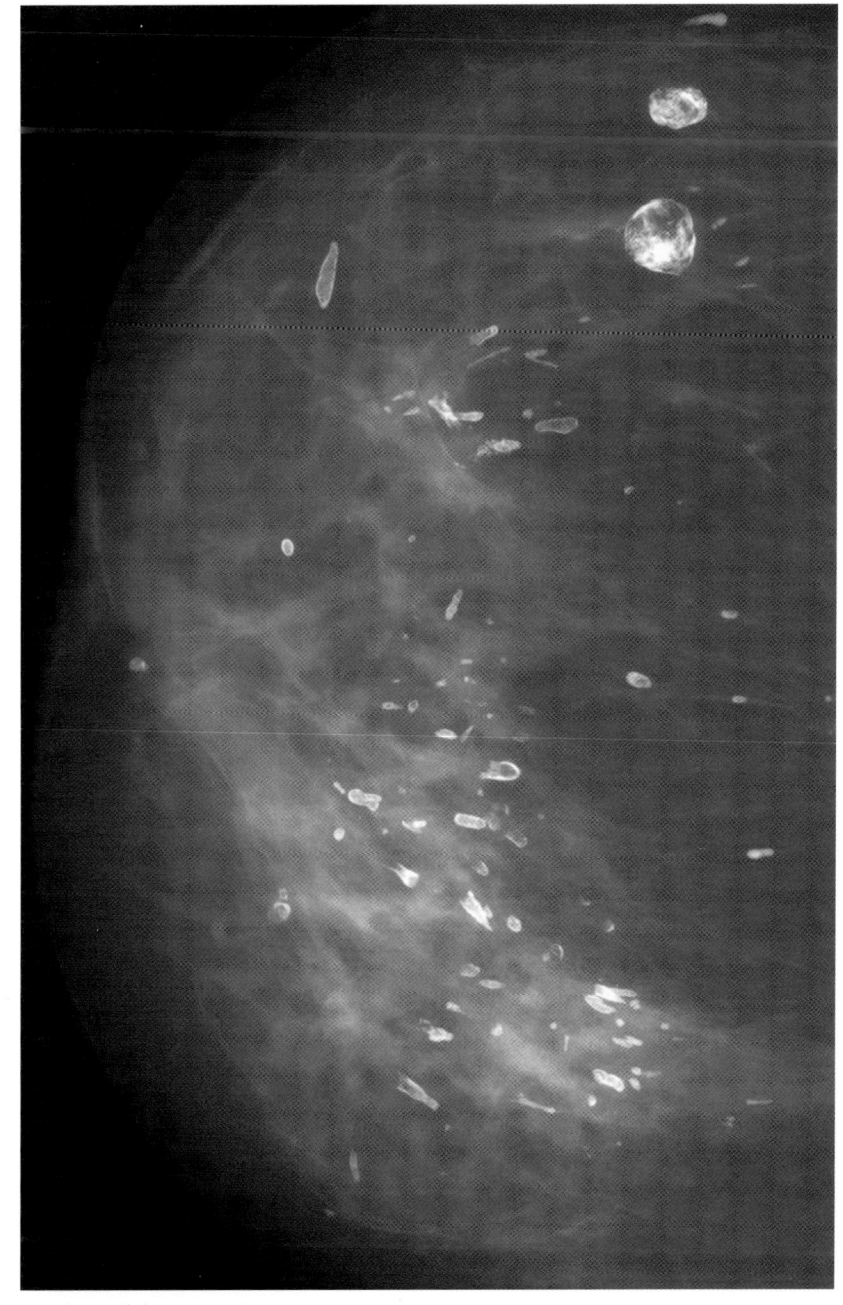

craniocaudal projection

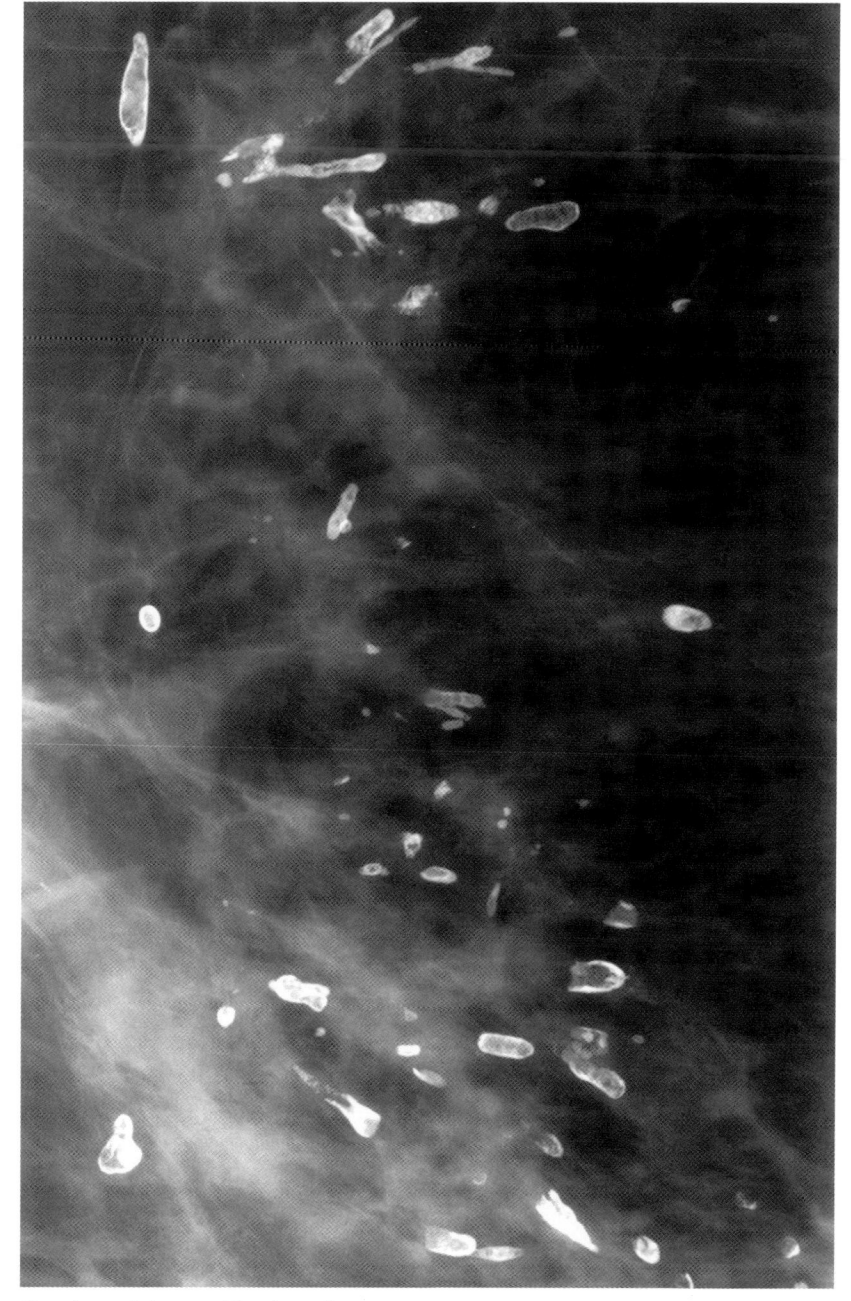

Craniocaudal magnification view

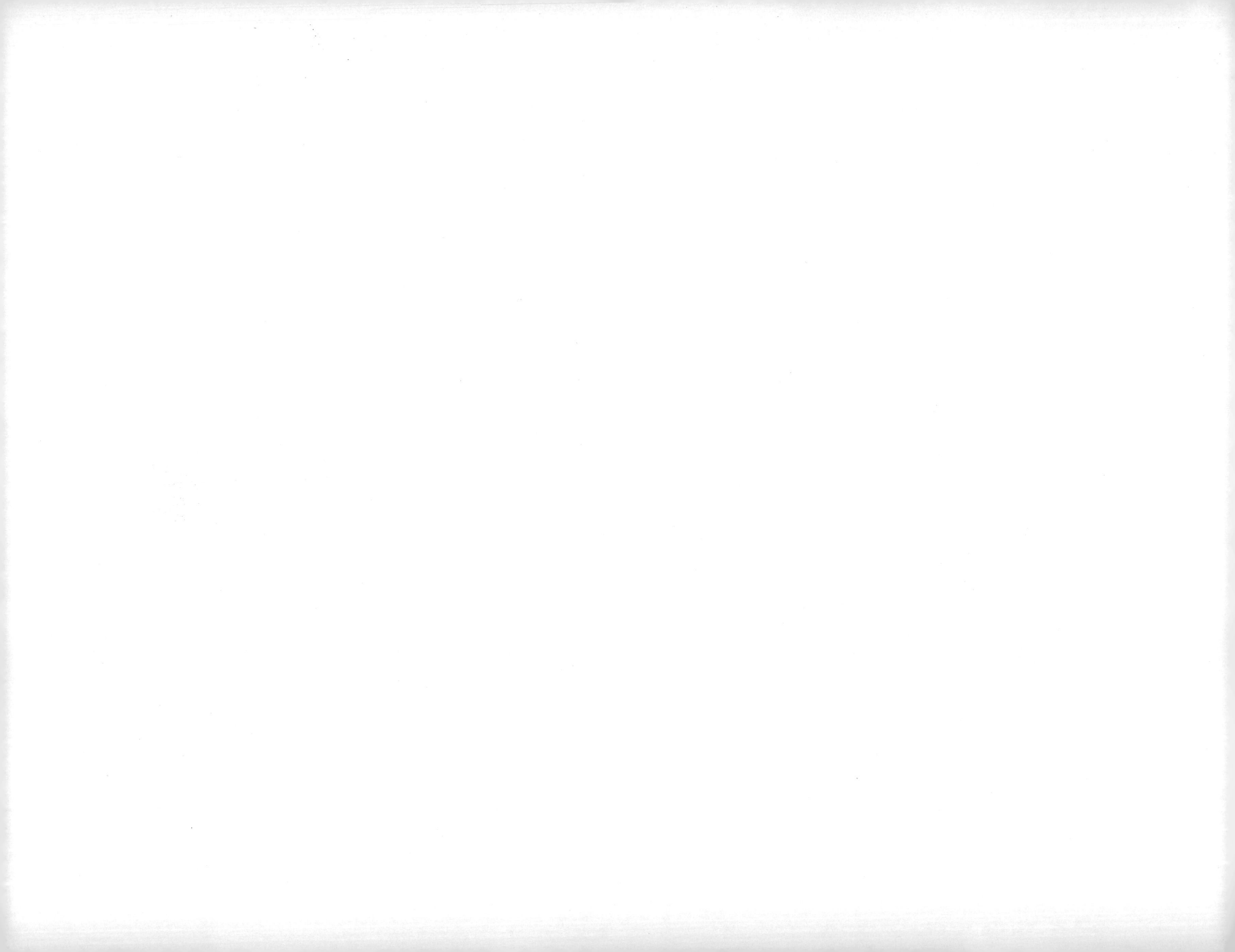

Coarse calcifications

These are patches of calcifications ("popcorn" or "candle-wax") of various shapes and sizes, generally around the edges of a lesion, sometimes covering it completely. They are usually coarse and markedly radiopaque and are distributed randomly throughout a circumscribed mass. They are compatible with calcifying fibroadenomas. Distinctly wavy, arc-shaped, continuous calcifications of variable density indicate the walls of cysts in the process of becoming calcified.

PROBABLY BENIGN CALCIFICATIONS

Coarse calcifications ("pop-corn", "candle-wax")

Several coarse calcifications are seen in a deep central location, within a circumscribed opacity with regular margins. This image is consistent with calcified fibroadenoma (A). Behind the areola there is a lobulated circumscribed opacity with clear margins, and coarse "blackberry-like" calcifications along the anterior profile, partly inside and partly outside the lesion (B).

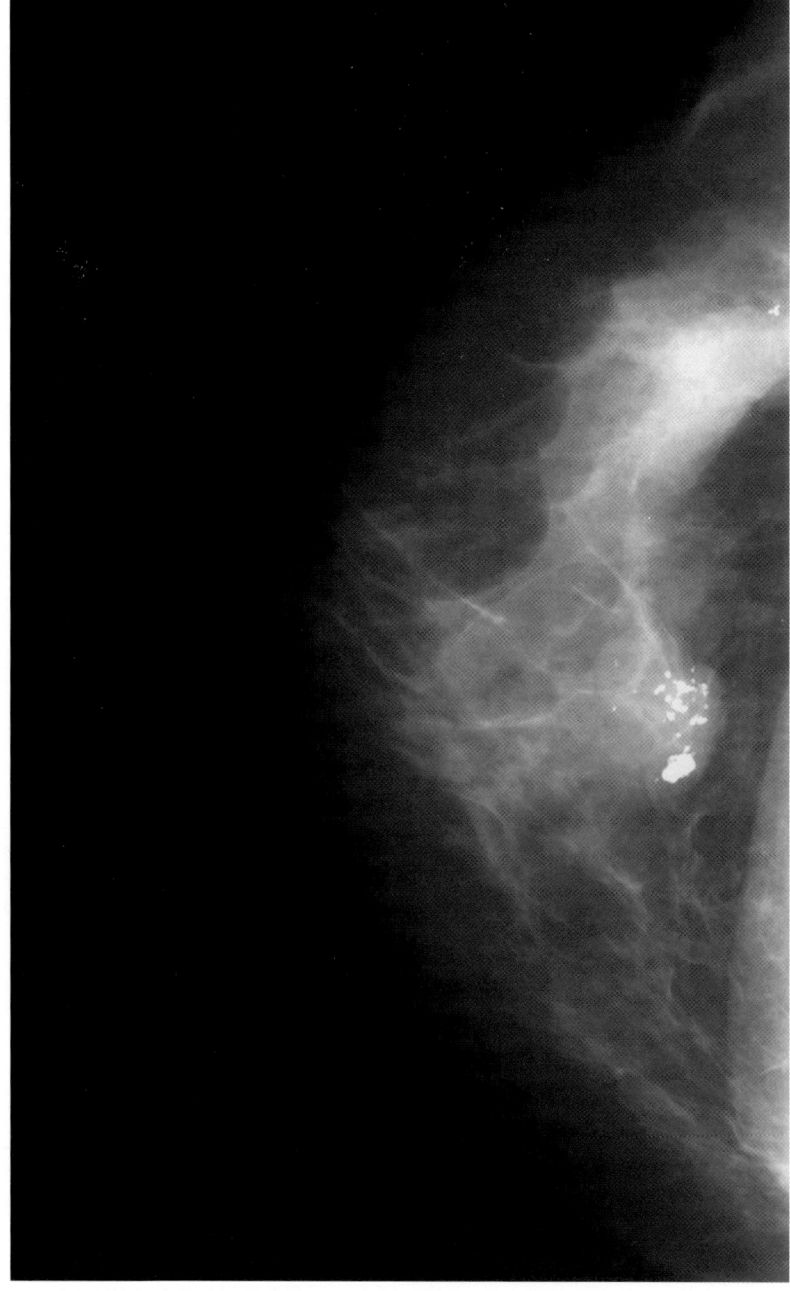

Craniocaudal projection (A)

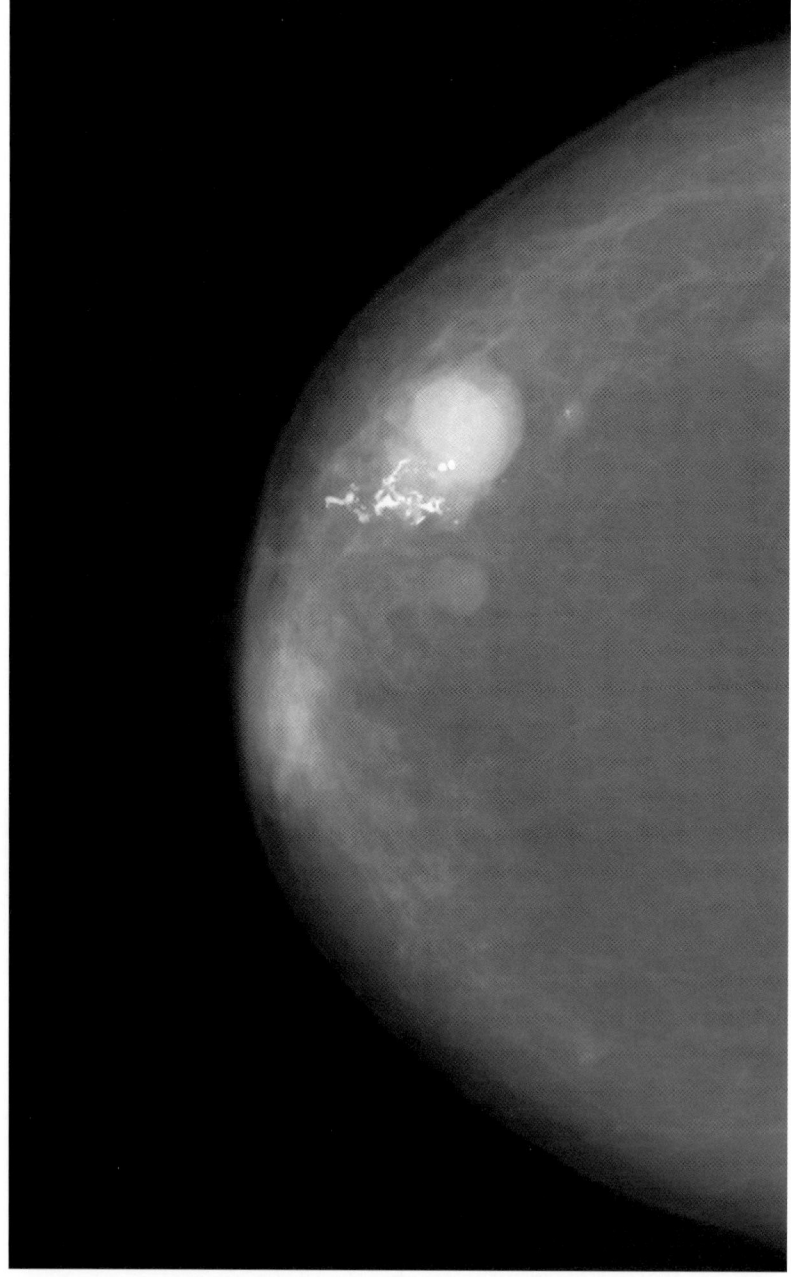

Craniocaudal projection (B)

PROBABLY BENIGN CALCIFICATIONS

Coarse calcifications ("pop corn", "candle-wax")

A markedly dense lobulated circumscribed opacity with sharp margins is visible in the outer retroareolar location, with coarse "blackberry-like" calcifications along the anterior profile, partly inside and partly outside the lesion. The magnification views clearly shows the intraductal pattern of the calcifications outside the lesion.

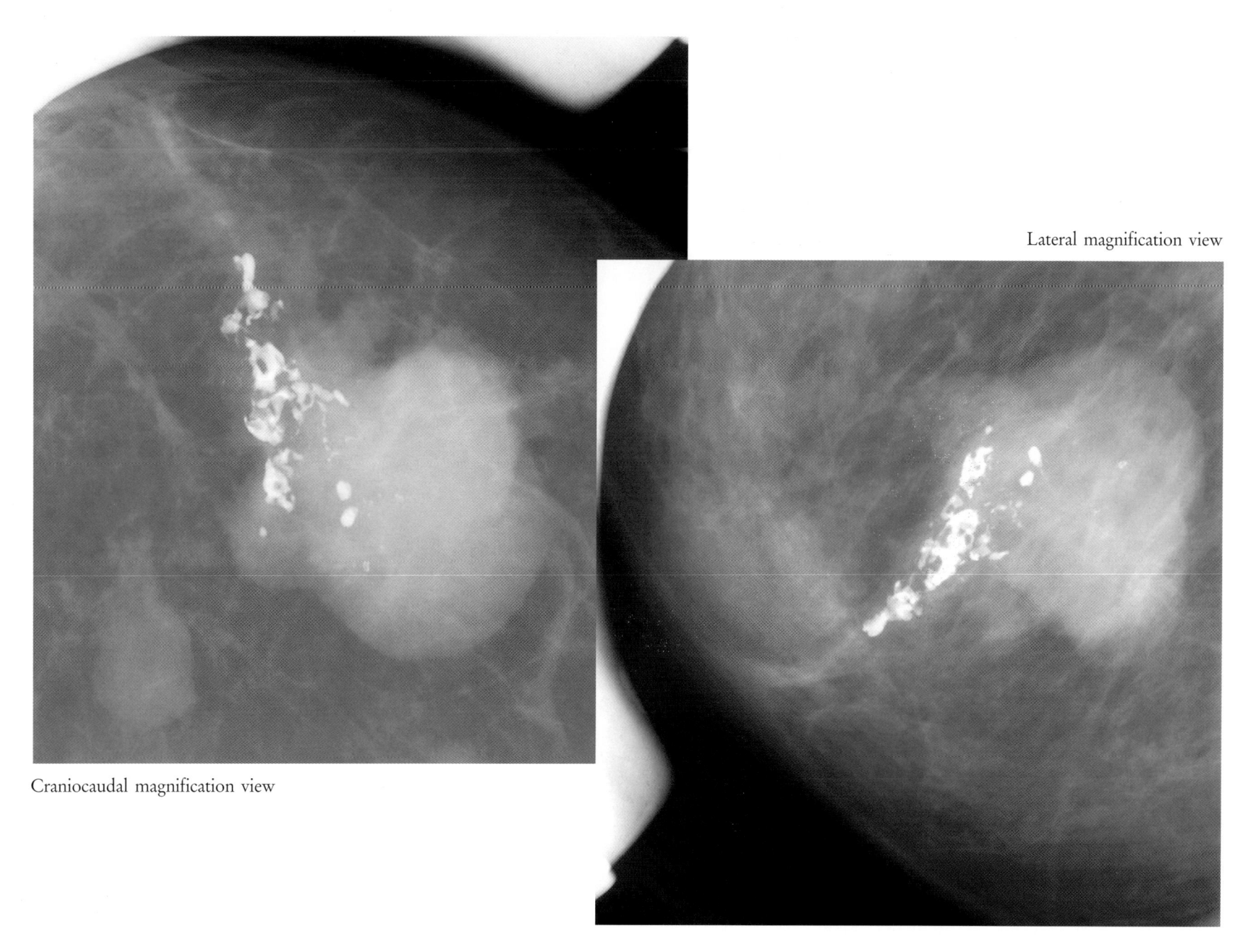

Lateral magnification view

Craniocaudal magnification view

Histological finding: multiple intraductal papillomas with foci of infiltrating papillary carcinoma

PROBABLY BENIGN CALCIFICATIONS

Coarse calcifications ("popcorn", "candle-wax")
Multiple circumscribed opacities are visible, with sharp margins and coarse calcifications varying in shape, size and density.

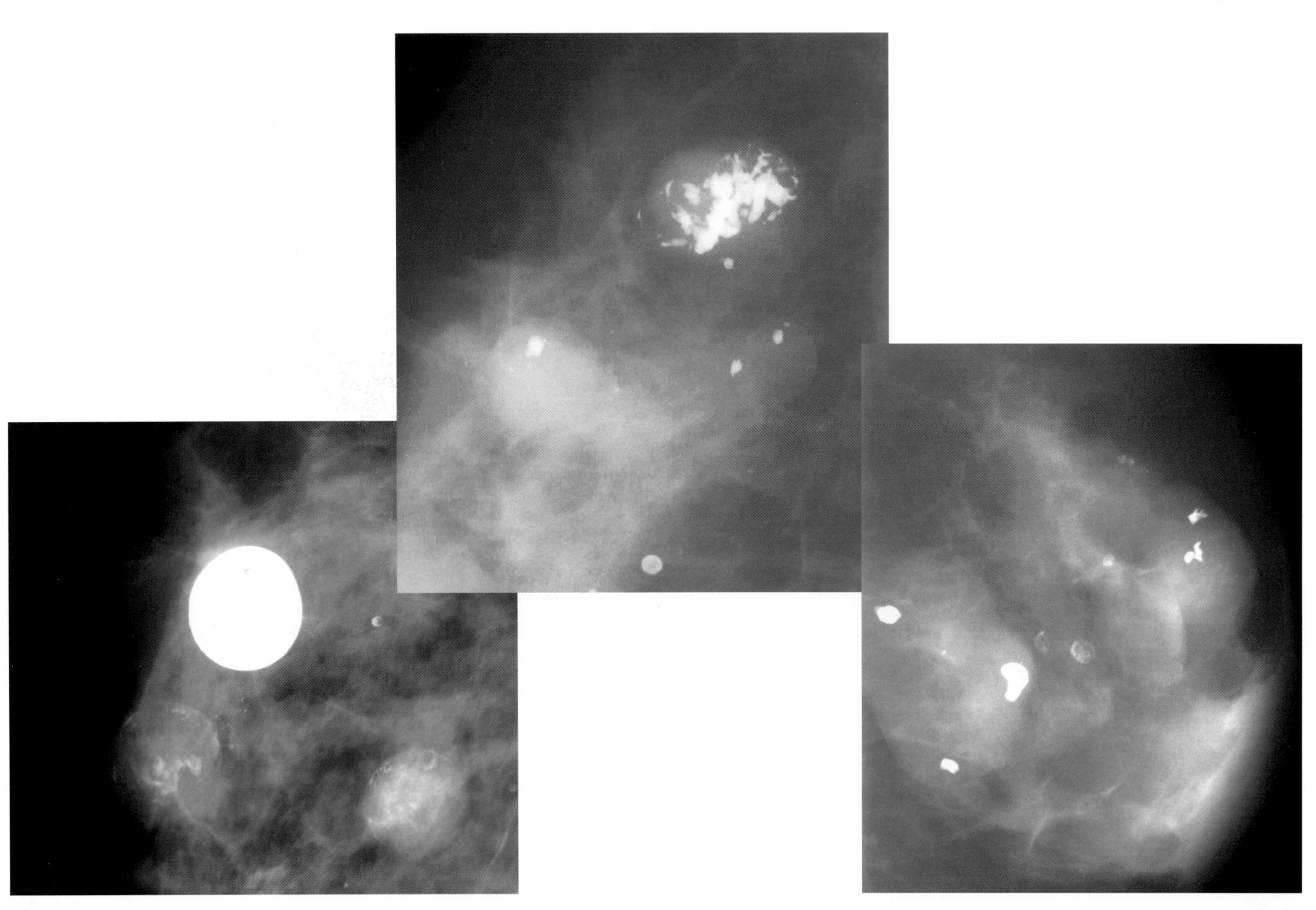

Vascular calcifications

Typically these give an image of one or two calcified lines along the vessel walls, giving rise to the characteristic "railway lines" pattern. Generally these calcifications are not difficult to interpret, unless only one wall is calcified, or only a single short segment of the vessel, with linear or pin-point calcifications which may be difficult to distinguish from "casting type" ductal calcifications.

PROBABLY BENIGN CALCIFICATIONS

Vascular calcifications

Multiple vessels in different stages of calcification are visible. In the upper area, there is a small, unevenly calcified twisted vessel. In the lower part, another vessel gives the characteristic "railway lines" pattern, with two thick calcified lines running along the vessel walls, in a tortuous "spiral" or "corkscrew" pattern.

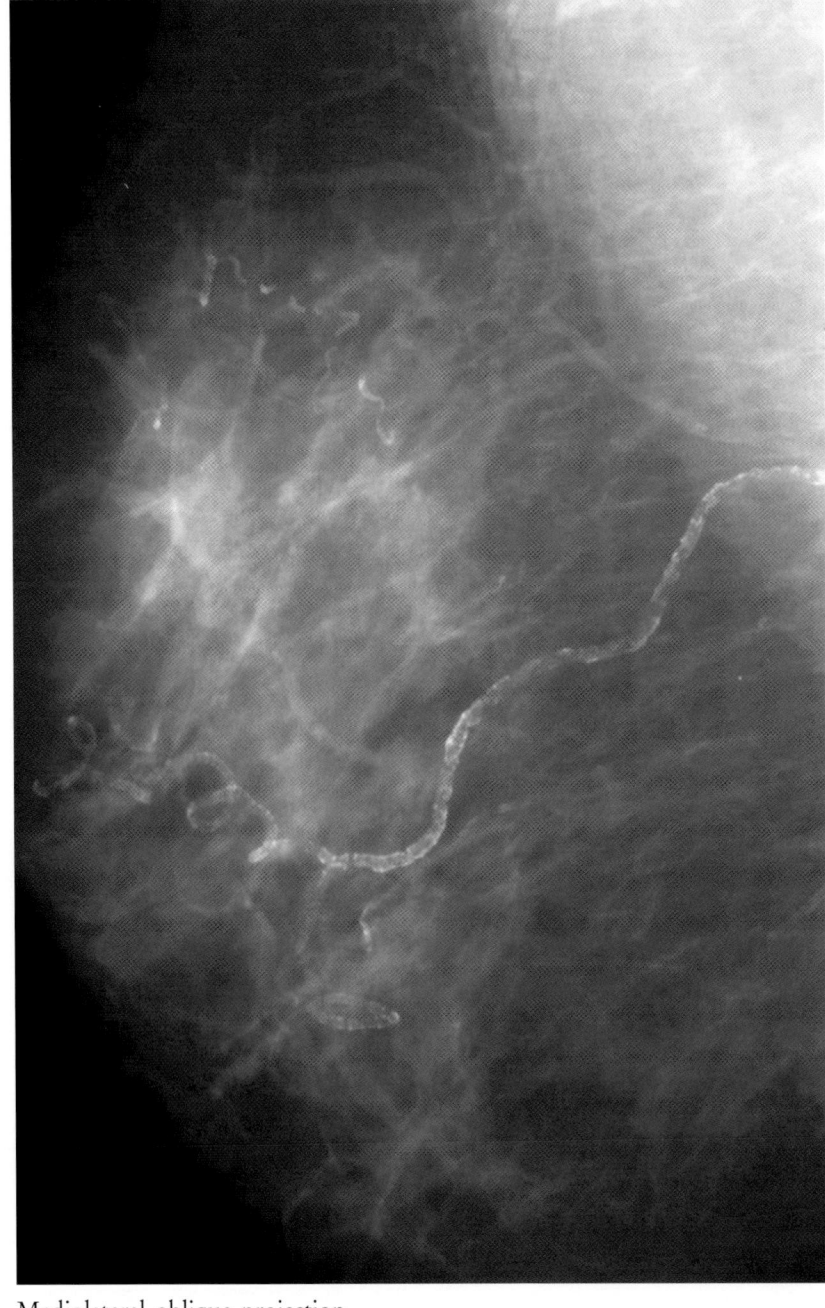

Mediolateral oblique projection

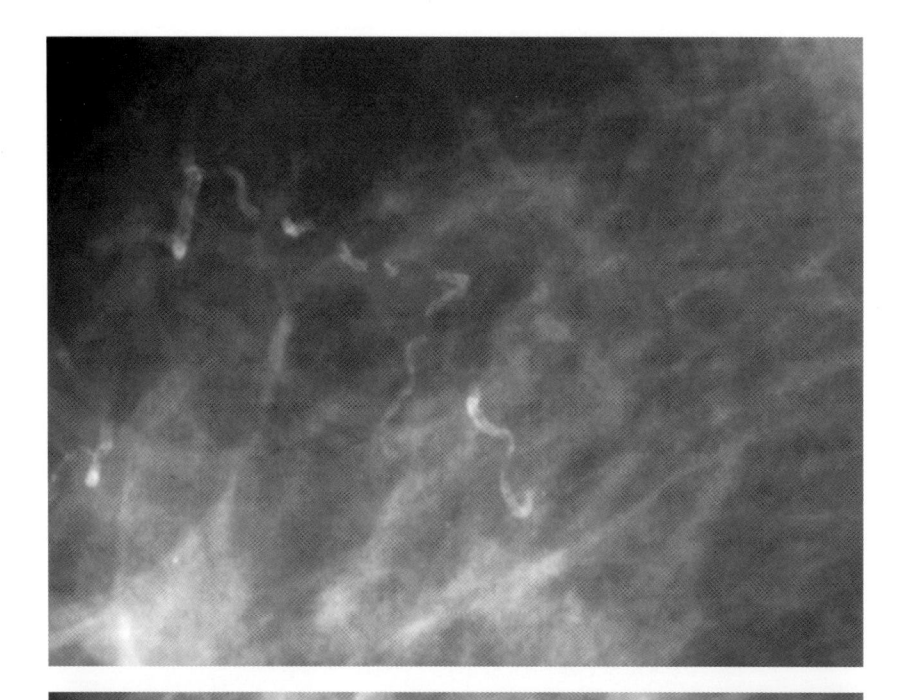

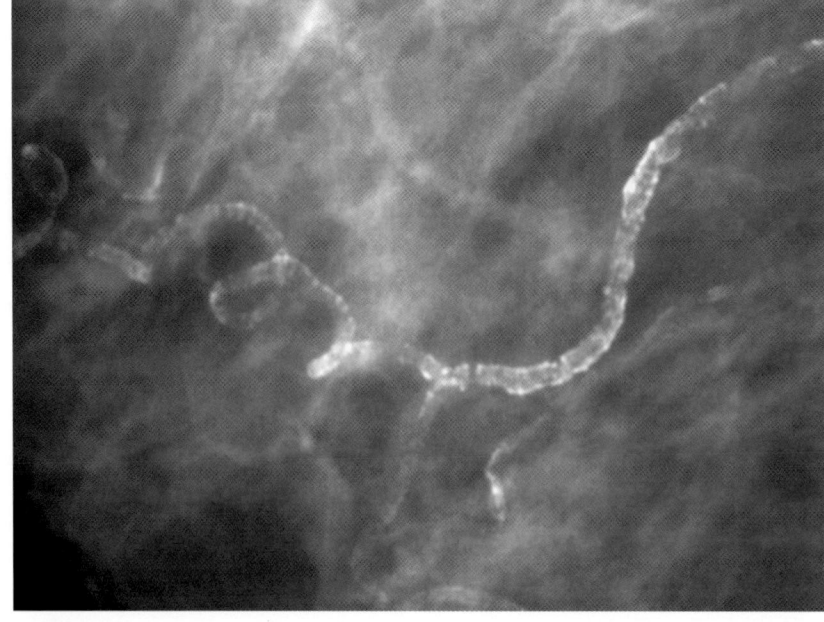

Magnification view

Dystrophic calcifications

These tend to vary in appearance and size: they may be elongated, rod-shaped, vermicular and hard to define, or large and coarse, and very easy to interpret. They can occur after radiotherapy or surgery.

PROBABLY BENIGN CALCIFICATIONS

Dystrophic calcifications
In the outer part of the breast a coarse calcification is visible, comprising several parts, seemingly surrounding a focus of fat necrosis. The largest calcified portion has the appearance of "lava flow" (A). The smaller ones are ring-like, with a lucent centre. Sequelae of Quart (Quadrantectomy and Radiotherapy).

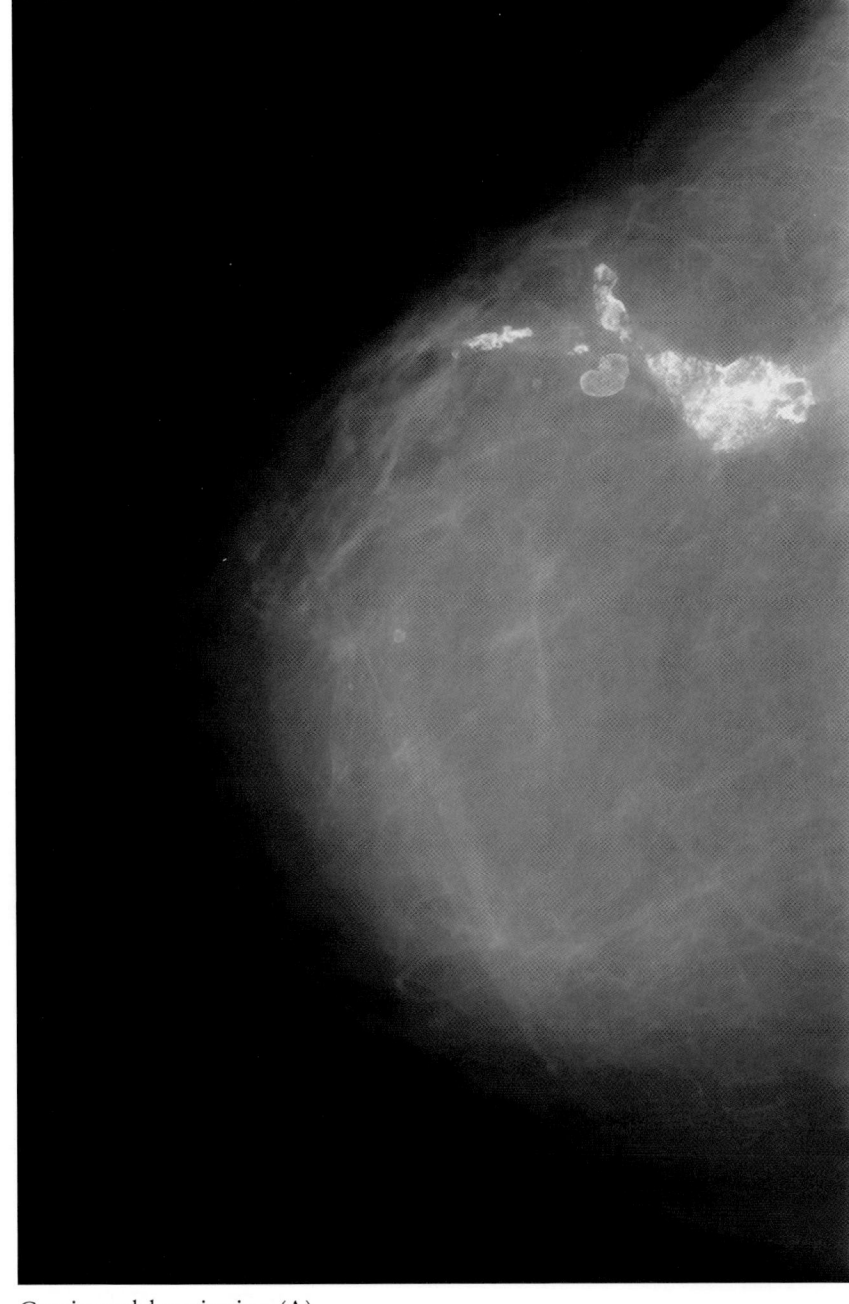

Craniocaudal projection (A)

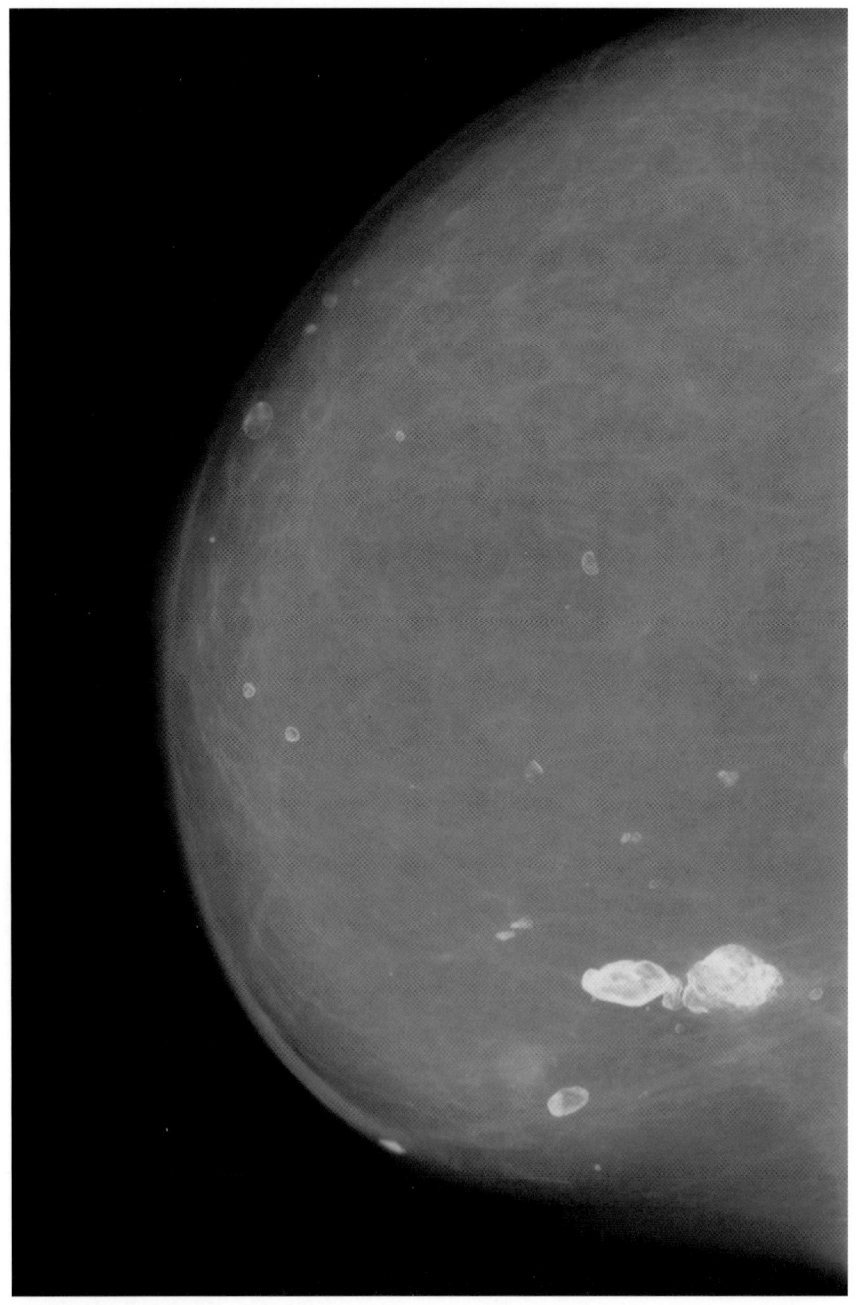

Craniocaudal projection (B)

Dystrophic calcifications

In the outer part of the breast a coarse calcification is visible, comprising several parts, seemingly surrounding a focus of fat necrosis. The largest calcified portion has the appearance of "lava flow" (A). The smaller ones are ring-like, with a lucent centre. Sequelae of QUART.

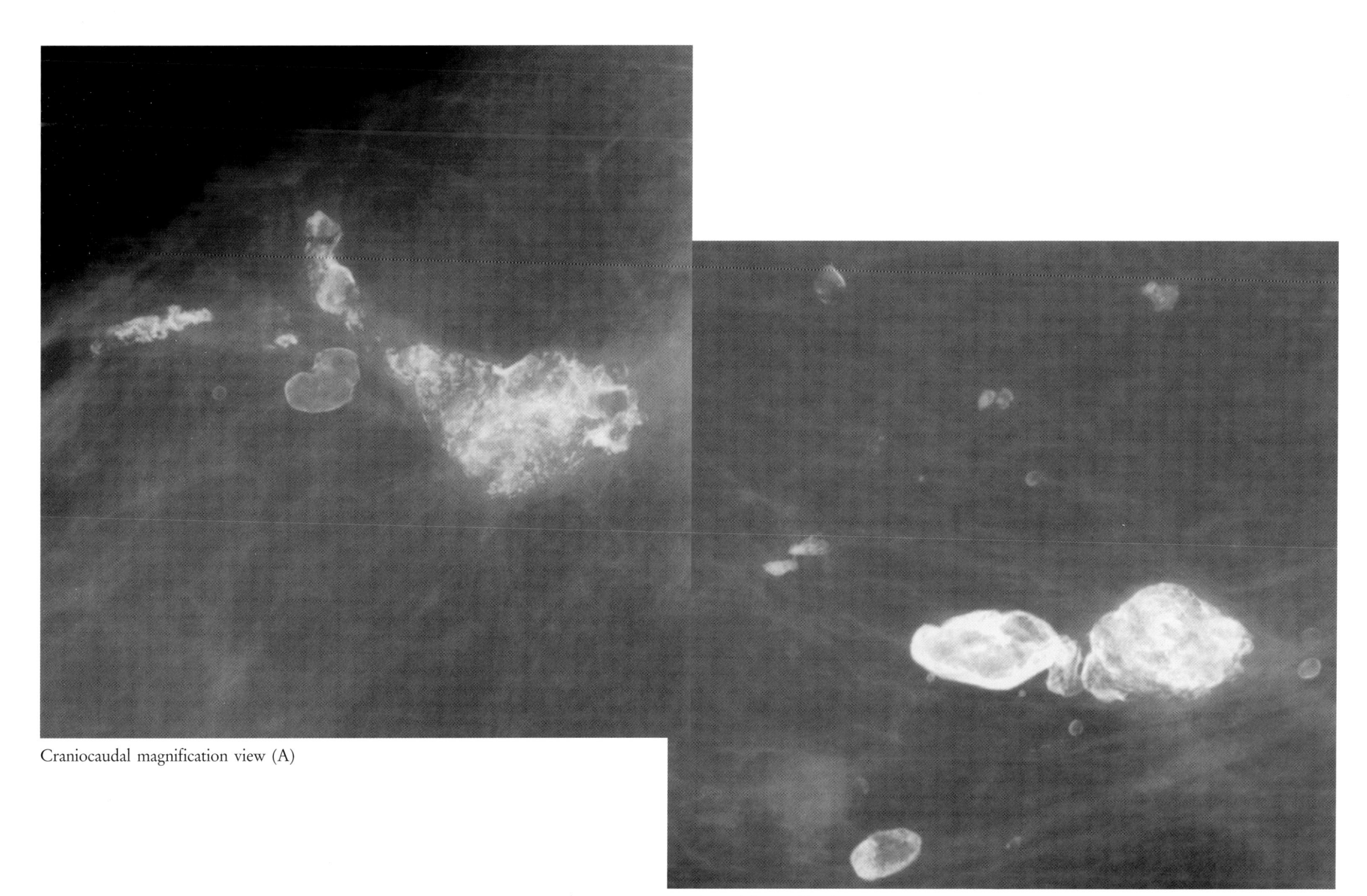

Craniocaudal magnification view (A)

Craniocaudal magnification view (B)

PROBABLY BENIGN CALCIFICATIONS

Dystrophic calcifications

A coarse calcification is visible in the retroareolar region, comprising several parts, seemingly surrounding a focus of fat necrosis, like a "string of beads". Multiple dystrophic calcifications; the smaller ones are ring-like, with a lucent centre. Sequelae of QUART.

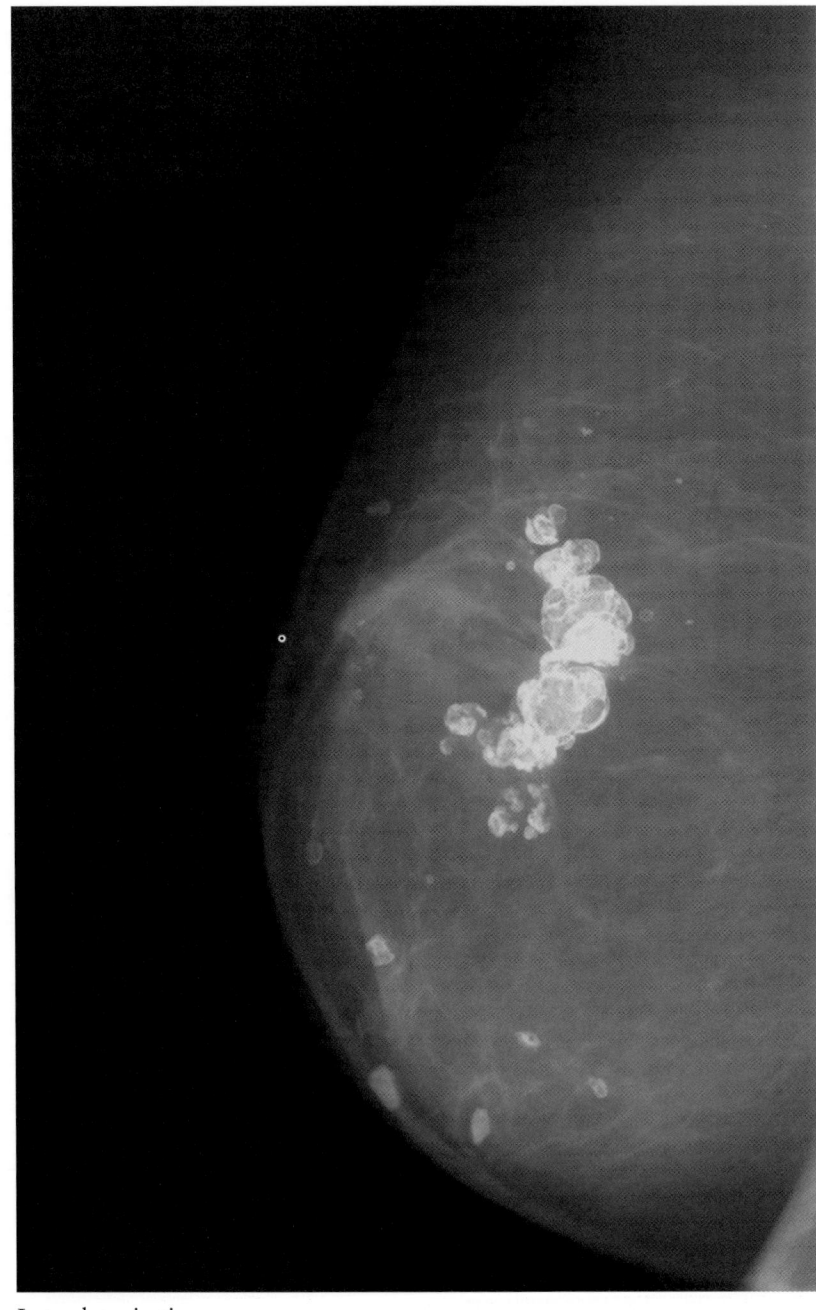

Lateral projection

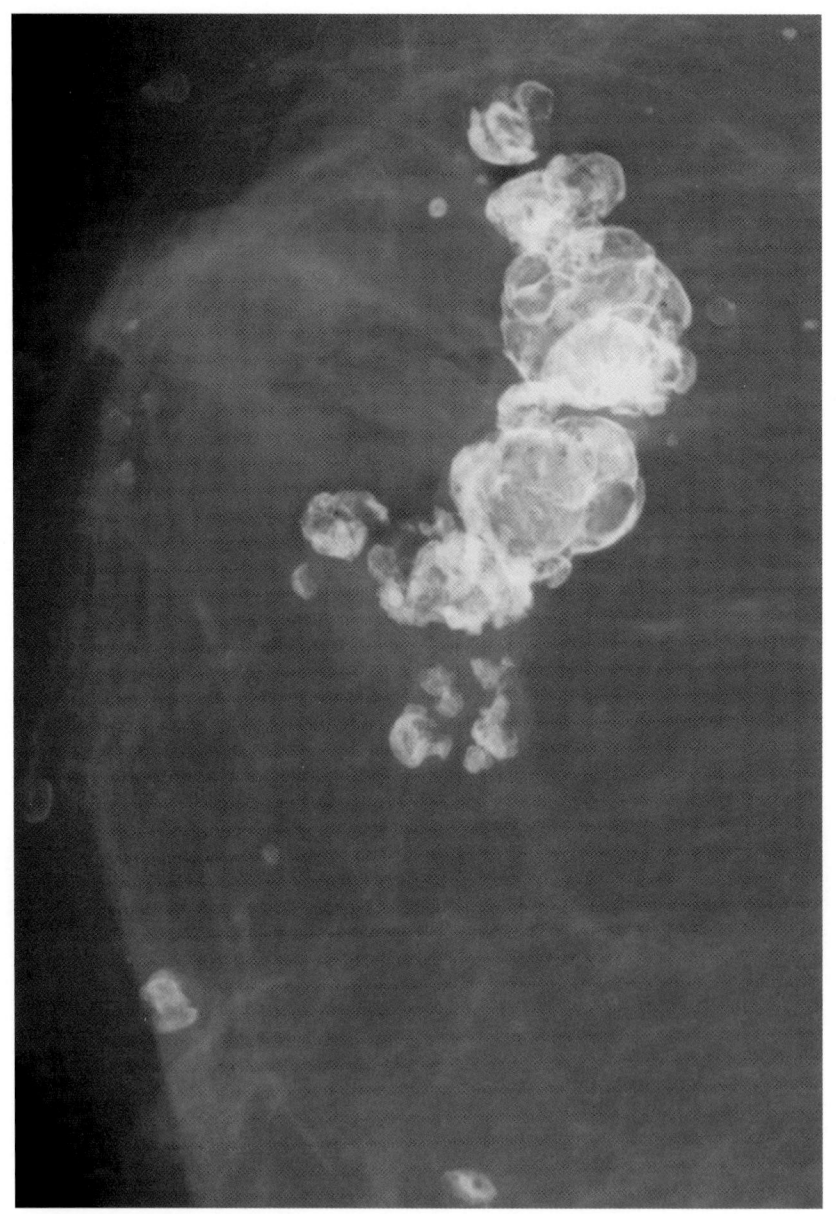

Lateral magnification view

Dystrophic calcifications

Numerous dystrophic calcifications are distributed in the lower quadrants, giving a "desert rose" image. Sequelae of QUART.

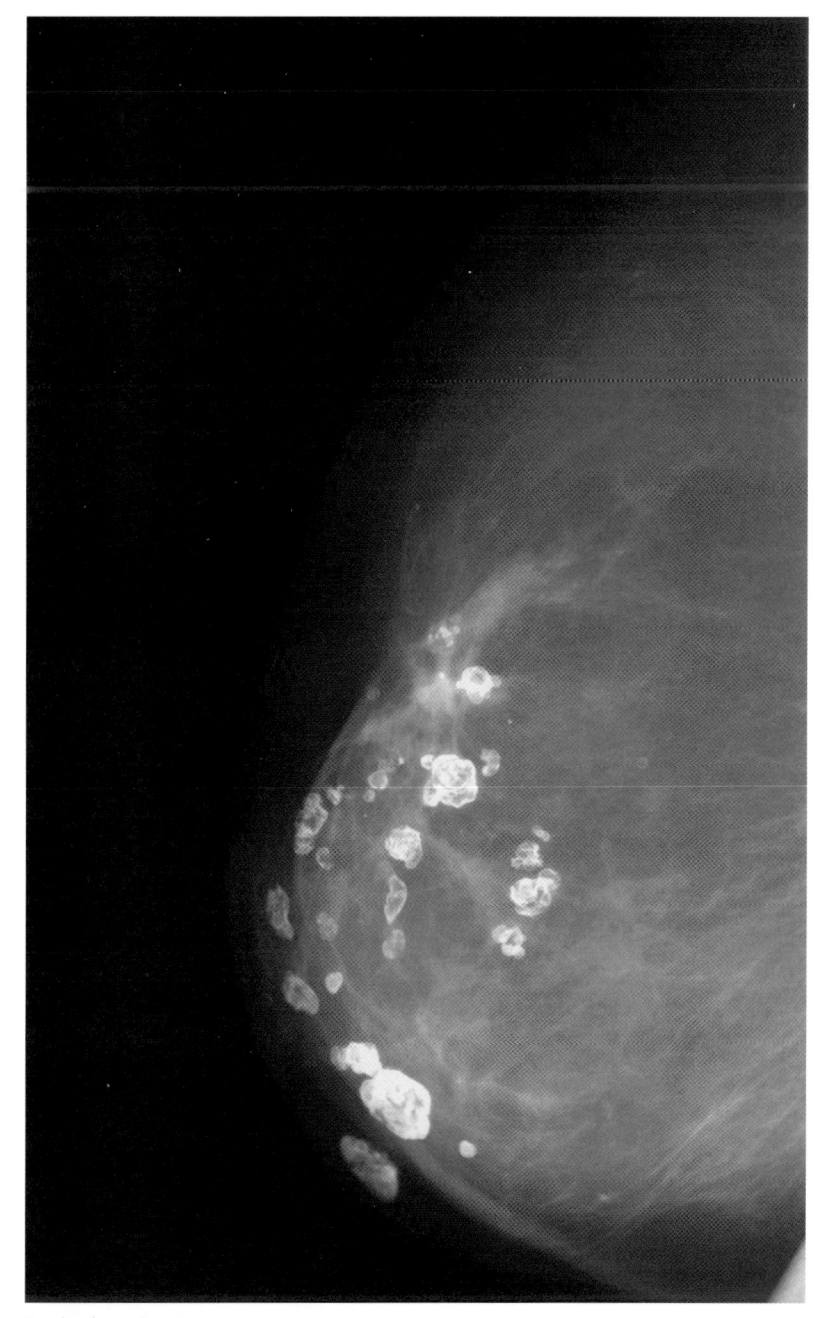

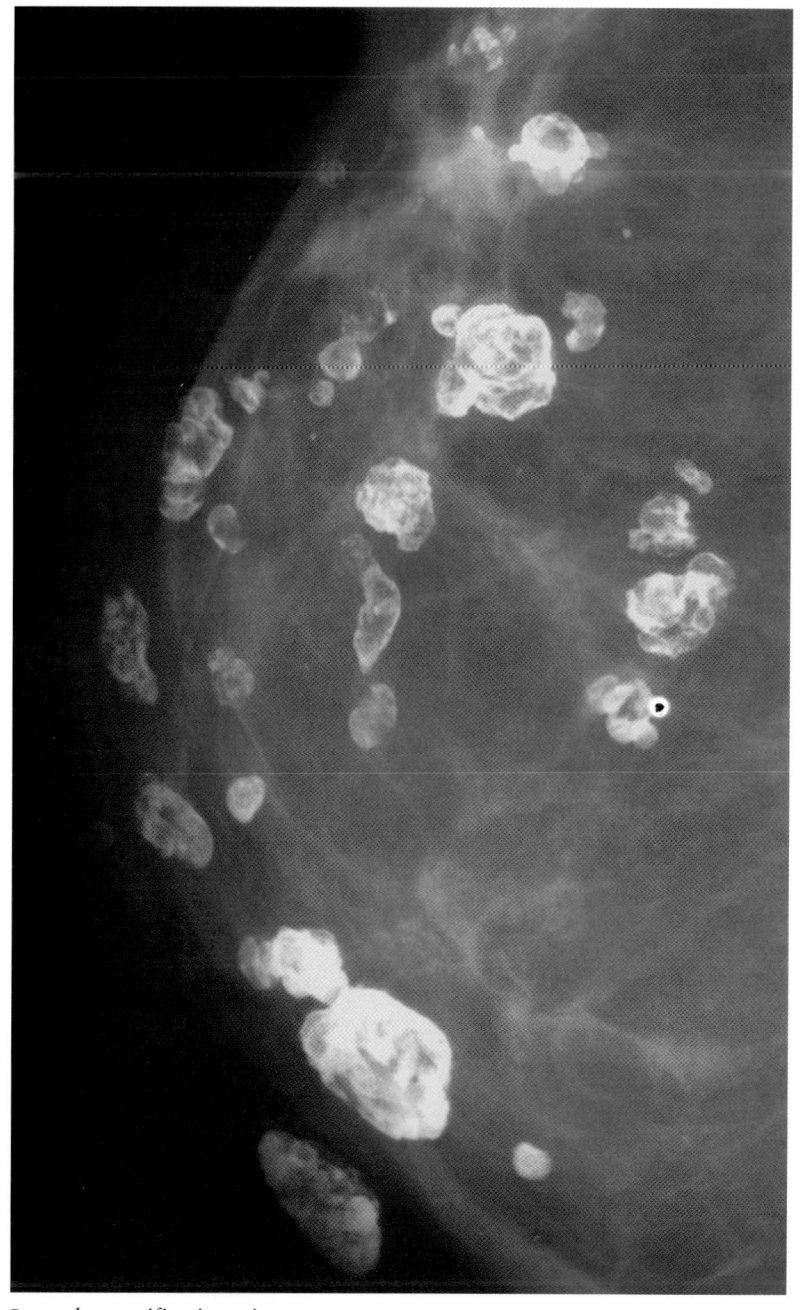

Lateral projection

Lateral magnification view

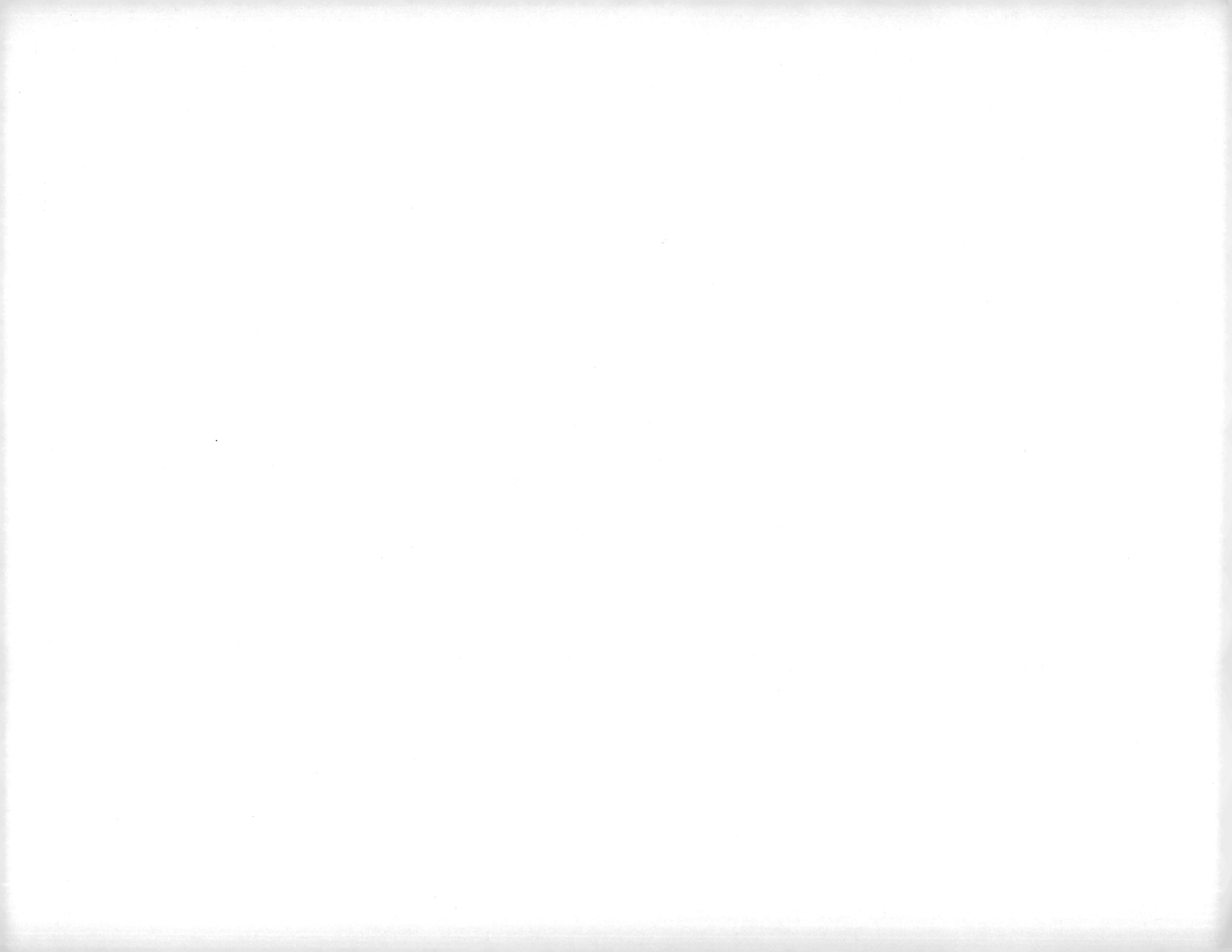

Skin calcifications

These may present as small calcified spheres measuring 1 or 2 mm or, more often, as ring-like, occasionally coalescing calcifications of "binocular" or "trifolium" appearance. The deposits are due to calcified sebaceous glands and are generally seen behind the areola, in the axilla, or peripherally in the medial quadrants, where they tend to project into the parenchyma rather than over the skin.
When these calcifications are clustered in small masses, tangential views of the skin may be useful.

PROBABLY BENIGN CALCIFICATIONS

Skin calcifications

Skin calcifications may present as small spheres measuring 1-2 mm or, more often, as ring-like, occasionally coalescing calcifications of "binocular" or "trifolium" appearance. In this case calcifications are visible peripherally in the medial quadrants, where they tend to project into the parenchyma rather than over the skin. When these calcifications are clustered in small masses, tangential views of the skin may be useful.

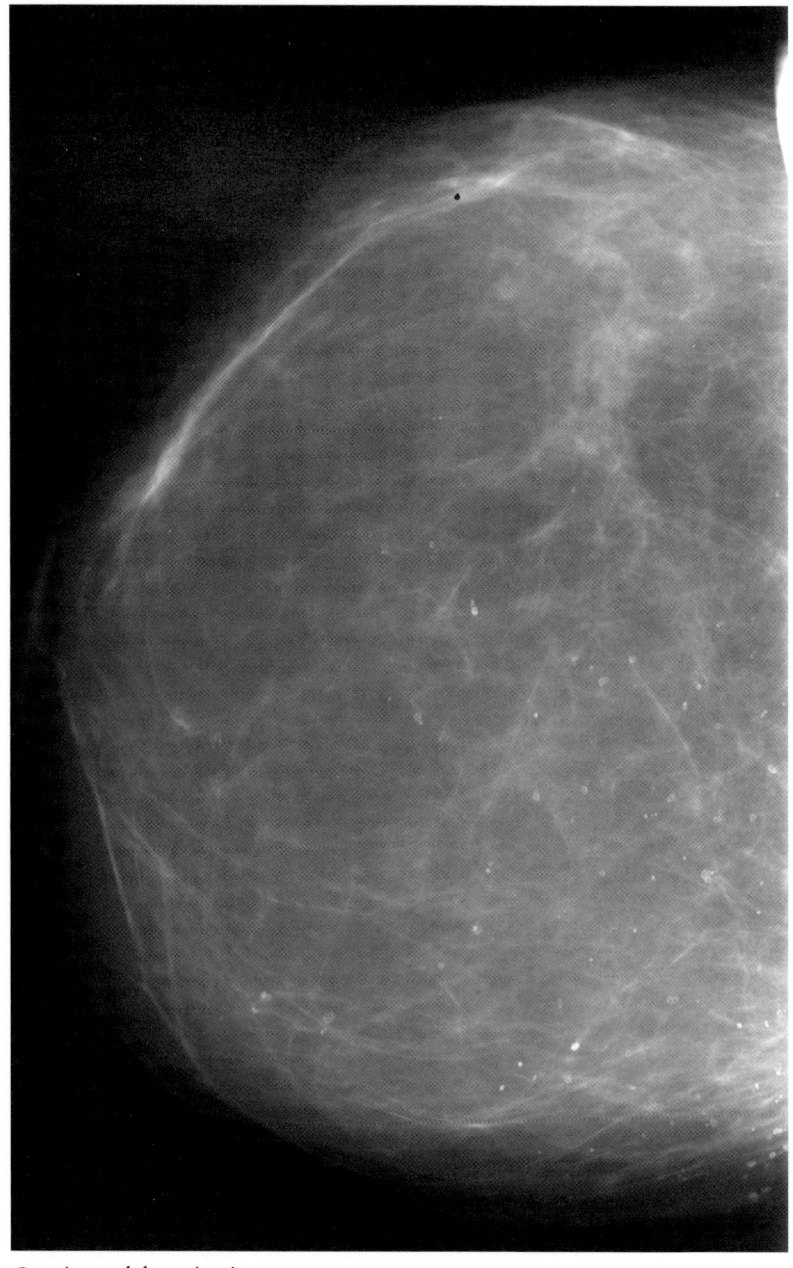

Craniocaudal projection

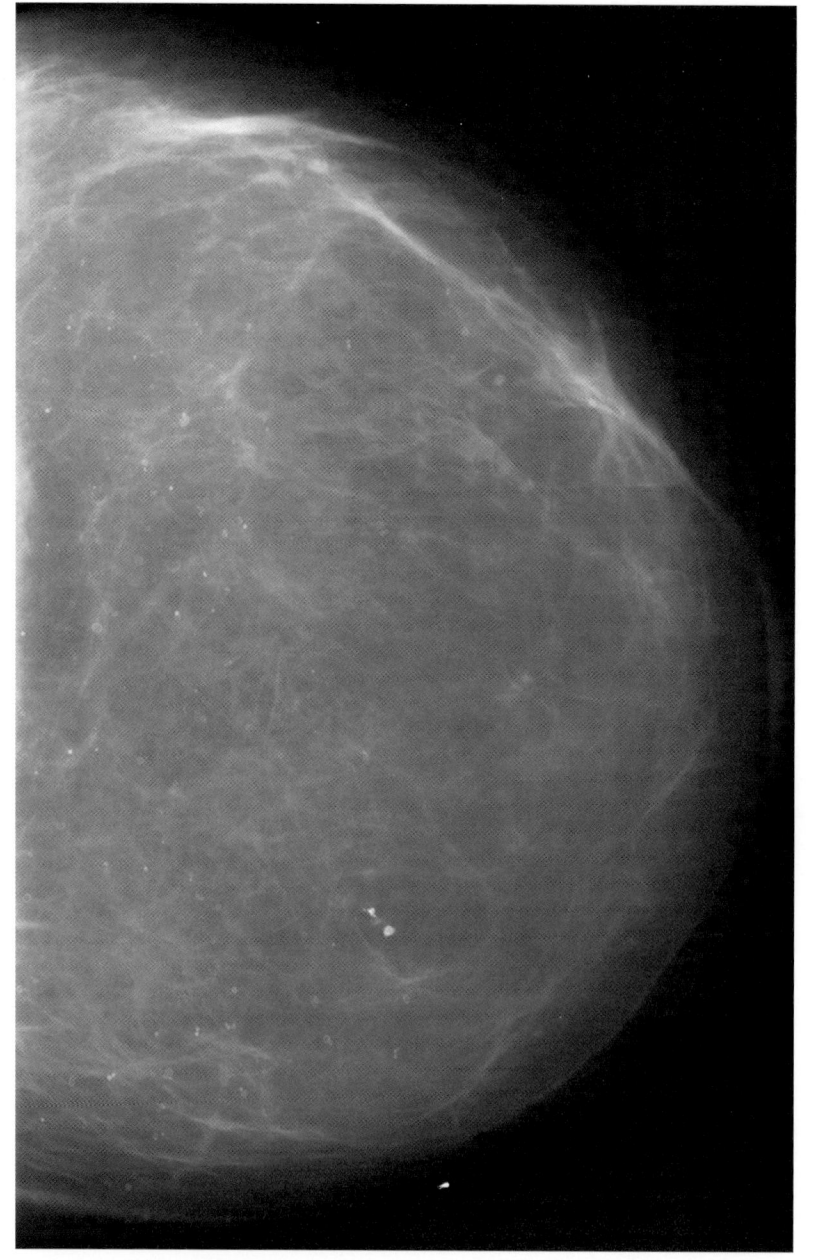

Craniocaudal projection

Skin calcifications

Skin calcifications may present as small spheres measuring 1-2 mm or, more often, as ring-like, occasionally coalescing calcifications of "binocular" or "trifolium" appearance. In this case calcifications are visible peripherally in the medial quadrants, where they tend to project into the parenchyma rather than over the skin. When these calcifications are clustered in small masses, tangential views of the skin may be useful.

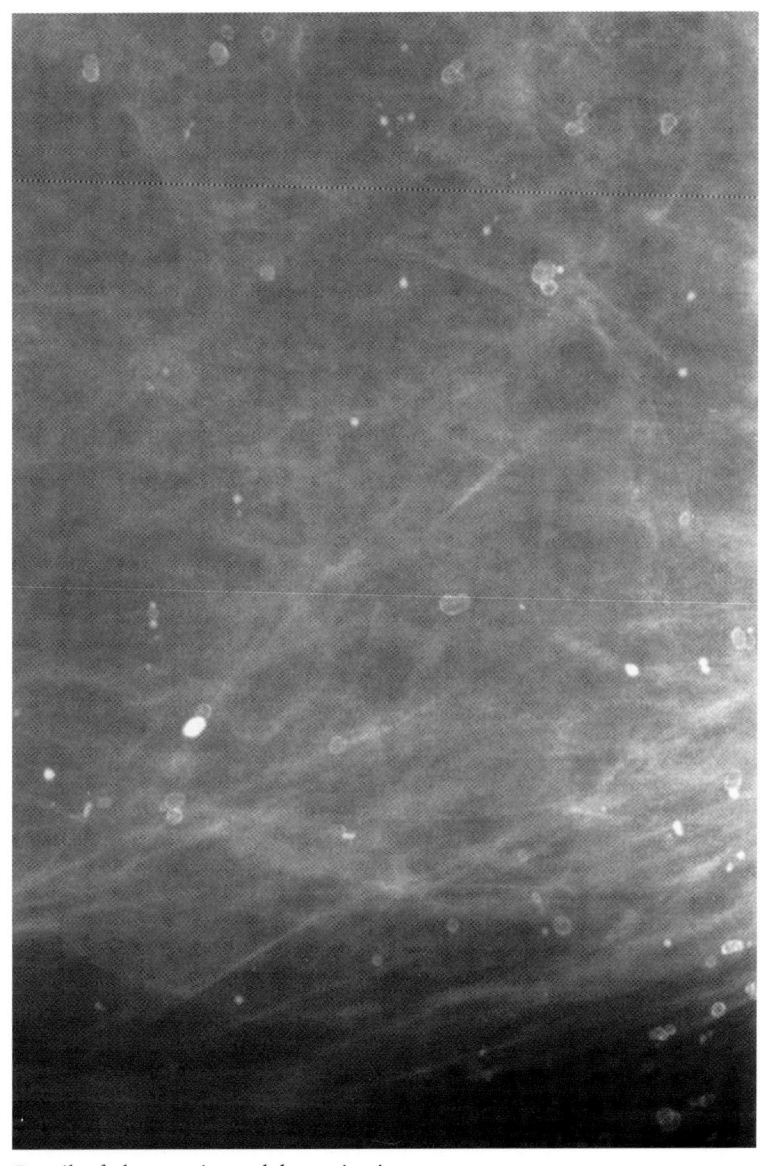

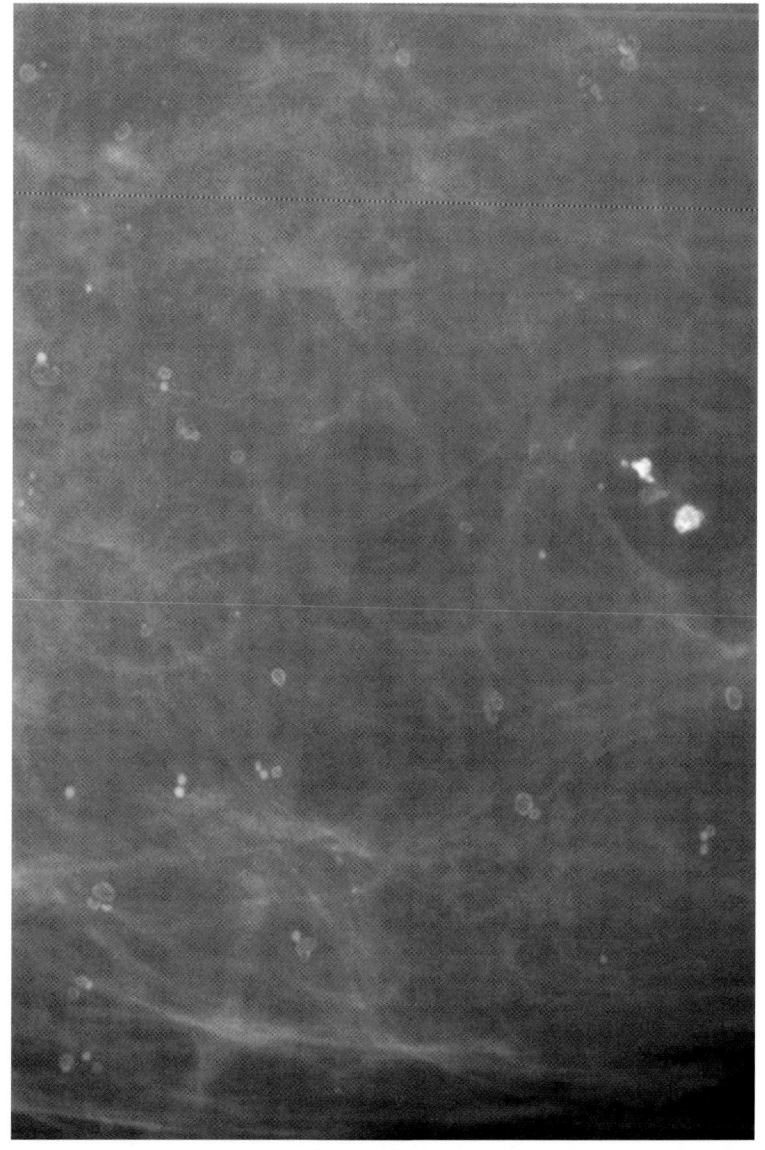

Detail of the craniocaudal projection

Detail of the craniocaudal projection

PROBABLY BENIGN CALCIFICATIONS

Skin calcifications

Small lucent-centred spheres, 1-2 mm wide with a "binocular" or "trifolium" appearance, occasionally coalescing, are visible at the periphery of the lower medial quadrant (A). These deposits, which are due to calcified sebaceous glands, project into the skin, as in these tangential views of the skin (B).

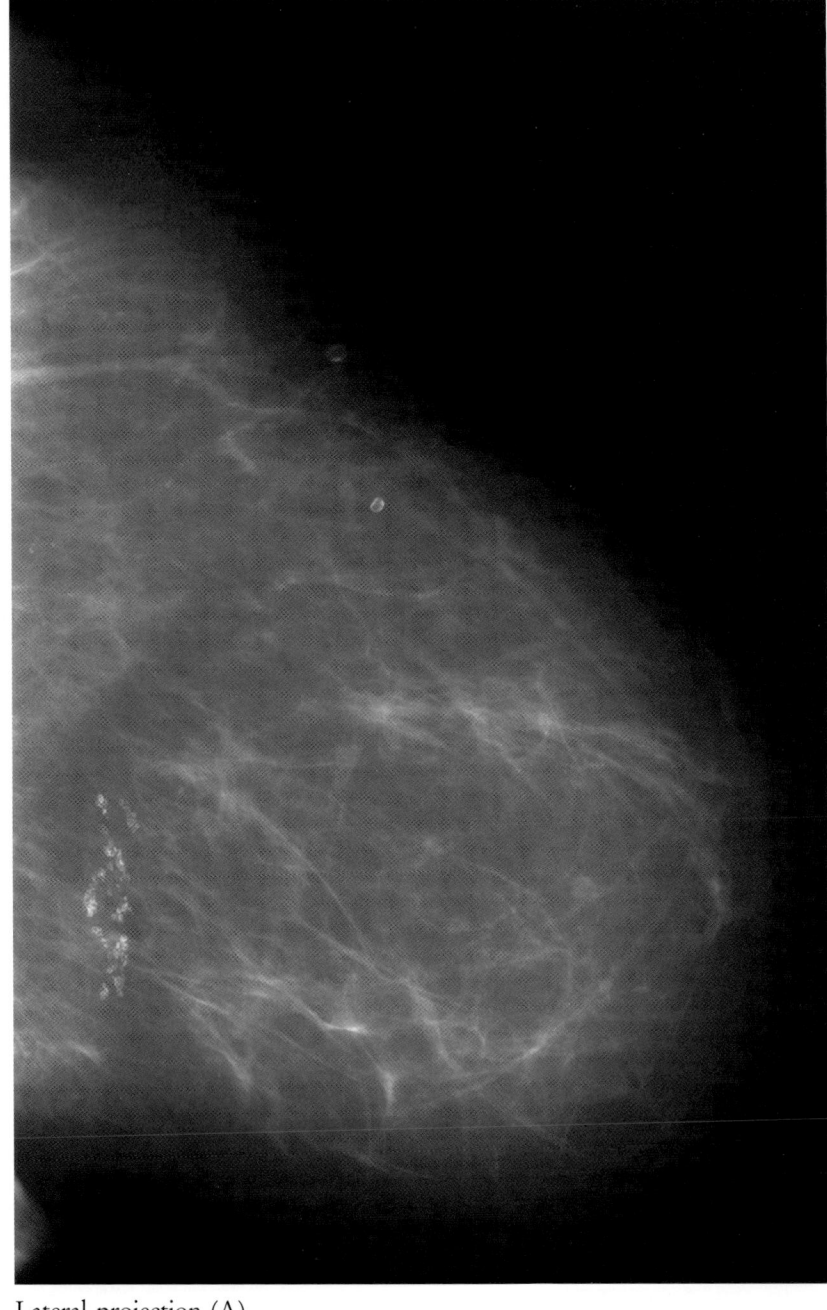

Lateral projection (A)

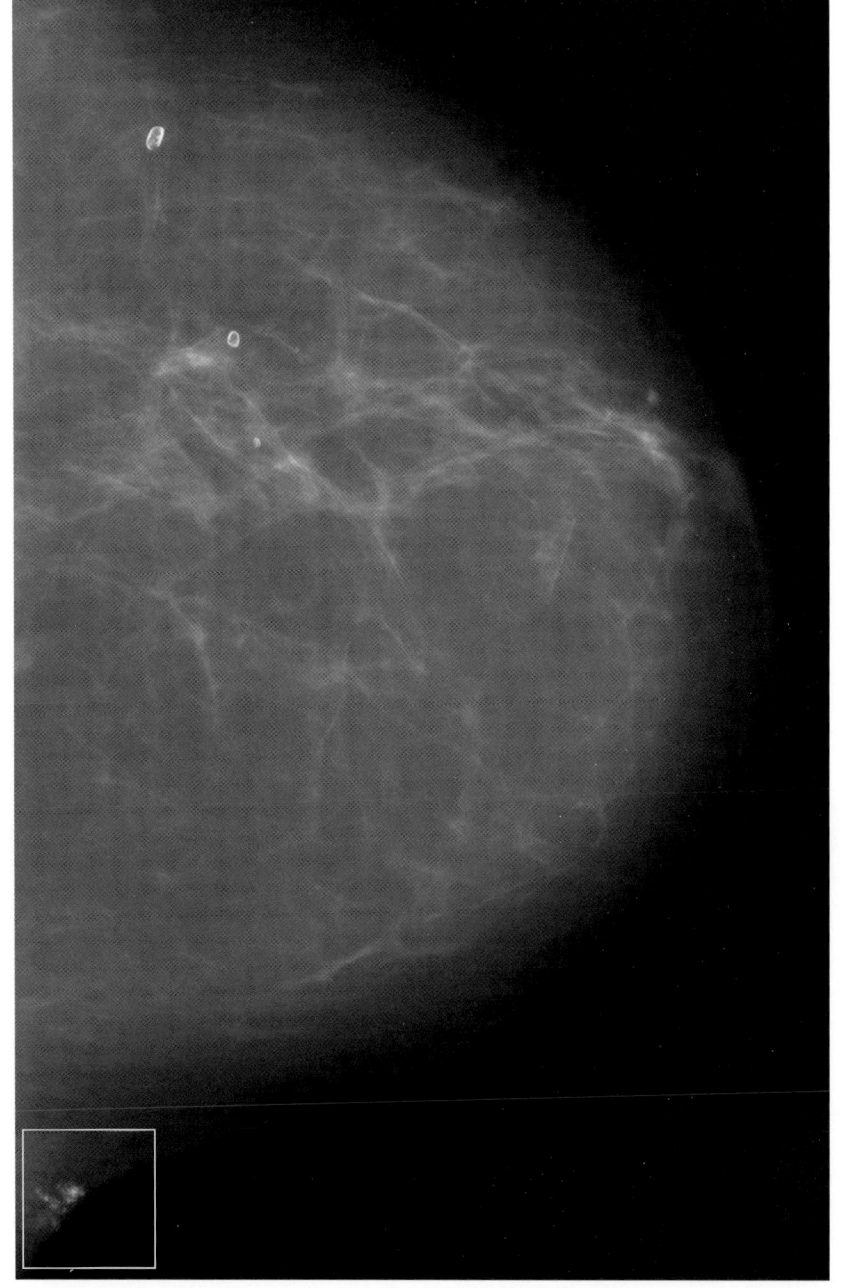

Lateral projection (B)

Skin calcifications

Small lucent-centred spheres, 1-2 mm wide with a "binocular" or "trifolium" appearance, occasionally coalescing, are visible at the periphery of the lower medial quadrant (A). These deposits, which are due to calcified sebaceous glands, project into the skin, as in these tangential views of the skin (B).

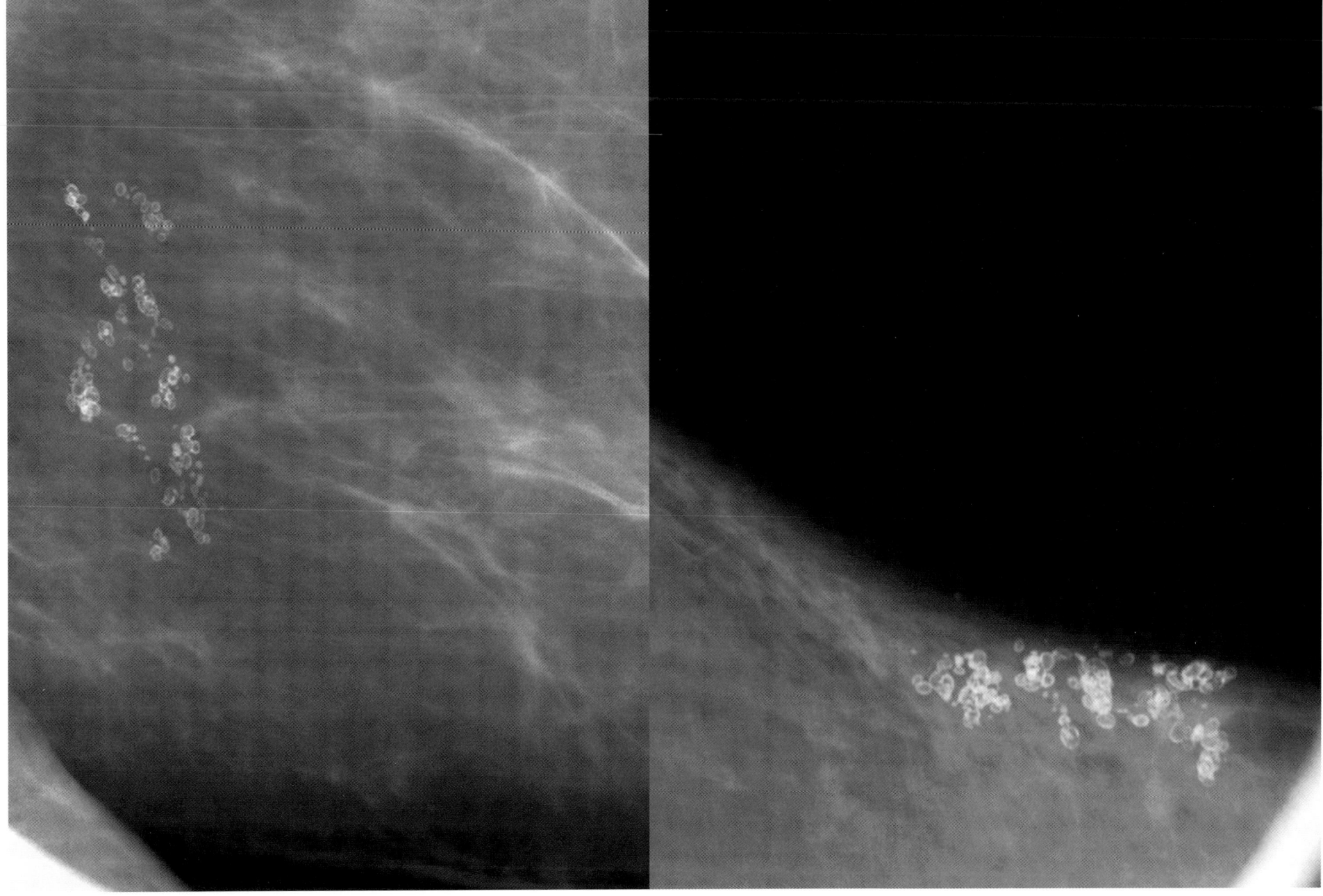

Lateral magnification view (A)

Tangential craniocaudal magnification view (B)

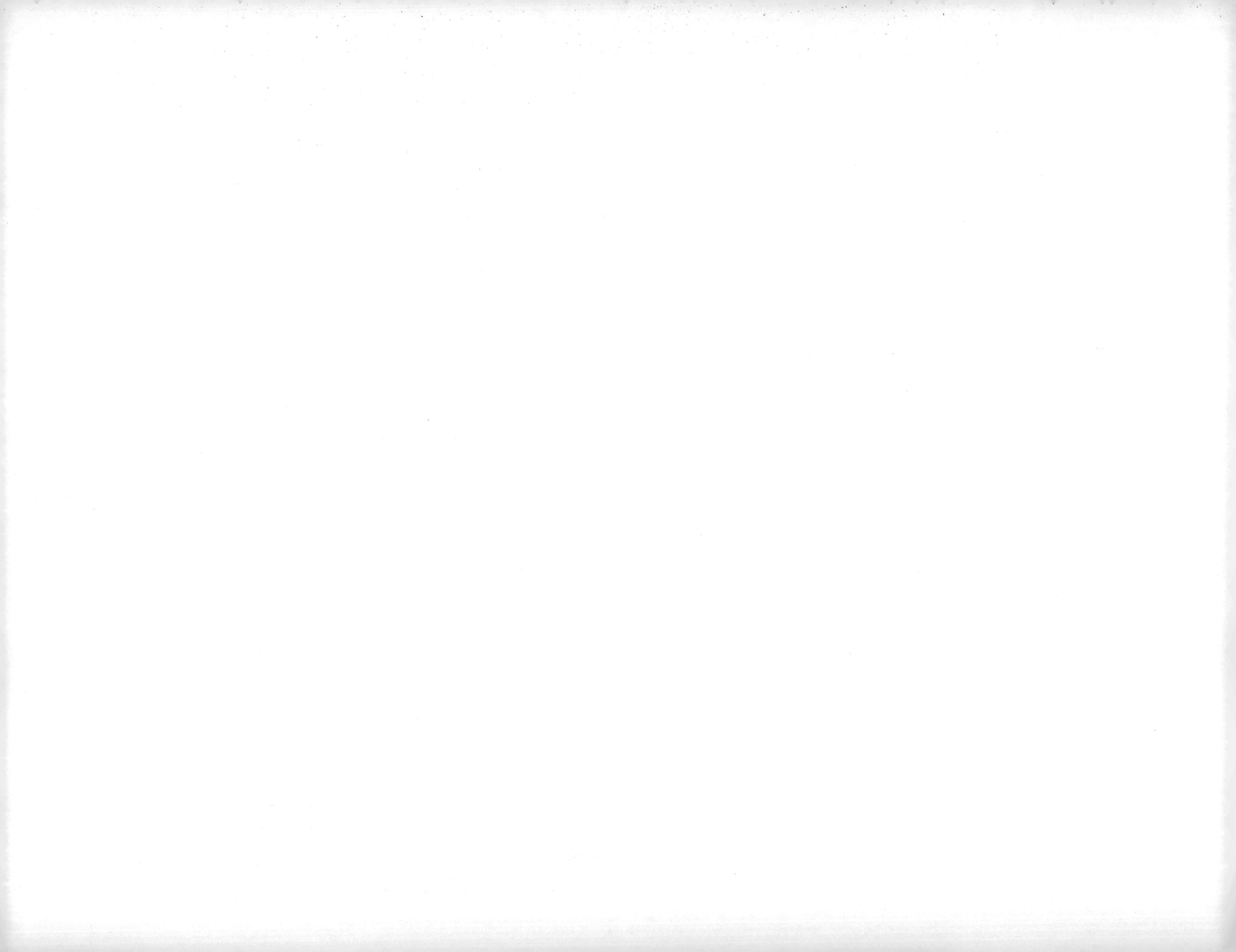

Pseudocalcifications

This group includes artifacts caused by: a) aluminium-based deodorizers in the armpit, b) talcum powder in the submammary groove or medial location area, c) particles of film emulsion caused by roller marks or spoiled chemicals and d) dust or scratches on the screen.

PROBABLY BENIGN CALCIFICATIONS

Pseudocalcifications
Numerous, small, low-density, flake-like calcified masses, occasionally coalescing, are seen deep in the lower inner quadrant, close to the submammary groove. These are caused by talcum powder.

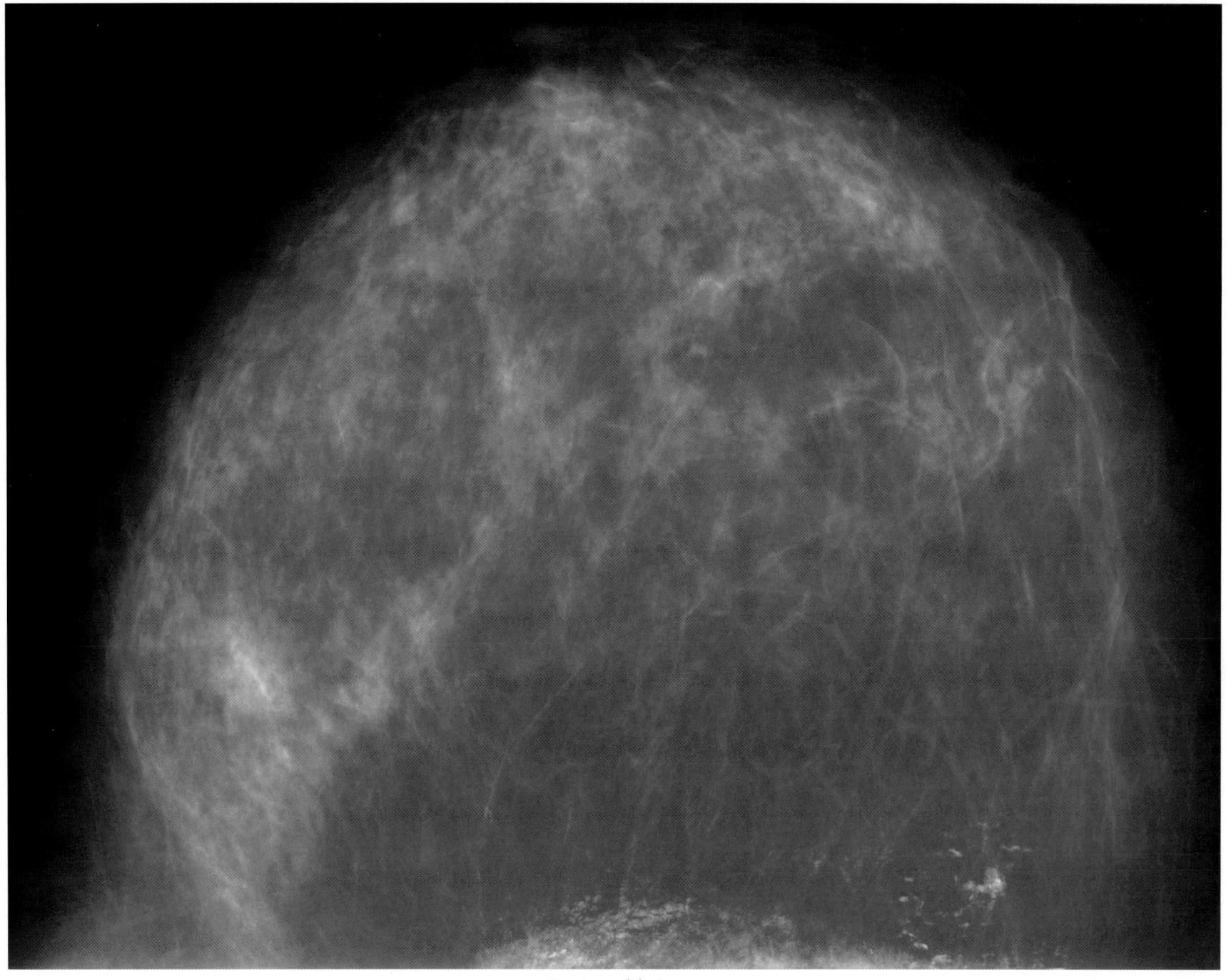

Craniocaudal view

Pseudocalcifications

Numerous, small, low-density, flake-like calcified masses, occasionally coalescing, are seen deep in the lower inner quadrant, close to the submammary groove. These are caused by talcum powder.

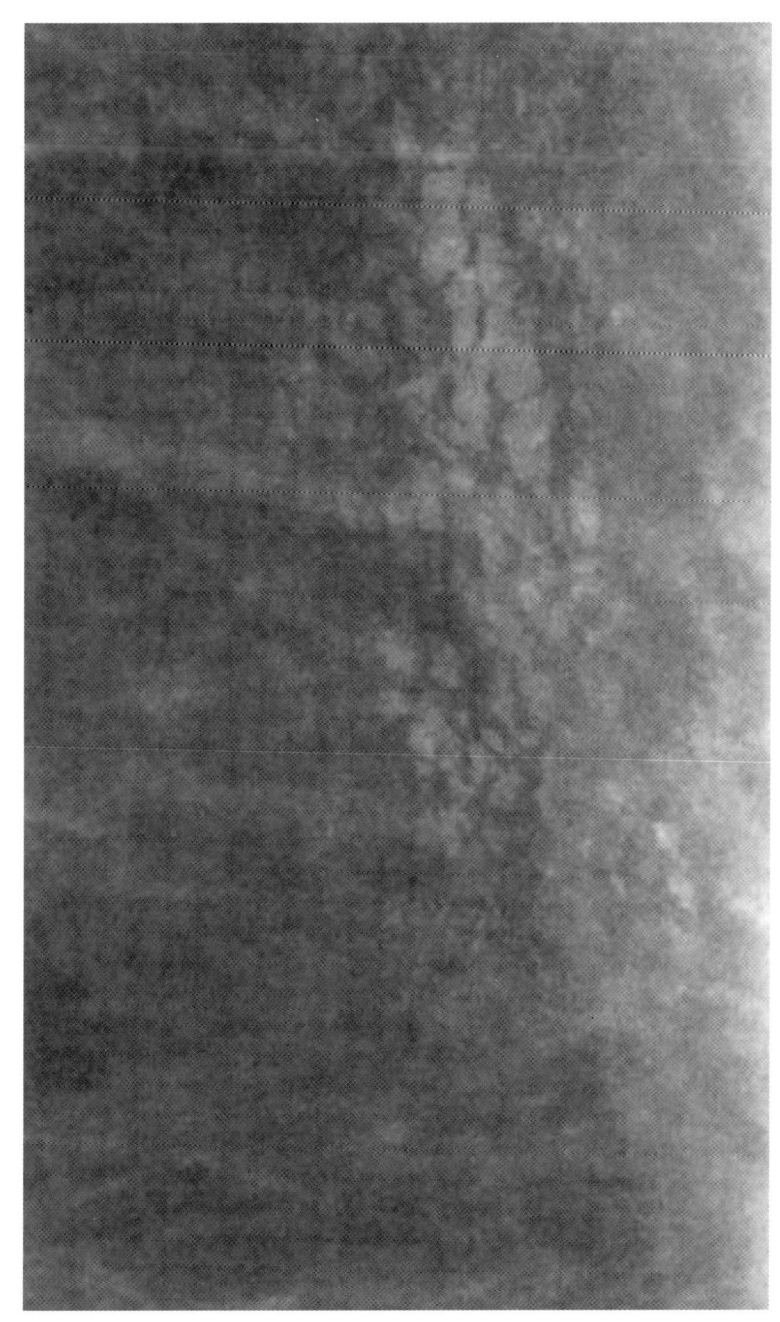

Craniocaudal magnification view

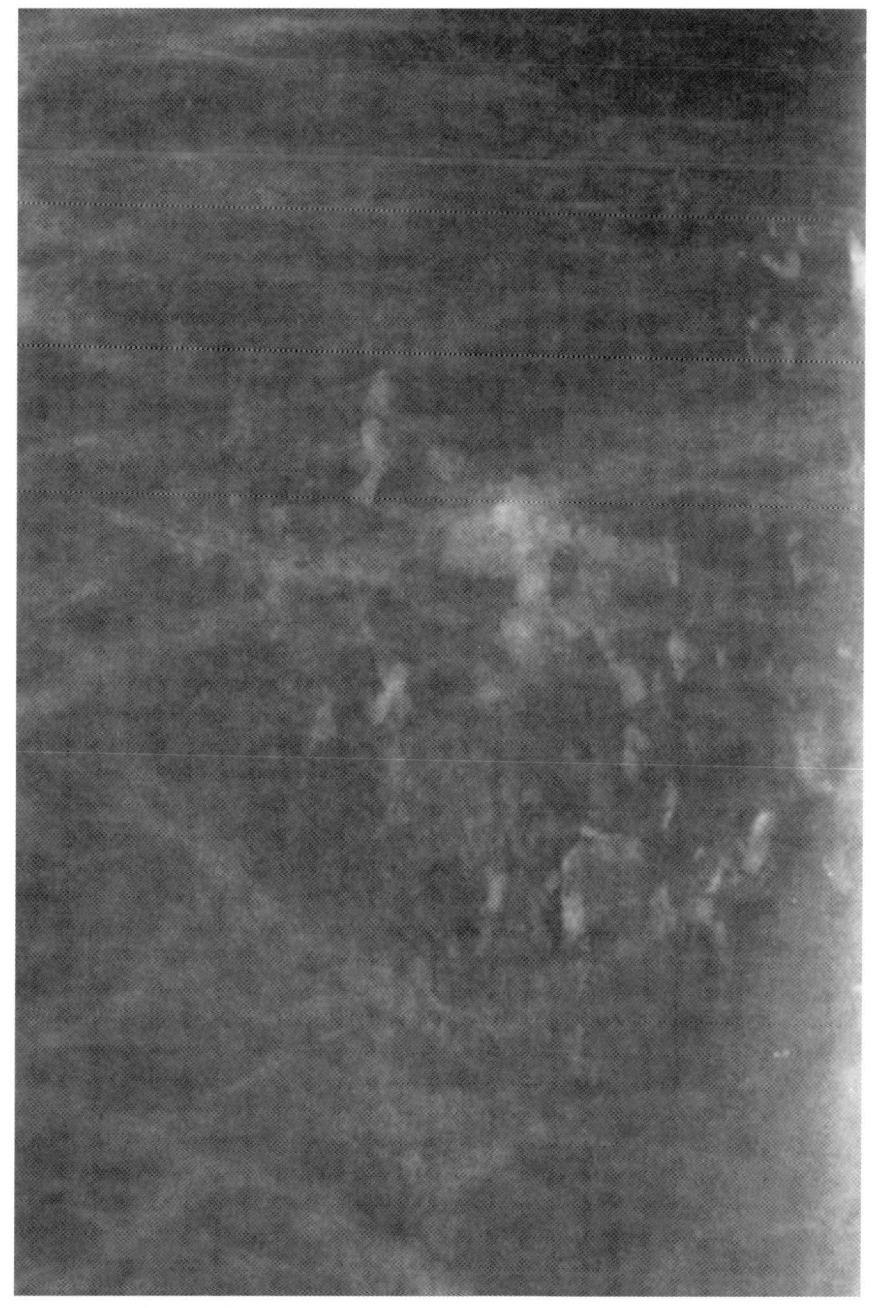

Craniocaudal magnification view

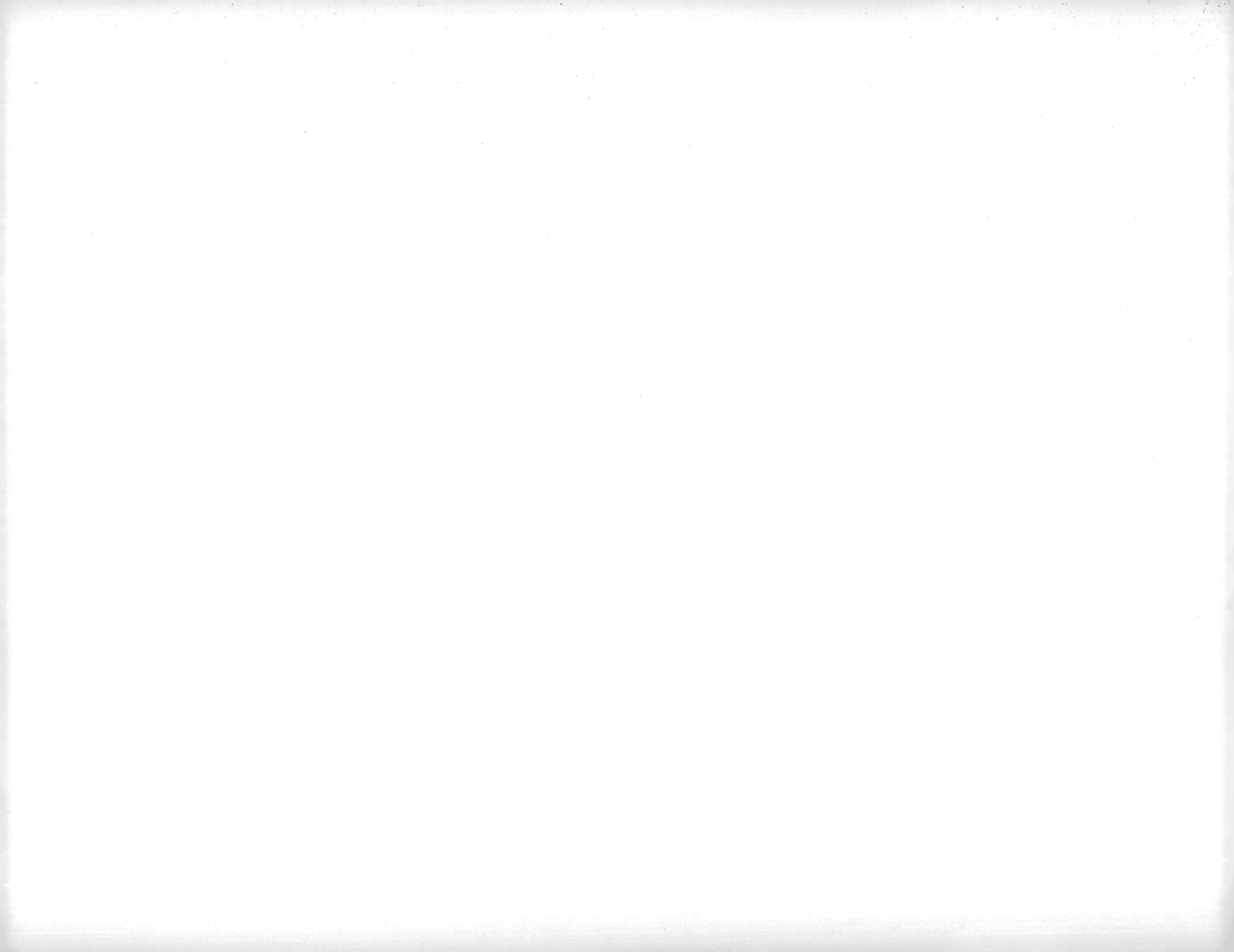

Doubtful or indeterminate calcifications

- *powdery or punctate*
- *round*
- *granular type*

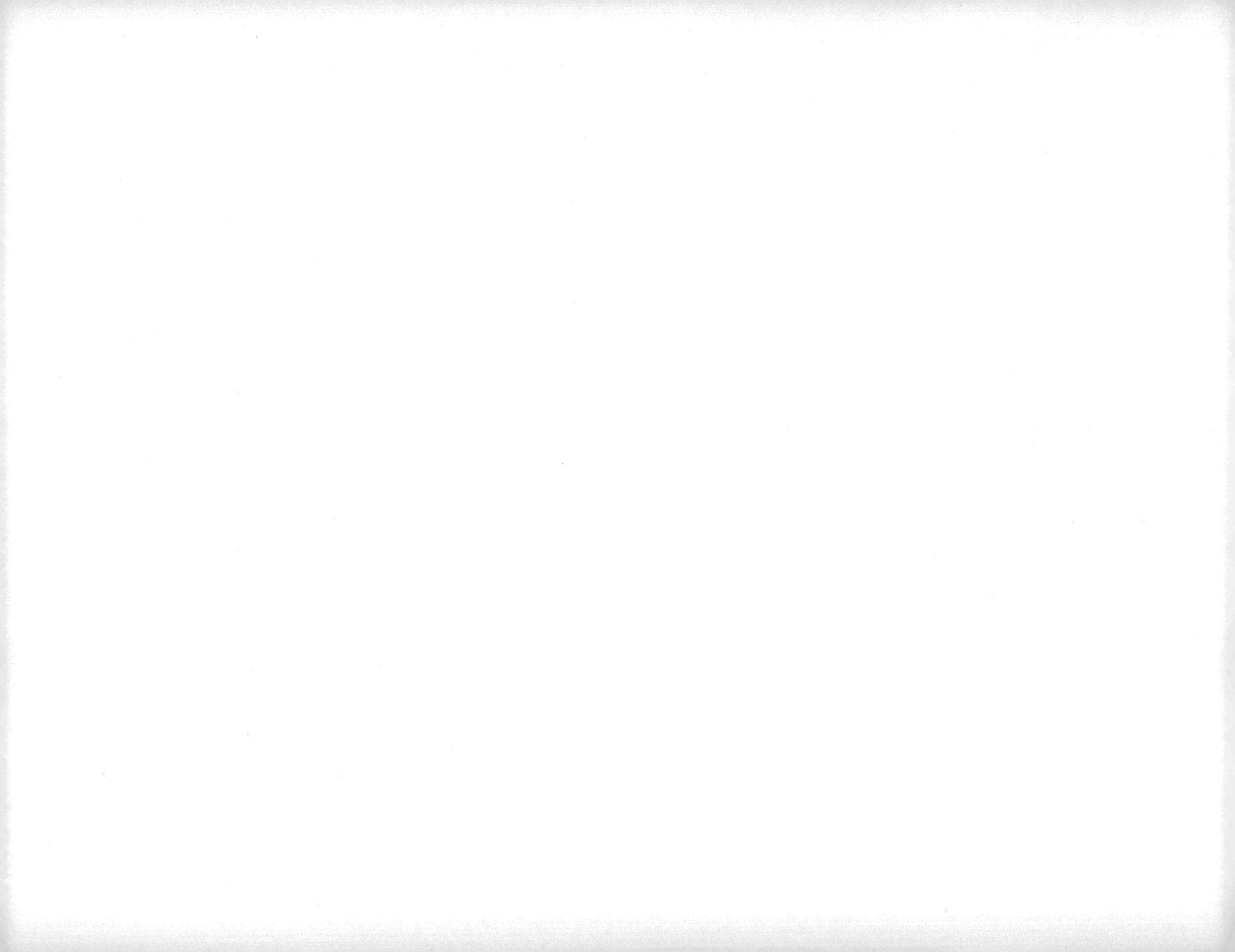

Powdery or punctate calcifications

Punctate calcifications are extremely small (less than 0.5 mm in diameter), often barely perceptible, round or oval, and of low density. They are usually sharply outlined, occur in clusters or are distributed regionally, and are less commonly diffuse or extensive. Magnification views may help differentiate punctate from granular type calcifications.
They may be found in the fibrous stroma with no certain aetiology. They rarely prove to be cancer or cancer-related.

DOUBTFUL OR INDETERMINATE CALCIFICATIONS

Powdery or punctate calcifications

There is a tiny cluster of barely perceptible punctate, powderish calcifications, in an anterior, upper paraareolar location. Due to their size, therefore, the difficulty of detecting these calcifications is added to the difficulty in classifying them as benign or malignant.

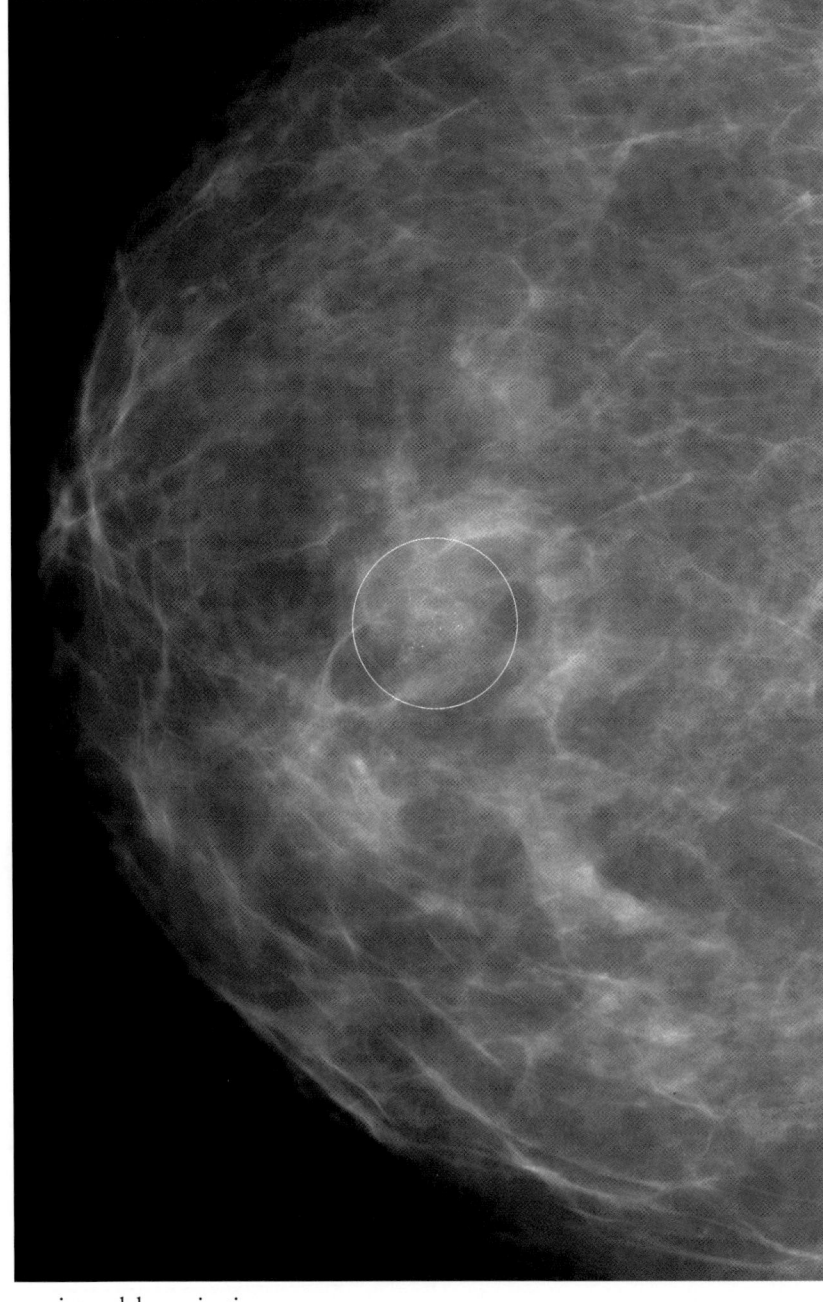

craniocaudal projection

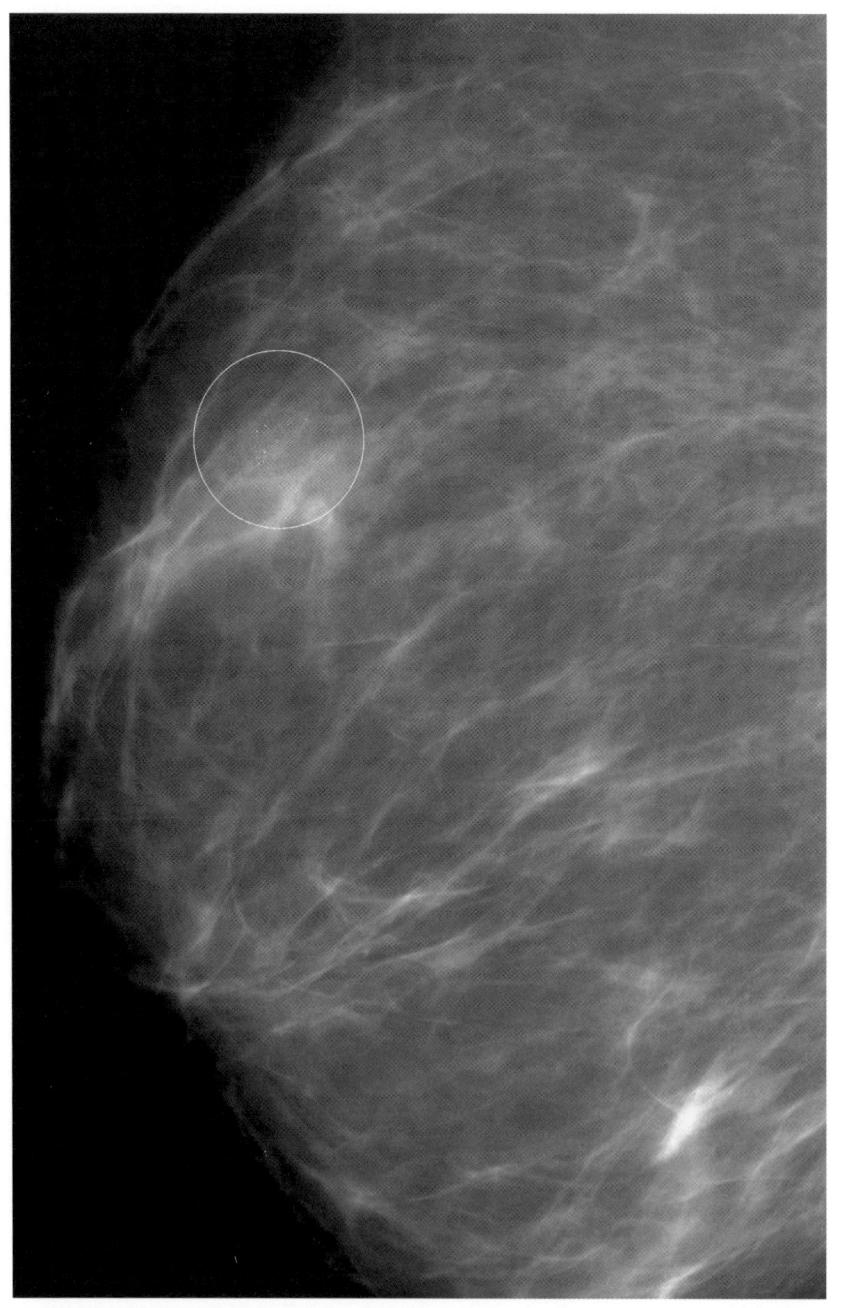

Lateral projection

DOUBTFUL OR INDETERMINATE CALCIFICATIONS

Powdery or punctate calcifications

There is a tiny cluster of barely perceptible, punctate calcifications, in an anterior, upper paraareolar location. The large number of calcified particles and the morphology and overall shape of the collection are best seen in the close-ups and the X-ray of the surgical specimen. Punctate calcifications are sometimes difficult to differentiate from granular type calcifications, but they are generally smaller and tend to coalesce.

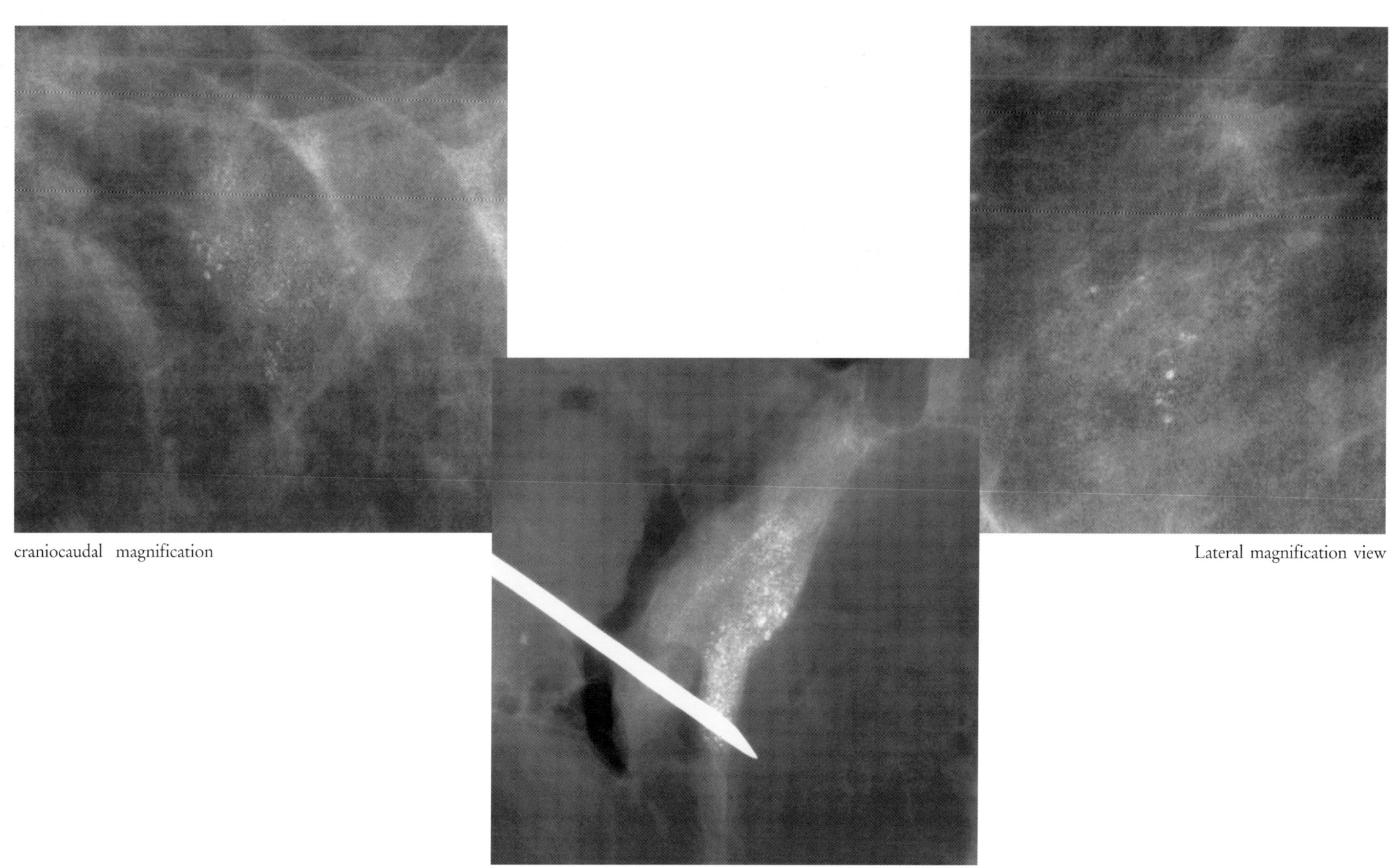

craniocaudal magnification

Lateral magnification view

View and X-ray of biopsy specimen

Histology: ductal hyperplasia without atypias

CALCIFICATIONS

DOUBTFUL OR INDETERMINATE CALCIFICATIONS

Powdery or punctate calcifications

In he medial anterior location there is a tiny cluster of barely visible punctate calcifications, apparently in an area of stromal thickening.

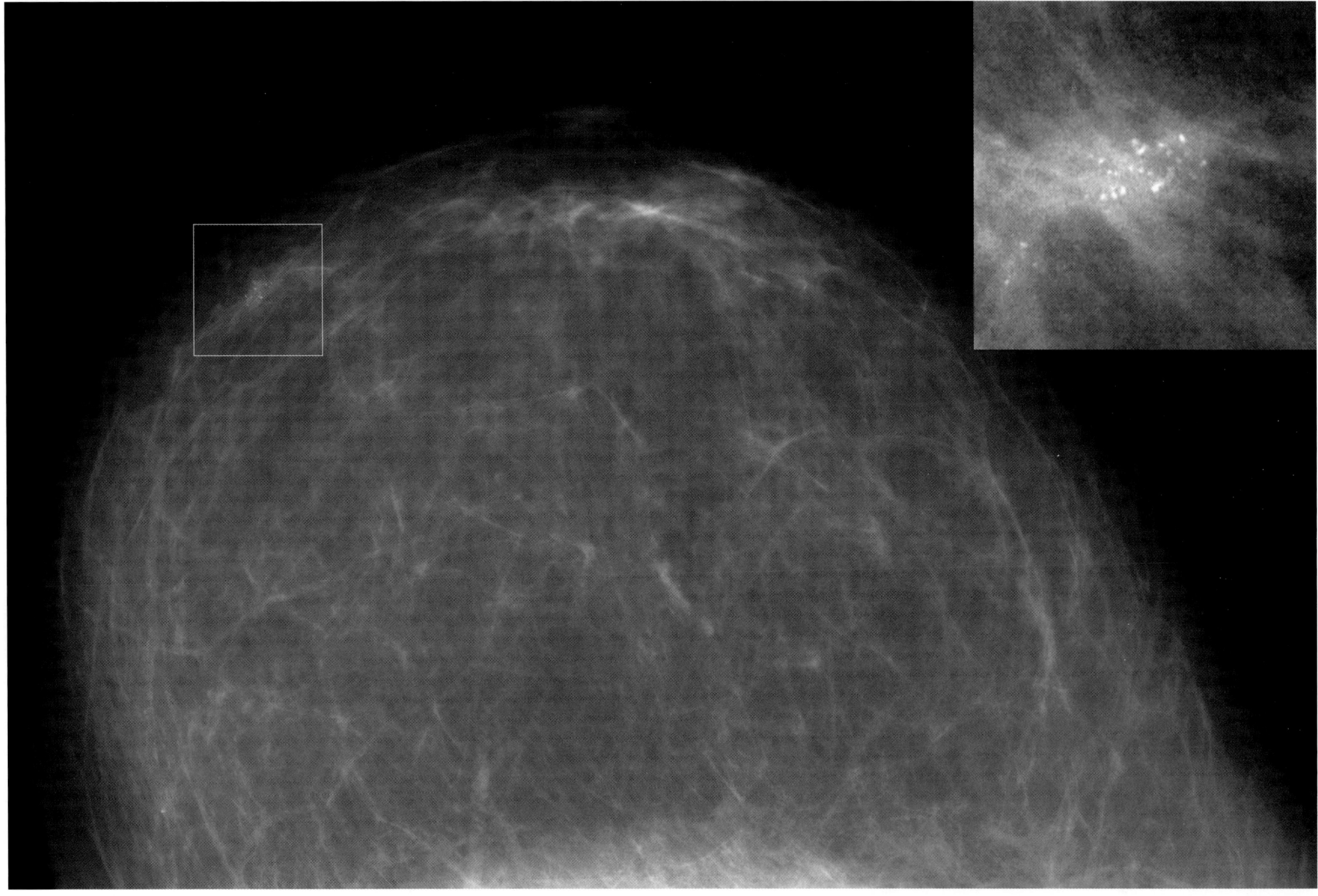

Craniocaudal projection

Powdery or punctate calcifications

This magnification detail shows more clearly the shape and density of these irregular, heterogeneous calcifications with ill-defined margins, located in a small irregularly shaped opacity. Only the size of the individual calcifications and of the cluster may help to distinguish them from granular type calcifications.

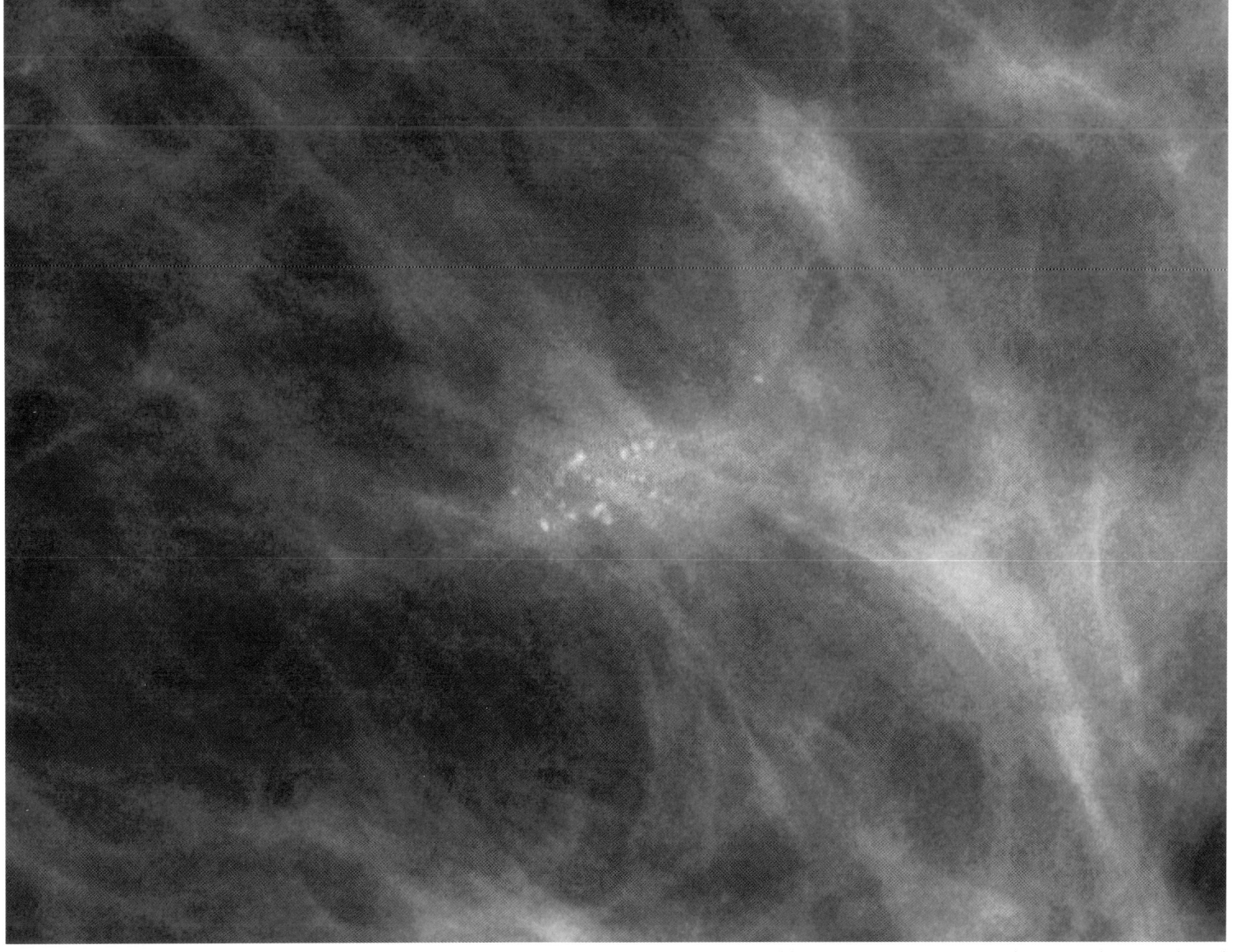

Magnification view

Histology: ductal infiltrating carcinoma, predominantly intraductal

DOUBTFUL OR INDETERMINATE CALCIFICATIONS

Powdery or punctate calcifications
An isolated cluster of punctate calcifications is visible centrally behind the areola.

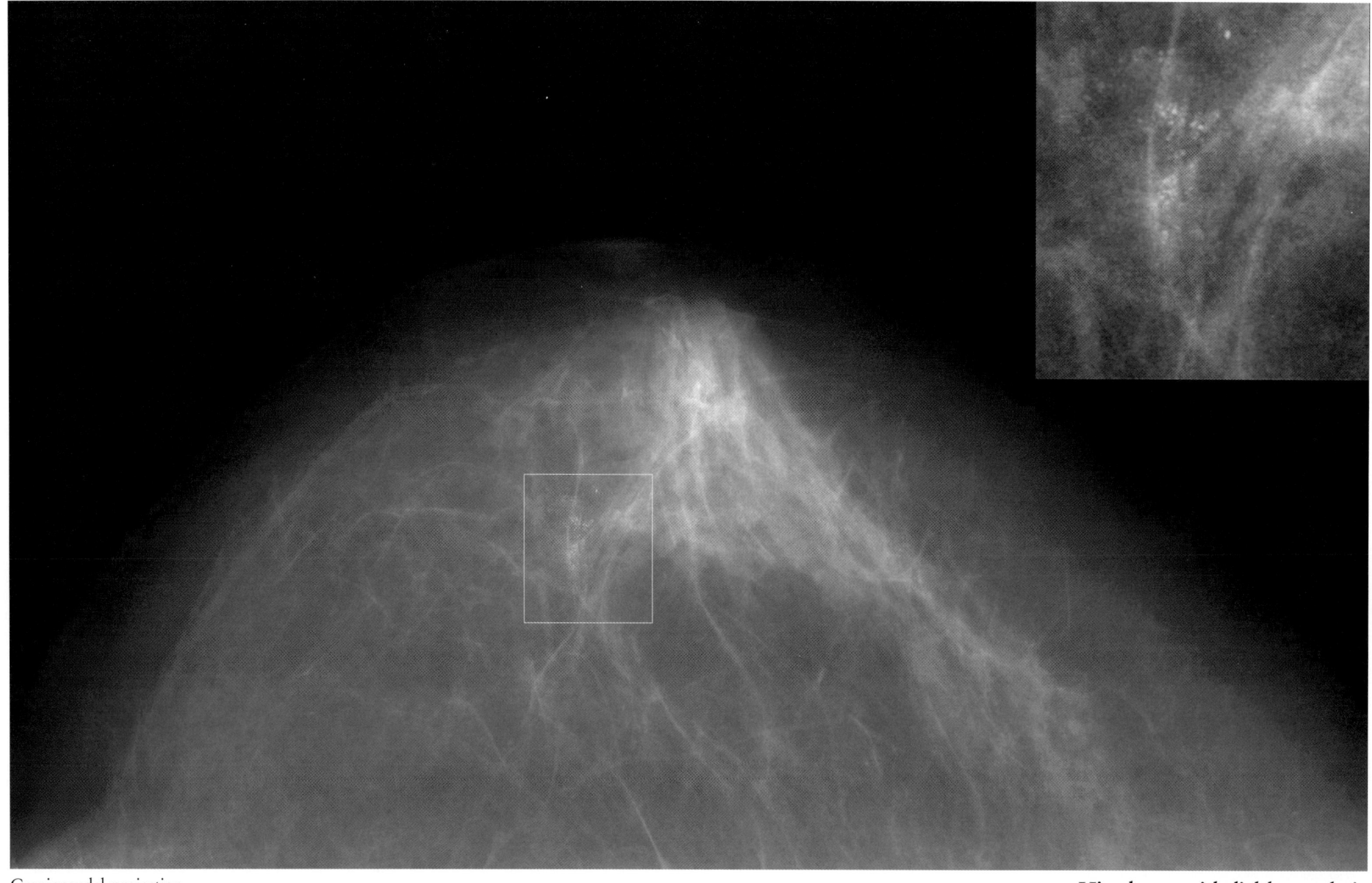

Craniocaudal projection

Histology: epithelial hyperplasia

Powdery or punctate calcifications

These magnification details show more clearly the large number and the morphology of the sharply outlined, spherical, uniformly dense calcified particles, and the shape of the whole cluster.

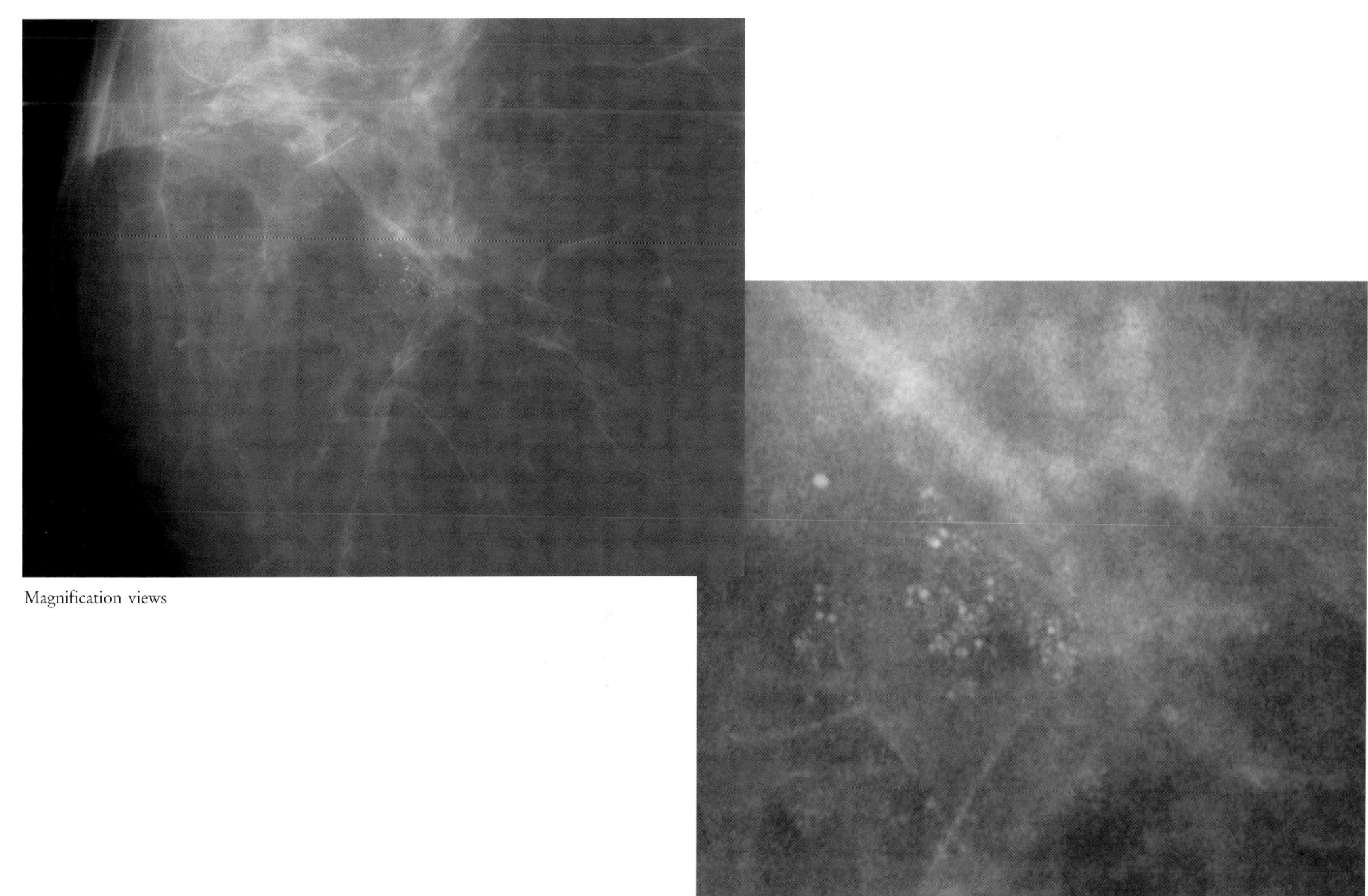

Magnification views

Histology: epithelial hyperplasia

DOUBTFUL OR INDETERMINATE CALCIFICATIONS

Powdery or punctate calcifications
Spread widely in the breast, behind the areola, are numerous barely perceptible punctate calcifications.

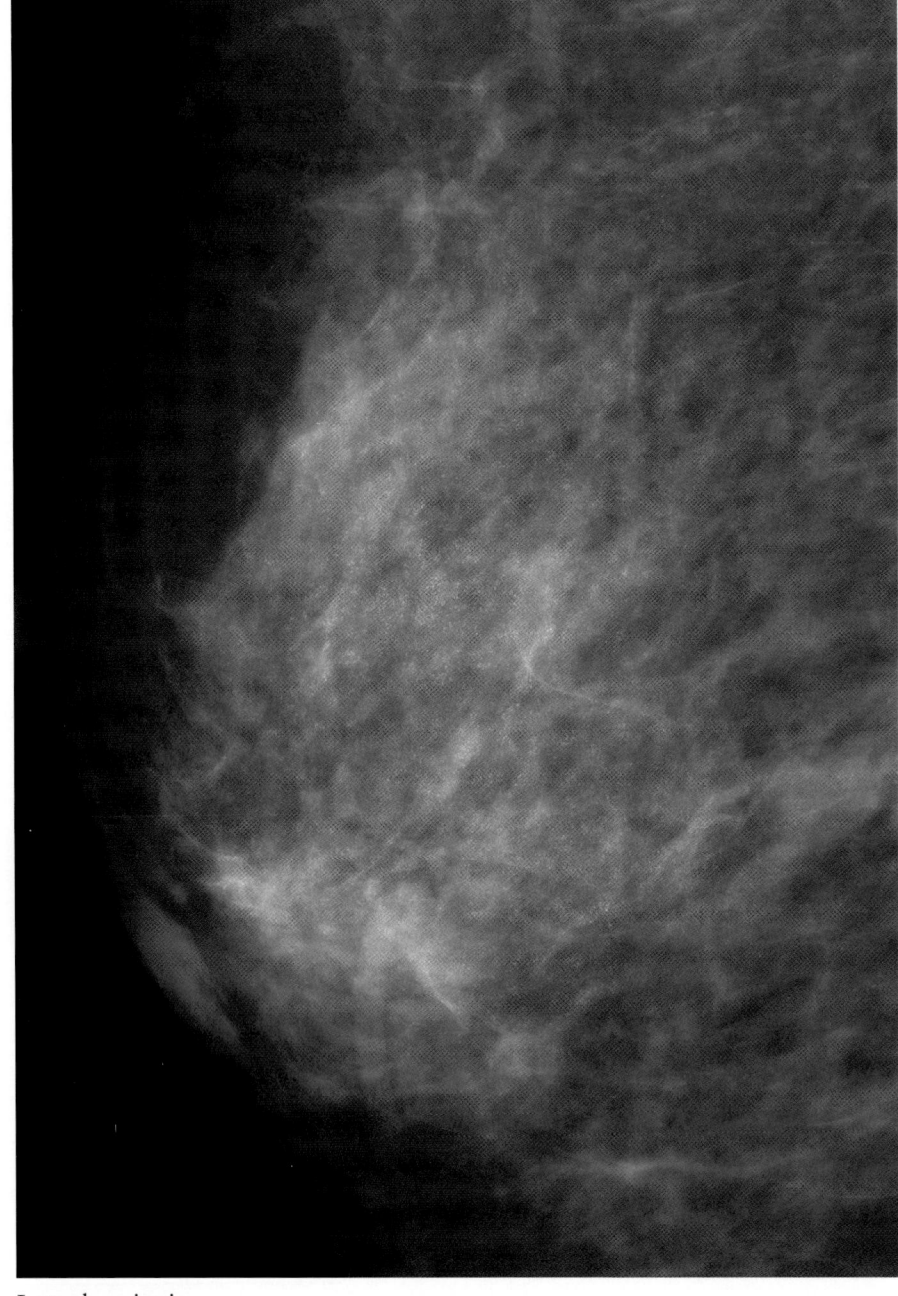

Lateral magnification view

Lateral projection

Round calcifications

Round, smooth sharply outlined, ("pearl-like") calcifications of various sizes are found in the acini of lobules, often grouped in clusters. When they are smaller than 0.5 mm they should be called "punctate" or "powderish".

DOUBTFUL OR INDETERMINATE CALCIFICATIONS

Round calcifications

Round calcifications varying in density and shape are scattered within the breast. In this a context, as seen in the magnification views, some areas show calcifications very difficult to classify.

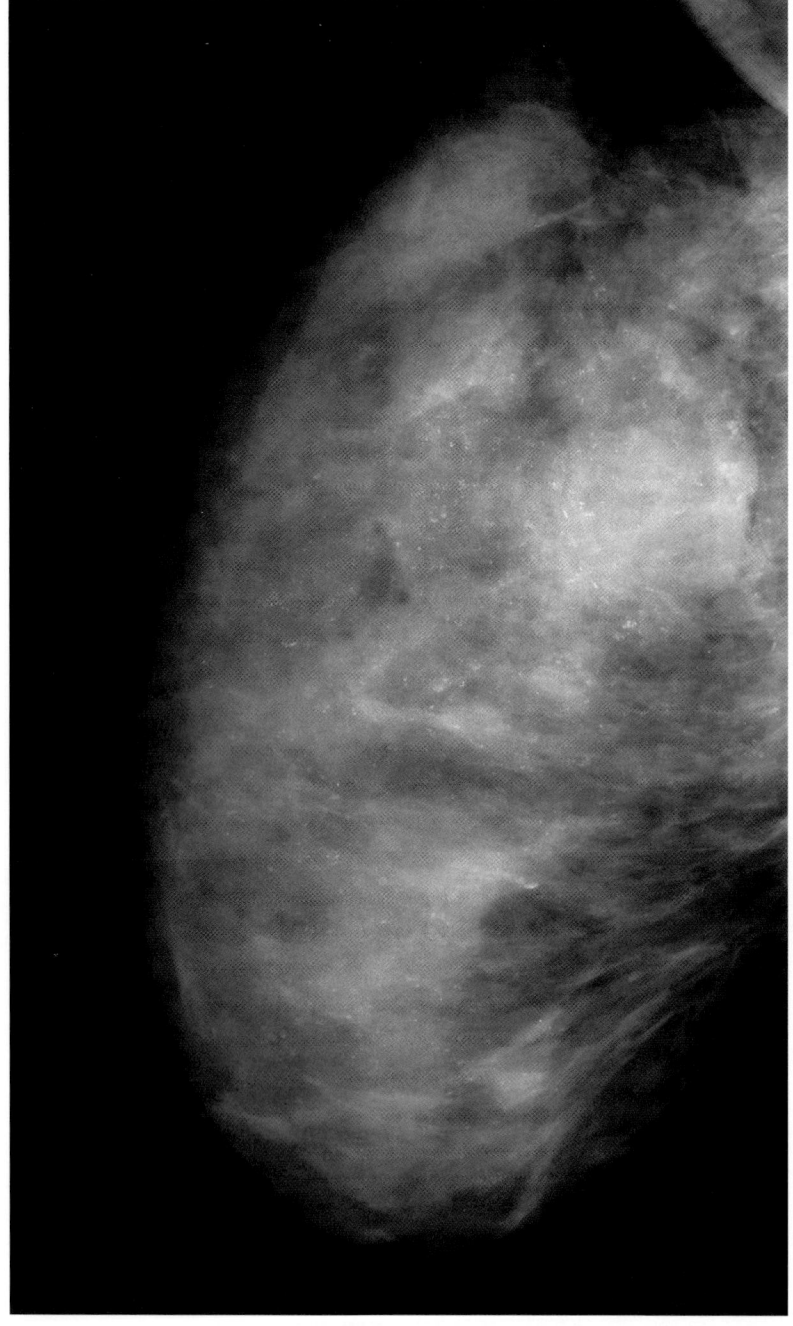

Lateral projection

Magnification views

DOUBTFUL OR INDETERMINATE CALCIFICATIONS

Round calcifications
Numerous round calcifications of varying density with regional distribution are seen in these magnification views.

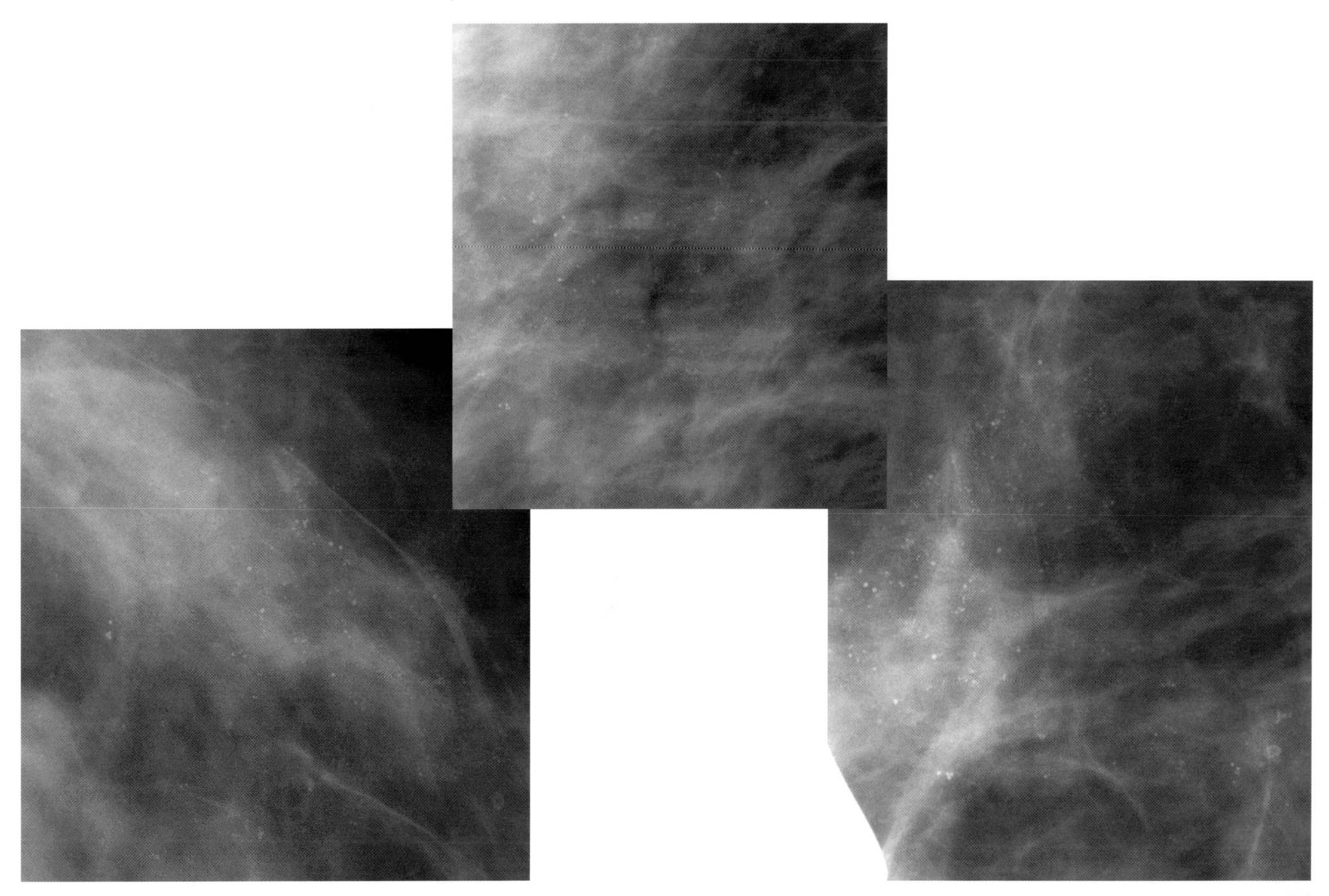

DOUBTFUL OR INDETERMINATE CALCIFICATIONS

Round calcifications

Roundish calcifications, variable in shape and density, appear to be clustered in the upper portion of the breast. A few elongated, crescent shaped calcifications are associated.

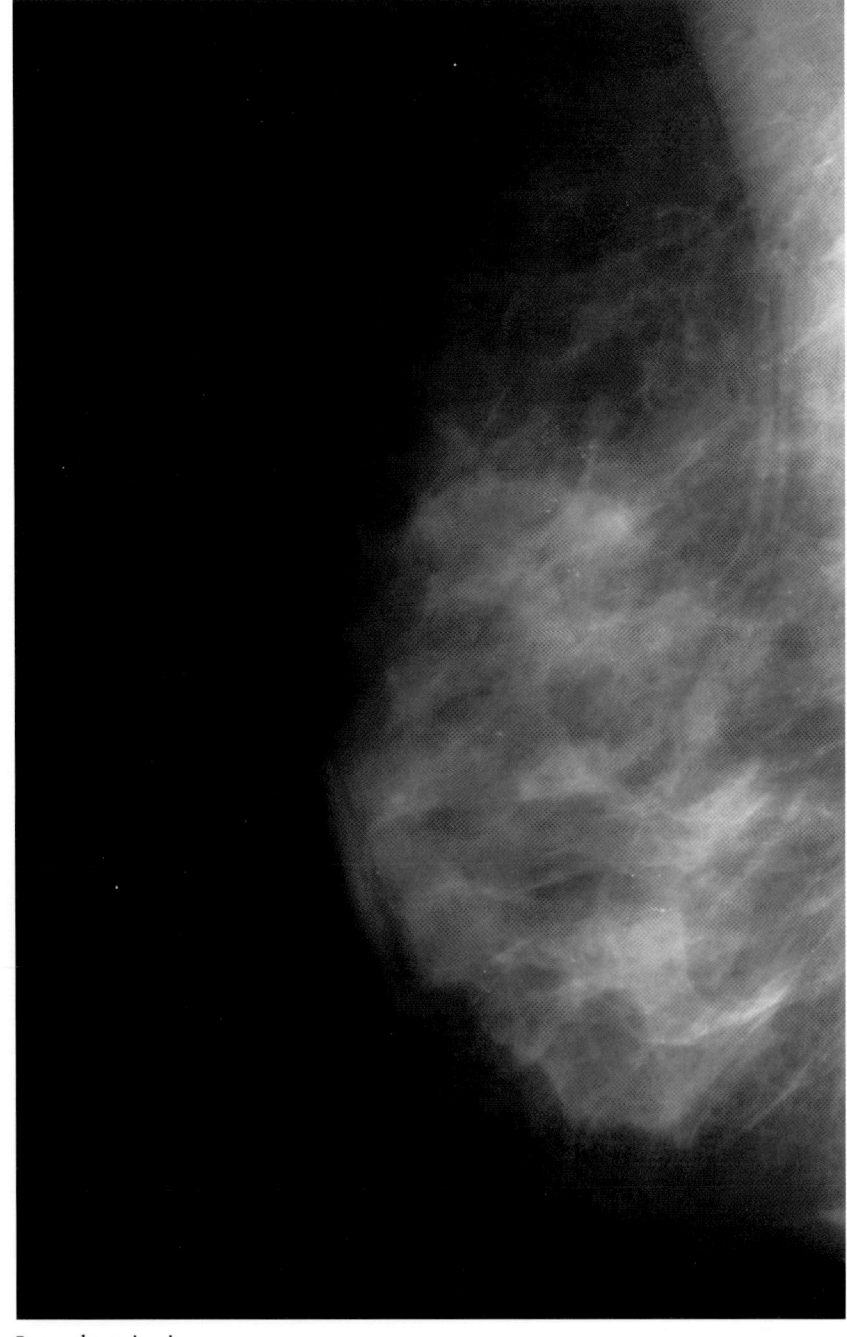

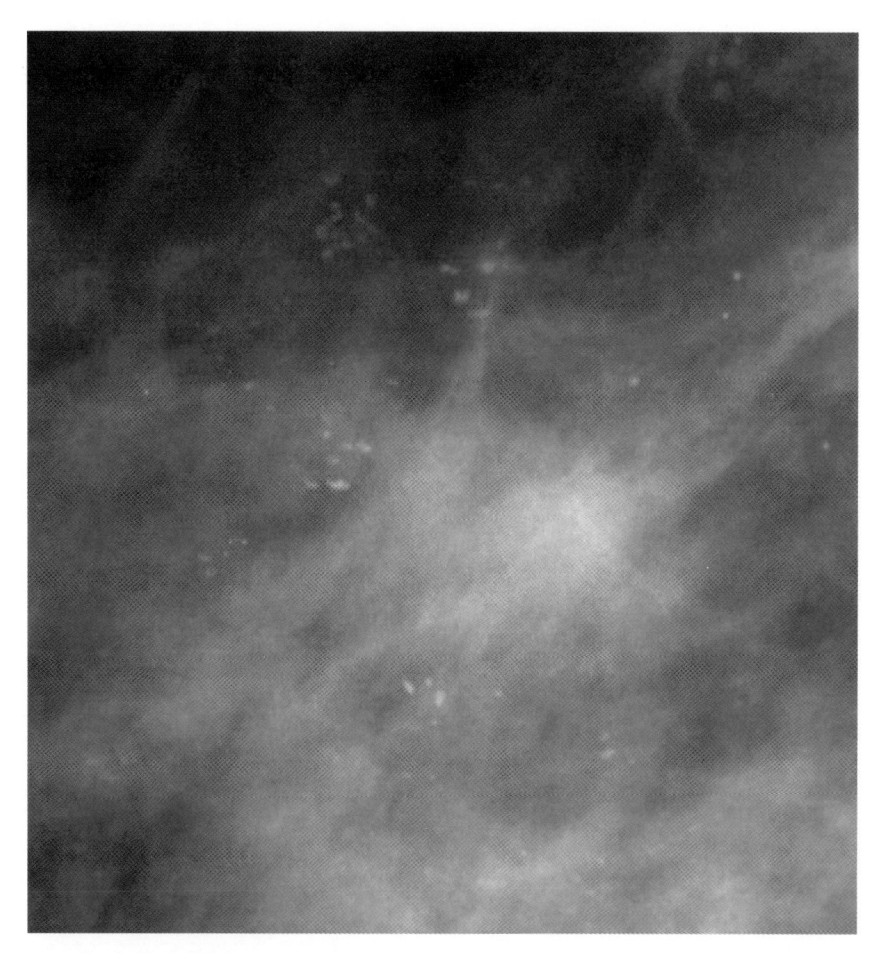

Detail of the lateral projection

Lateral projection

Round calcifications

These magnification details show calcifications varying in shape from round to granular and "milk-of-calcium". This finding is not easy to interpret. Follow-up at two years shows no morphological or structural changes.

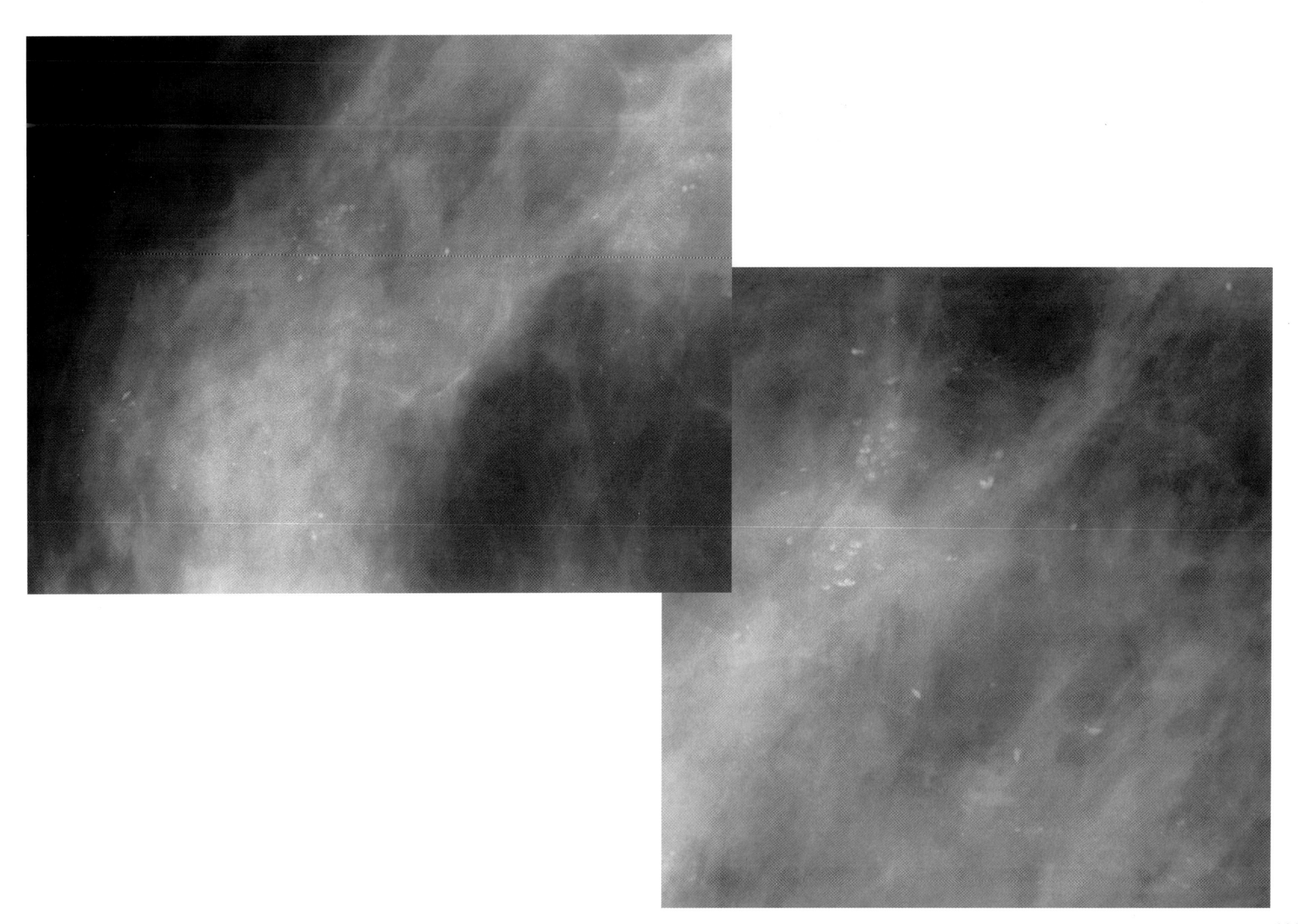

DOUBTFUL OR INDETERMINATE CALCIFICATIONS

Round calcifications
Diffuse, round calcifications, varying in density and morphology. In the lowerouter quadrant in a posterior location there appear to be clustered calcifications, not easy to classify. A circumscribed, oval opacity with coarse calcifications along the contour is visible in the upper outer quadrant.

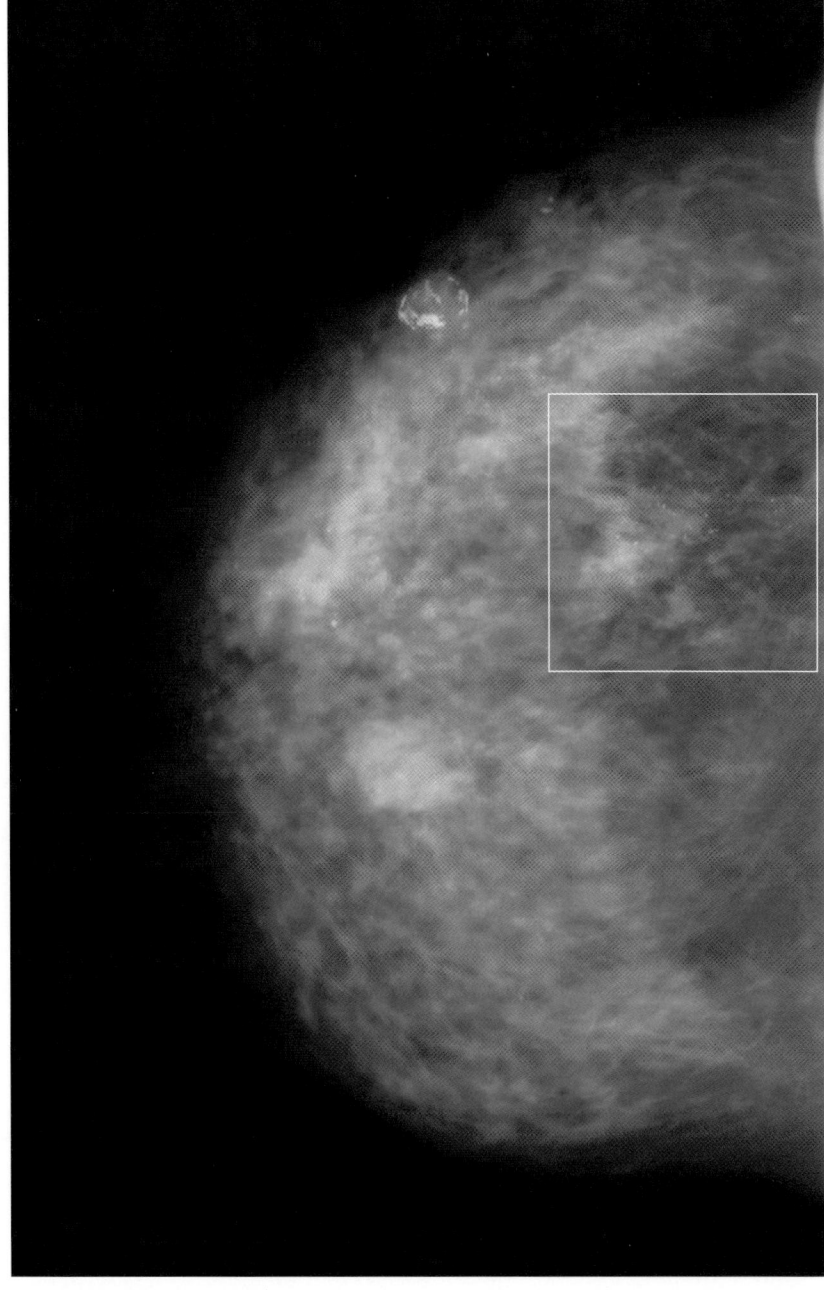

Craniocaudal projection

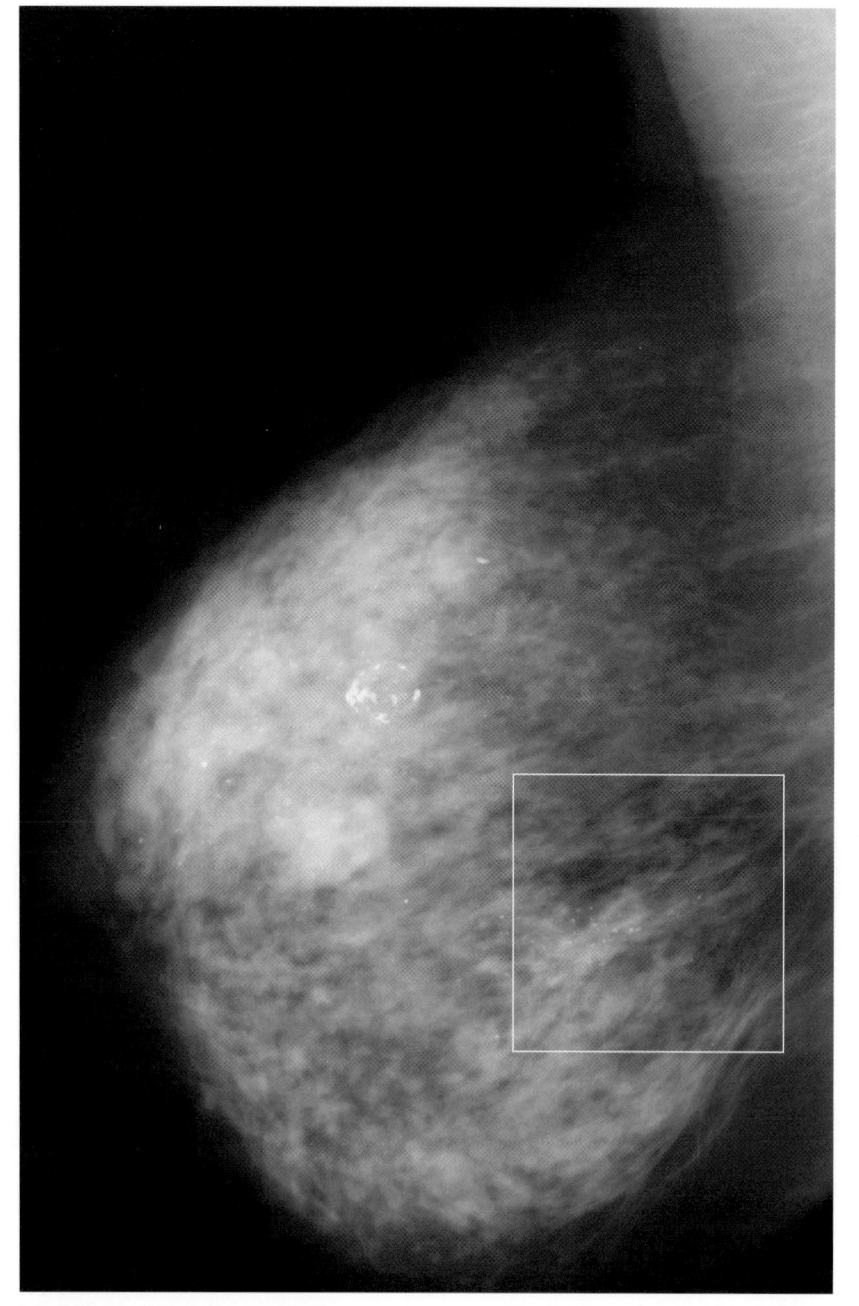

Mediolateral oblique projection

DOUBTFUL OR INDETERMINATE CALCIFICATIONS

Round calcifications

These magnification details show calcifications varying in shape from round to granular type and "milk-of-calcium", with distribution that to be more likely regional. This finding is not easy to interpret. Follow-up at three years shows no morphological or structural changes.

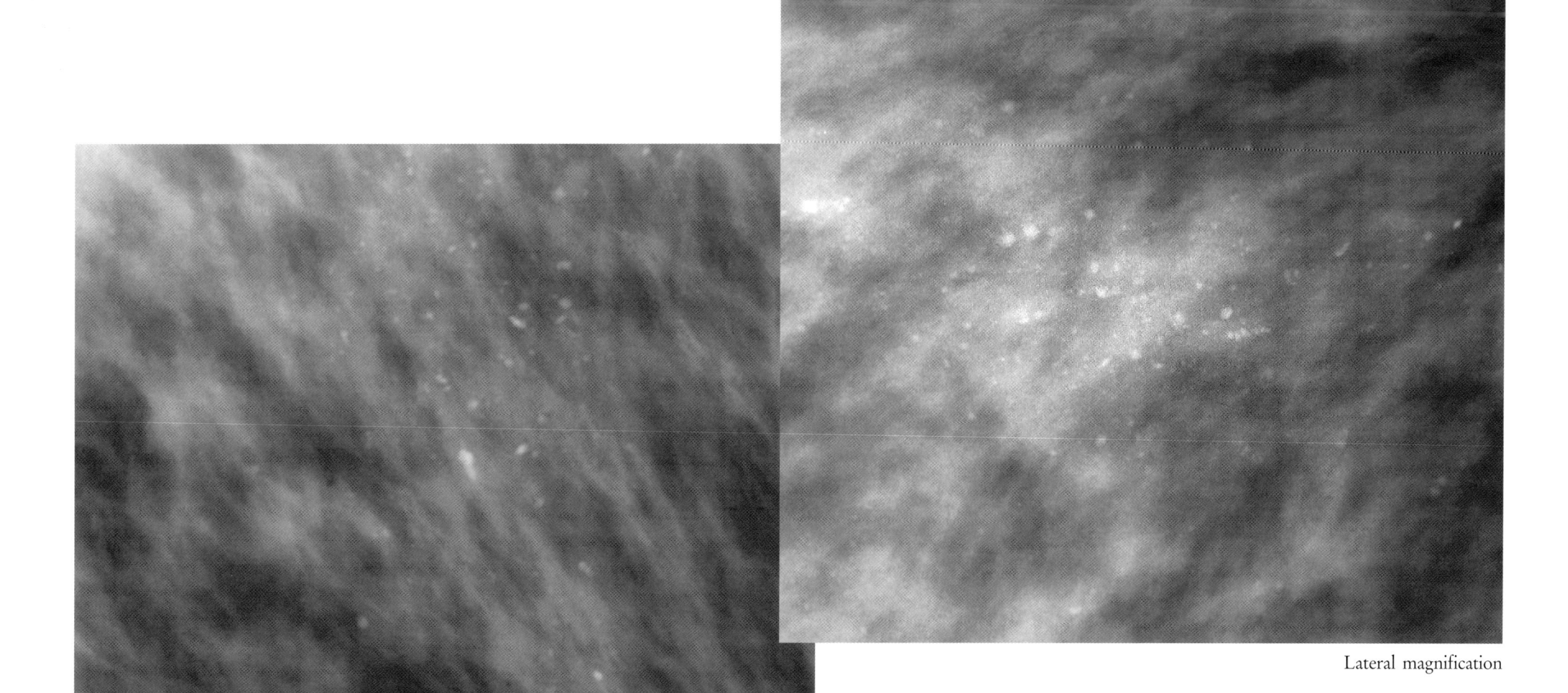

Lateral magnification

Craniocaudal magnification

Histology: epithelial hyperplasia

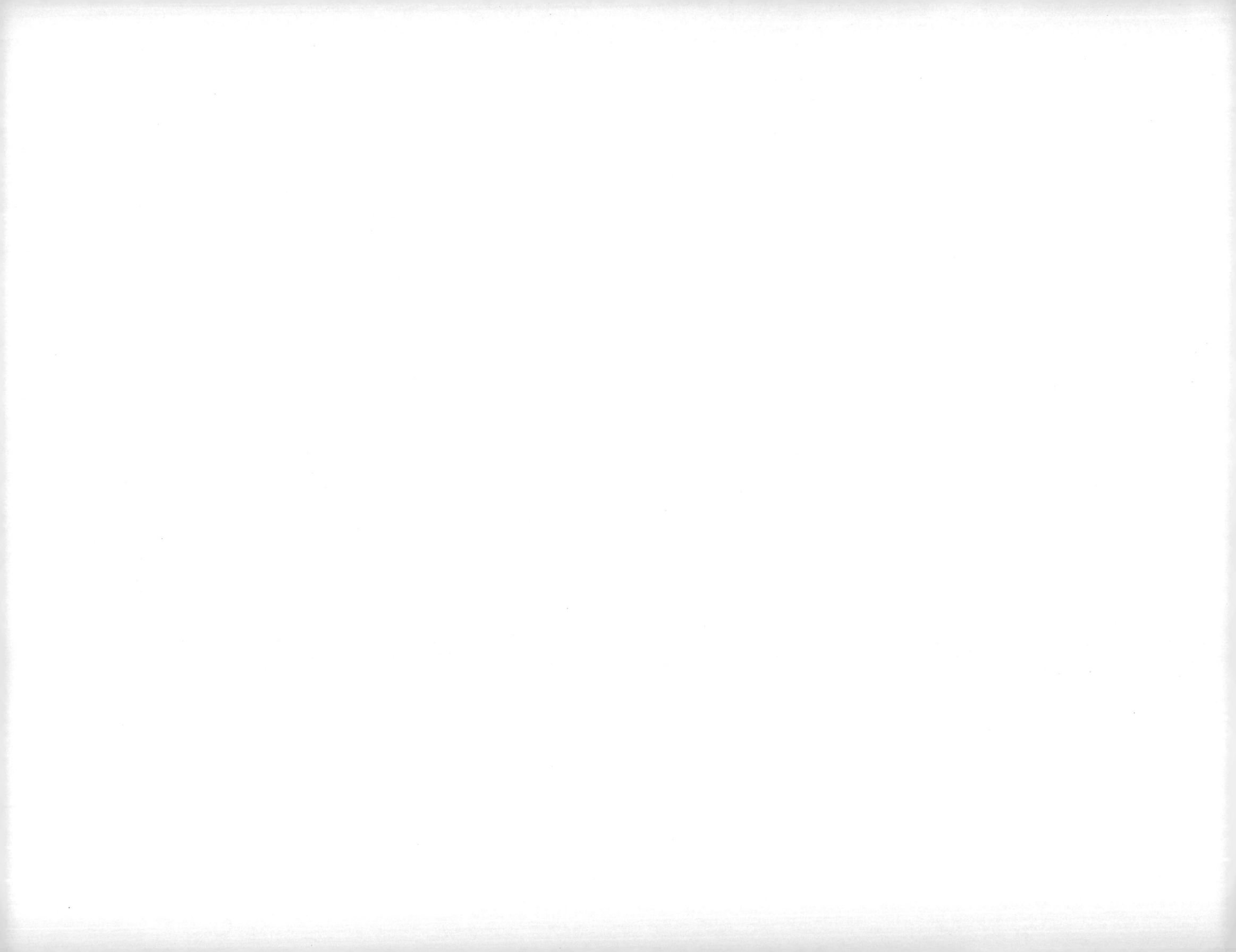

Granular type calcifications

Granular type calcifications (BI-RADS: pleomorphic, heterogeneous) are irregular, highly dense and may look like "crushed stones", "iron filings", or fine "grains of salt". They generally form in clusters, sometimes multiple groupings. When their distribution is segmental or diffusely scattered, they may not be readily distinguishable from dysplastic calcifications. When their density is somehow lower and morphology relatively homogeneus, they often cannot be differentiated from round or "milk-of-calcium" calcifications.

DOUBTFUL OR INDETERMINATE CALCIFICATIONS

Granular type calcifications
Posteriorly in the lower inner quadrant there is a tightly packed cluster of high-density, heterogeneous granular type calcifications, within an ill-defined opacity of the same density as the surrounding parenchyma. Two more similar tiny clusters are visible anteriorly and superiorly. This radiological finding is not easy to interpret.

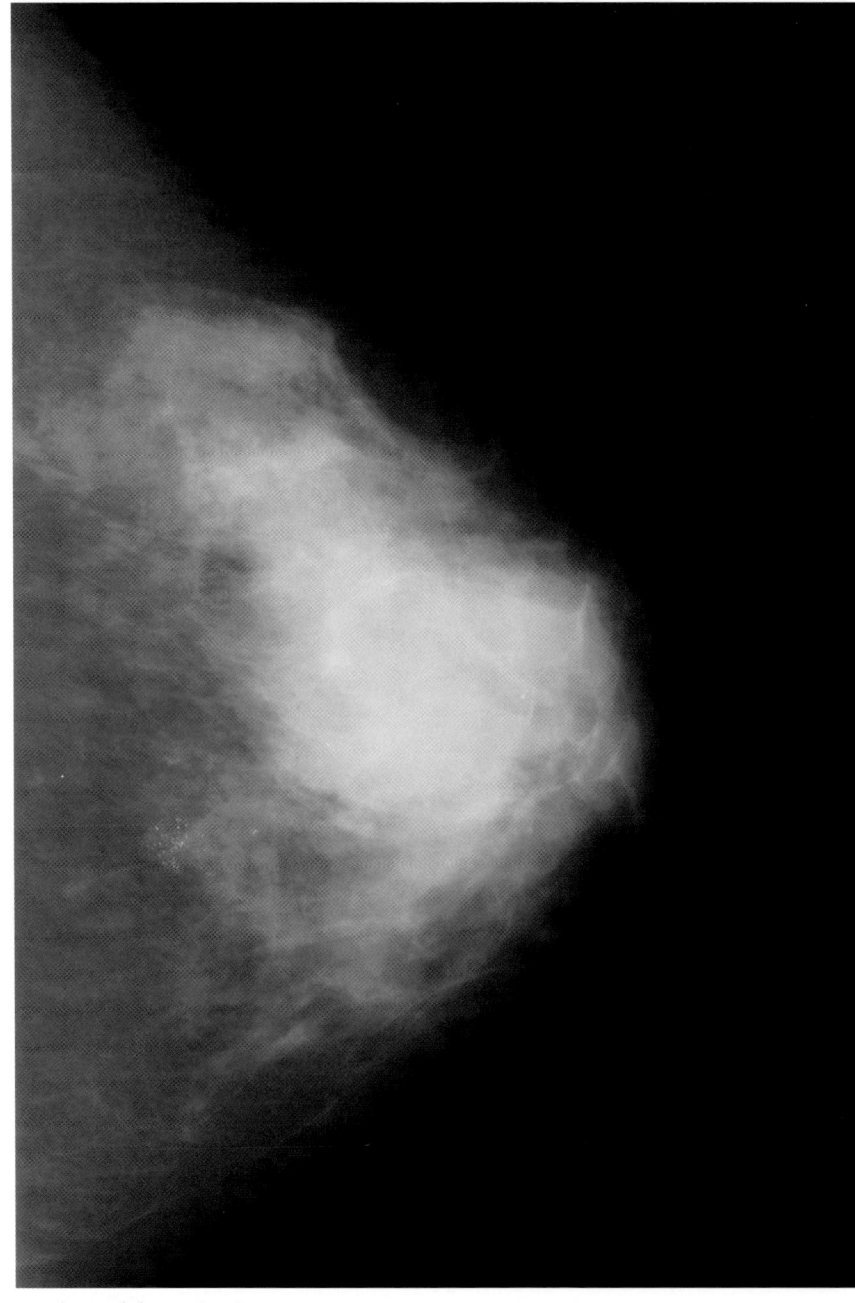

craniocaudal projection

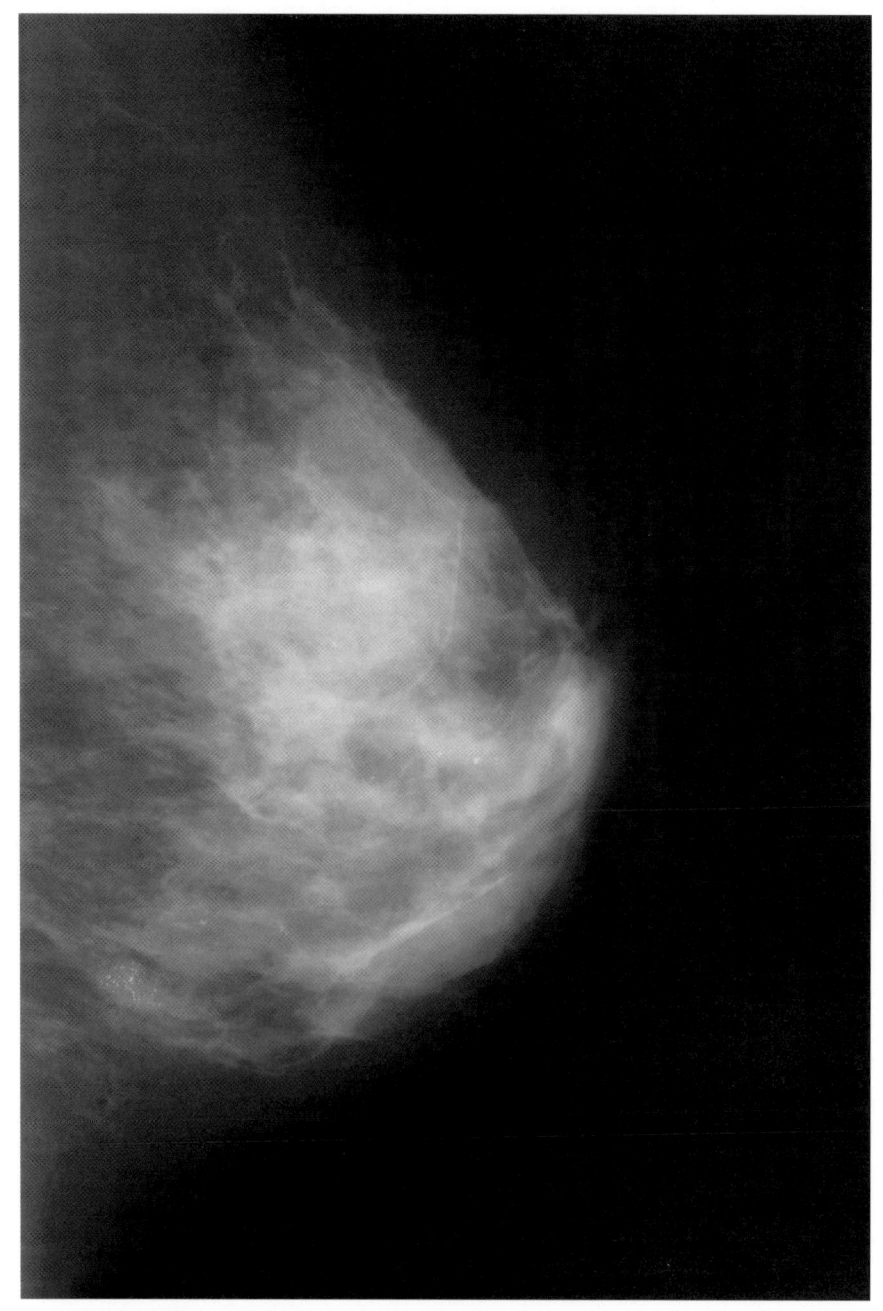

Lateral projection

Granular type calcifications

The tightly packed clusters of high-density, heterogeneous granular type calcifications, within an ill-defined opacity of the same density as the surrounding parenchyma, not visible in all the projections. Two more similar tiny clusters are visible. This radiological finding is not easy to interpret.

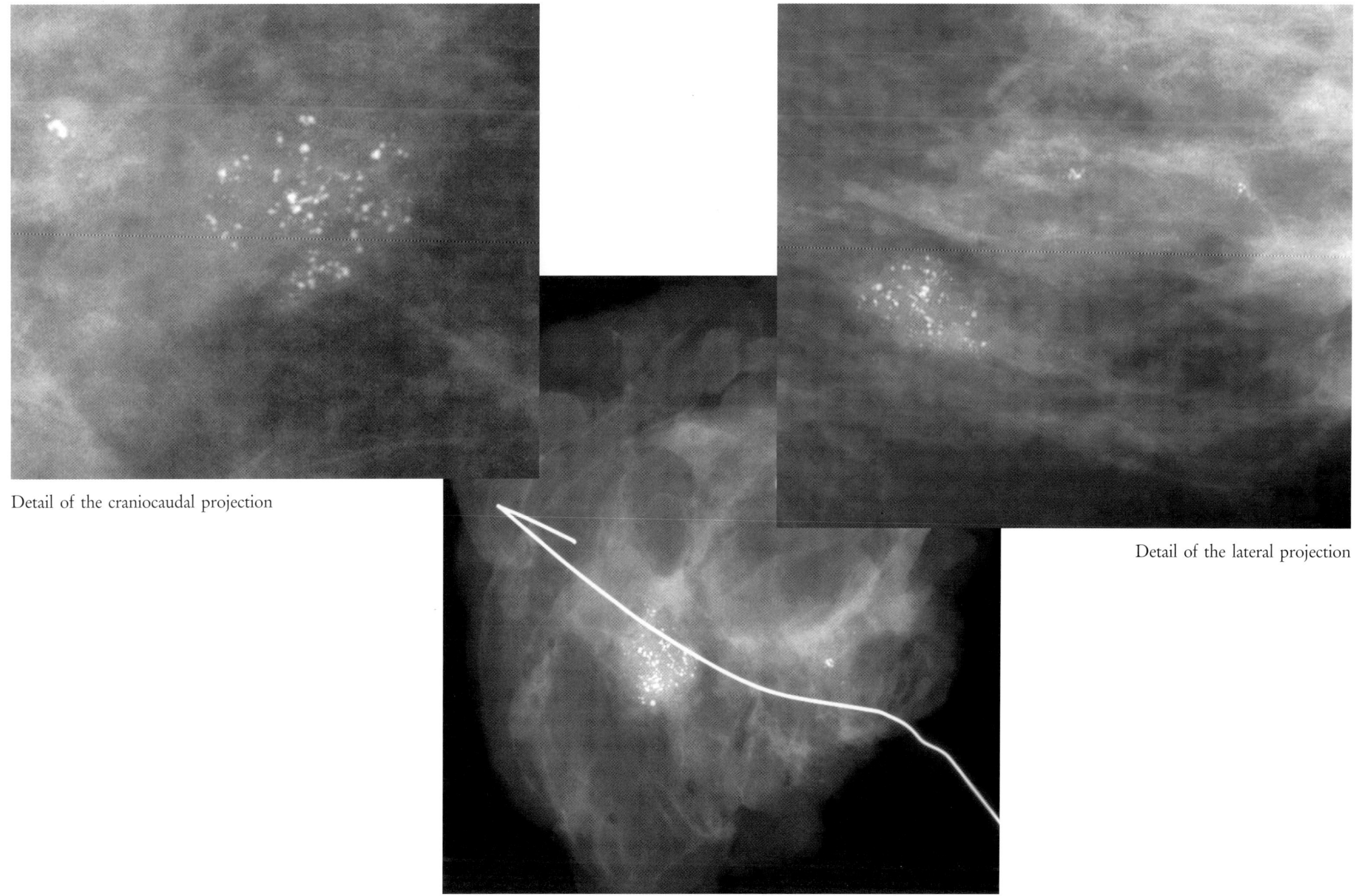

Detail of the craniocaudal projection

Detail of the lateral projection

X-ray of the surgical specimen

Histology: sclerosing adenosis

DOUBTFUL OR INDETERMINATE CALCIFICATIONS

Granular type calcifications
A cluster of predominantly granular type calcifications is seen posteriorly in an upper central location. It is barely detectable in the craniocaudal projection.

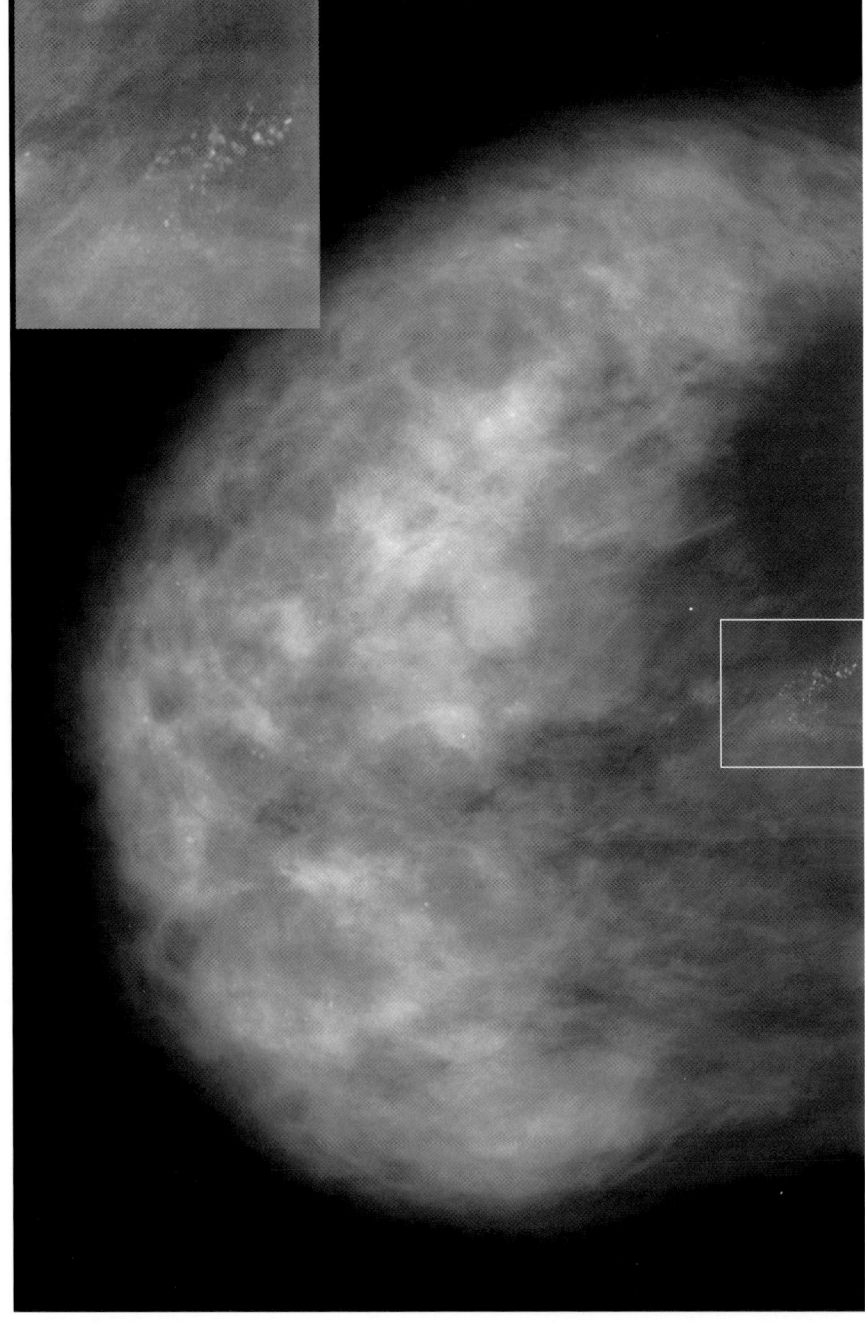

Craniocaudal projection

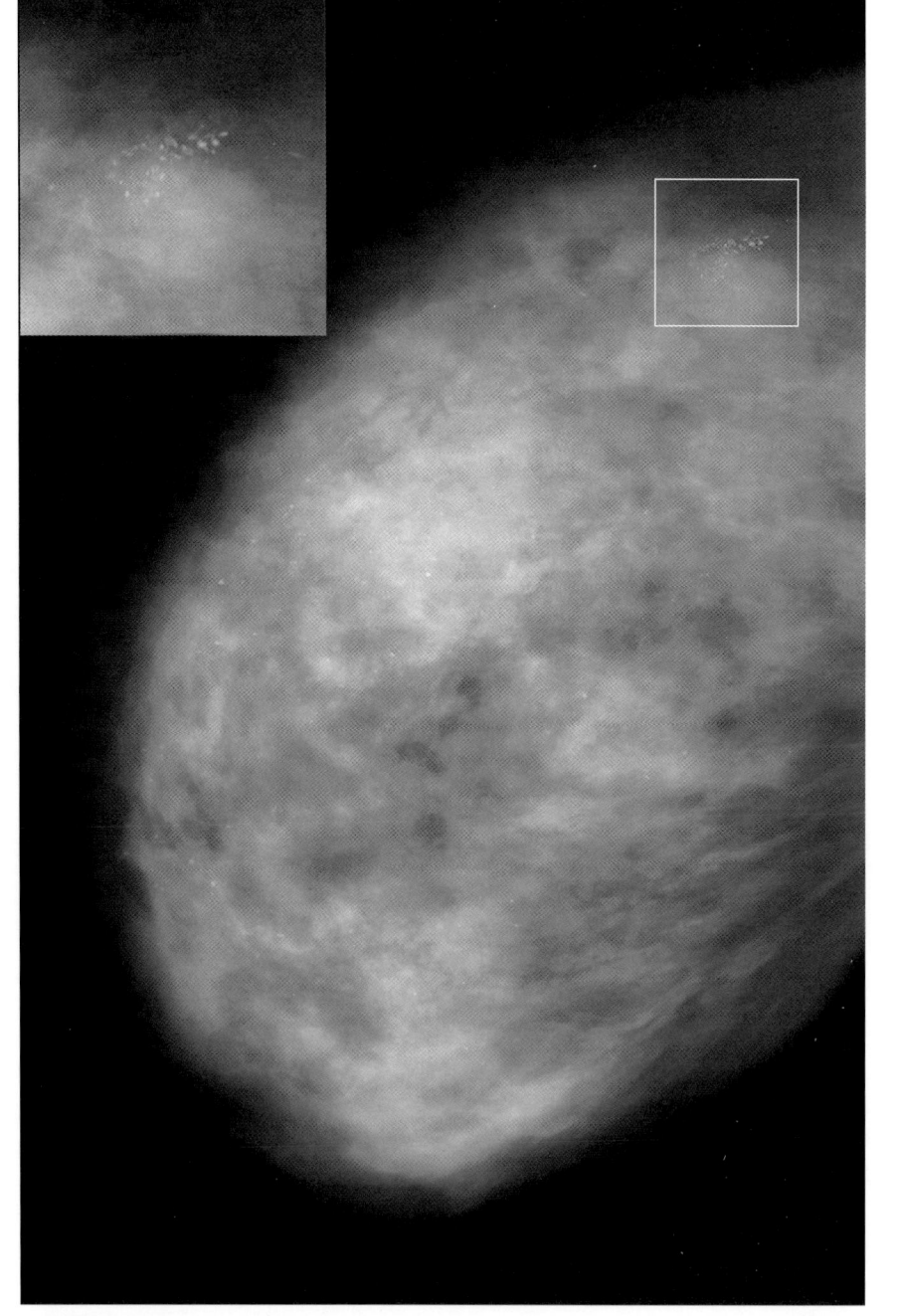

Lateral projection

DOUBTFUL OR INDETERMINATE CALCIFICATIONS

Granular type calcifications

The magnification views show granular type calcifications, varying in density and shape and possibly leading to different interpretations. The radiography of the surgical specimen clearly shows an irregular pattern of calcifications, some of them branching, which arouse a suspicion of malignancy.

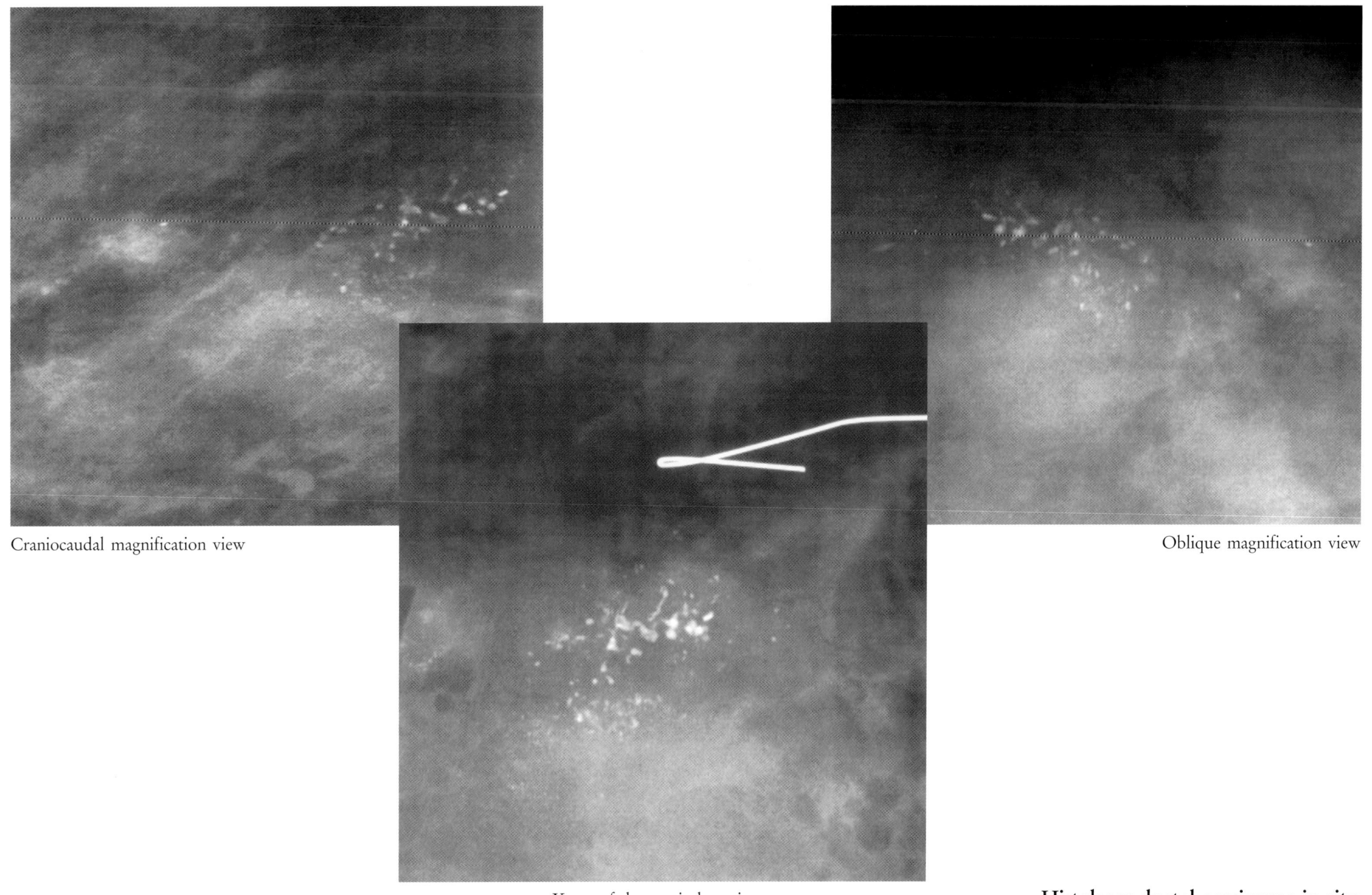

Craniocaudal magnification view

Oblique magnification view

X-ray of the surgical specimen

Histology: ductal carcinoma in situ

DOUBTFUL OR INDETERMINATE CALCIFICATIONS

Granular type calcifications

In the anterior outer part of the breast granular type calcifications seem to have a segmental distribution. In the magnification views these polymorphic entities can be seen more clearly: some granular type, some roundish, some branching. Interpretation of this specimen is not straightforward.

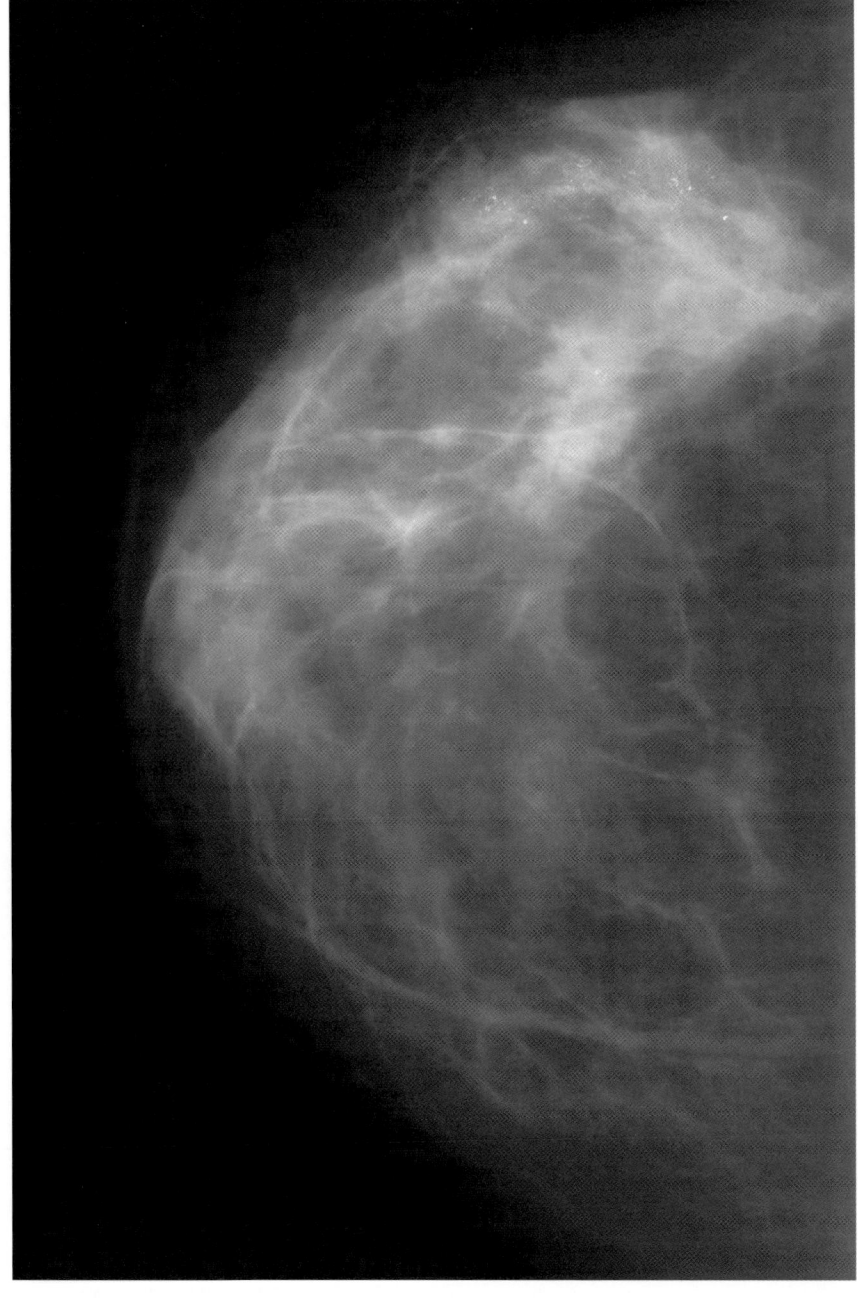

Detail of the craniocaudal projection

Craniocaudal projection

Histology: atypical ductal hyperplasia

Probably malignant calcifications

- *casting type*
- *granular type*
- *mixed*

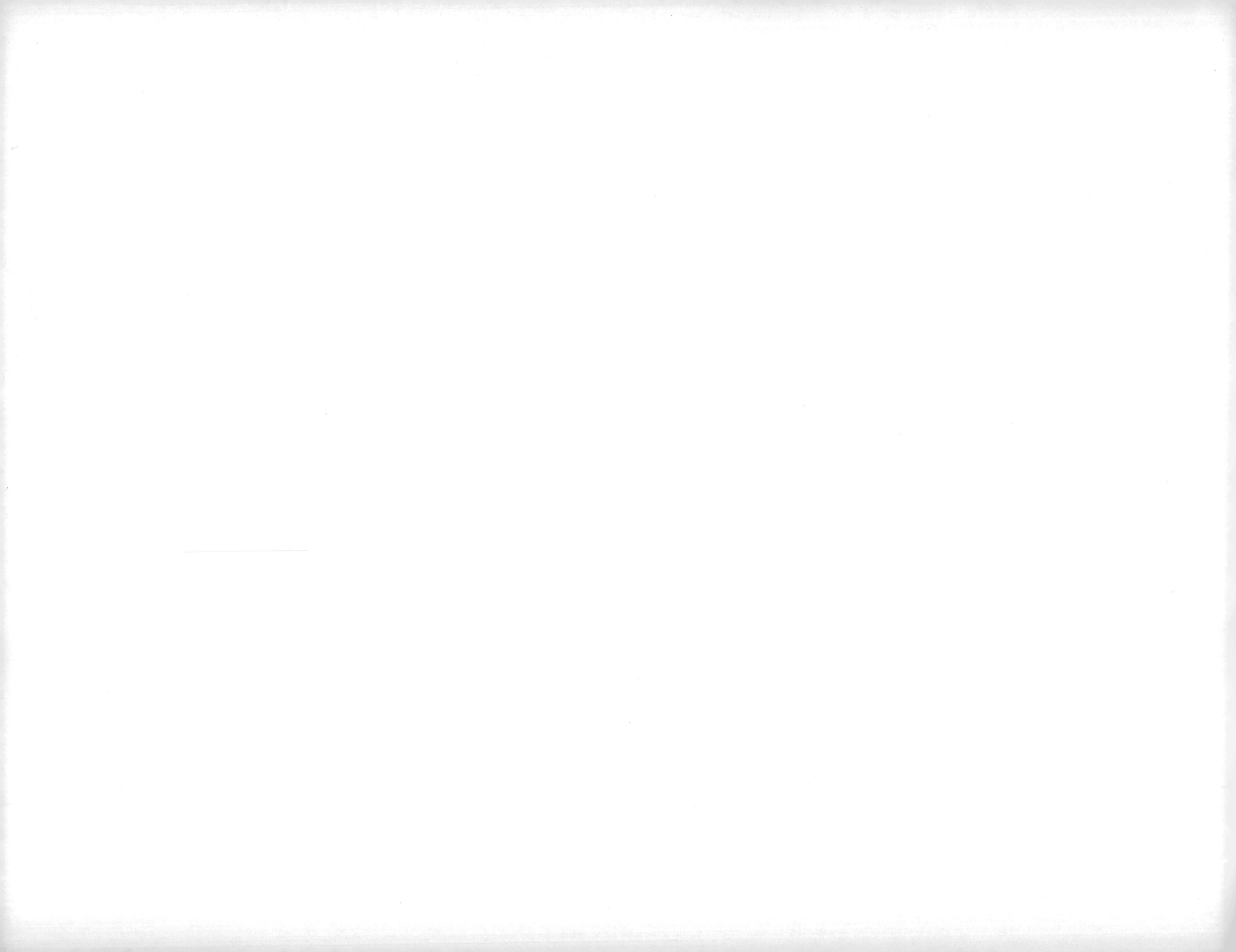

Casting type calcifications

These calcifications are limor and irregularly shaped, giving a high-density image. They fill the ducts and their branches, giving a distinctive linear or fragmented pattern. The necrotic cellular fragments give rise to the cast of the dilated ductal lumen.
They are usually easily distinguishable from rod-like calcifications which are typically regular and following a radiating pattern.

PROBABLY MALIGNANT CALCIFICATIONS

Casting type calcifications
Elongated, irregular, high-density, casting type calcifications fill a duct in a retroareolar location, and follow a linear distribution pattern in the underlying parenchyma.

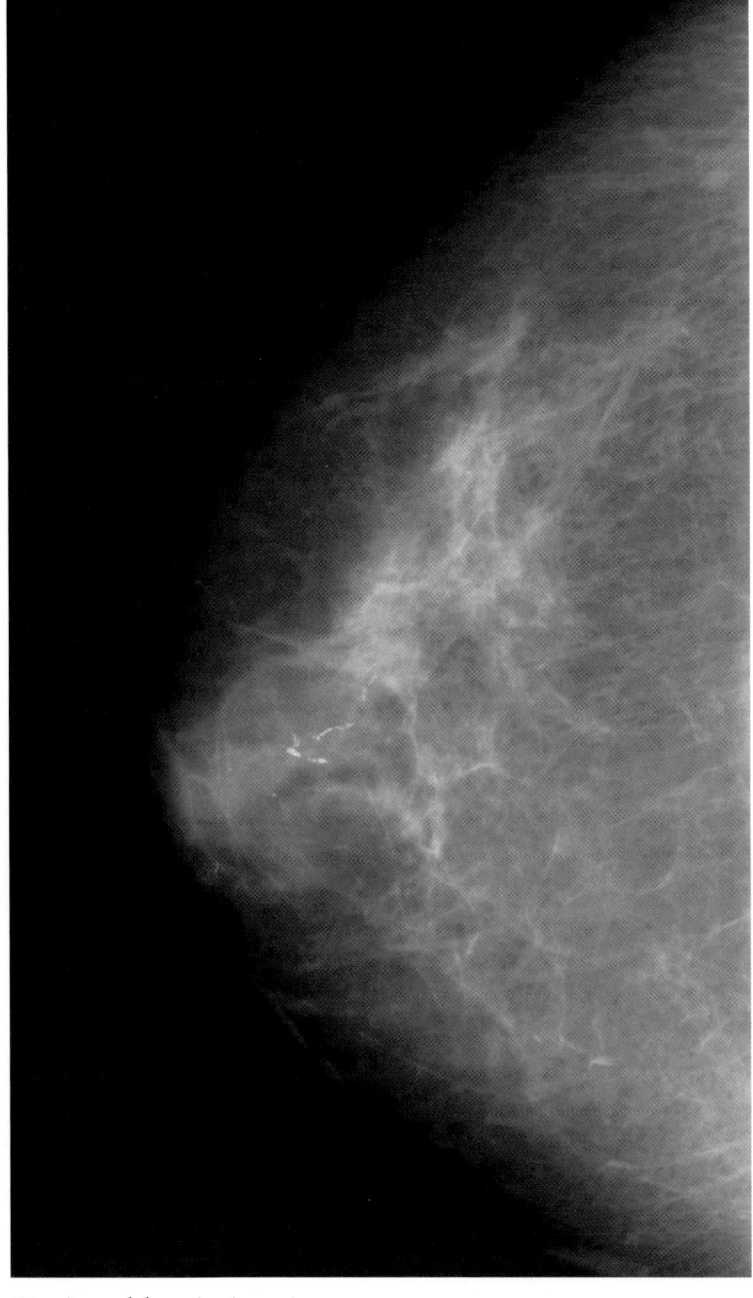

Craniocaudal projection

Craniocaudal magnification view

Histology: Paget's carcinoma

Casting type calcifications

Closely-packed, elongated, irregularly shaped, branching type calcifications follow the course of the duct (A), reproducing its anatomy perfectly. Note the thickening of the portion involved by the neoplasia, which is larger than the cluster of calcifications (B).

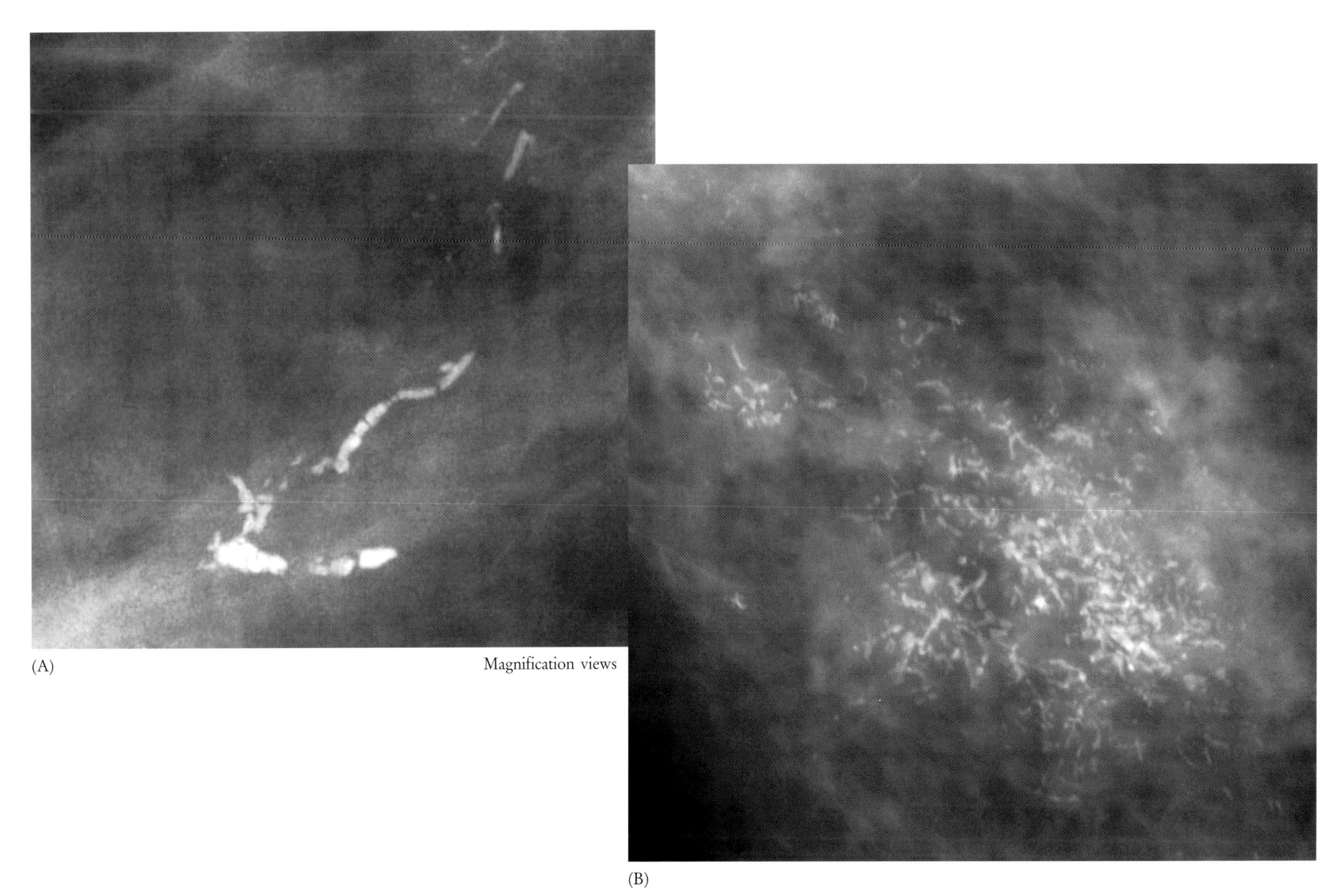

(A)

Magnification views

(B)

PROBABLY MALIGNANT CALCIFICATIONS

Casting type calcifications
Linear, branching, irregular intraductal calcifications mimic the morphology of the ducts involved by the carcinoma in the lower medial quadrant. The calcifications follow a linear distribution and involve several ducts of a lobe, across a roughly triangular area.

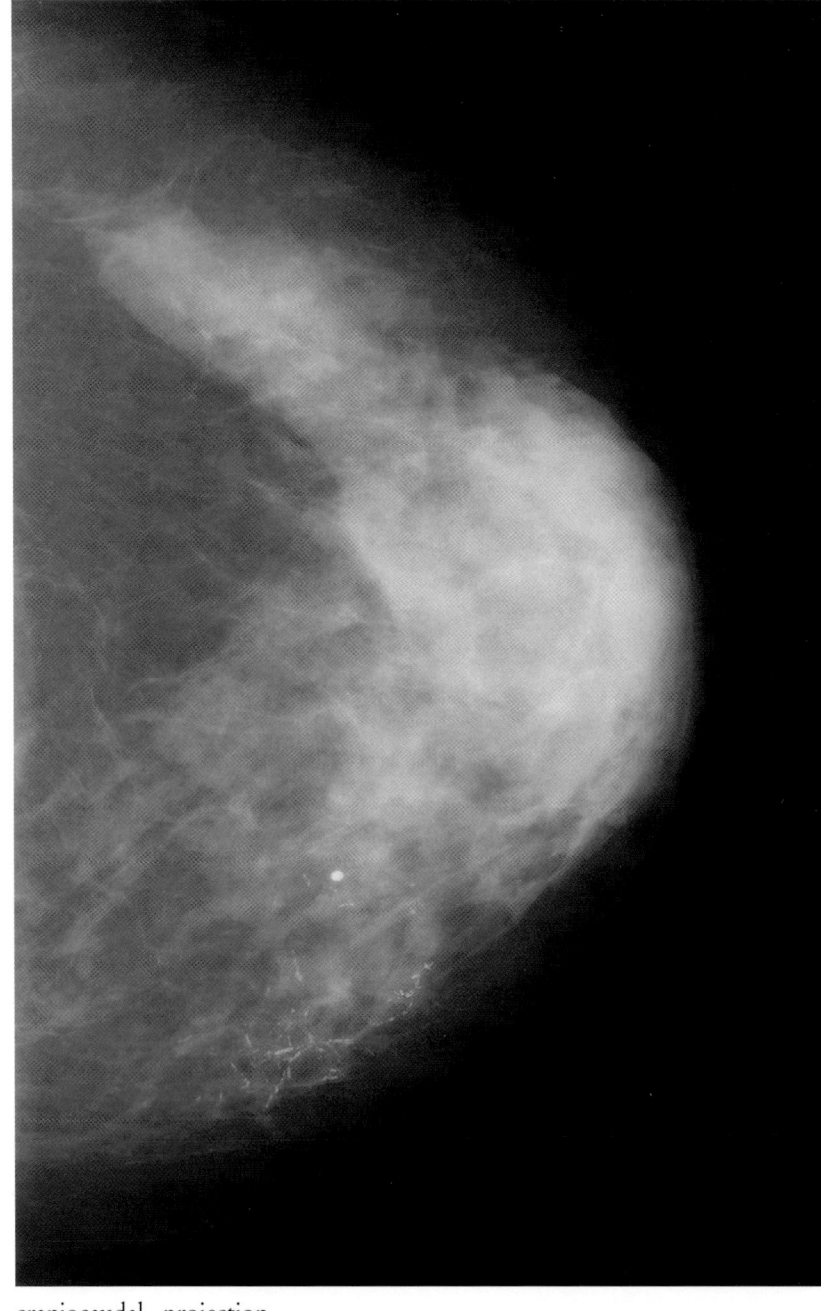

craniocaudal projection

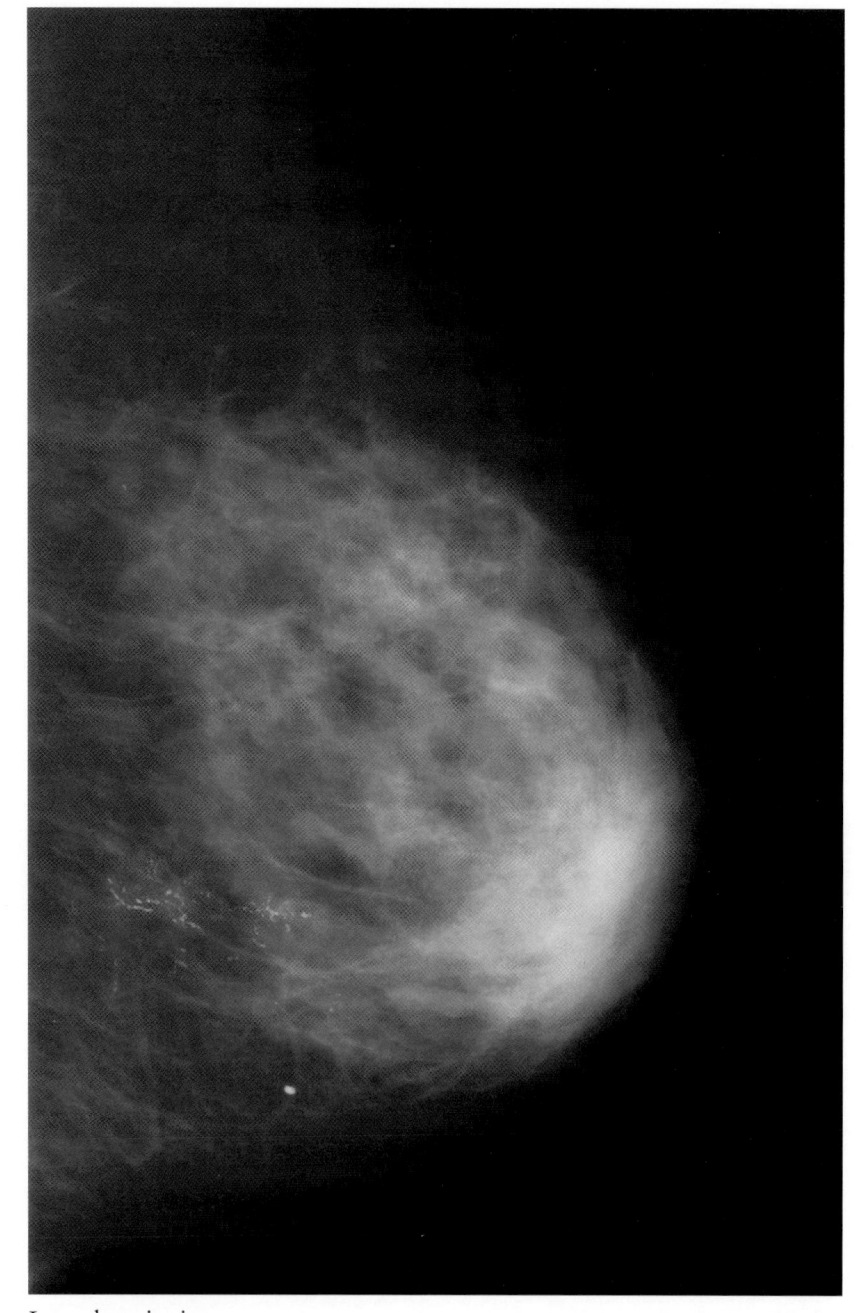

Lateral projection

Casting type calcifications
Linear, branching, irregular intraductal calcifications mimic the morphology of the ducts involved by breast cancer in the lower medial quadrant. The calcifications follow a linear distribution and involve several ducts of a lobe.

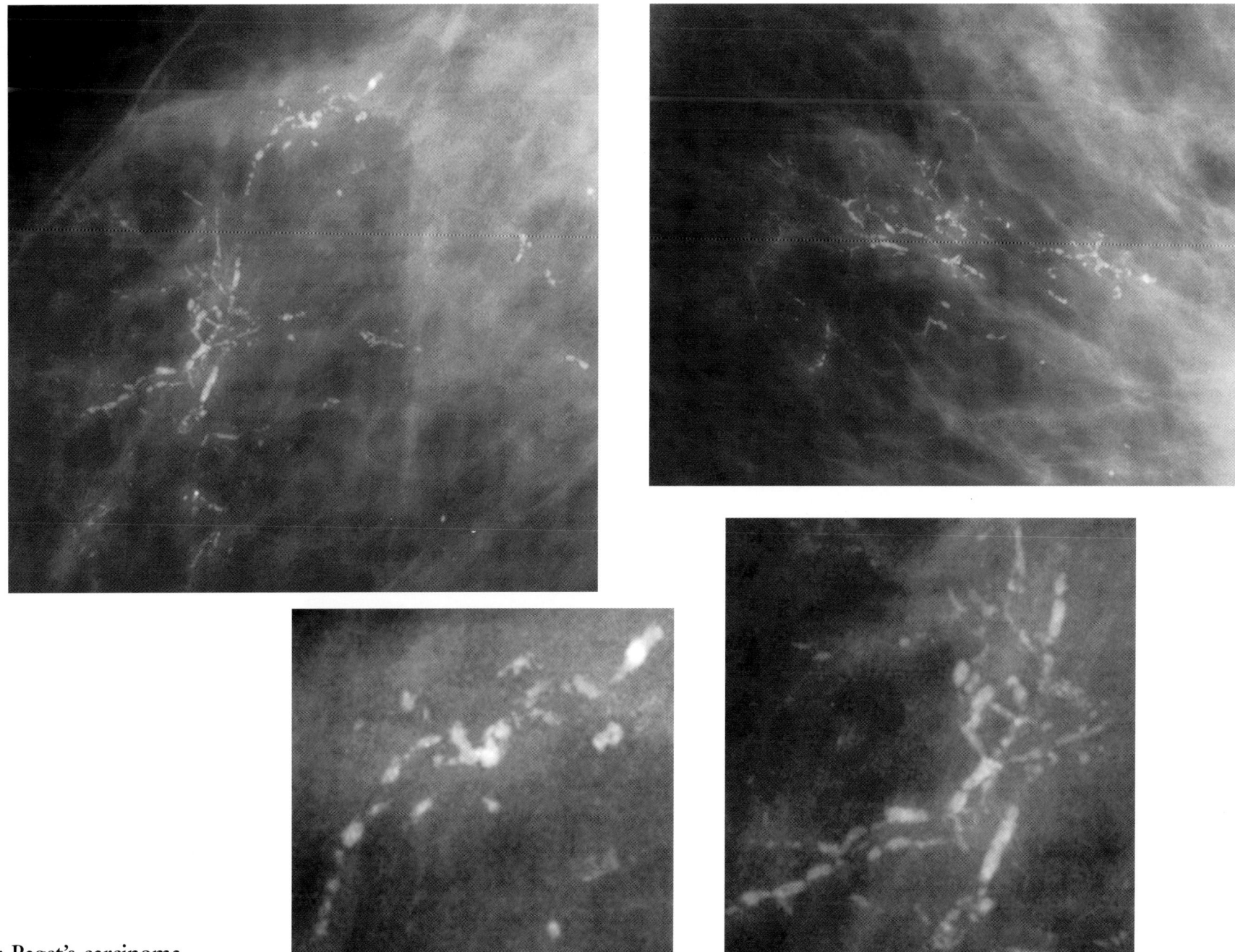

Histology: Paget's carcinoma

PROBABLY MALIGNANT CALCIFICATIONS

Casting type calcifications
Here there is pronounced thickening of the skin of the areola, with swelling due to diffuse oedema. Tightly-packed casting type calcifications are distributed segmentally behind the areola and centrally, together with multiple clusters of granular type calcifications.

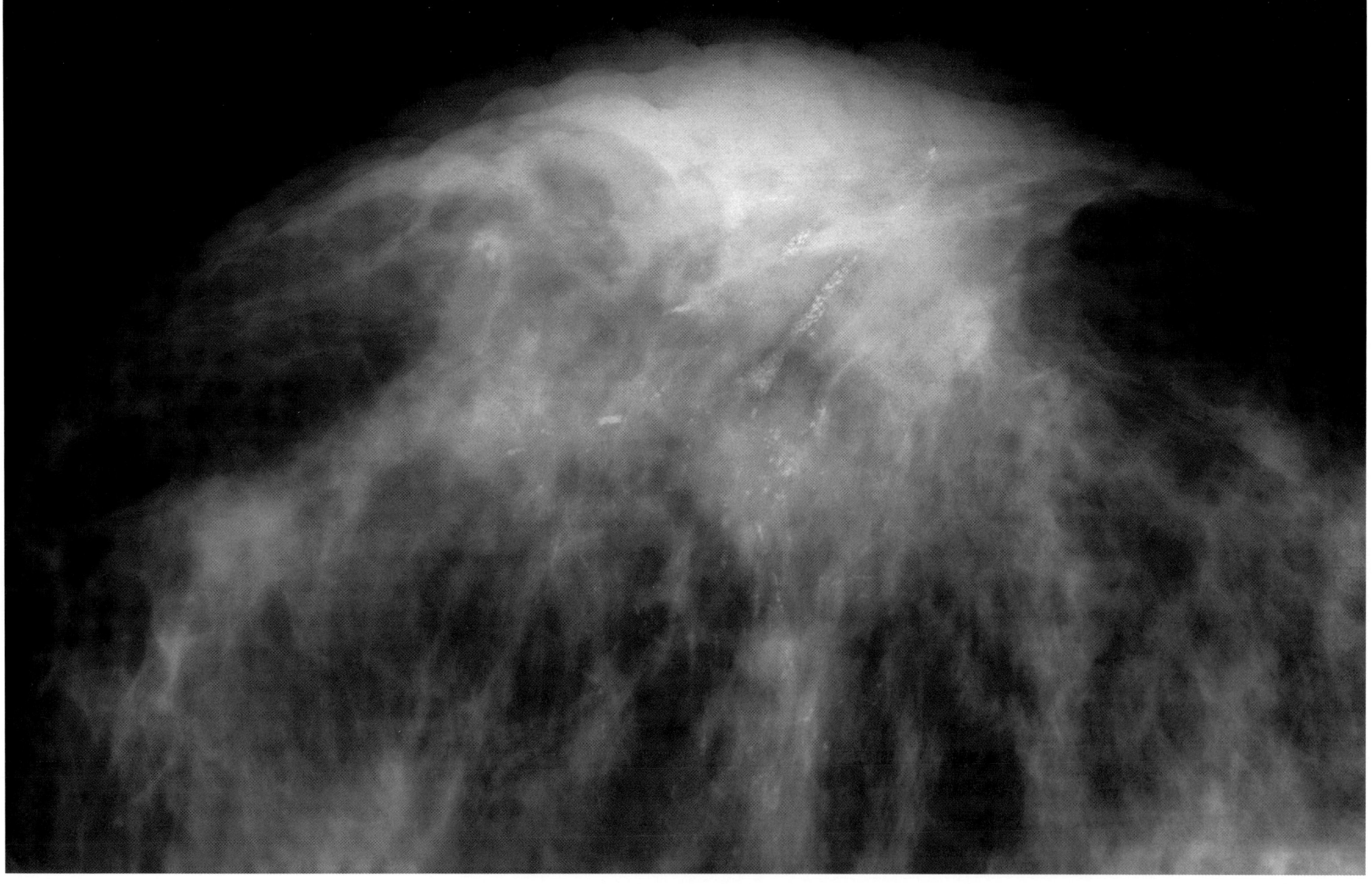

Craniocaudal projection

PROBABLY MALIGNANT CALCIFICATIONS

Casting type calcifications

These magnification views clearly show retroareolar ducts containing casting type calcifications at different stages of formation; some ducts are completely full of calcifications. The multiple clusters of granular type or mixed calcifications indicate a multifocal lesion.

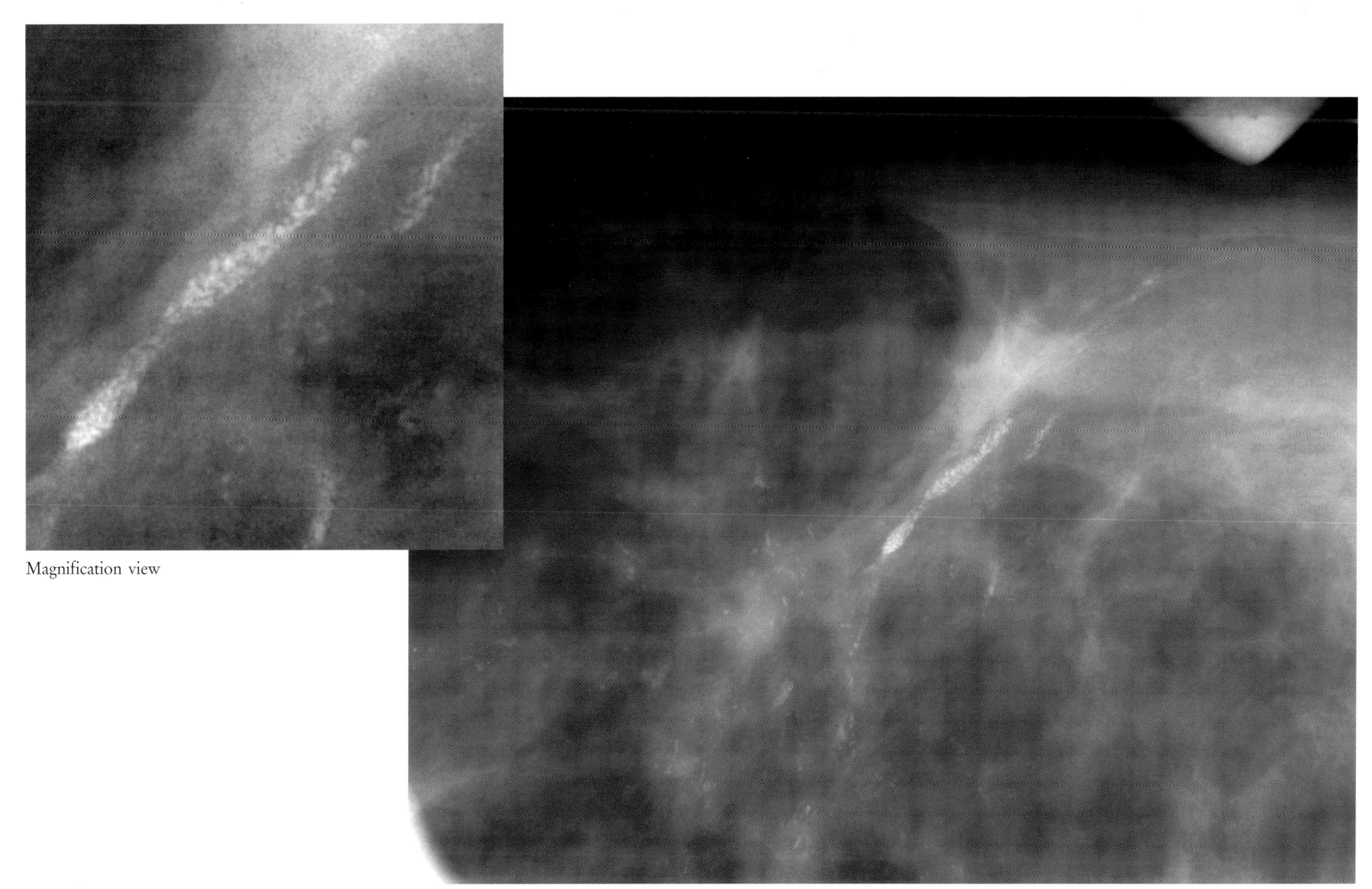

Magnification view

Histology: inflammatory carcinoma with an extensive intraductal component

Craniocaudal projection

PROBABLY MALIGNANT CALCIFICATIONS

Casting type calcifications
These calcifications are extensively distributed along the ducts, spreading through one or more lobes and raising the possibility of multifocal or multicentric breast cancer. Such a distribution may, however, commonly be found in secretory disease or late in "plasma cell mastitis".

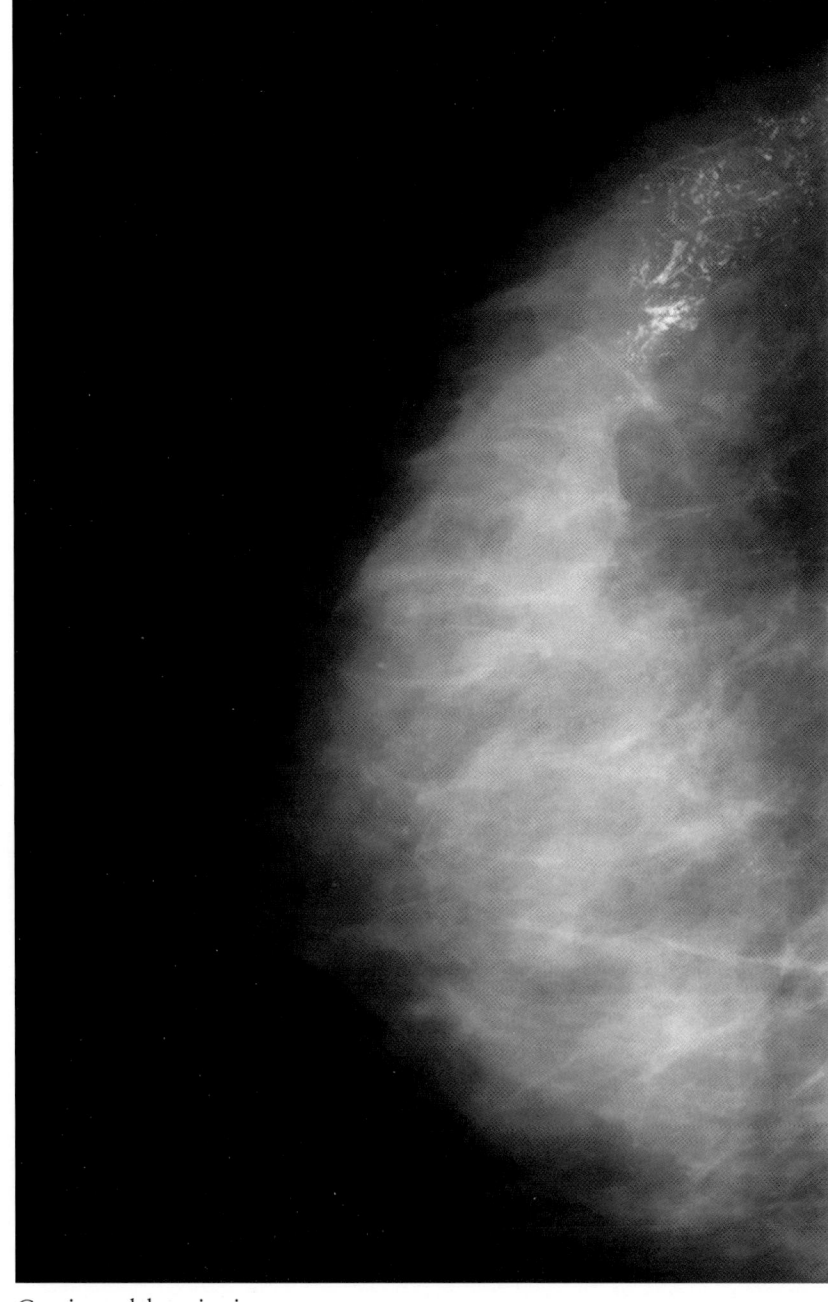

Craniocaudal projection

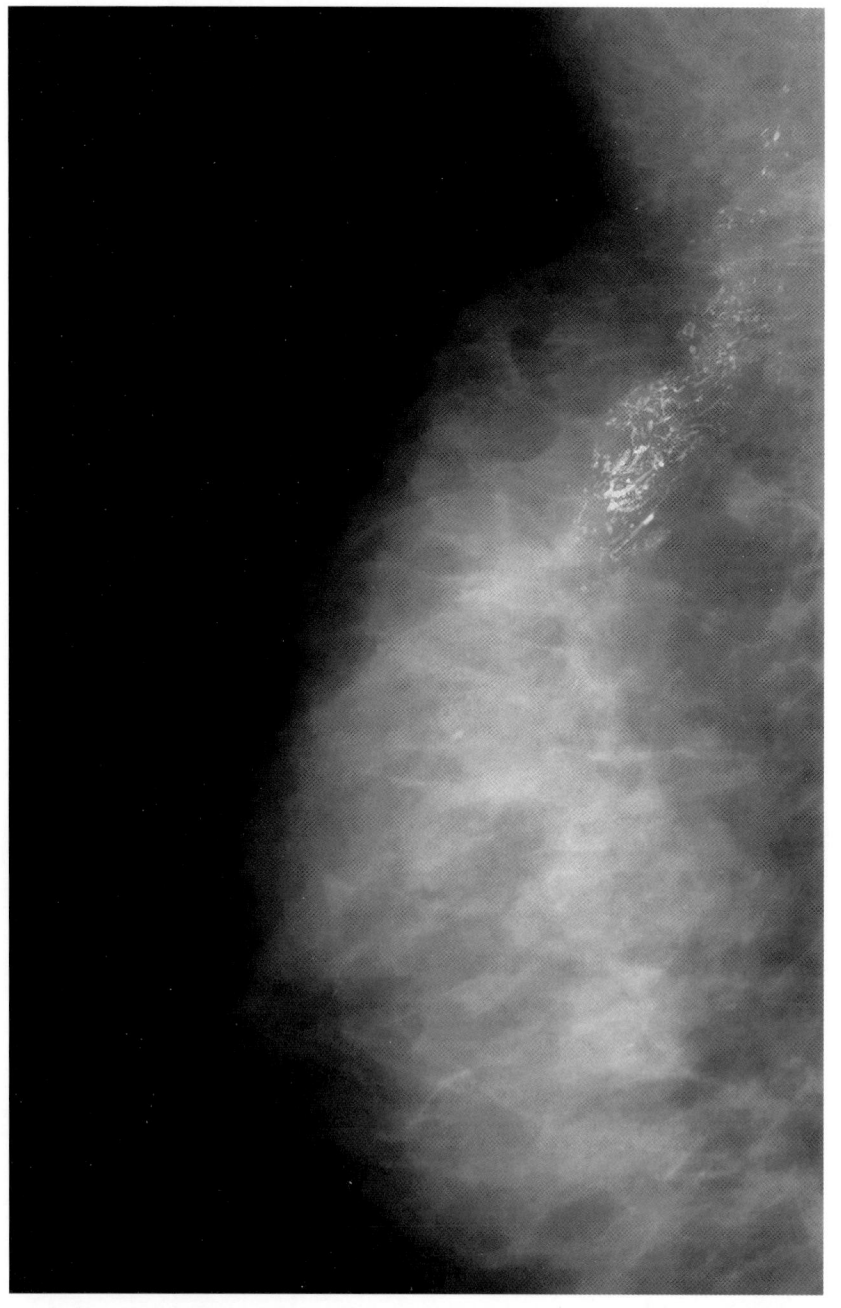

Mediolateral oblique projection

Casting type calcifications

These calcifications are extensively distributed along the ducts, spreading through one or more lobes and raising the possibility of multifocal or multicentric breast cancer. Such a distribution may, however, commonly be found in secretory disease or late in "plasma cell mastitis".

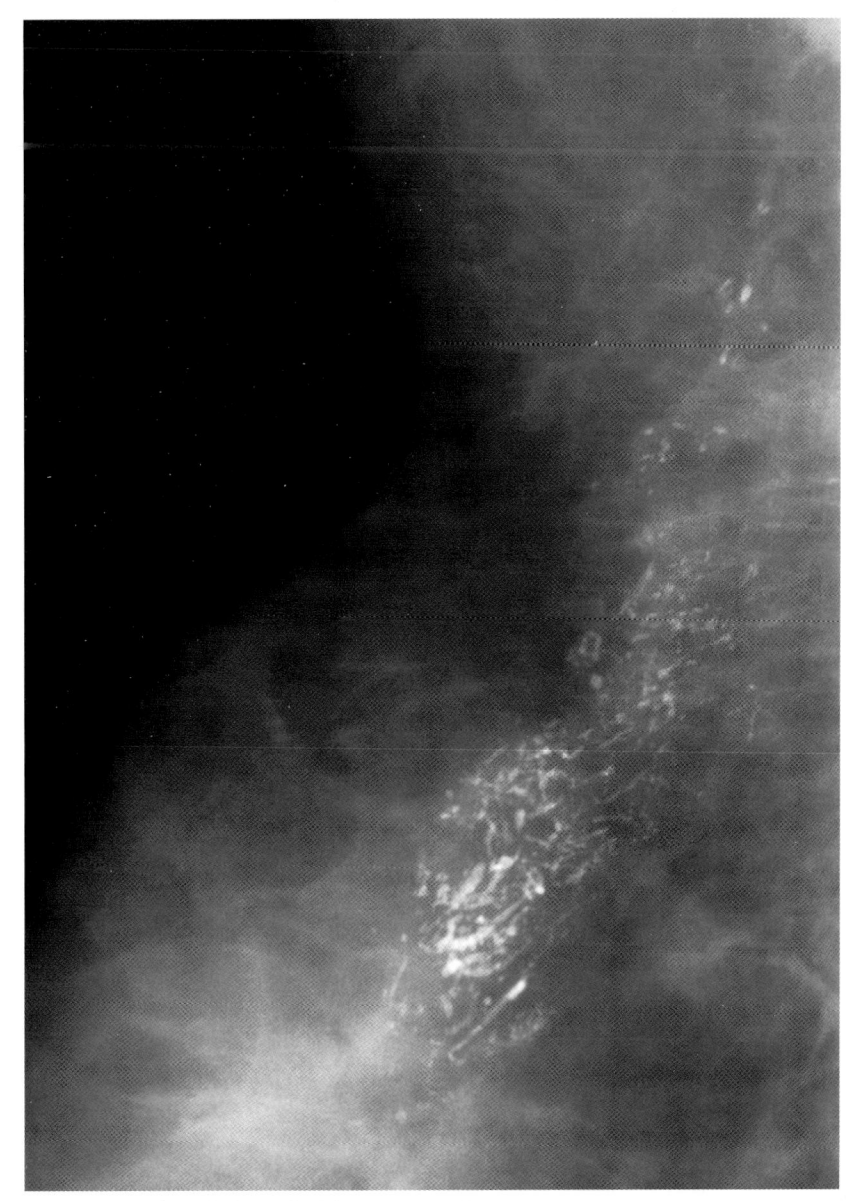

Detail of the mediolateral oblique projection

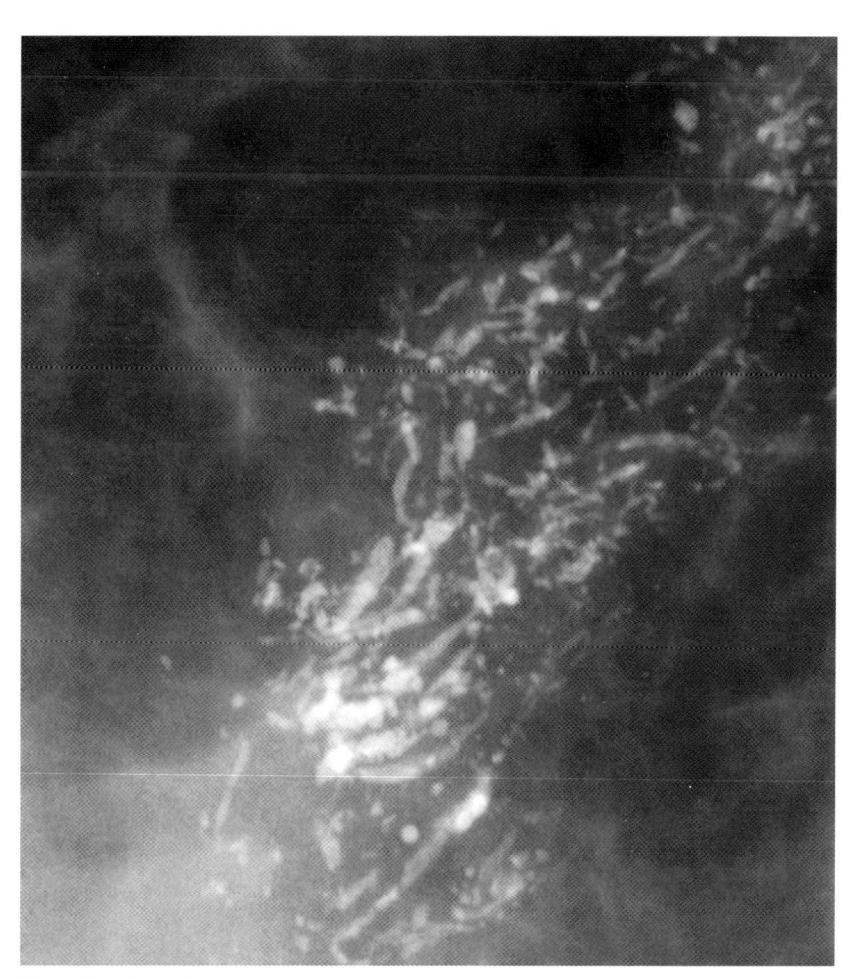

Magnification view

Histology: inflammatory carcinoma with an extensive intraductal component

Granular type calcifications

Granular type calcifications have irregular shape, high density and may look like gravel, crushed stones iron filings, or fine grains of salt. They generally have a clustered distribution, sometimes multiple groupings. When they are scattered segmentally or diffusely, they are not readily distinguishable from dysplastic calcifications. When their density and morphology are heterogeneous, they often cannot be differentiated from round or "milk-of-calcium" calcifications.

PROBABLY MALIGNANT CALCIFICATIONS

Granular type calcifications
A small cluster of granular type calcifications is visible medially in the upper outer quadrant. The calcifications vary in shape and density and resemble crushed stones, iron filings and fine grains of salt.

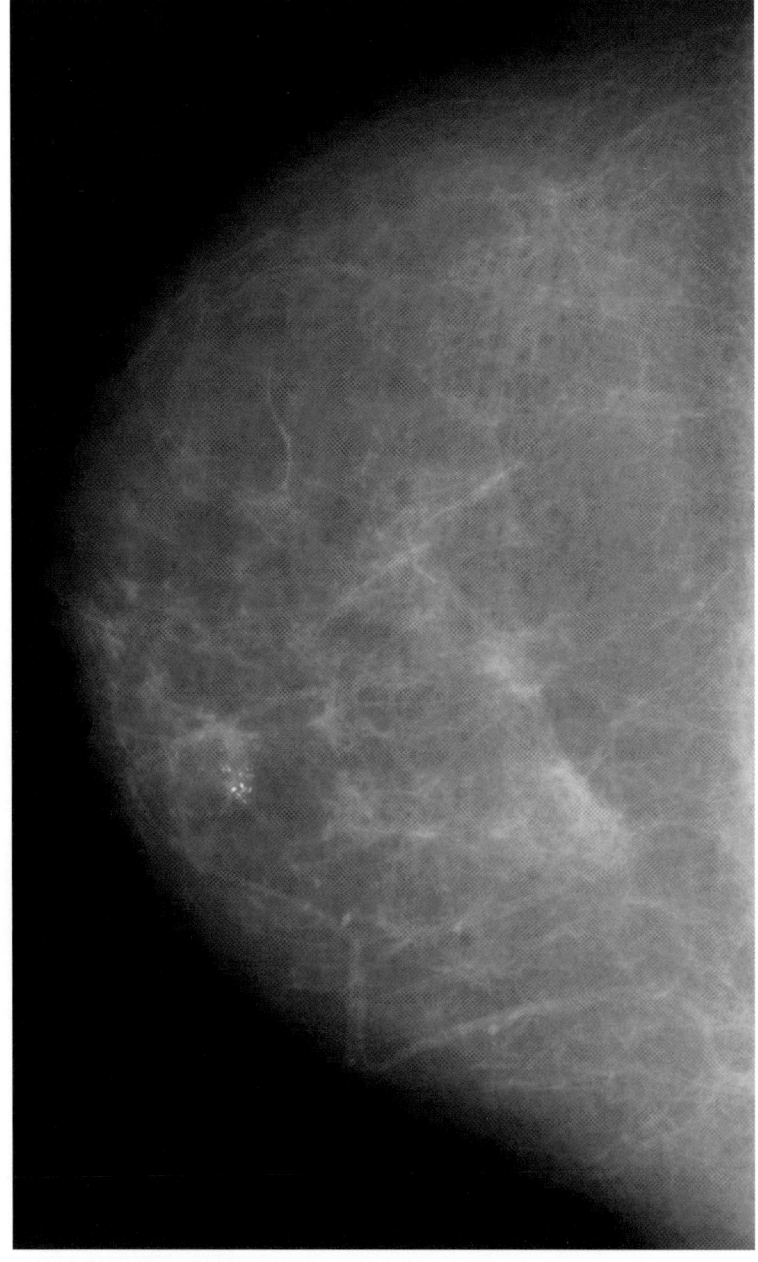

Craniocaudal projection

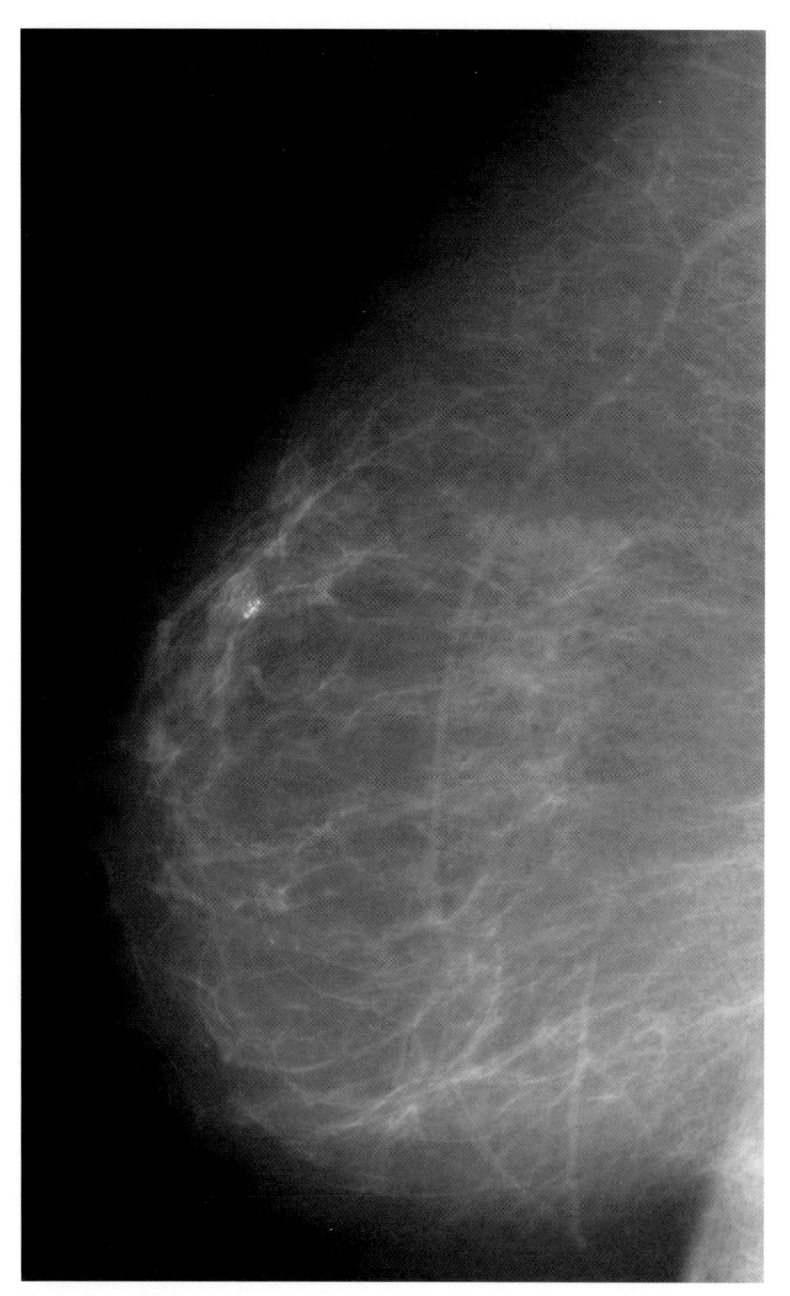

Lateral projection

Histology: ductal carcinoma in situ

PROBABLY MALIGNANT CALCIFICATIONS

Granular type calcifications

A small cluster of granular type calcifications is visible medially in the upper outer quadrant. The calcifications vary in shape and density and resemble crushed stones, iron filings and fine grains of salt.

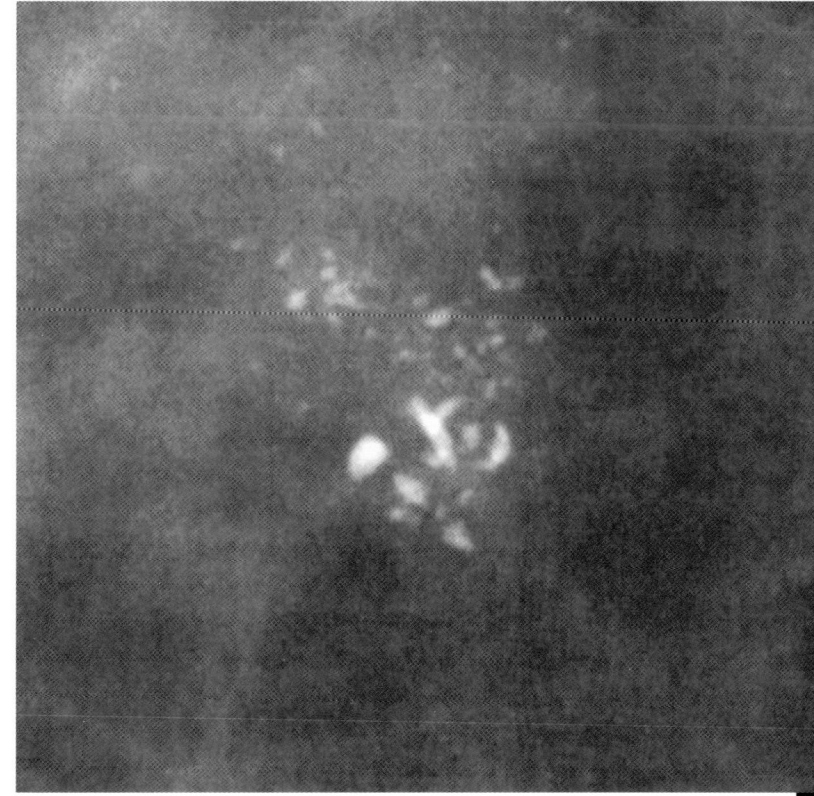

Craniocaudal magnification view

X-ray of the surgical specimen

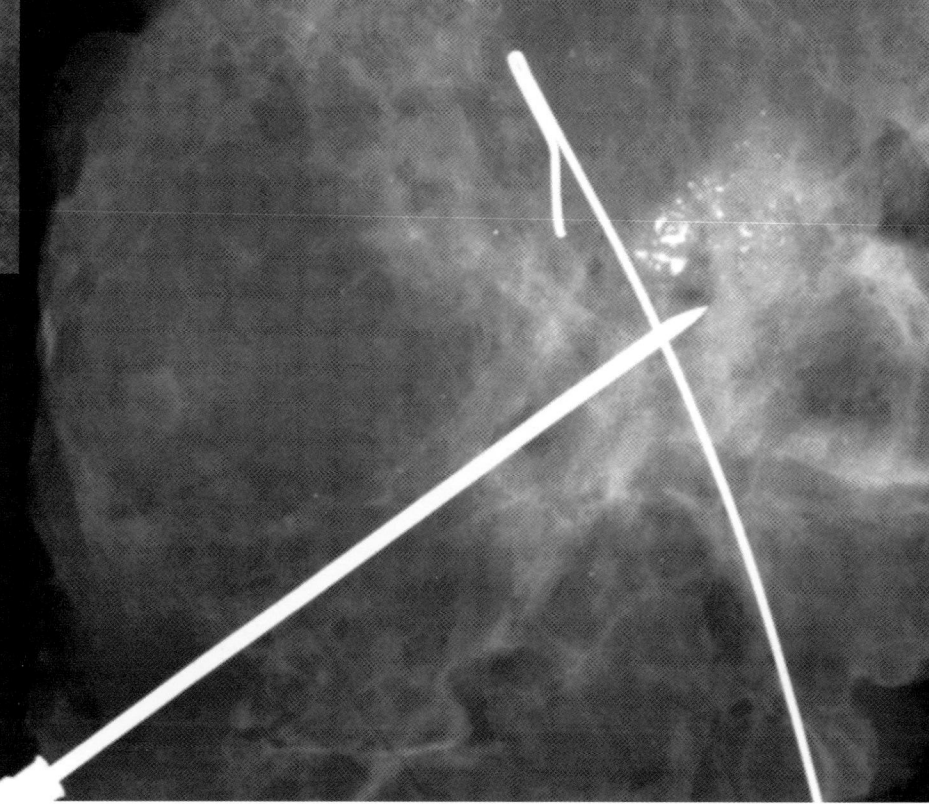

PROBABLY MALIGNANT CALCIFICATIONS

Granular type calcifications
Foci of intraductal microcalcifications, heterogeneous in density and morphology, resembling crushed stones, iron filings and fine grains of salt.

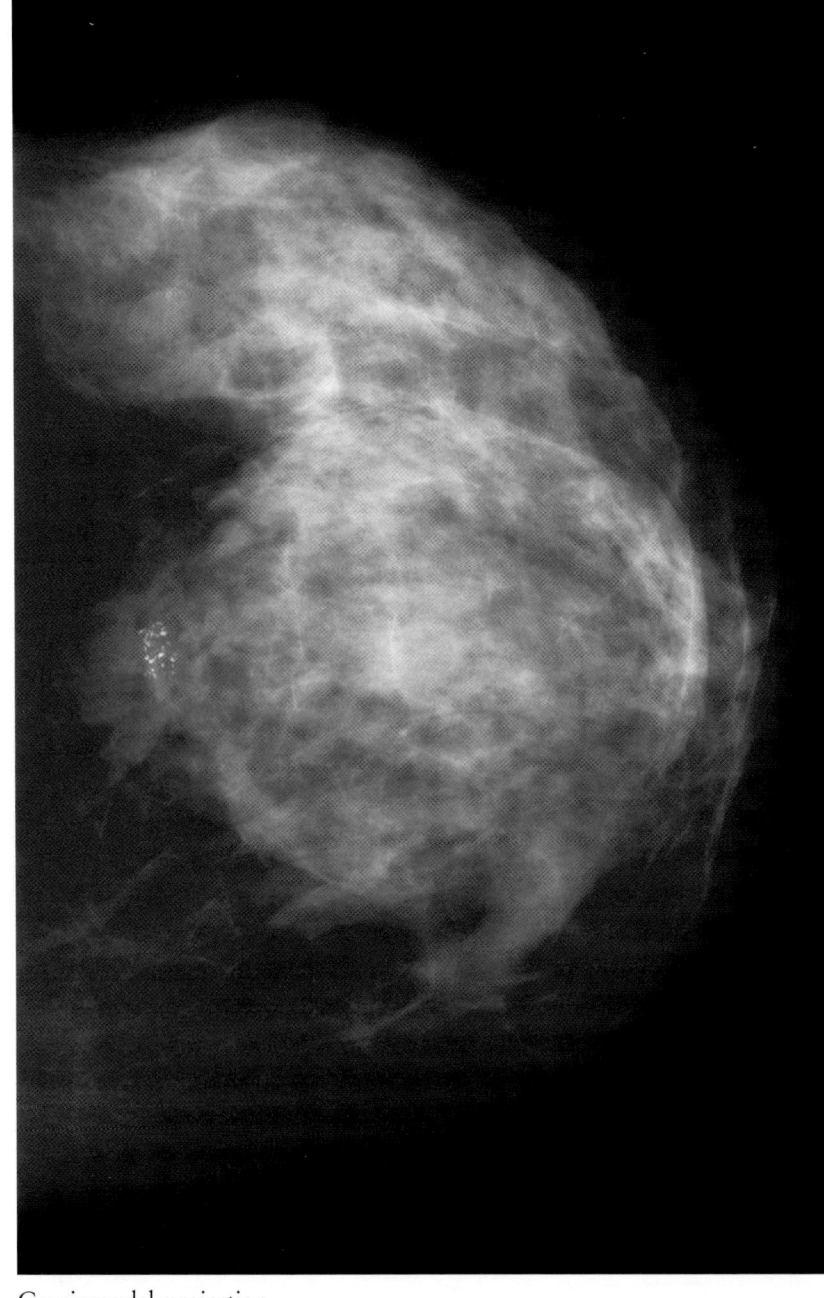

Craniocaudal projection

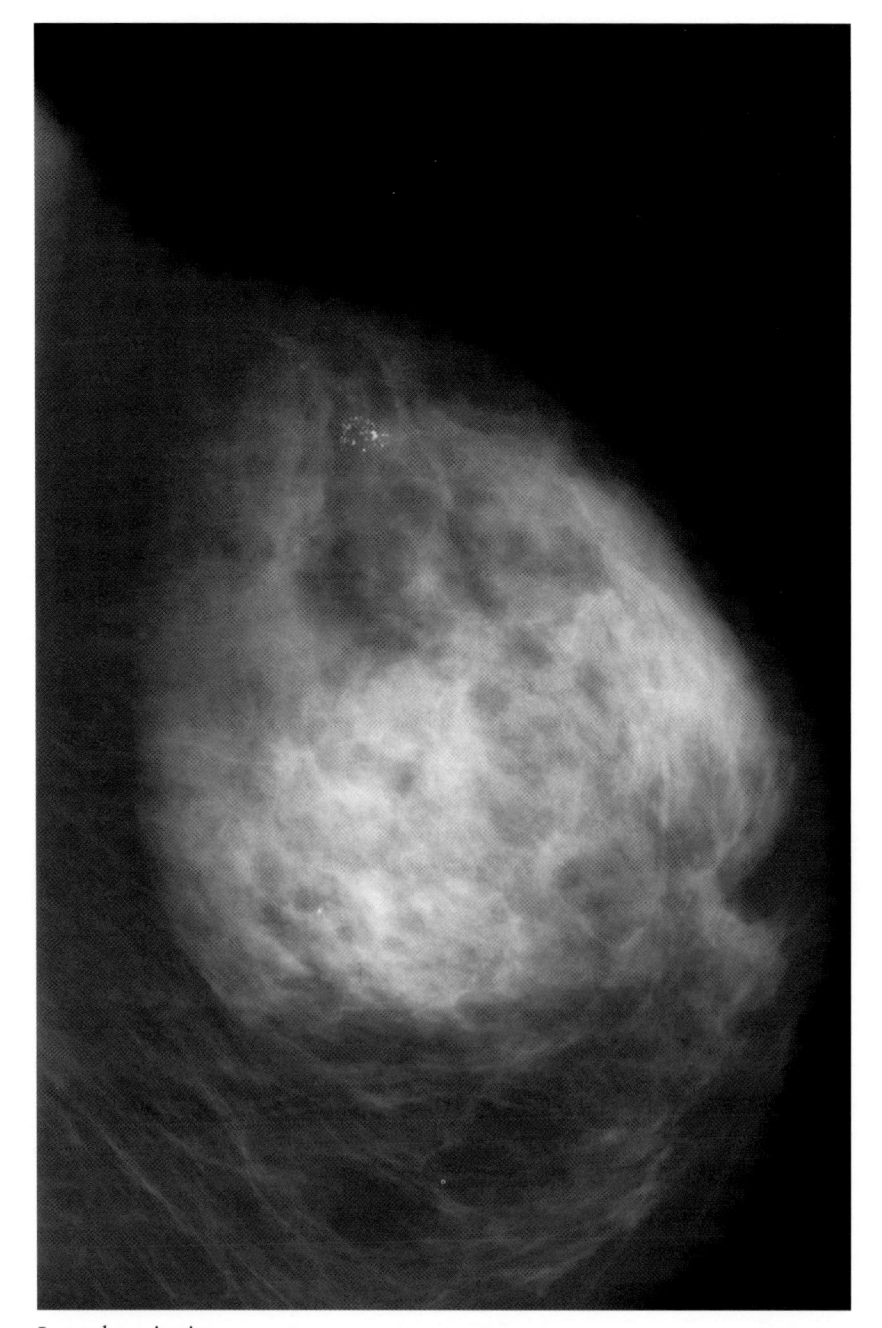

Lateral projection

Granular type calcifications
Foci of intraductal calcifications, heterogeneous in density and morphology, resembling crushed stones, iron filings and fine grains of salt.

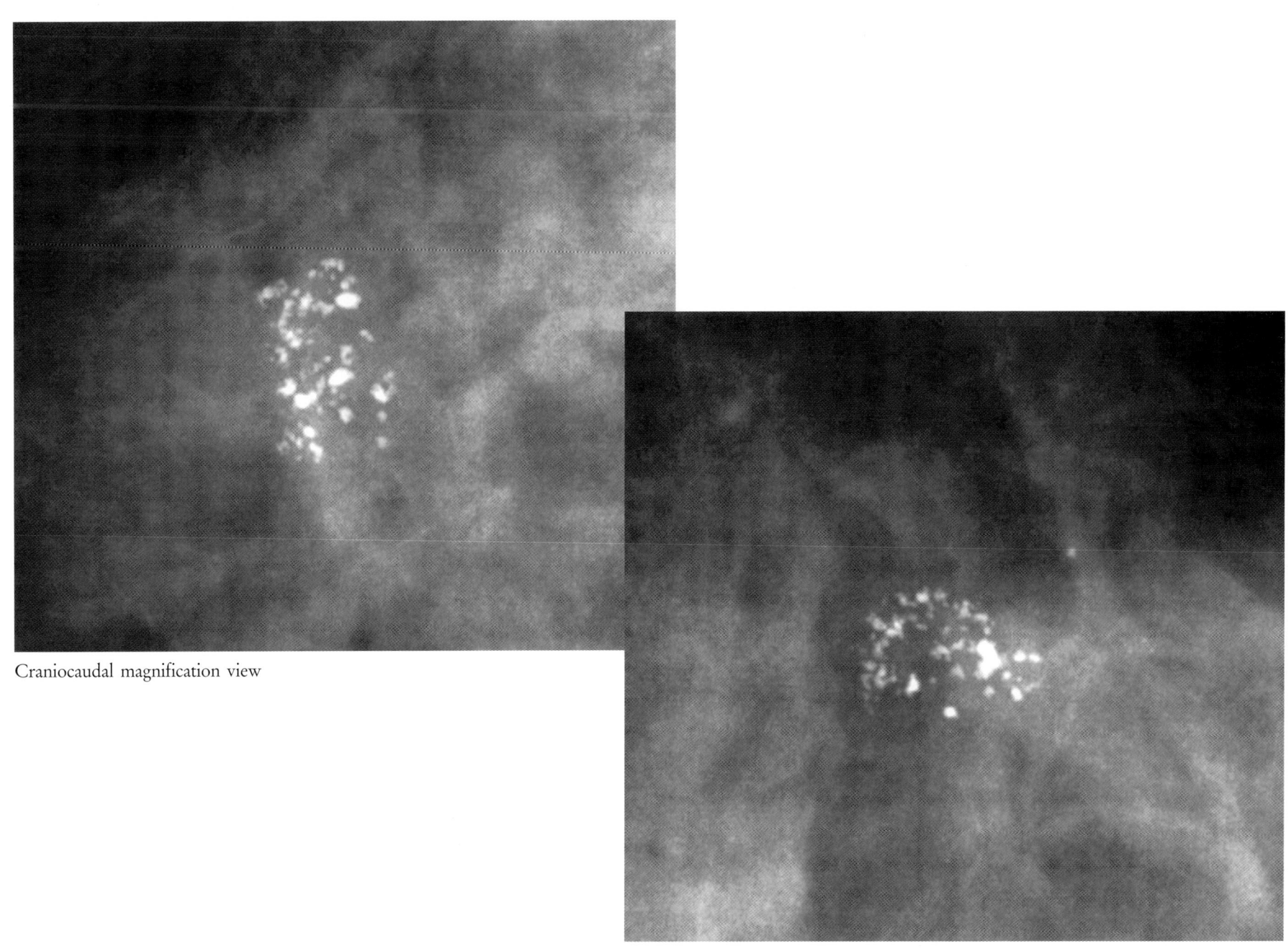

Craniocaudal magnification view

Lateral magnification view

Histology: fibroadenoma

PROBABLY MALIGNANT CALCIFICATIONS

Granular type calcifications
This tightly-packed cluster of irregularly shaped, high-density granular type calcifications lies within an opacity that is heterogeneous in density with irregular and ill defined margins. Contiguously is another small opacity, similar in appearance, indicating the multifocality of the neoplasia.

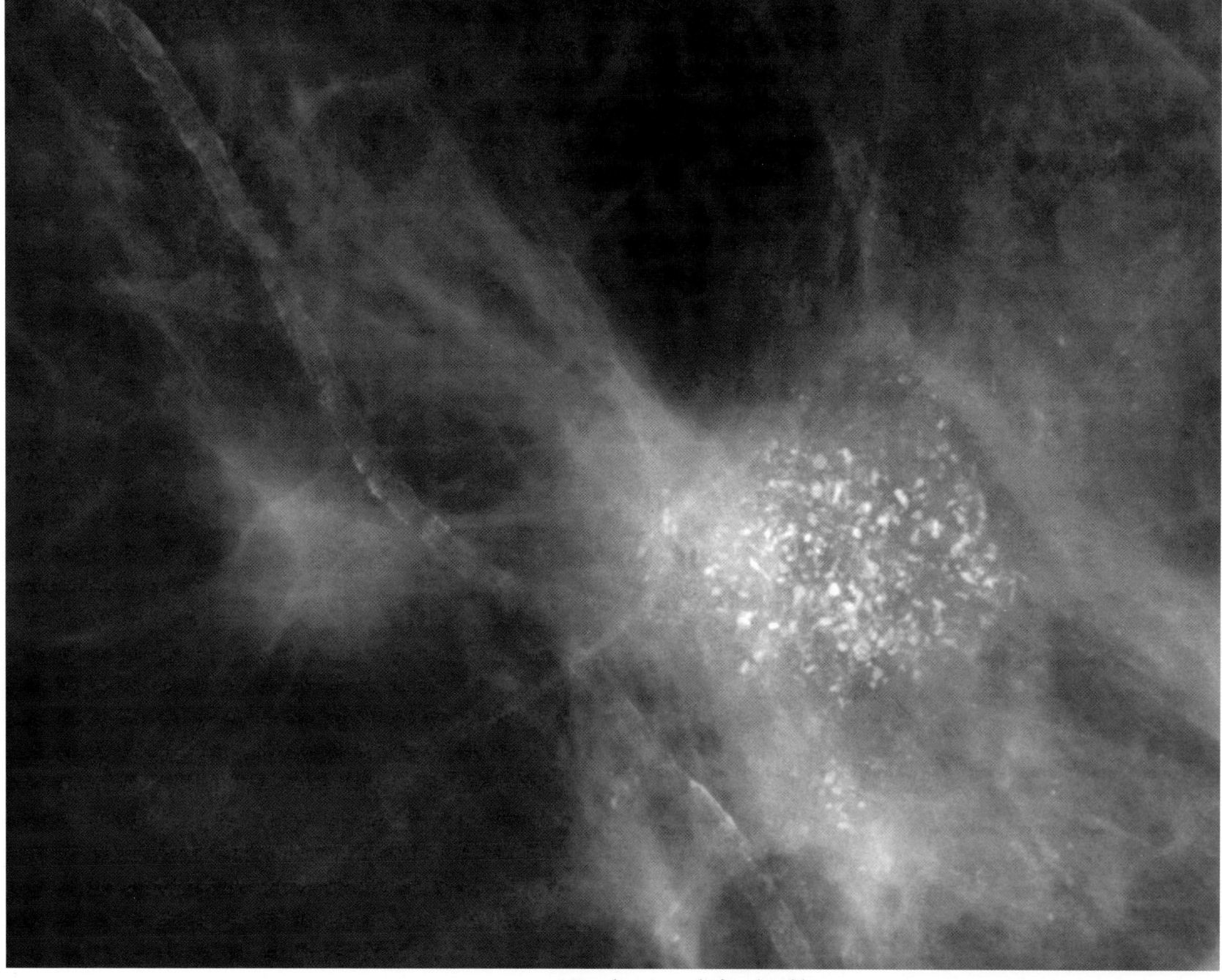

Histology: multifocal infiltrating carcinoma, with an extensive intraductal component

Granular type calcifications
Irregularly shaped, high-density, heterogeneous calcifications resembling crushed stones, iron filings and fine grains of salt.

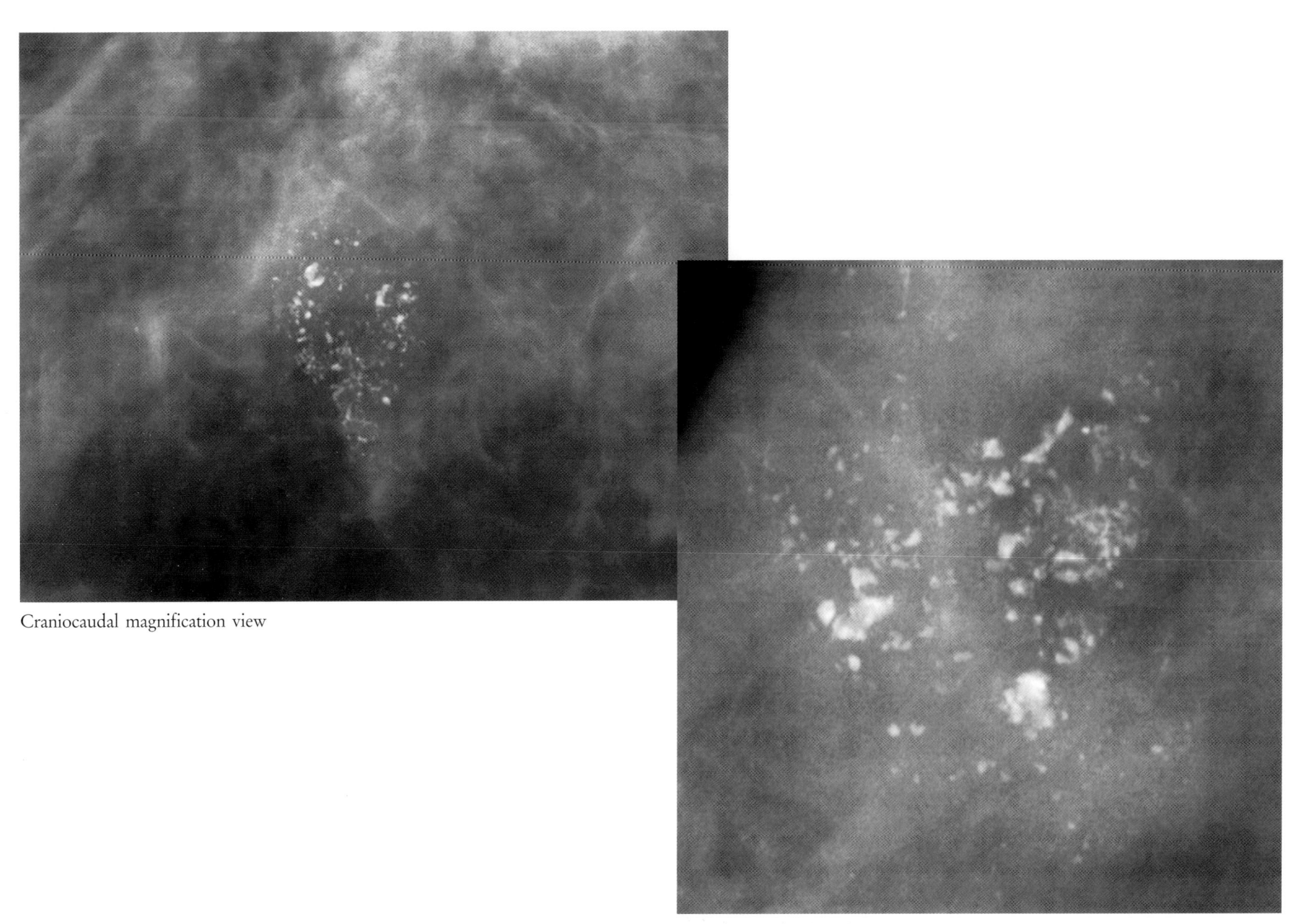

Craniocaudal magnification view

Lateral magnification view

Histology: infiltrating ductal carcinoma

PROBABLY MALIGNANT CALCIFICATIONS

Granular type calcifications
Multiple clusters of granular type calcifications are seen in the outer areolar area of the breast, some filling an ectactic retroareolar duct.

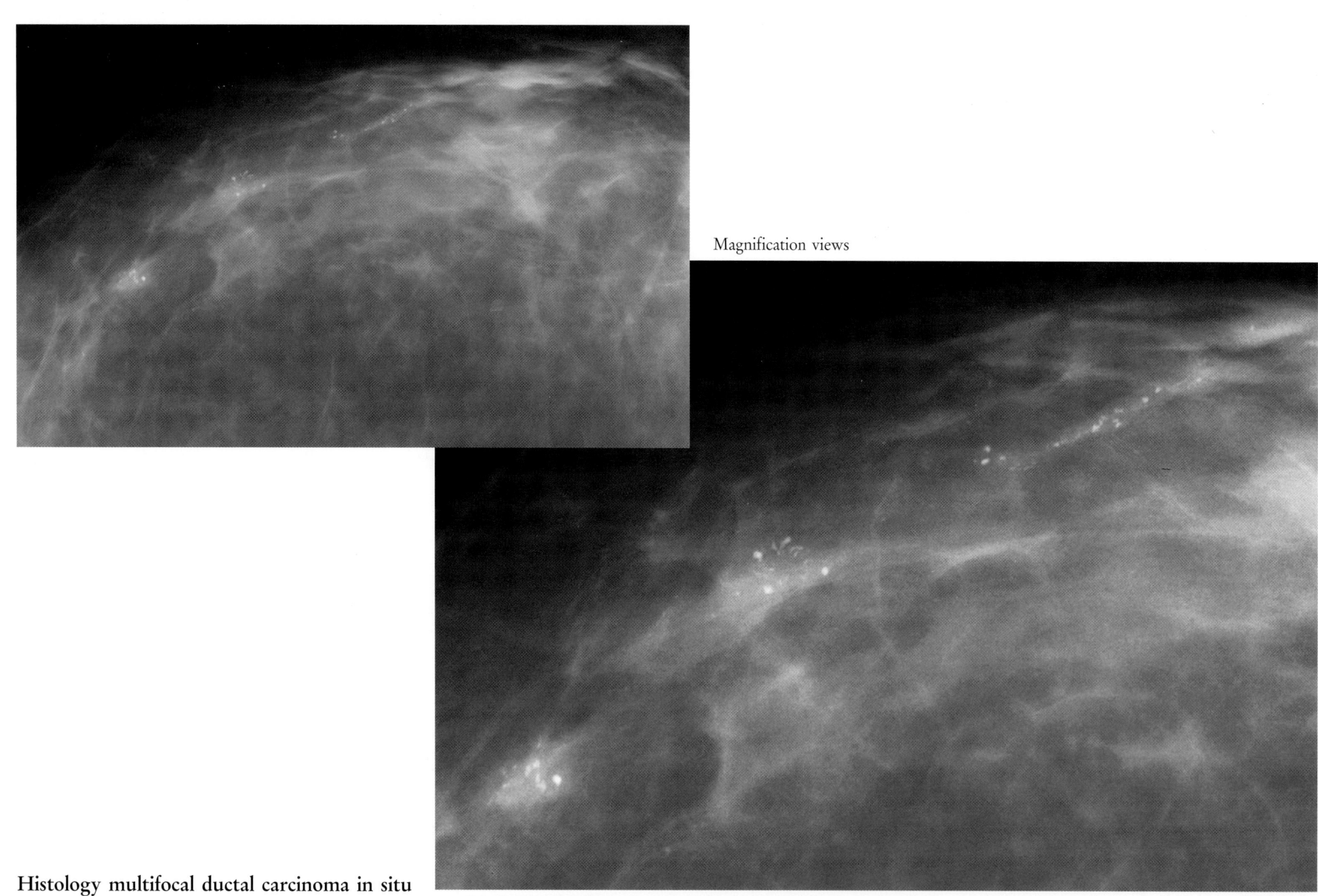

Magnification views

Histology multifocal ductal carcinoma in situ

Mixed calcifications

Mixed calcifications present variably as granular type formations or casting type. Their distribution is generally diffuse or segmental. They are diagnostic of a malignant process.

PROBABLY MALIGNANT CALCIFICATIONS

Mixed calcifications
Diffuse granular type and cast-like calcifications associated with malignancy are visible anteriorly.

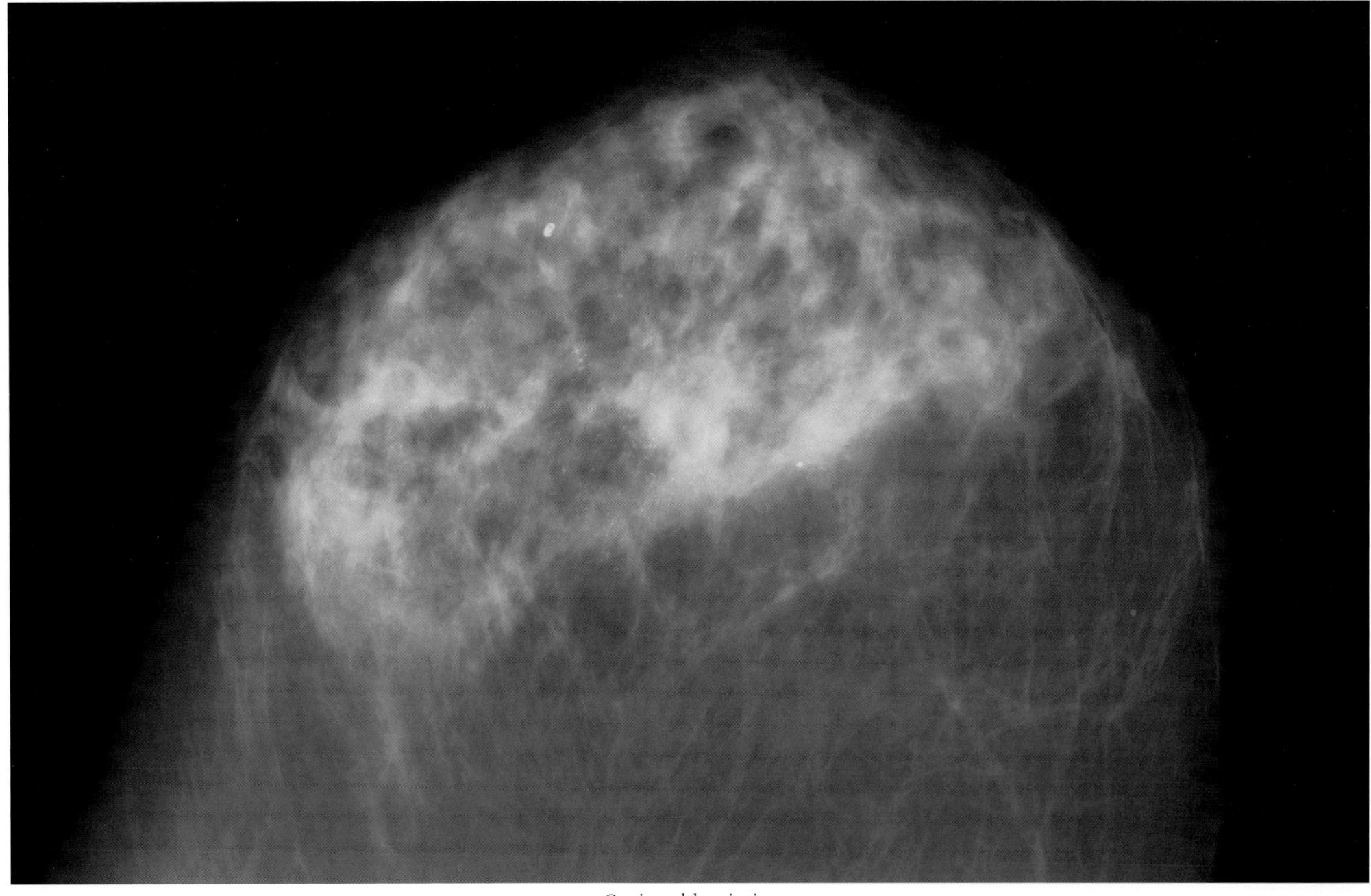

Craniocaudal projection

Mixed calcifications

Diffuse mixed calcifications, granular type associated with cast-like ones, are visible anteriorly, highly consistent with malignancy.

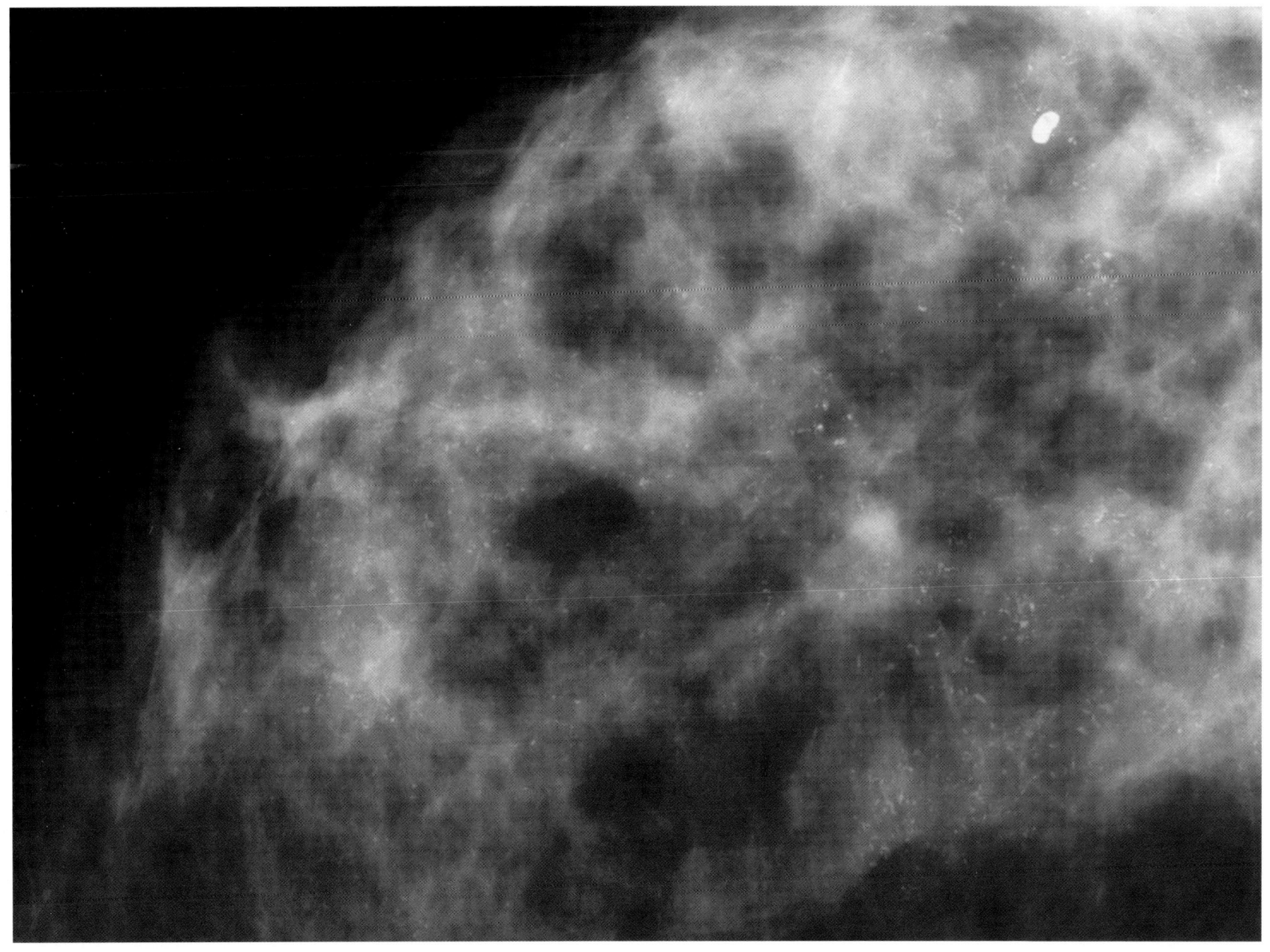

Craniocaudal magnification view

Histology: multifocal infiltrating carcinoma, with an extensive intraductal component

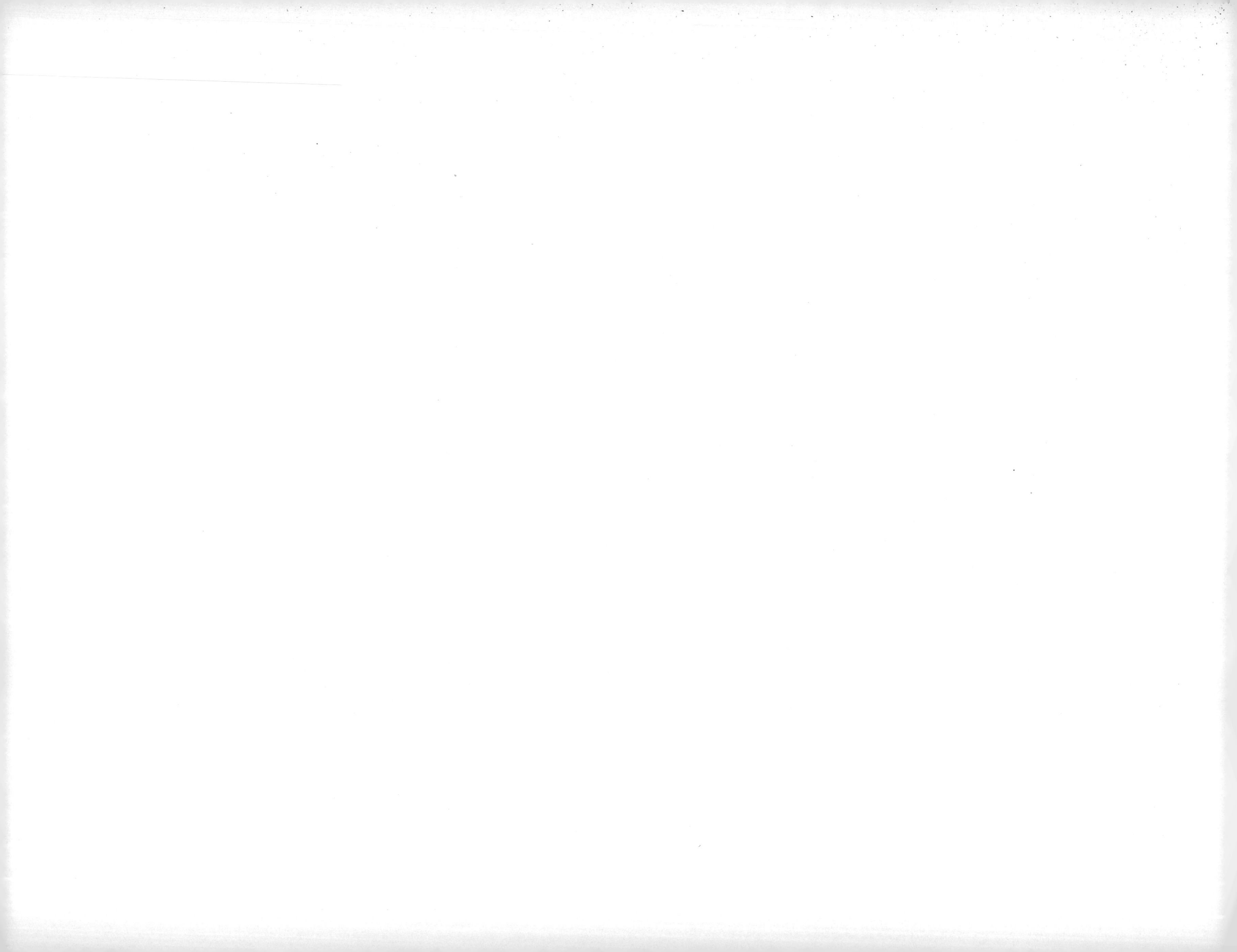

Radiolucency

A sharp-edged radiolucent mass may be seen, with a radiopaque rim that is generally complete or only partly broken. Varying in size and sometimes occupying the whole breast, these may be round, oval or more rarely lobulated. They are usually caused by lipomas, pseudolipomas and foci of fat necrosis.

Radiolucency

A large, round, radiolucent mass is visible in the upper part, occupying most of the breast and surrounded for two thirds by a radiopaque rim that gradually fades into the background (A). This oval mass has a radiopaque capsule that can be seen clearly only in the lower portion, proximal to the submammary groove, and contains another lobular radiolucent mass with a contiguous coarse calcification (B).

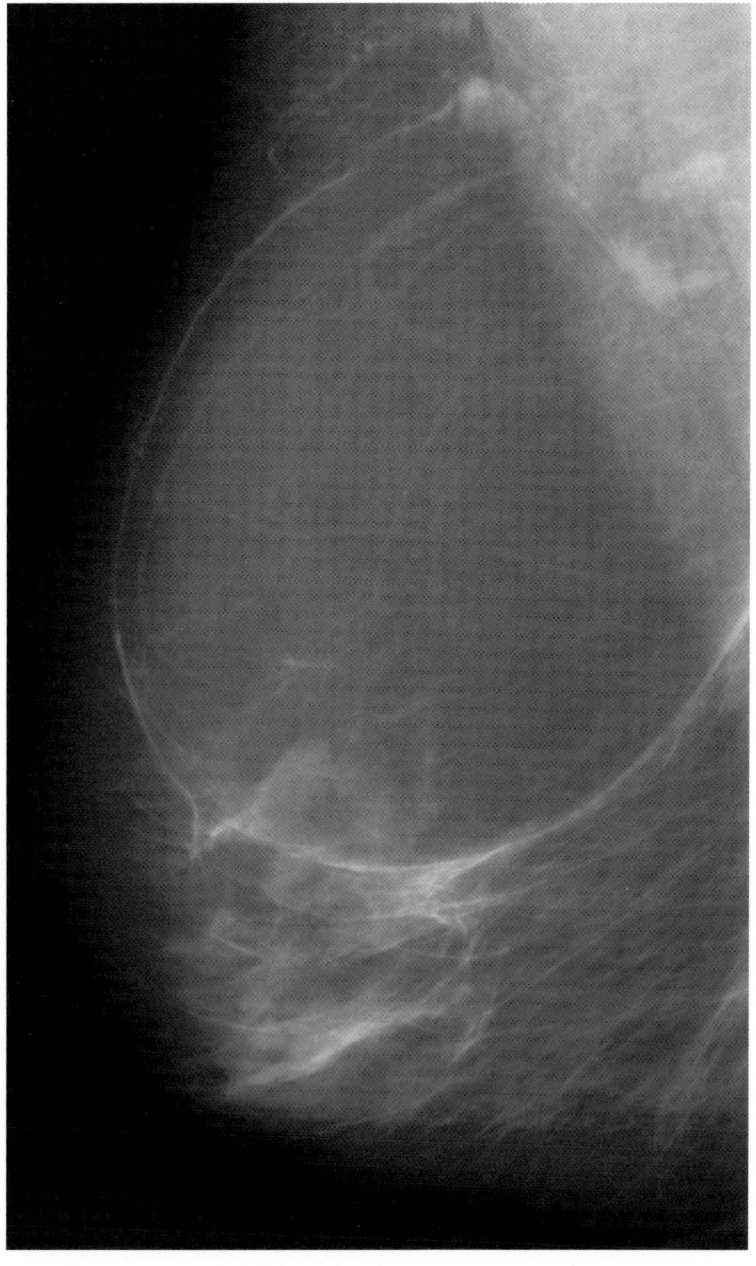

Mediolateral oblique projection (A)

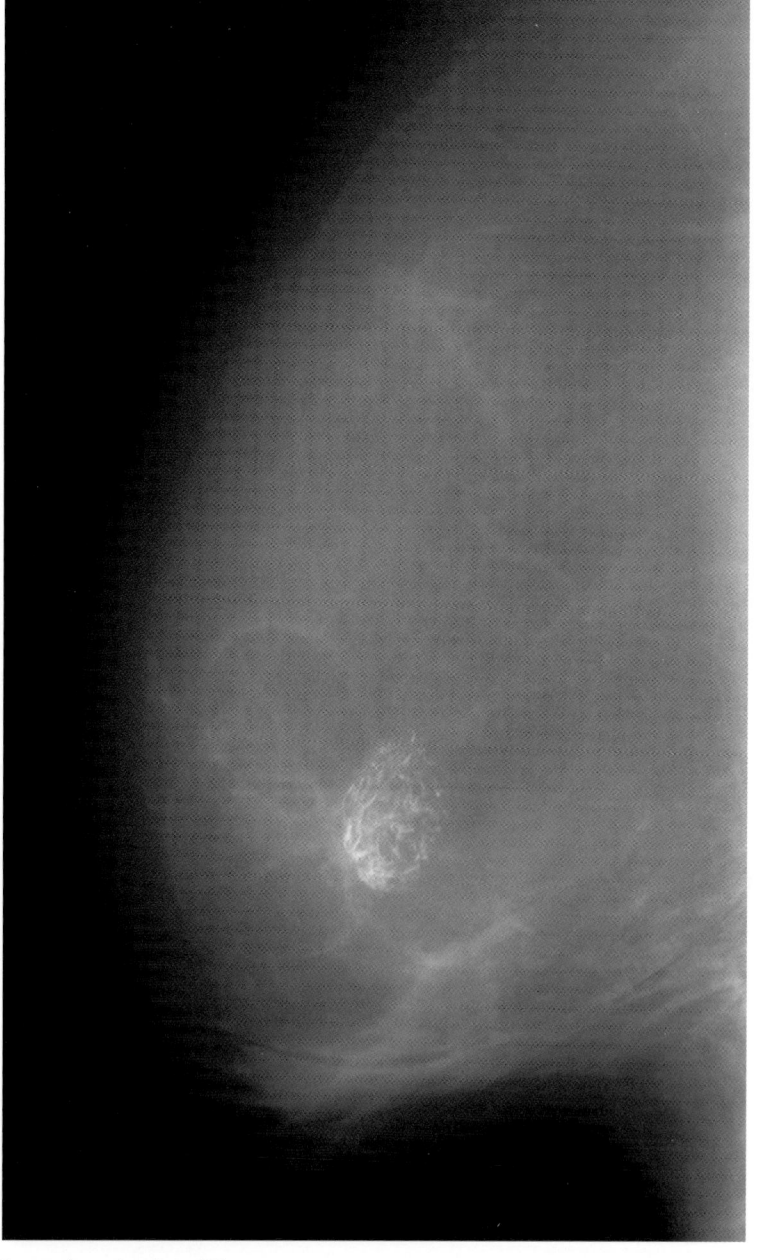

Lateral projection (B)

Radiolucency

These spot magnification views show inferiorly, near the submammary groove, the radiopaque capsule which seems to run parallel to the thin halo rim of the mass (A). More clearly visible is the lobulated radiolucent mass, with its fine, low-density radiopaque ring. The contiguous coarse oval calcification seems to delimit another radiolucent mass (B). Both structures are probably the result of fat necrosis, partly calcified.

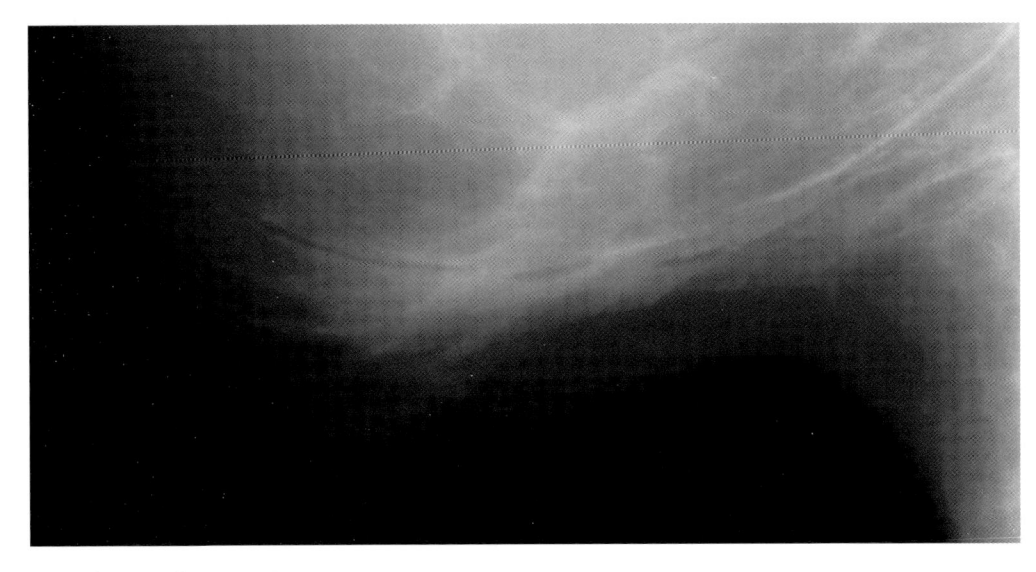

Lateral magnification view (A)

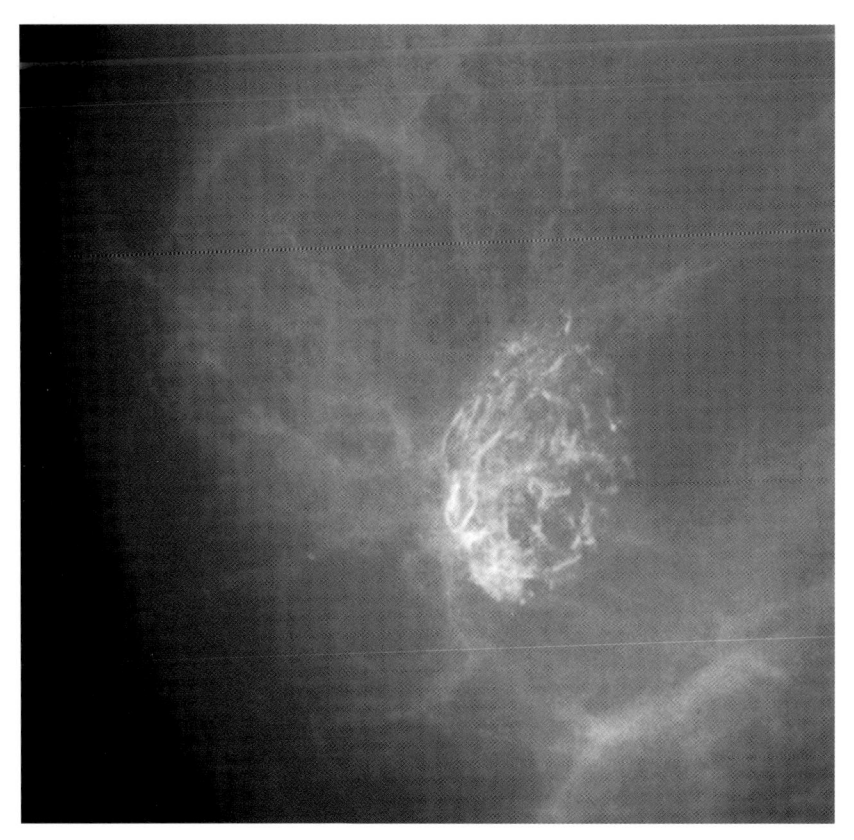

Lateral magnification view (B)

Radiolucency

An oval radiolucent mass, surrounded by a thin radiopaque ring, is seen posteriorly in the lower outer quadrant. In the oblique projection (A) it seems to contain multiple, sharply outlined, oval, circumscribed opacities, suggestive of fibroadenolipoma. The craniocaudal projection (B) clearly shows the opacities are outside the lesion. The finding is consistent with lipoma.

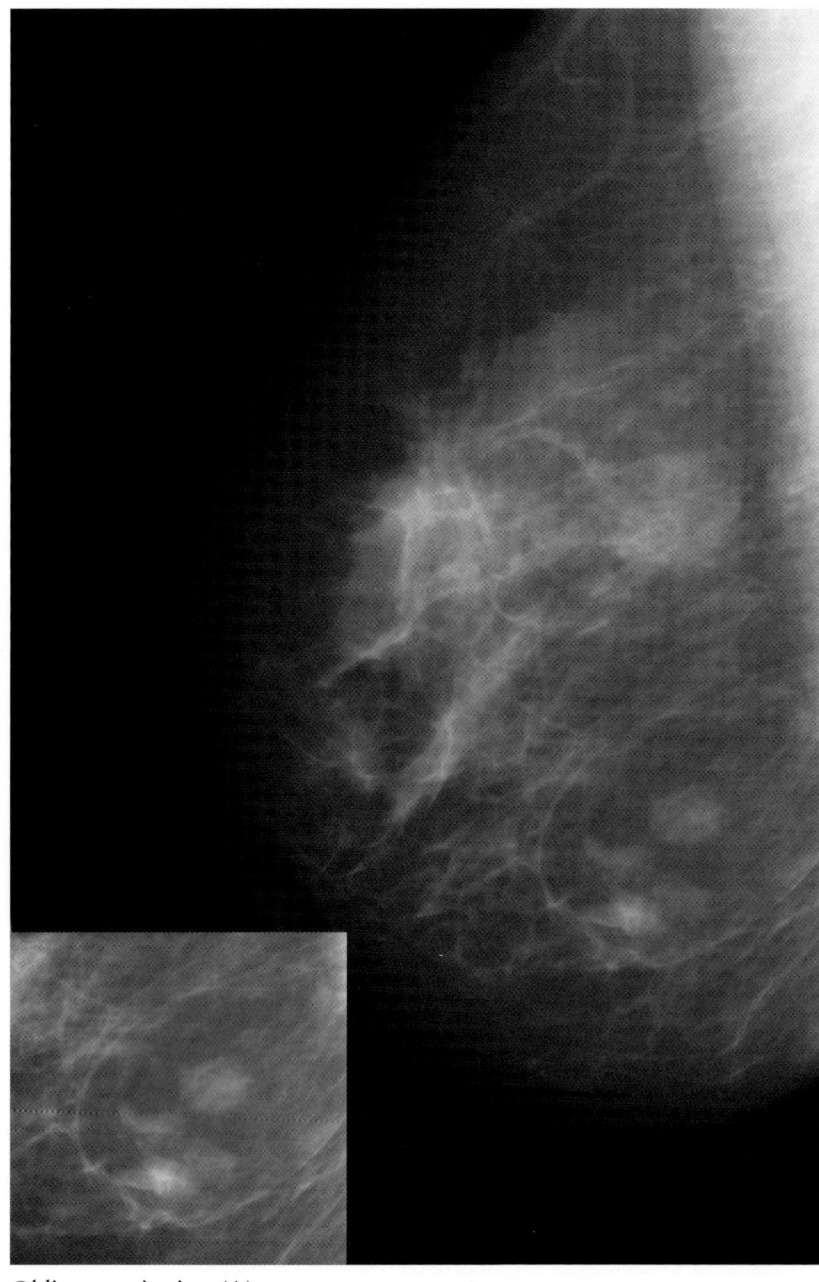

Oblique projection (A)

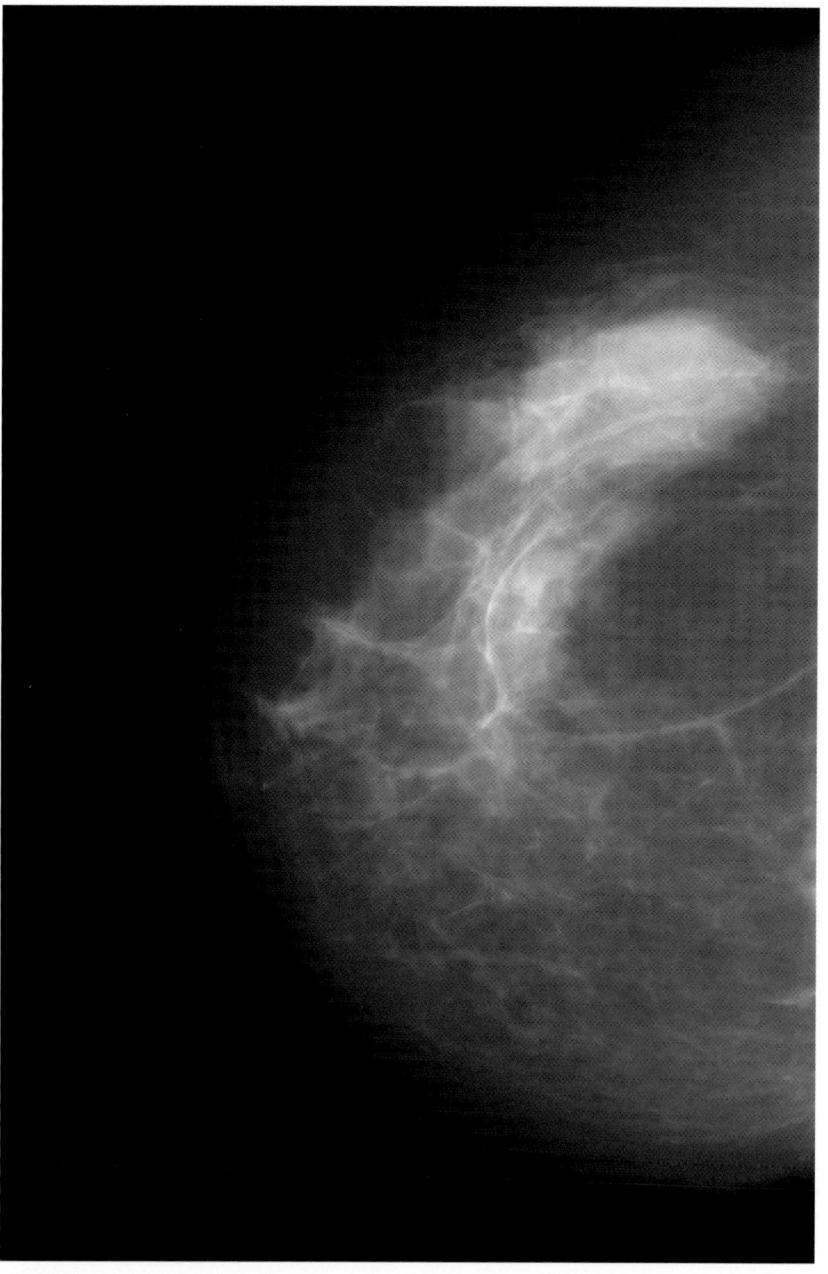

Craniocaudal projection (B)

Radiolucency

A huge, oval, radiolucent mass, occupying most of the breast and surrounded by a thin radiopaque line, is seen on the oblique (A) and craniocaudal projections (B). The finding is consistent with lipoma.

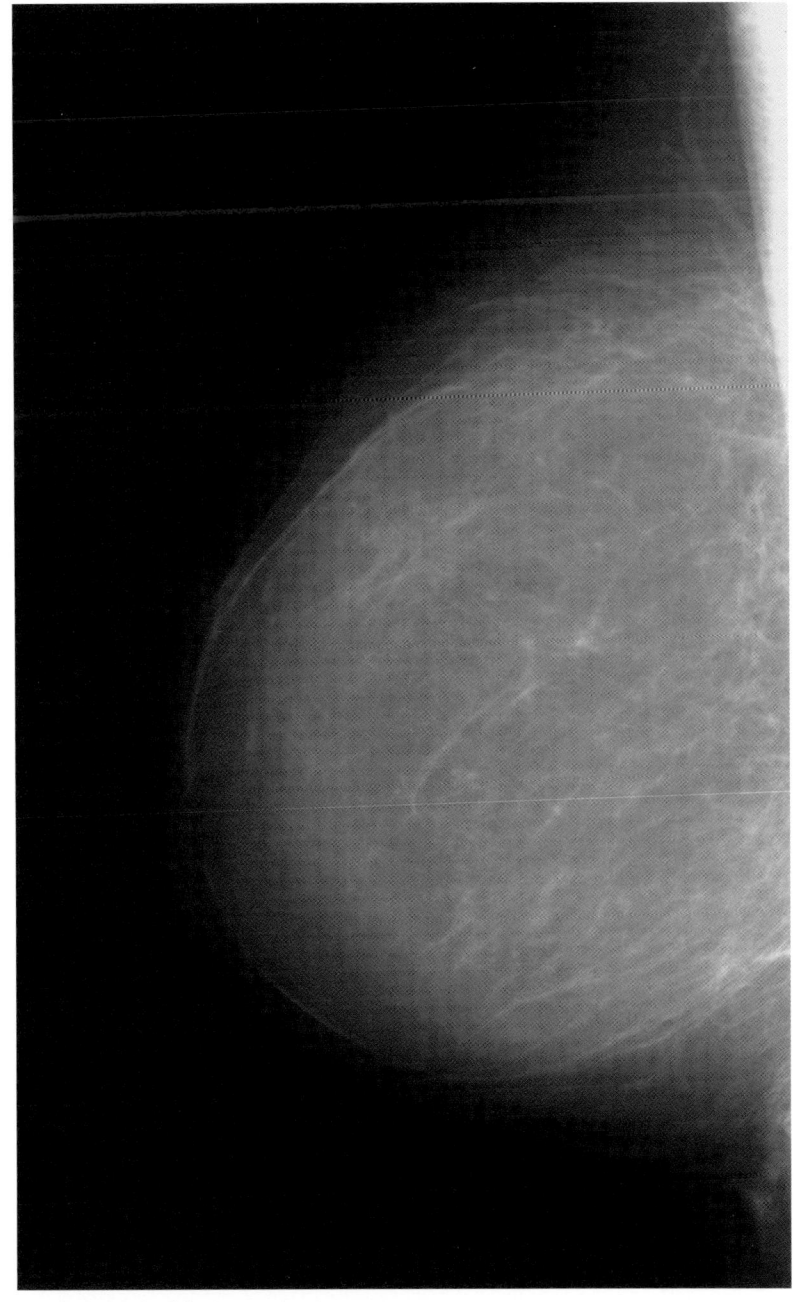

Mediolateral oblique projection (A)

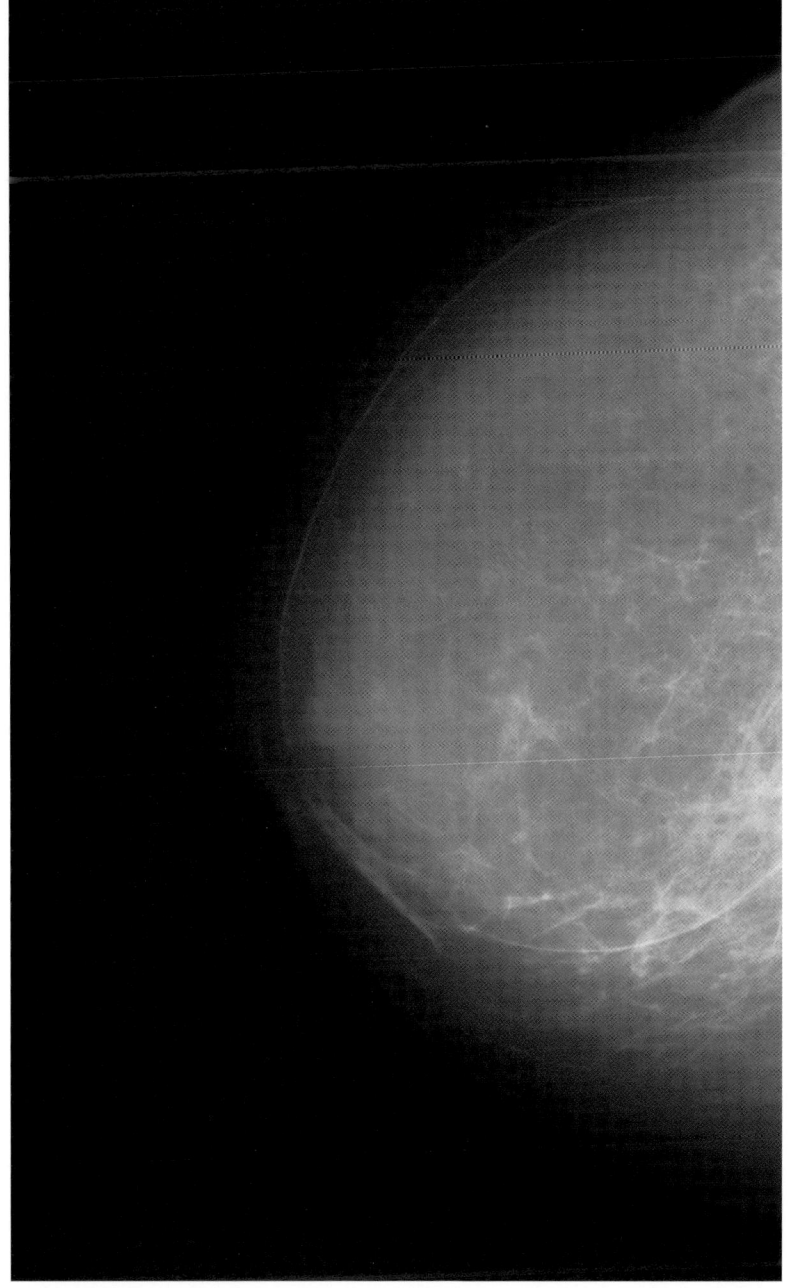

Craniocaudal projection (B)

Radiolucency

An oval radiolucent mass is seen posteriorly in the upper quadrant with a clear-cut posterior outline and an ill-defined anterior margin fading into the surrounding parenchyma (A). An oval, well-delineated radiolucent mass is seen centrally in the upper quadrant (B). Neither formation has a radiopaque rim. The finding is consistent with pseudolipomas.

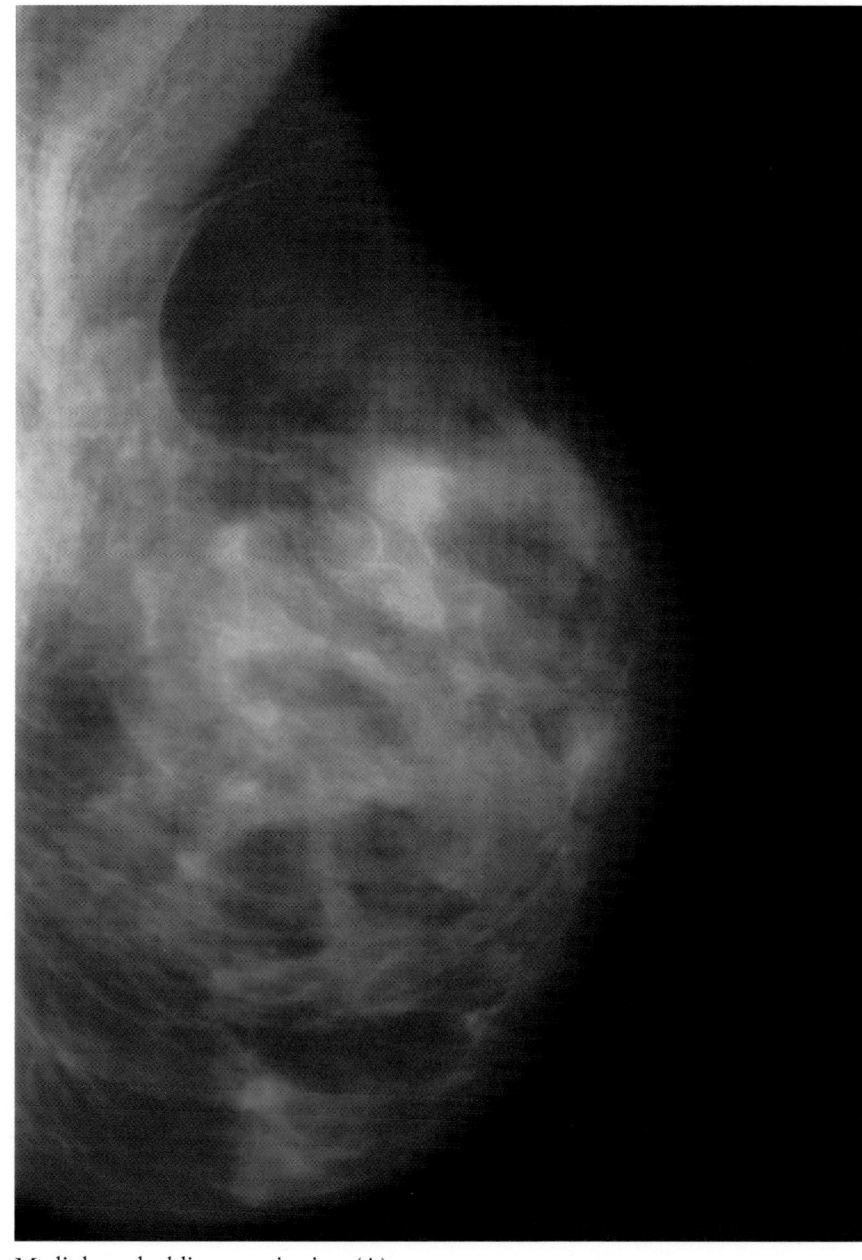

Mediolateral oblique projection (A)

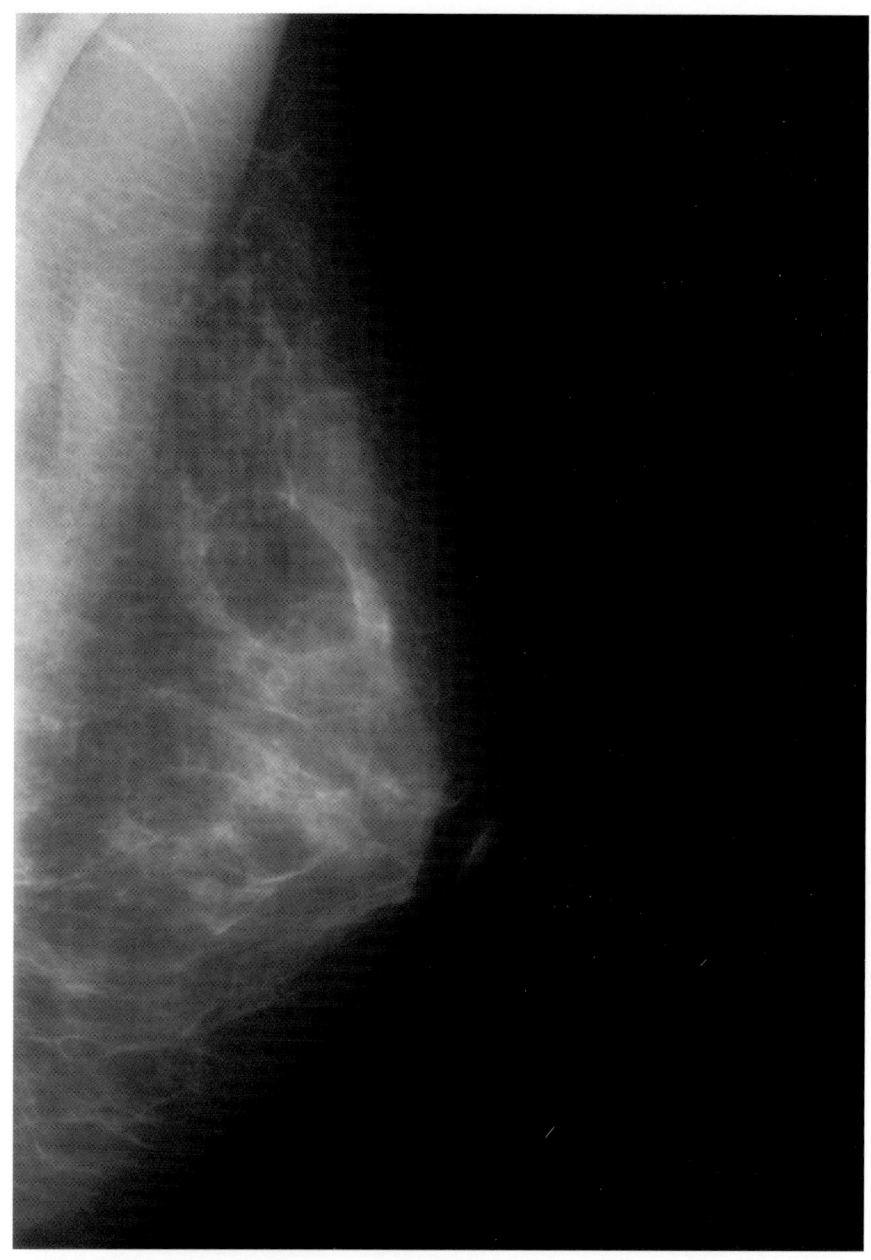

Craniocaudal projection (B)

Radiolucency

A lobulated, radiolucent mass is apparent anteriorly in the upper quadrant, surrounded by an unevenly thick radiopaque rim, with partial septa inside. A hard nodular mass with an irregular contour is palpable at clinical examination. This finding points to traumatic fat necrosis.

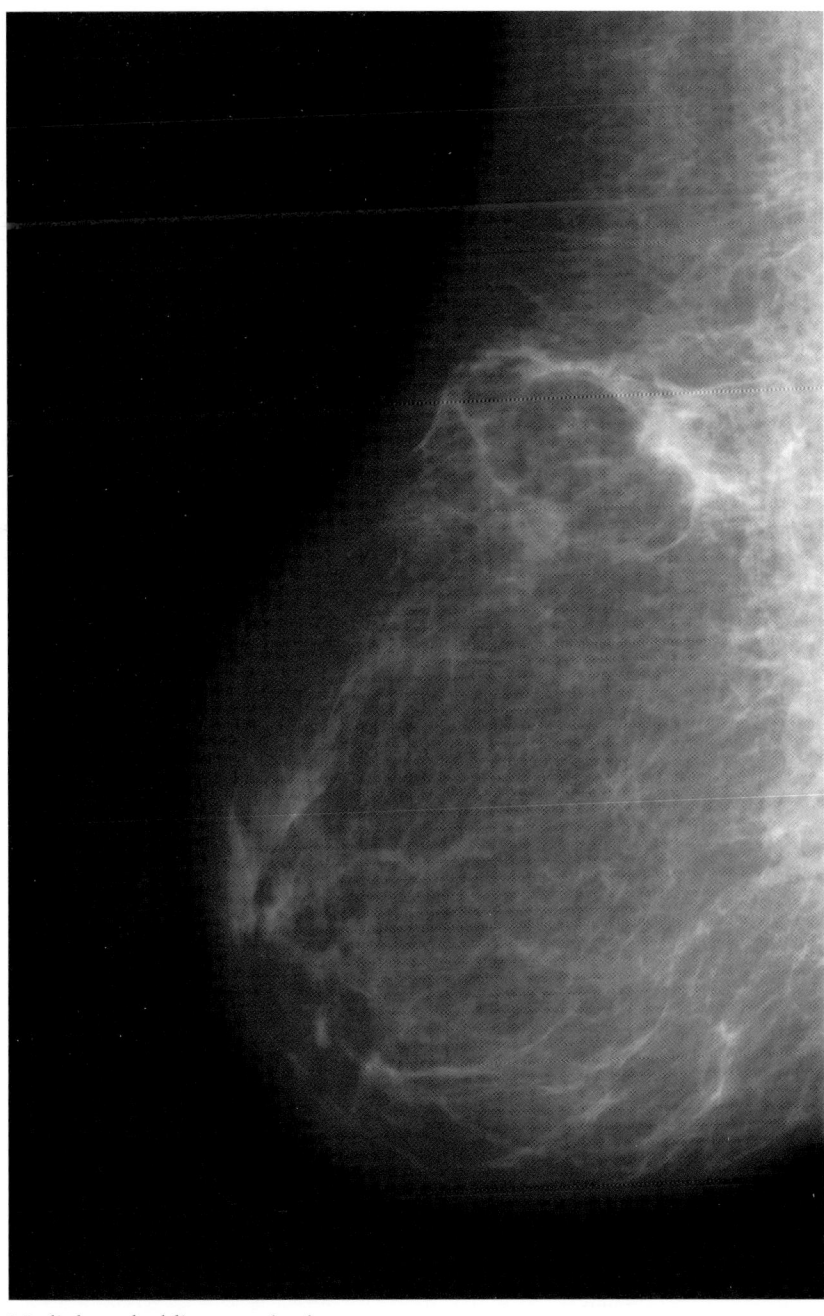

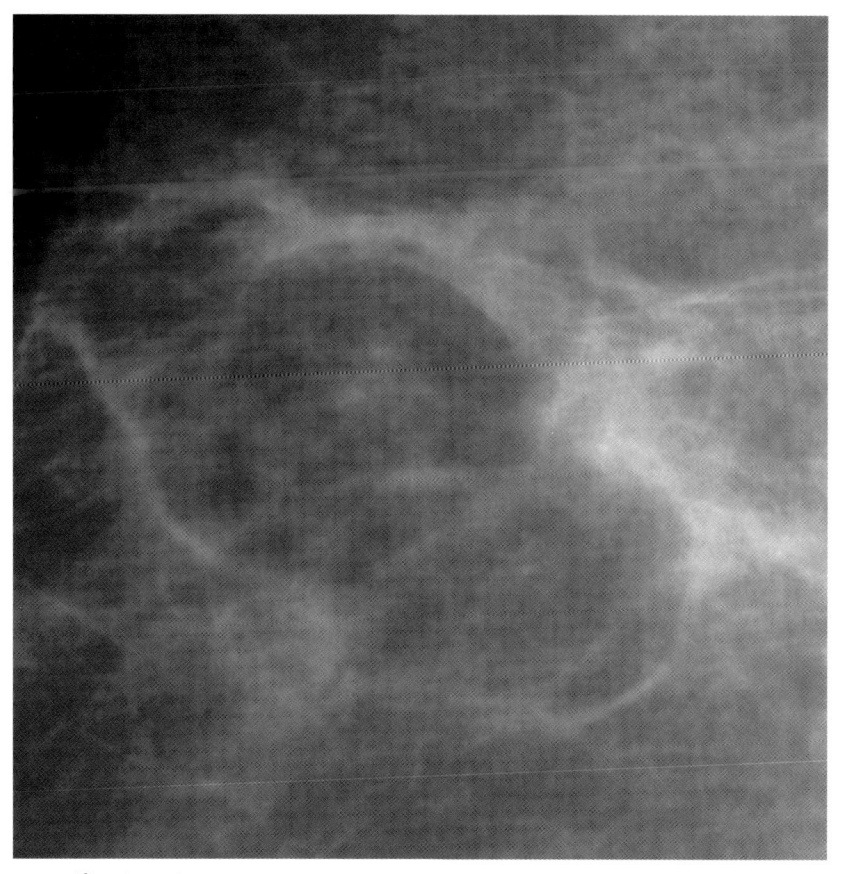

Magnification view

Mediolateral oblique projection

RADIOLUCENCY

Radiolucency

An oval radiolucent mass, surrounded by an unevenly thick radiopaque rim, is seen posteriorly in a central location in the breast (B). This image was taken six months after nodulectomy for an opacity in the same place (A). The diagnostic finding is consistent with traumatic fat necrosis.

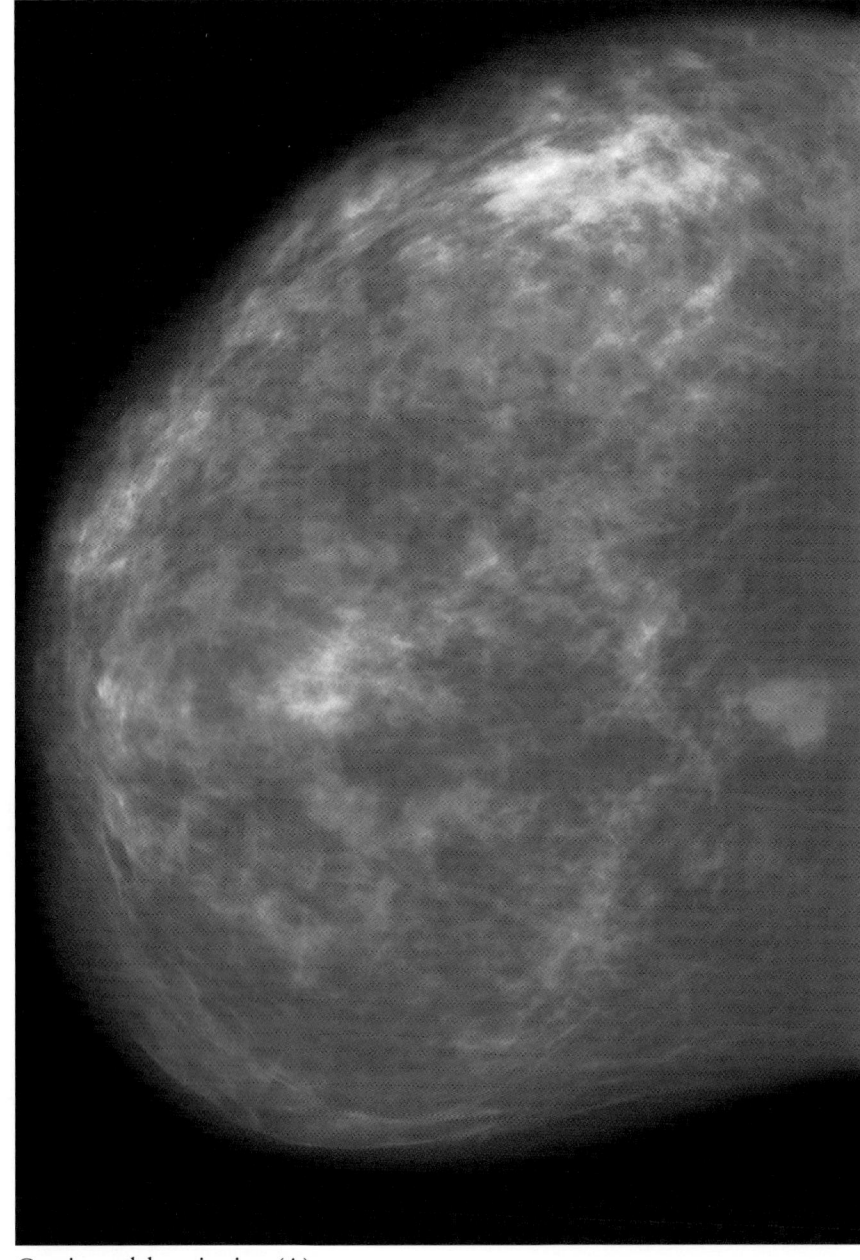

Craniocaudal projection (A)

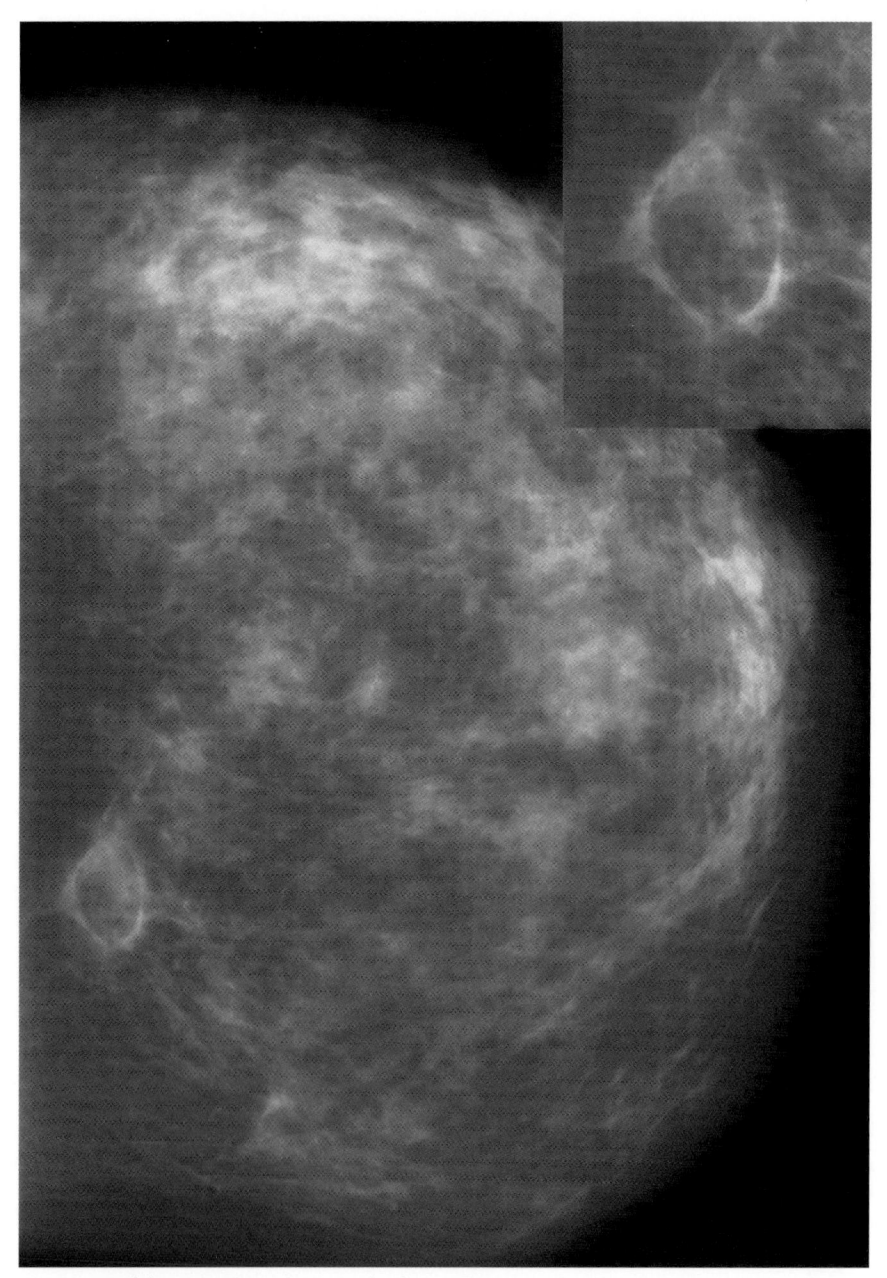

Craniocaudal projection six months later (B)

Asymmetric breast tissue

Significant areas of fibroglandular tissue on one side that appear different compared with the contralateral breast, because they are either of greater extent or of higher density. If there are no other abnormalities, this is simply a normal variant of breast structure.

ASYMMETRIC BREAST TISSUE

Parenchymal asymmetry
In the upper outer quadrant the density of the parenchymal tissue is higher than in the controlateral breast, as shown in both the oblique and craniocaudal views, with no signs of focal pathology.

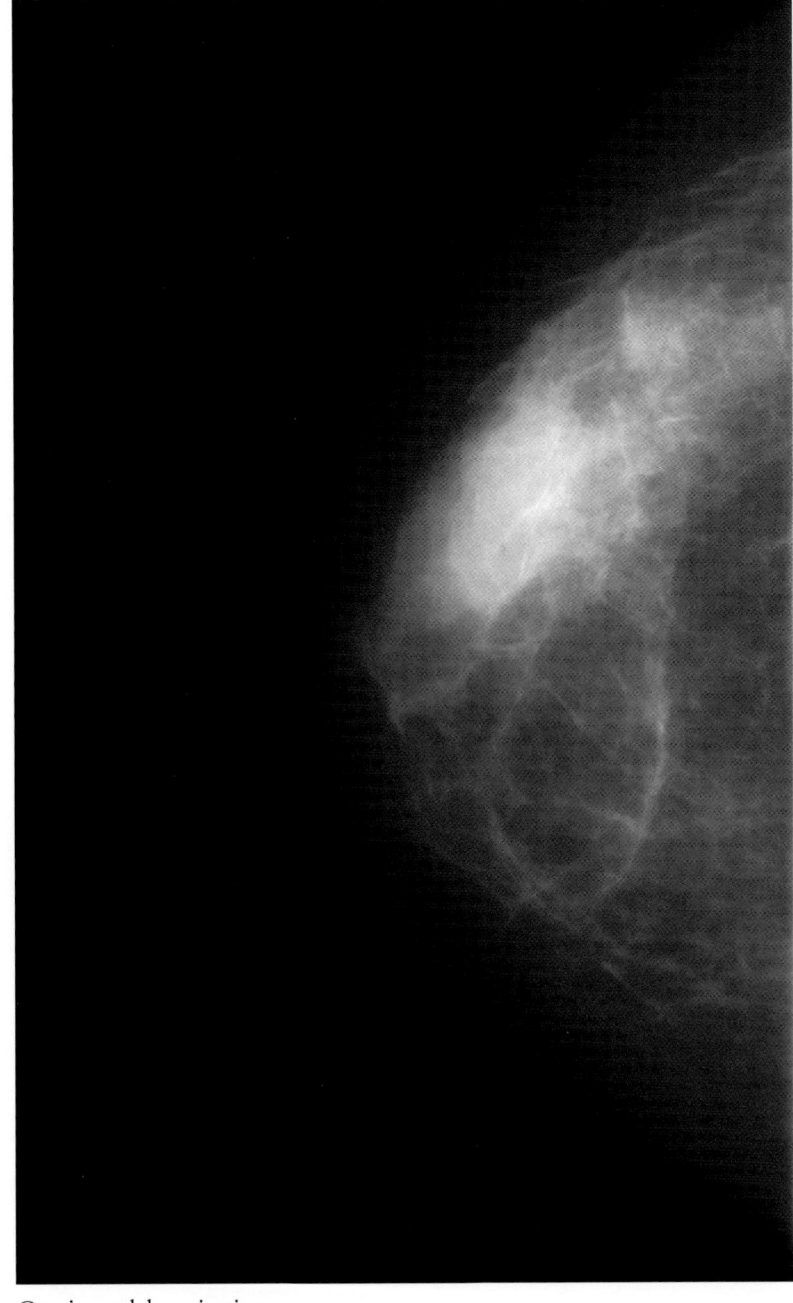

Craniocaudal projection

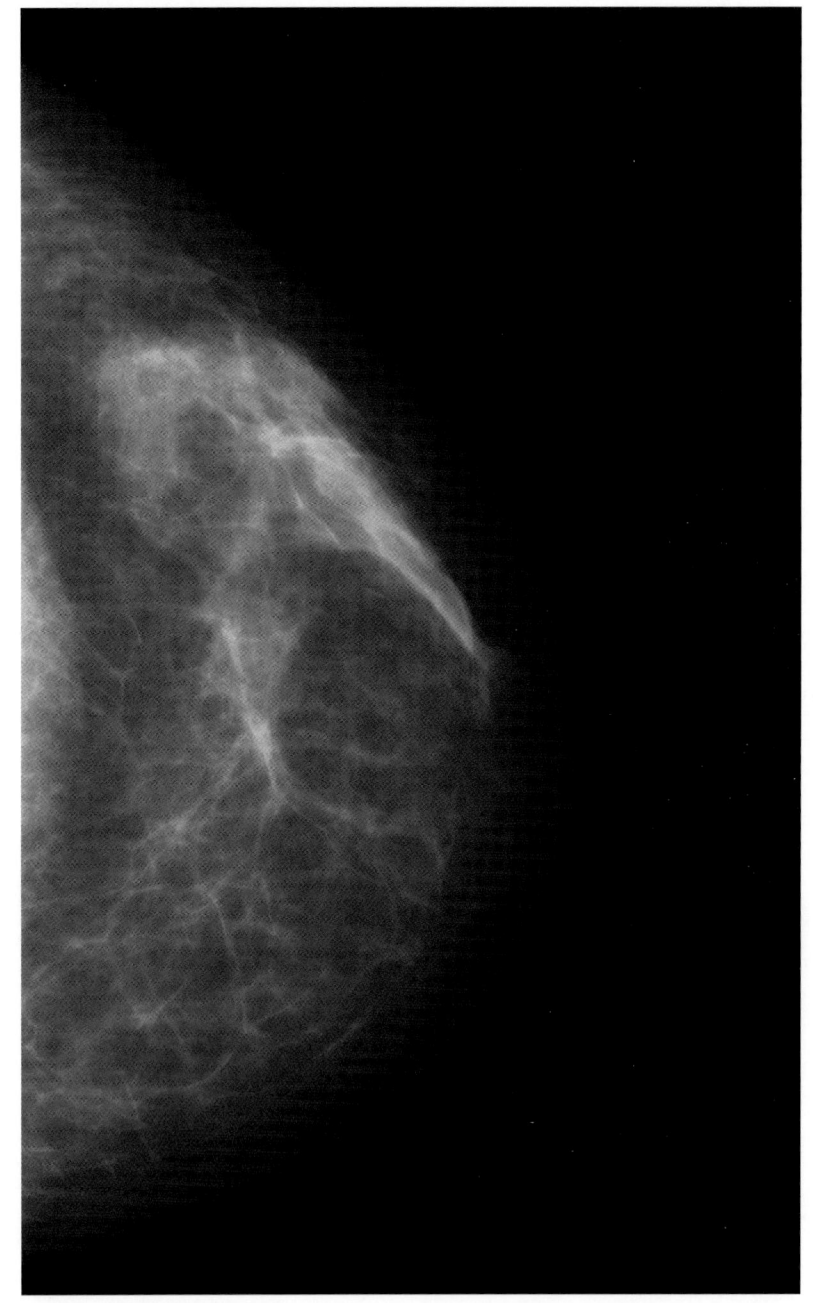

Craniocaudal projection

Parenchymal asymmetry

In the upper outer quadrant the density of the parenchymal tissue is greater than in the controlateral breast, as shown in both the oblique and craniocaudal views, with no signs of focal pathology.

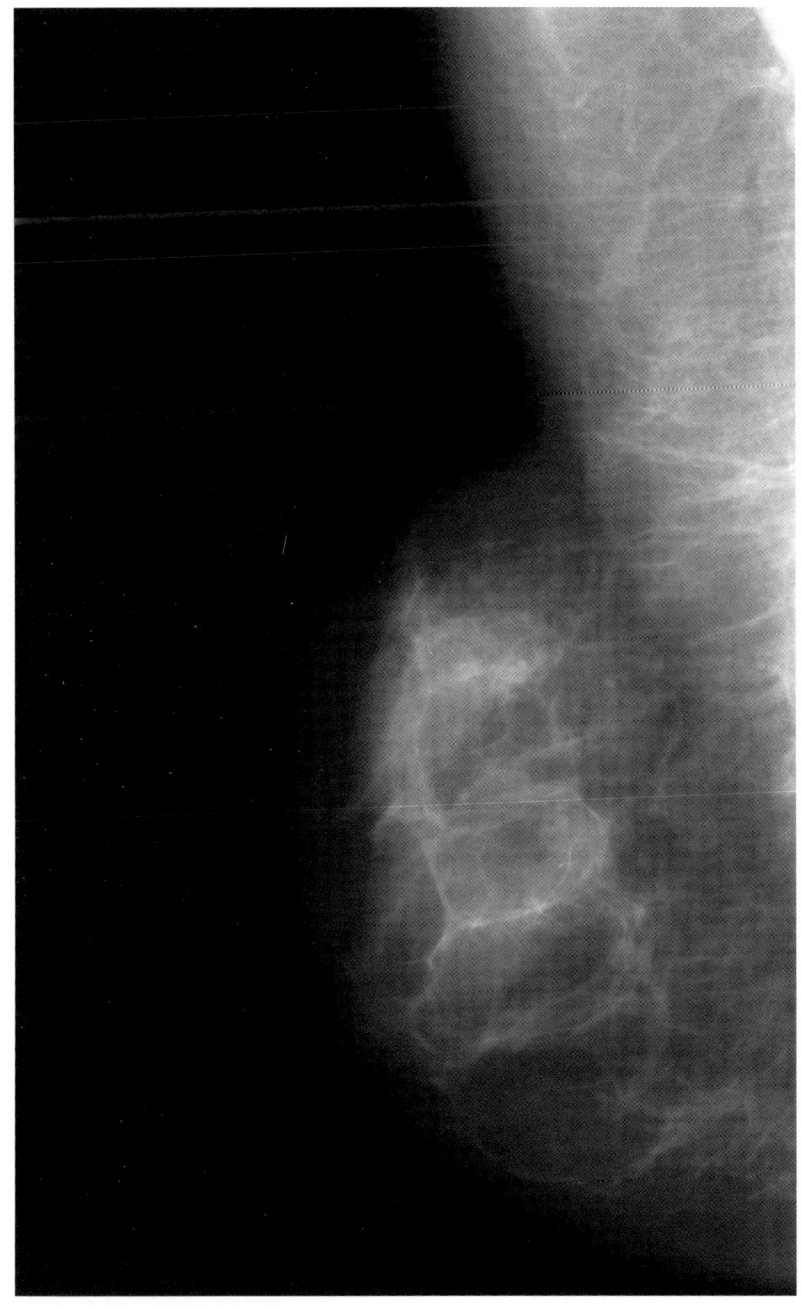

Mediolateral oblique projection

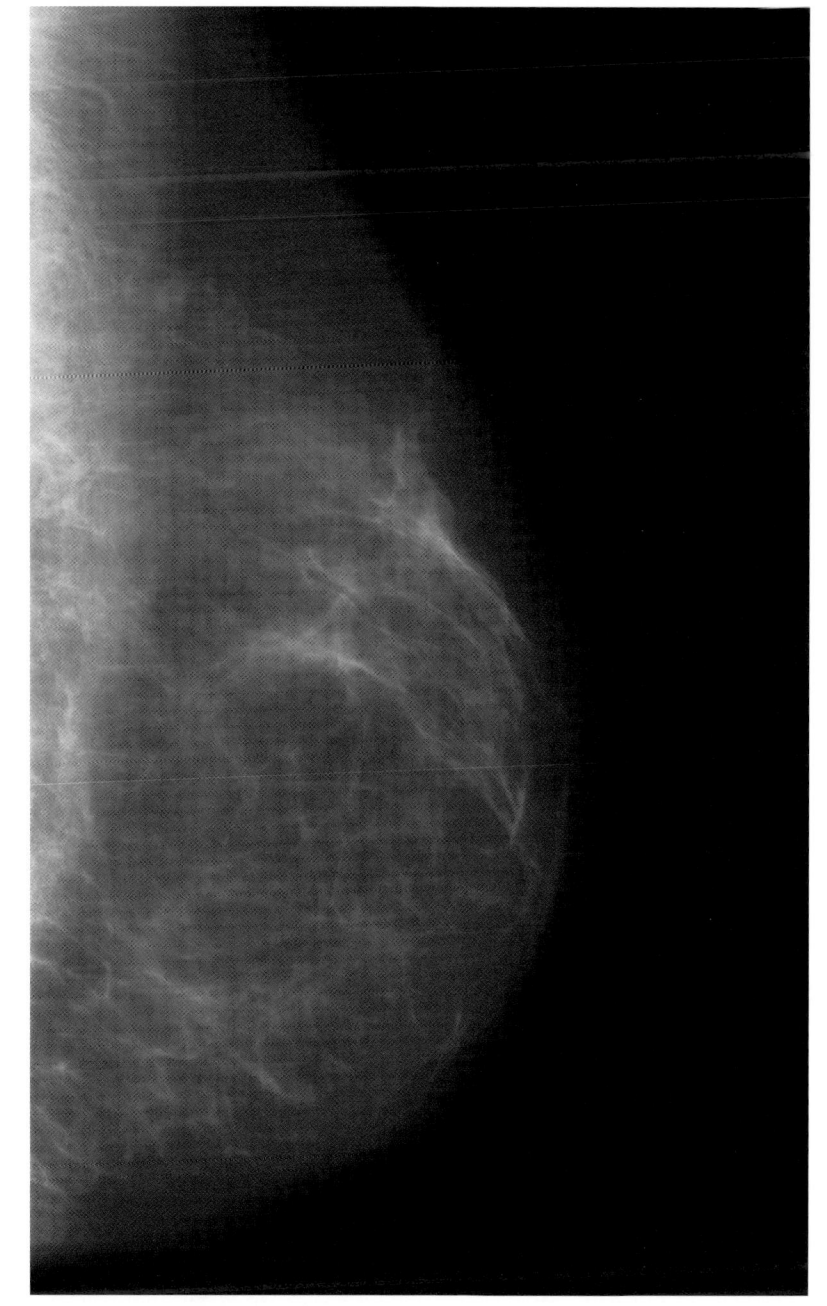

Mediolateral oblique projection

ASYMMETRIC BREAST TISSUE

Parenchymal asymmetry
The breast parenchyma on the left seems more voluminous than the other one, with no signs of focal pathology.

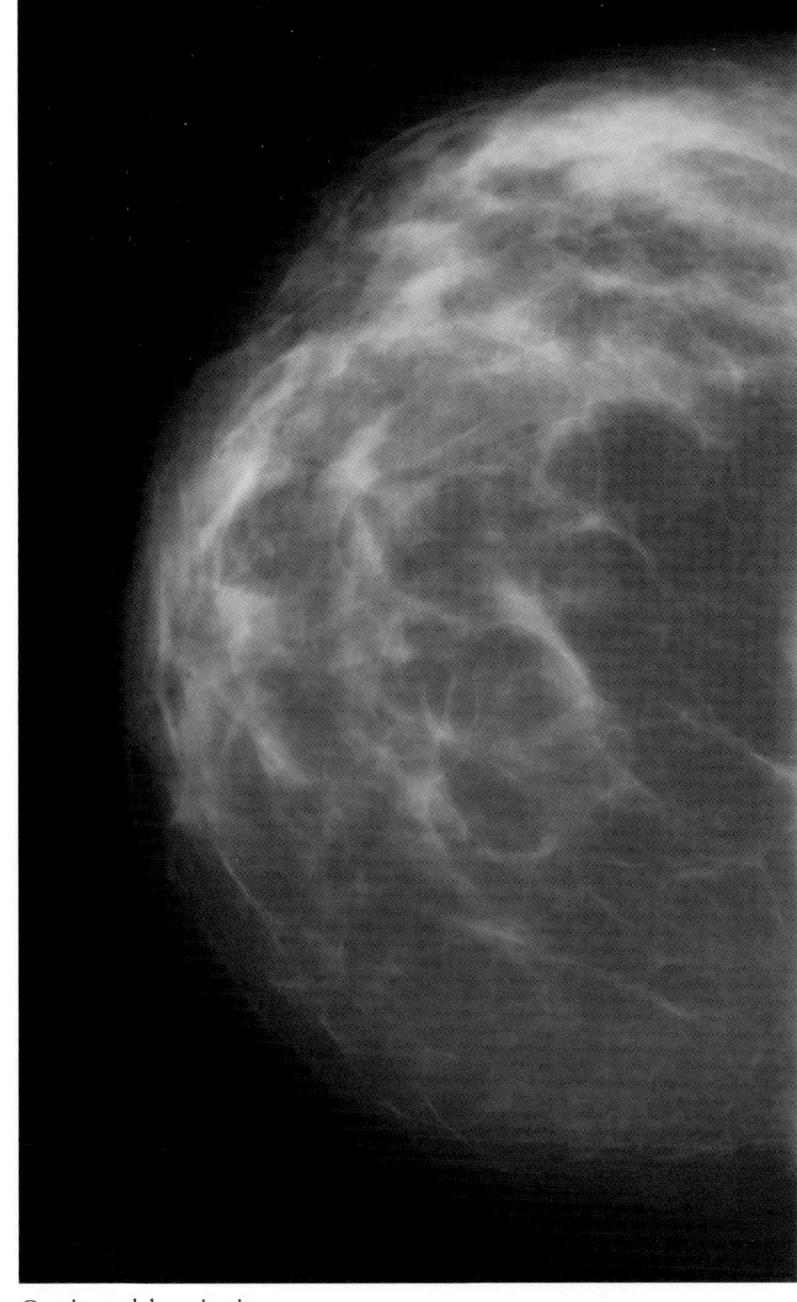

Craniocaudal projection

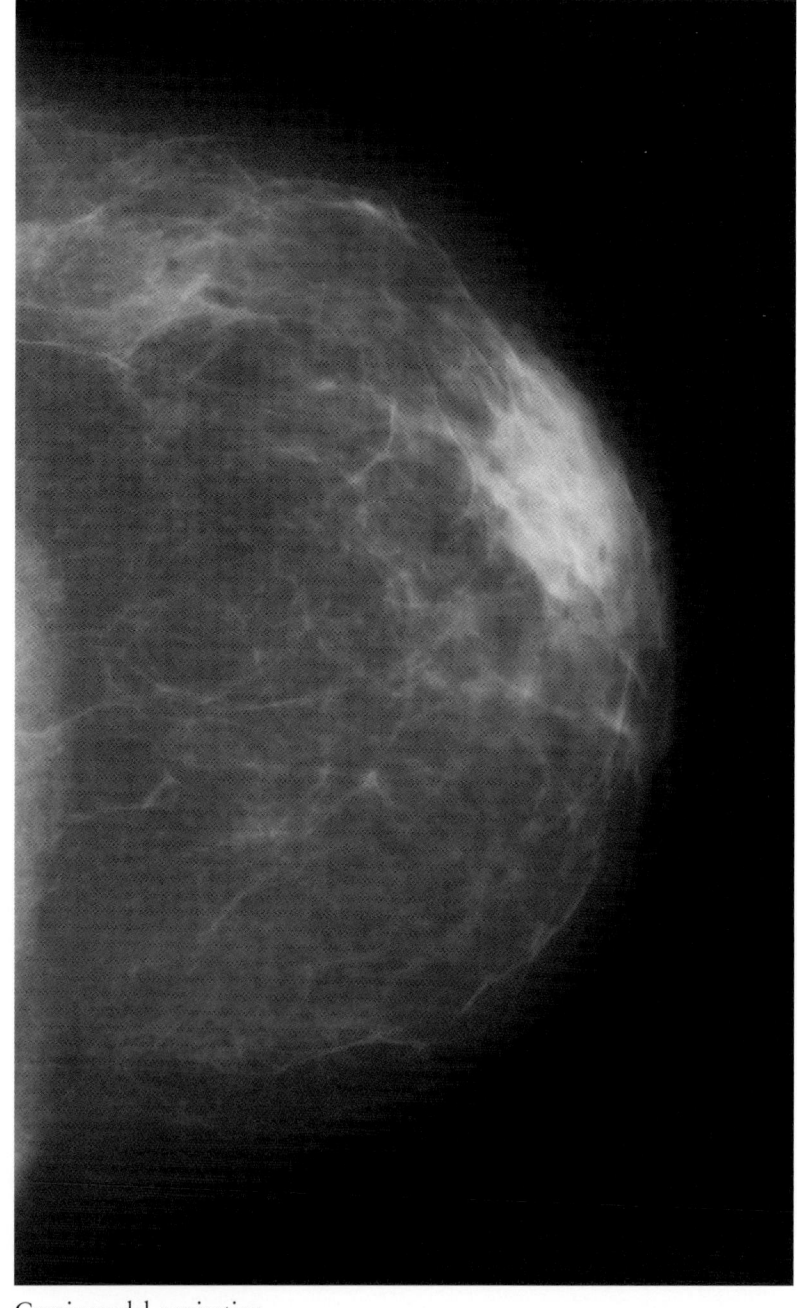

Craniocaudal projection

Focal asymmetry

Areas of glandular tissue without the characteristics of a true mass, but recognizable with similar appearance in the craniocaudal, lateral and oblique projection. These may simply be normal local asymmetries but further investigation is justified, with targeted magnification views and if necessary ultrasound.

FOCAL ASYMMETRY

Focal asymmetry

In the right upper outer quadrant there is a visible area of parenchymal tissue of higher density than the other breast, with a similar appearance in both the oblique and craniocaudal views, with no signs of focal pathology.

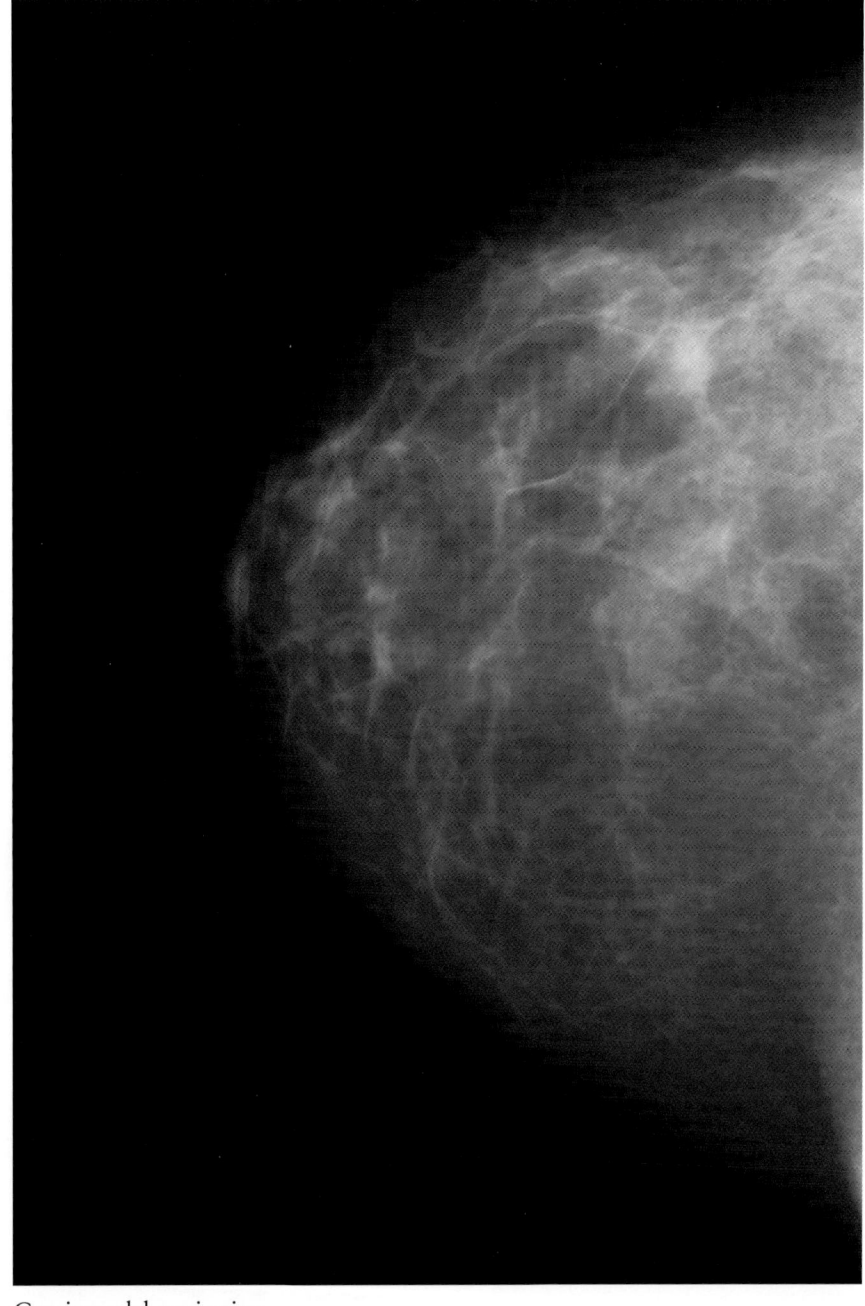

Craniocaudal projection

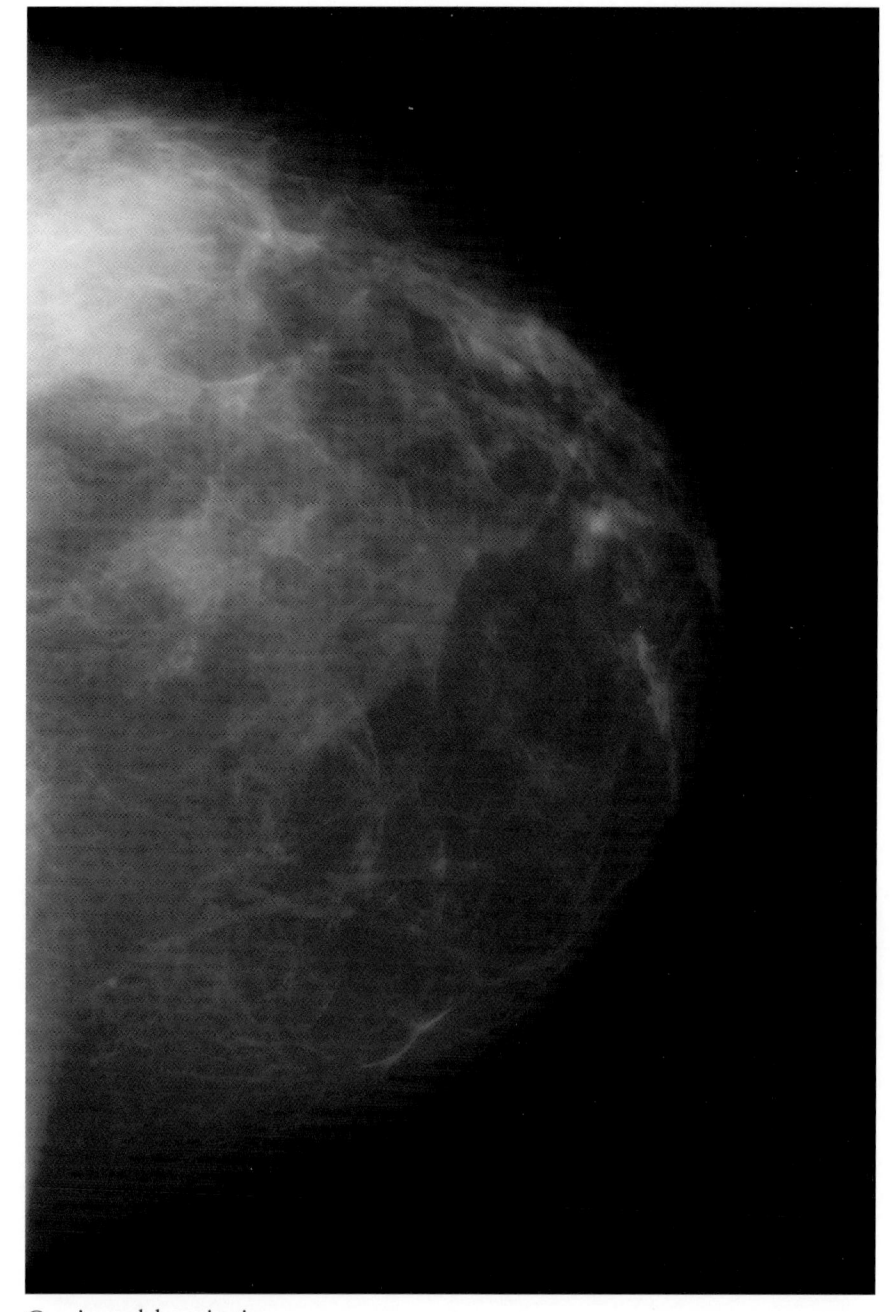

Craniocaudal projection

Focal asymmetry

In the right upper outer quadrant there is a visible area of parenchymal tissue of higher density than the other breast, with a similar appearance in both the oblique and craniocaudal views, with no signs of focal pathology.

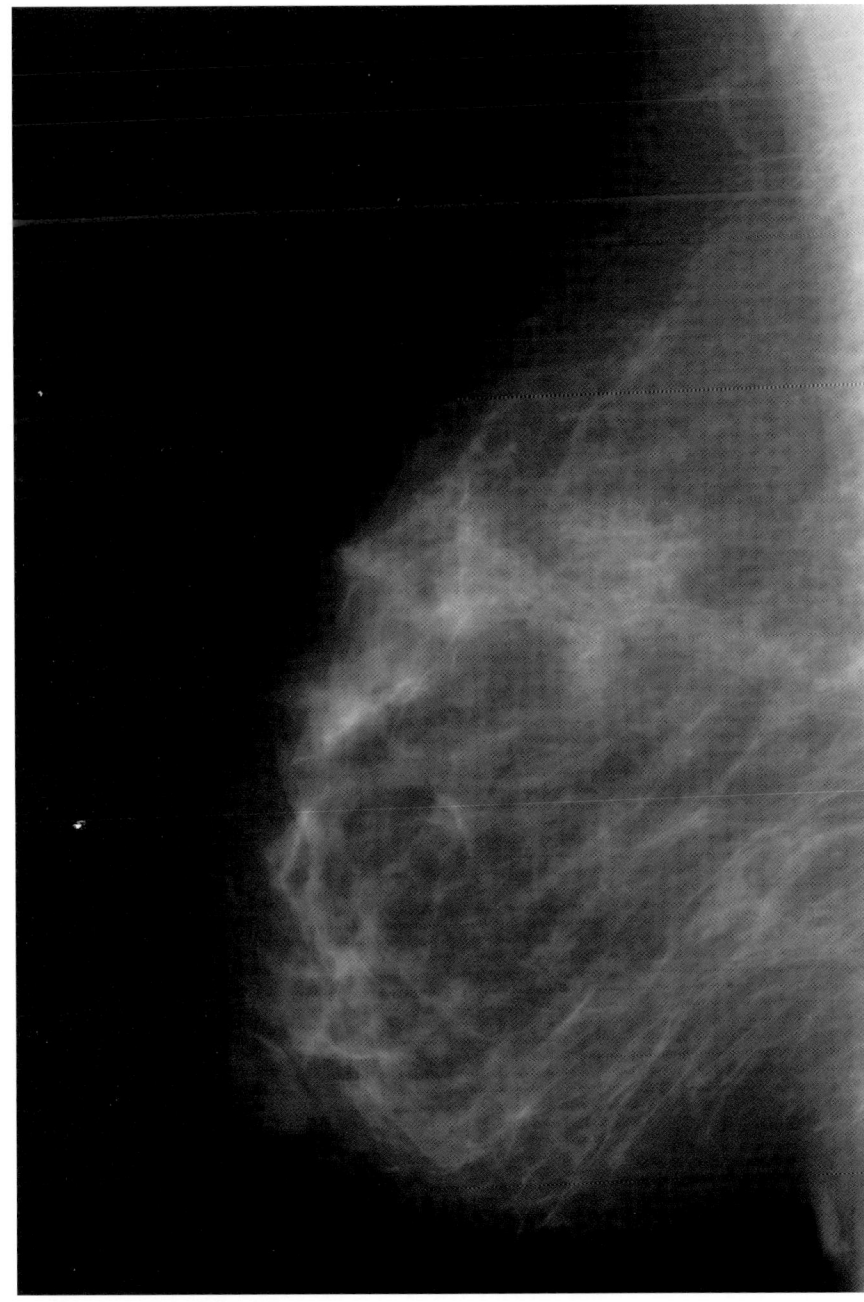

Mediolateral oblique projection

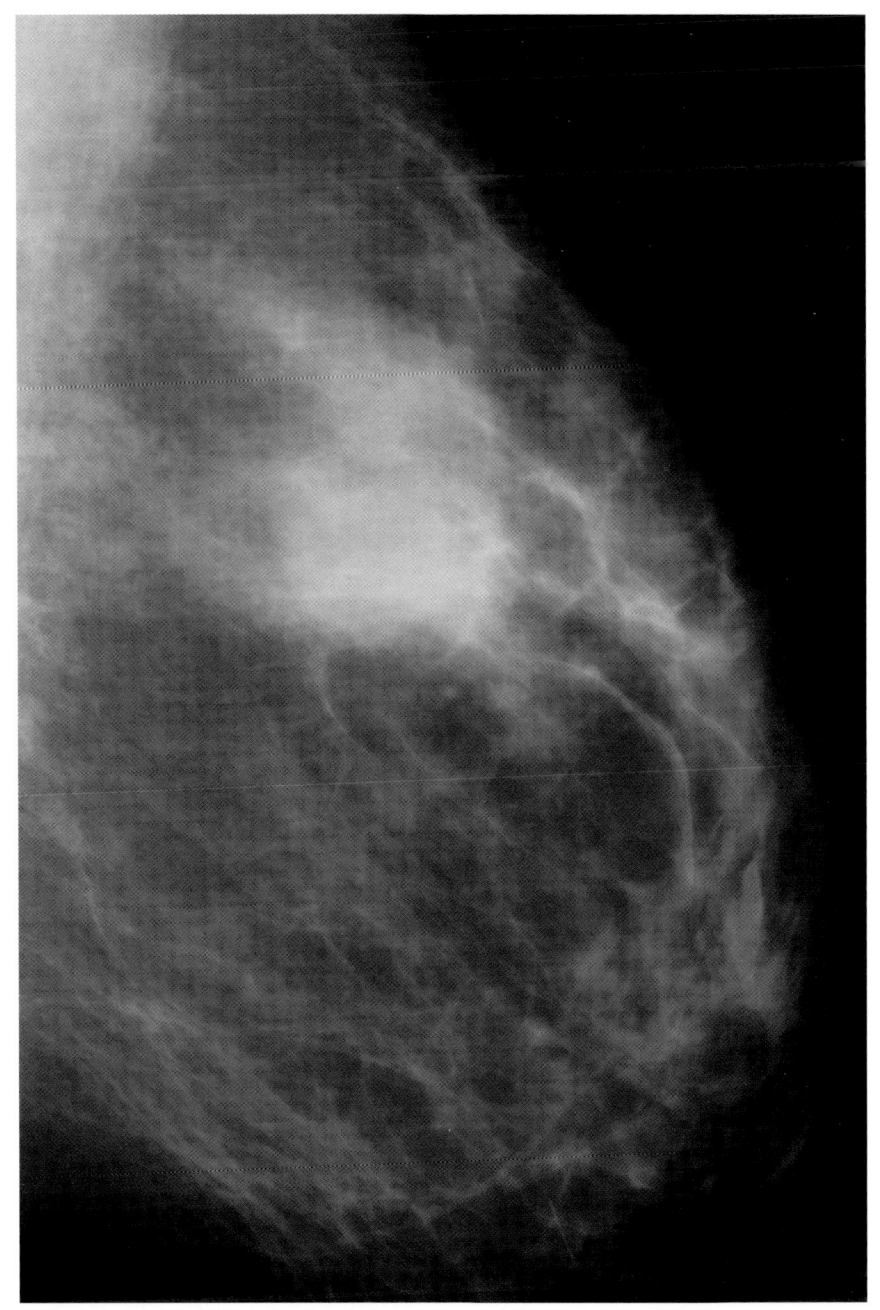

Mediolateral oblique projection

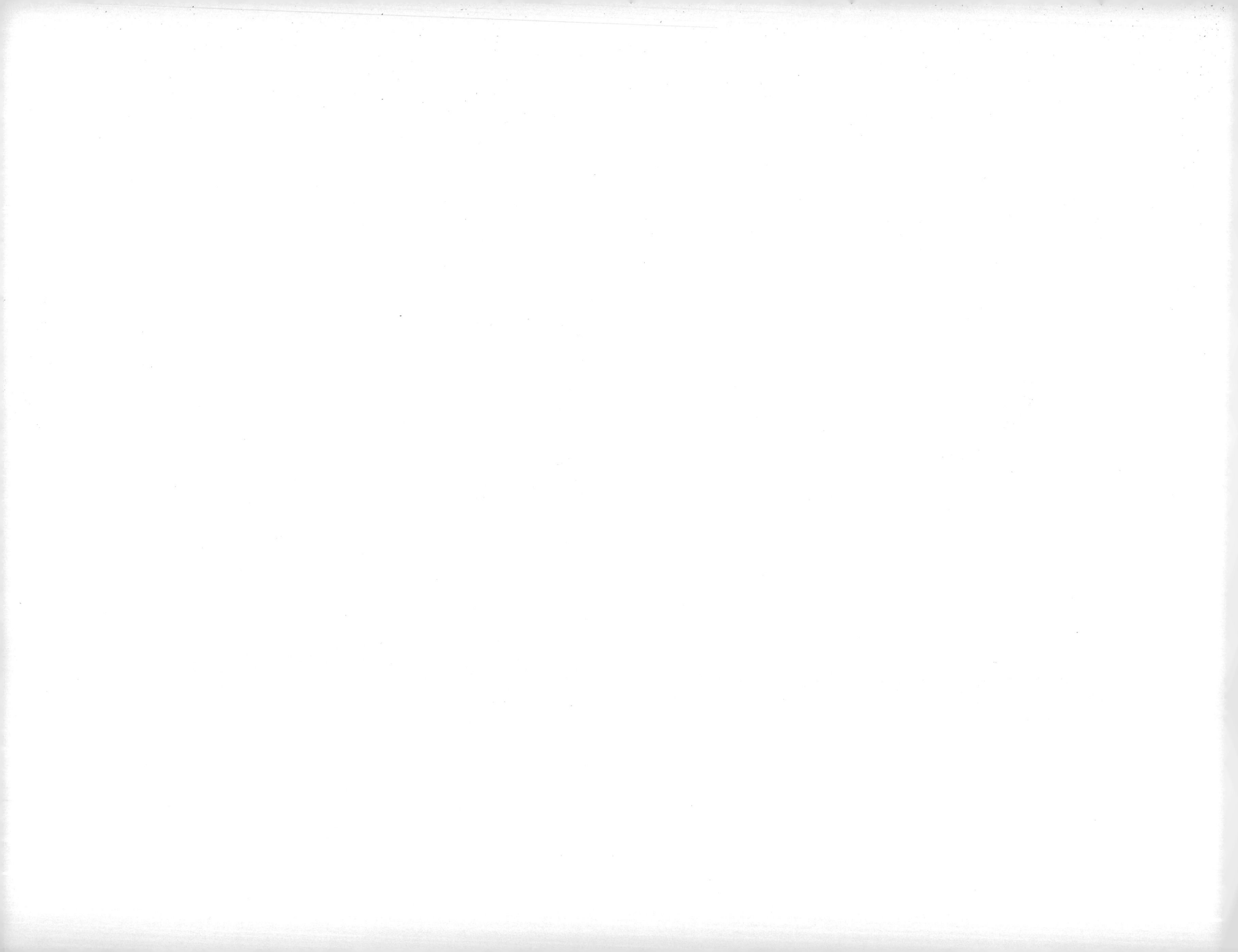

Skin thickening and retraction

Skin thickening and retraction can be diffuse or focal. Skin thickening, or even ulceration, can occur as a result of tumour direct invasion or through thickening and retraction of Cooper's ligaments.
Skin changes can result from a contiguous malignancy, infection or inflammation, primary skin disorders, lymphatic or vascular obstruction, and systemic diseases affecting the skin. Post-surgical scarring and fat necrosis can also cause skin thickening and retraction.

Skin thickening and retraction

A high density, stellate opacity with radiating spicules into the surrounding parenchyma is seen in the inner subareolar location with thickened and retracted overlying areolar skin.

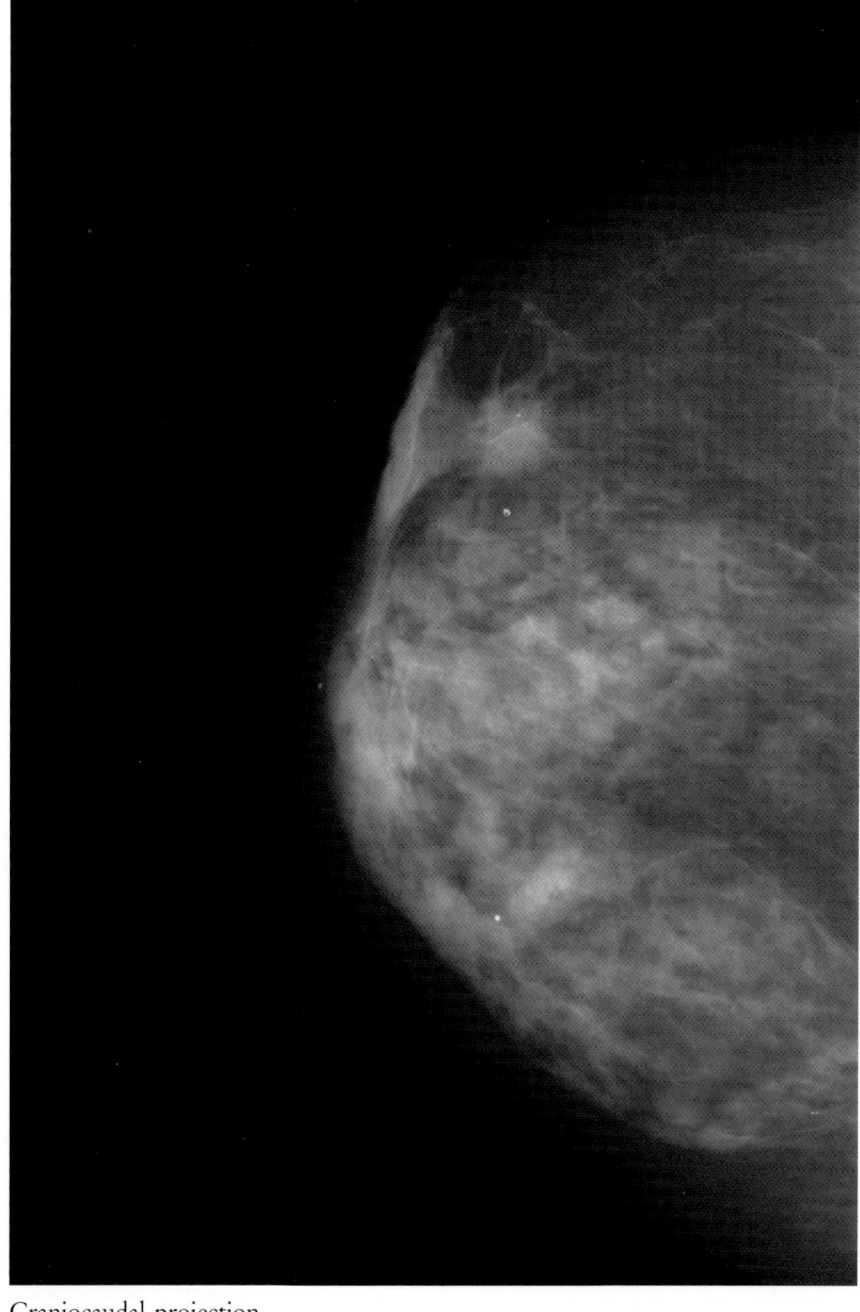

Craniocaudal projection

Craniocaudal magnification view

Skin thickening and retraction

In the outer retroareolar location a roundish radiolucent mass with a radiopaque rim is contiguous with the thickened and retracted areolar skin. This appears to be the result of traumatic fat necrosis which produces a clinically detectable hard lump with unclear edges mimicking a malignancy.

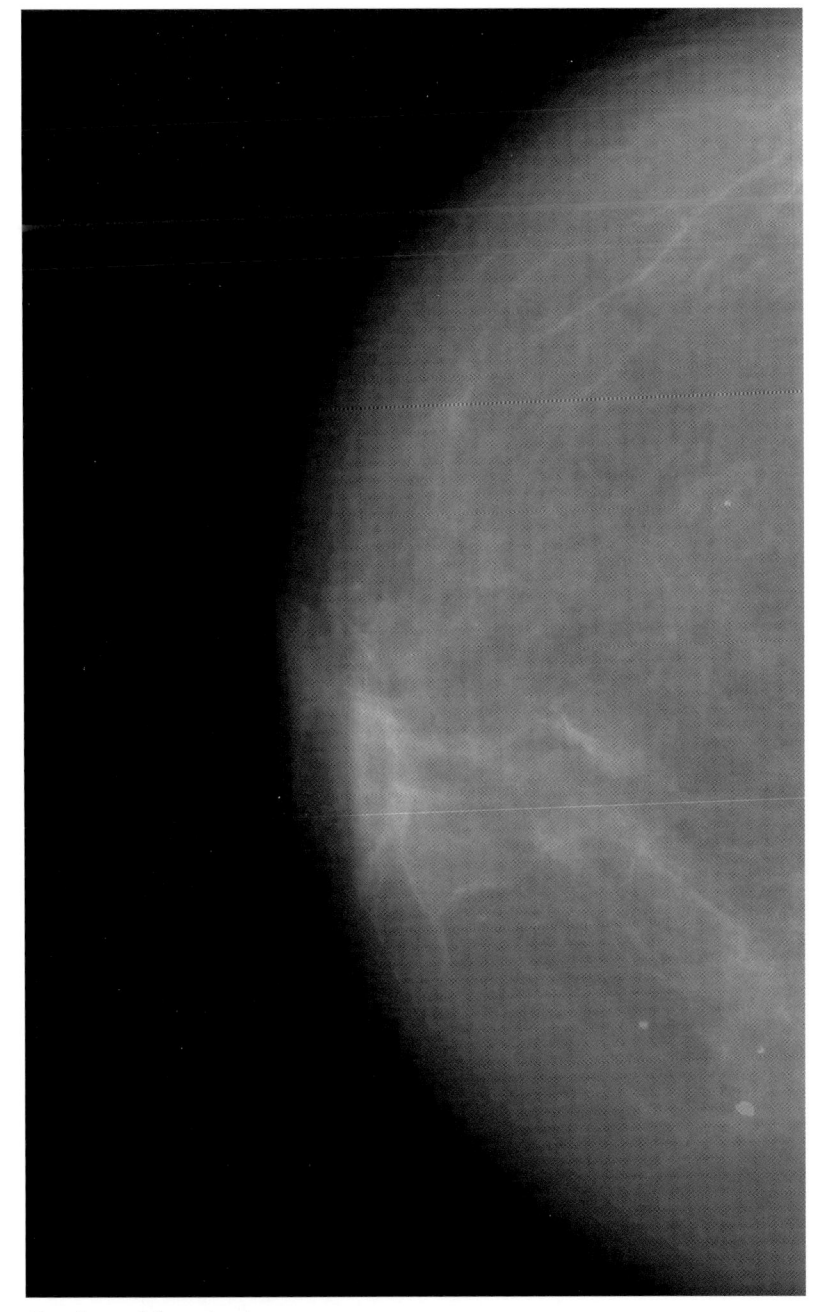

Craniocaudal projection

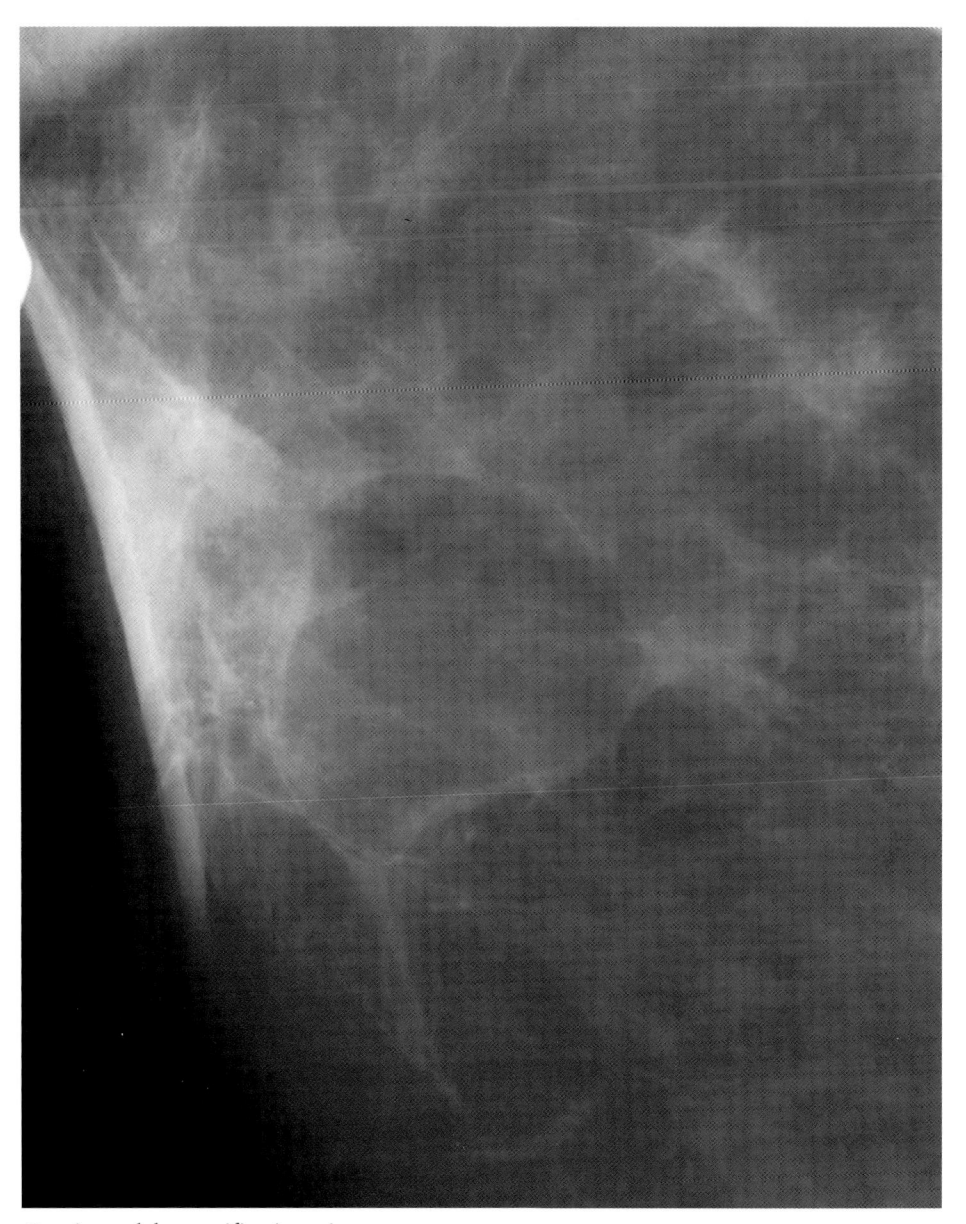

Craniocaudal magnification view

SKIN THICKENING AND RETRACTION

Skin thickening and retraction

Anterior marginal distortion in the outer quadrant is visible with fine spicules radiating into the subcutaneous fat and toward the thickened and retracted skin.

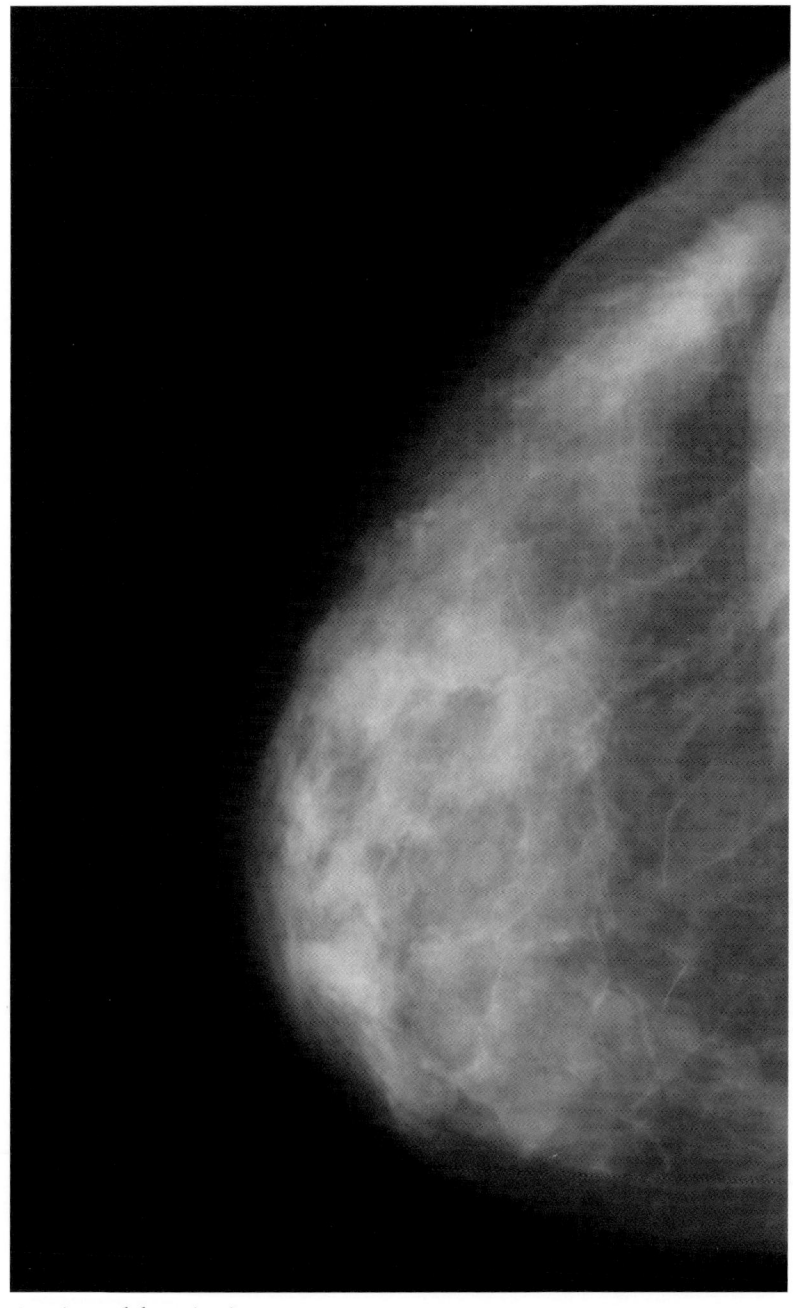

Craniocaudal projection

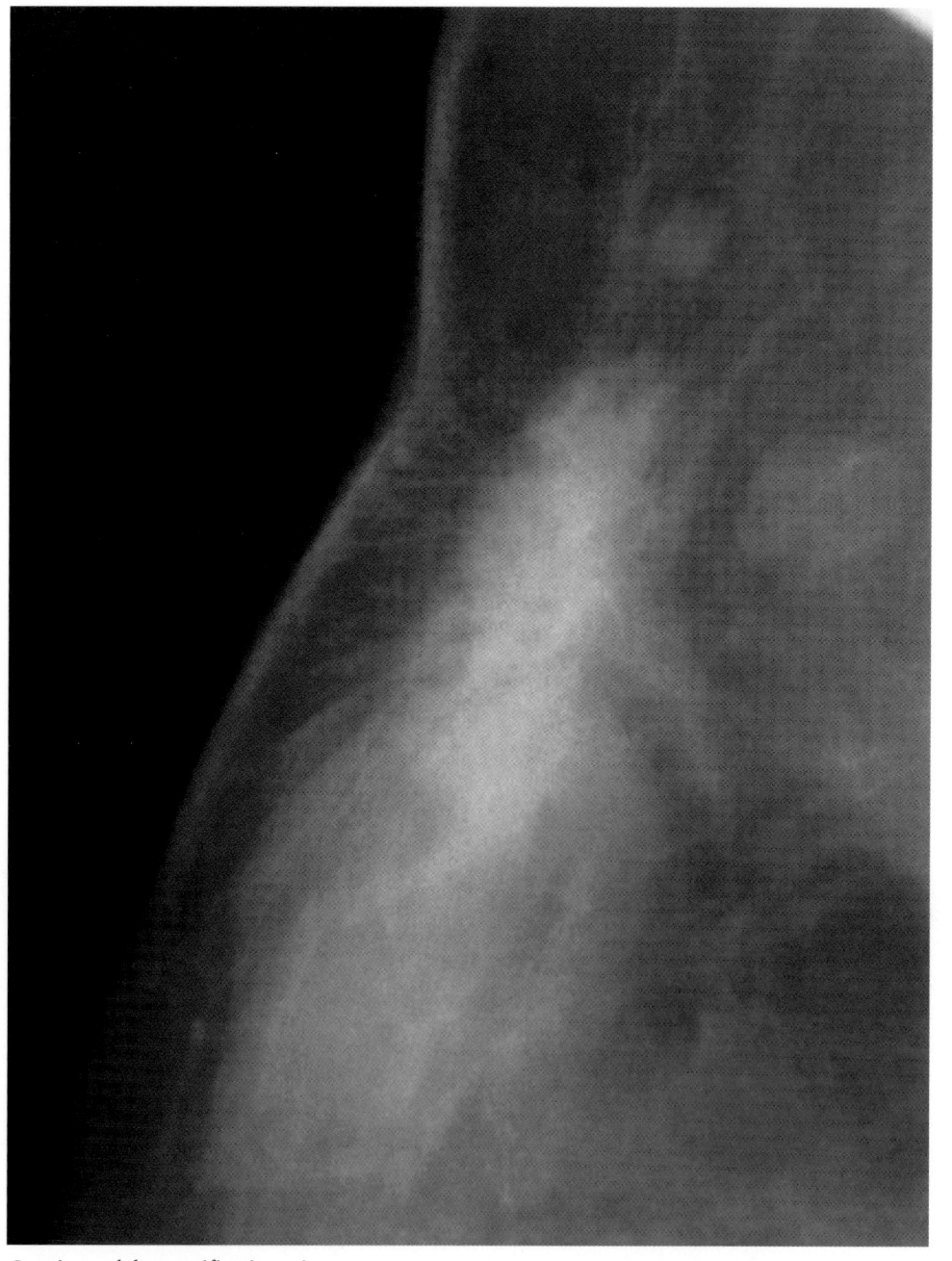

Craniocaudal magnification view

Oedema

Diffuse oedema causes generalized thickening of the trabecular stromal net, comprising Cooper's ligaments and the retinacula cutis, with dilated satellite lymphatics. There may also be thickening of the skin.
This finding is typical of benign processes such as mastitis, post-radiotherapy changes and congestive heart failure secondary to kidney failure. Thickened skin also invariably accompanies inflammatory carcinoma in which a focal opacity may be visible mammographically. Post-therapy follow-up may be advisable in these cases, to permit a differential diagnosis.

OEDEMA

Oedema

Diffuse oedema with thickening of the trabecular stromal net; the whole breast appears "blurred". The lateral projection clearly shows thickening of the skin of the areola and surrounding skin, down to the lower quadrants.

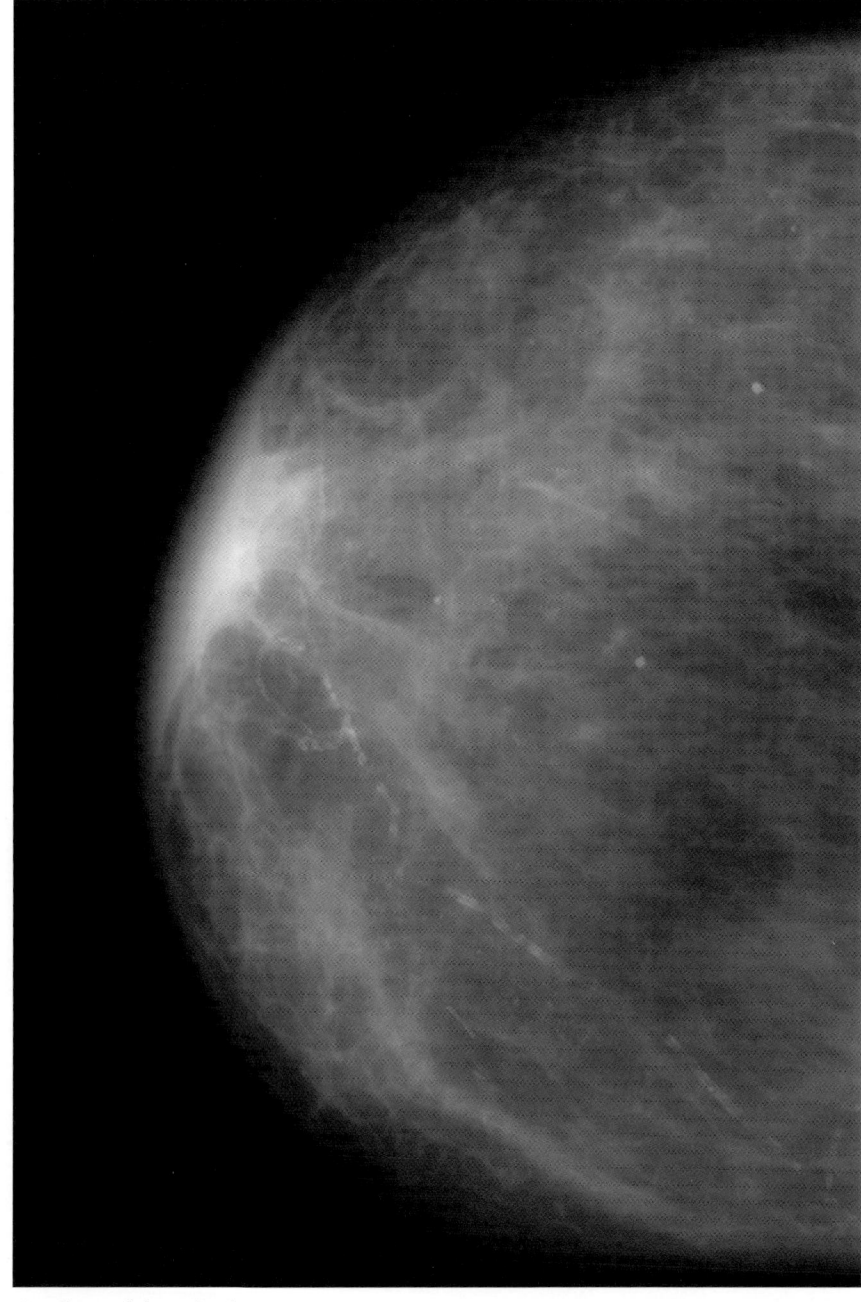

Craniocaudal projection

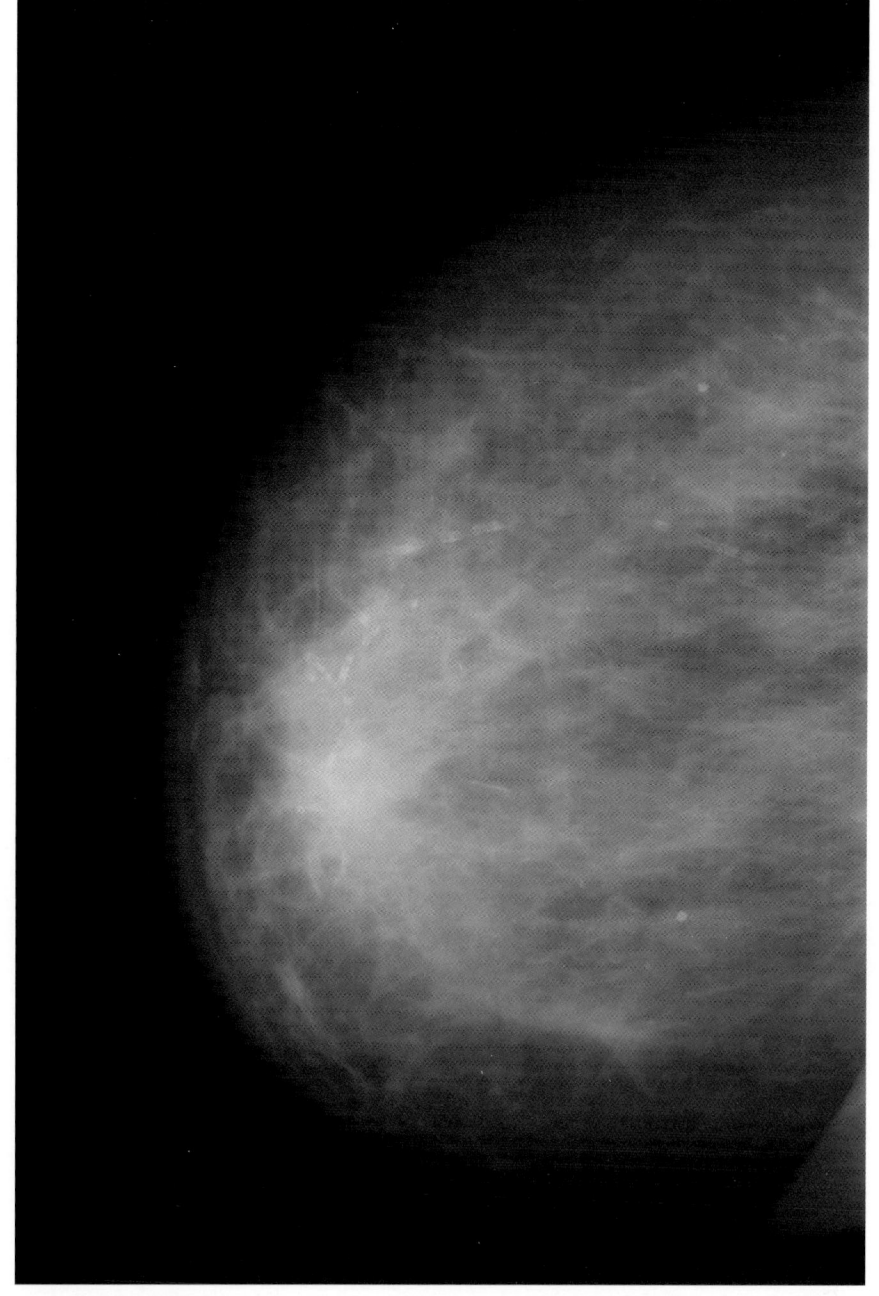

Lateral projection

Oedema

Diffuse oedema with thickening of the trabecular stromal net and "blurring" of the whole breast. The lateral projection clearly shows thickening of the skin of the areola and surrounding skin, down to the lower quadrants. The magnification view illustrates the "trabecular" appearance of the premammary fatty tissues as a result of the accumulated fluid in inframammary lymphatics.

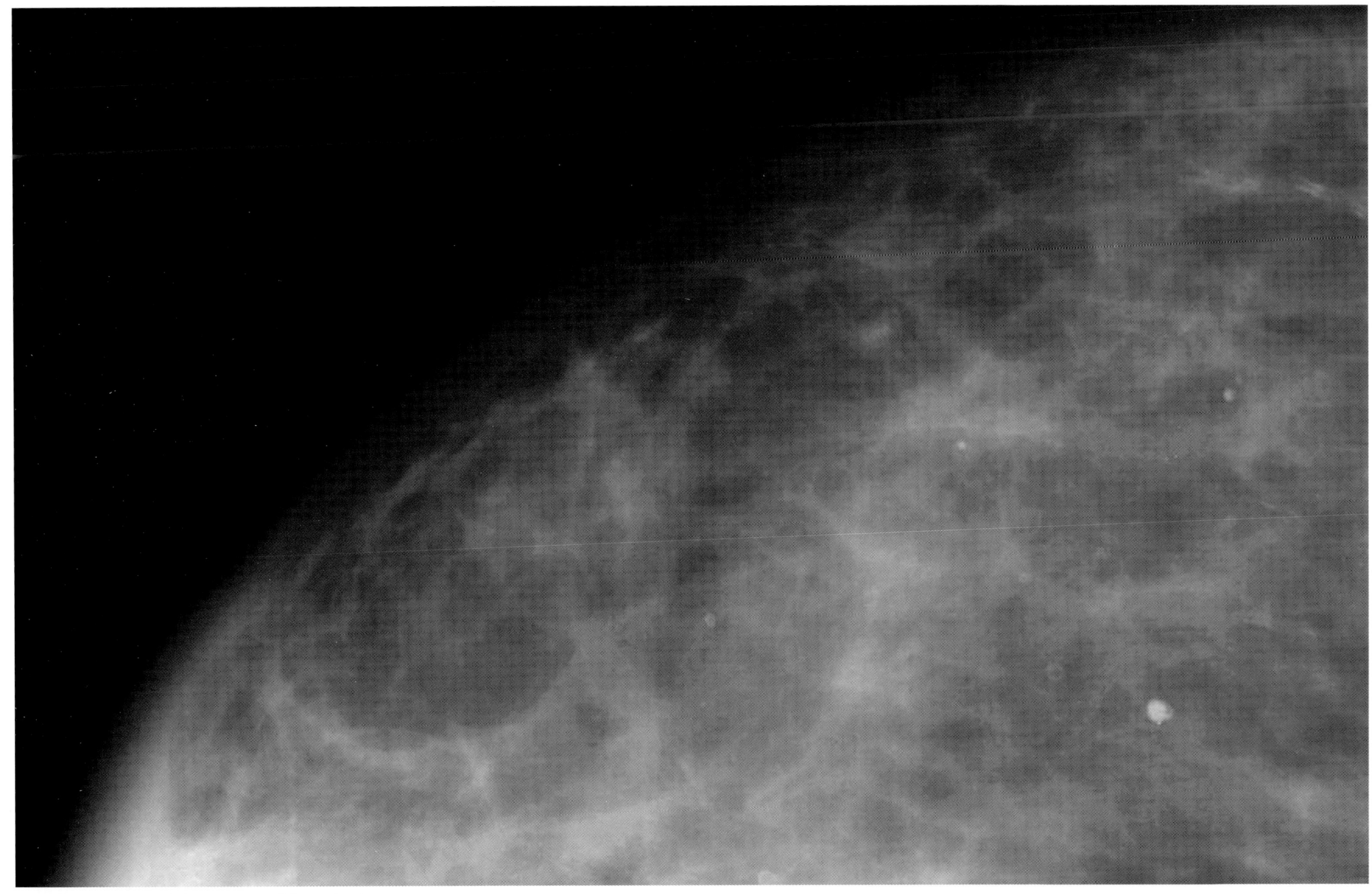

Magnification view of the craniocaudal projection

Oedema

Diffuse oedema with thickening of the trabecular stromal net and "blurring" of the whole breast. The lateral projection also clearly shows thickening of the skin of the areola and surrounding skin, down to the lower quadrants. The magnification view illustrates the "trabecular" appearance of the premammary fatty tissues as a result of the accumulated fluid in inframammary lymphatics.

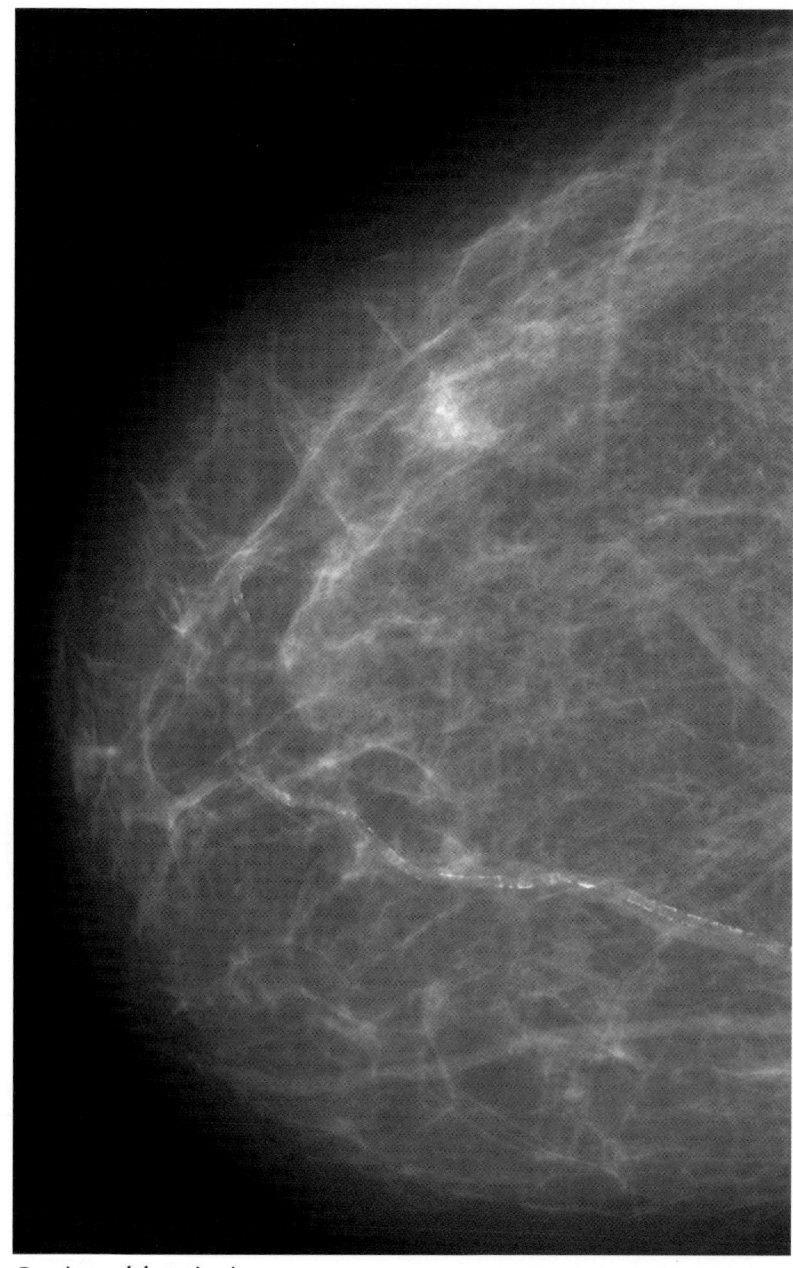

Craniocaudal projection

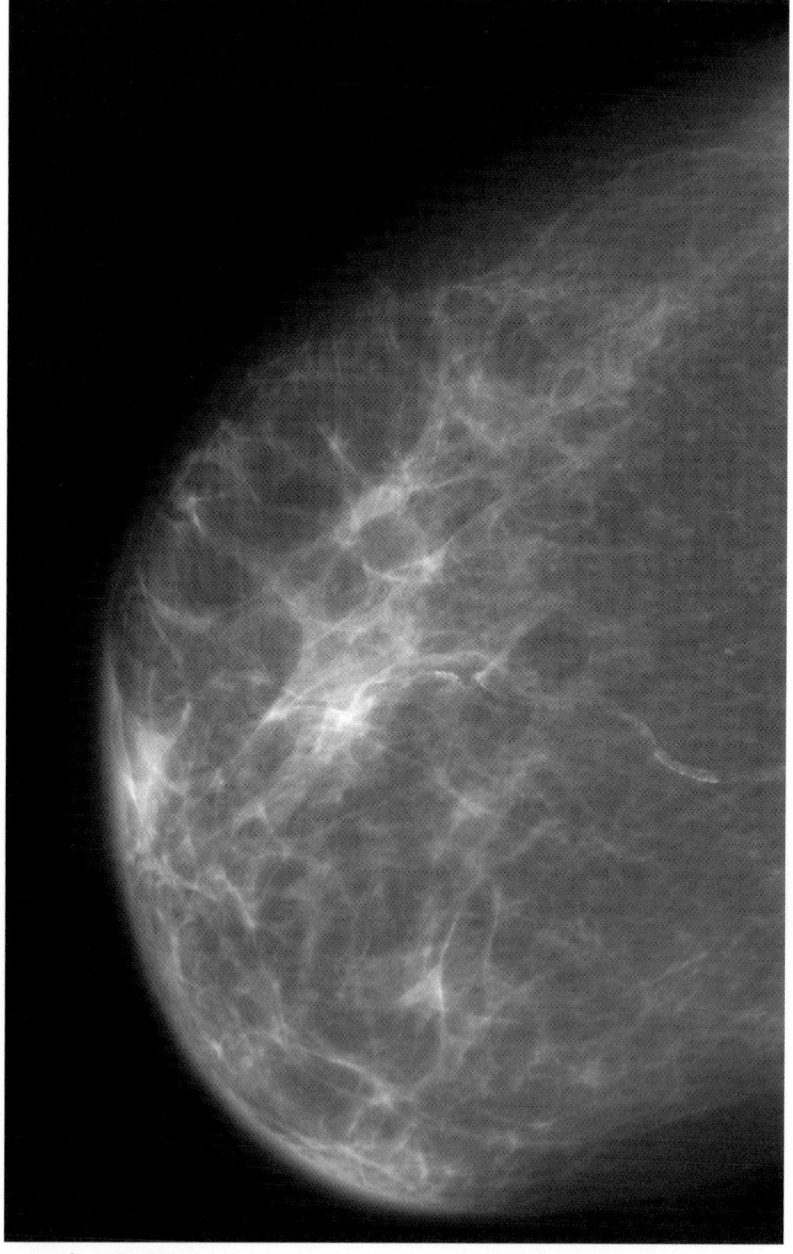

Lateral projection

Oedema

This magnification view clearly shows the thickening of the skin of the areola and surrounding skin, down to the lower quadrants. It illustrates the "trabecular" appearance of the premammary fatty tissues as a result of the accumulated fluid in Cooper's ligaments and inframammary lymphatics.

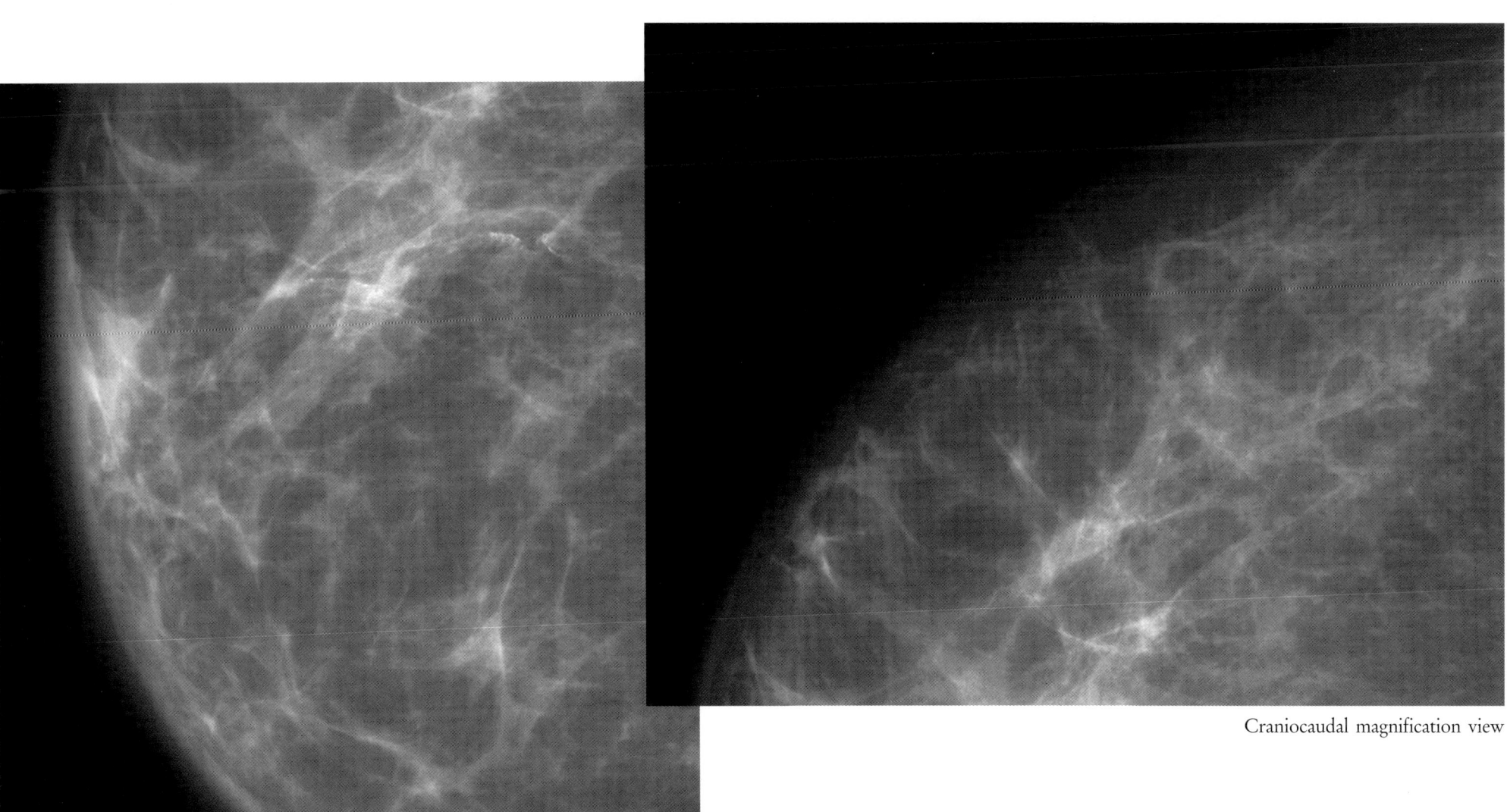

Craniocaudal magnification view

Craniocaudal magnification view

Oedema

Diffuse oedema with thickening of the the trabecular stromal net and "blurring" of the whole breast. This image also clearly shows thickening of the skin of the areola and surrounding skin, down to the lower quadrants.

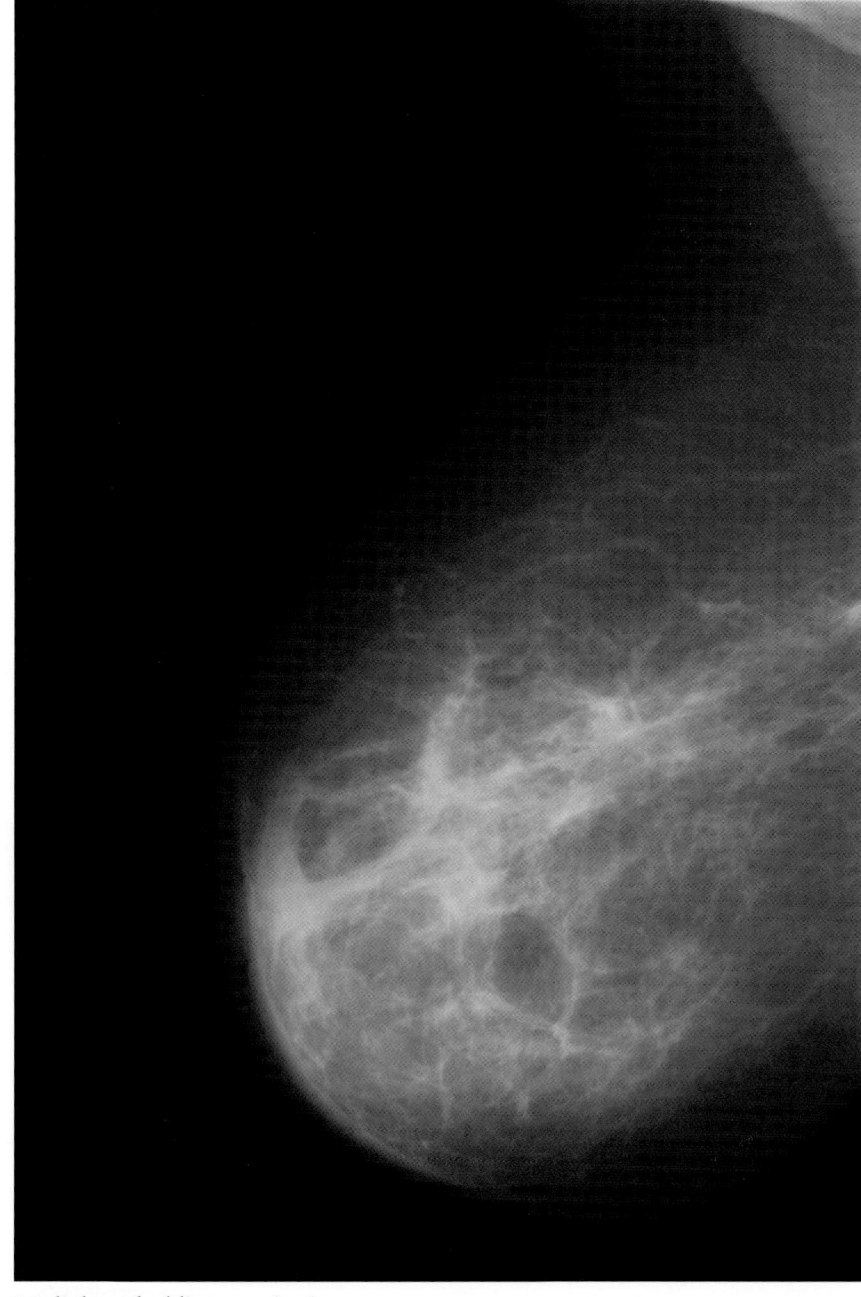

Mediolateral oblique projection

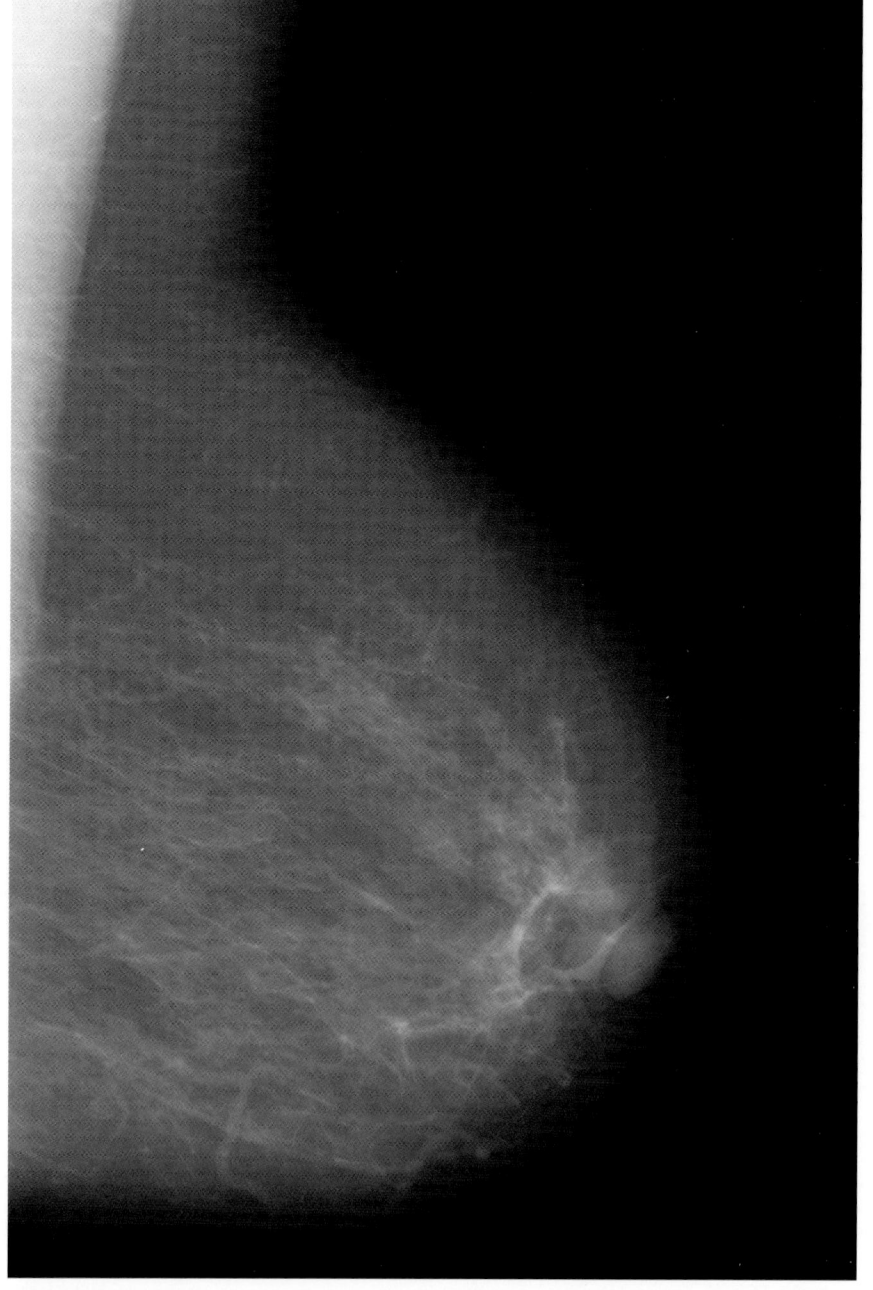

Mediolateral oblique projection

Asymmetrically dilated ducts

Linear, ribbon-like, tubular or branching, single or multiple opacities, parallel and radiating in the retroareolar space. This appearance is typical of ectactic ducts and, less commonly, of intraductal papilloma or carcinoma.

Asymmetrically dilated ducts

In the retroareolar location a circumscribed roundish, radiolucent mass of low density is visible, seemingly contiguous with the areolar skin (A). Galactography shows an ectactic main duct contiguous anteriorly with a lobulated mass filling the duct lumen and posteriorly with the opacity previously described (B). The retroareolar duct is straight up to a few centimetres from the areolar skin (C).

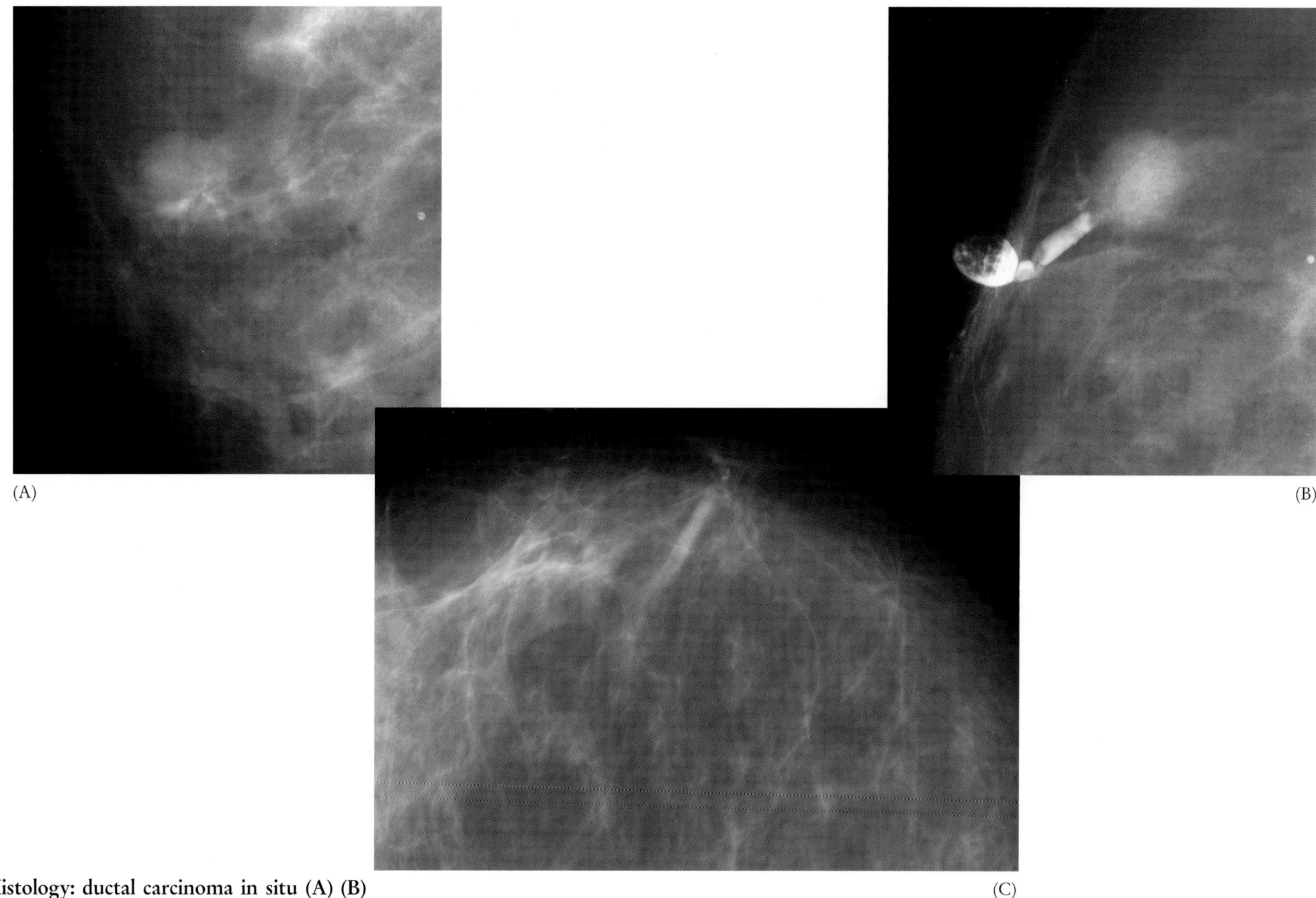

(A)

(B)

(C)

Histology: ductal carcinoma in situ (A) (B)

Part 2

INTERPRETING AND REPORTING

INTERPRETING AND REPORTING

"The report is an X-ray of the radiologist"

The report formally describes the professional service rendered by a radiologist and expresses his or her diagnostic assessment and suggestion of action to be taken. The two basic components of a mammogram report are interpretation and language.

INTERPRETATION

The interpretation phase of a mammogram follows a logical sequence of key steps leading automatically to a systematic process comprising the following:

a) Image quality control

Quality standards for mammography are well known and cover the proper performance and acquisition of the images and their correct identification.

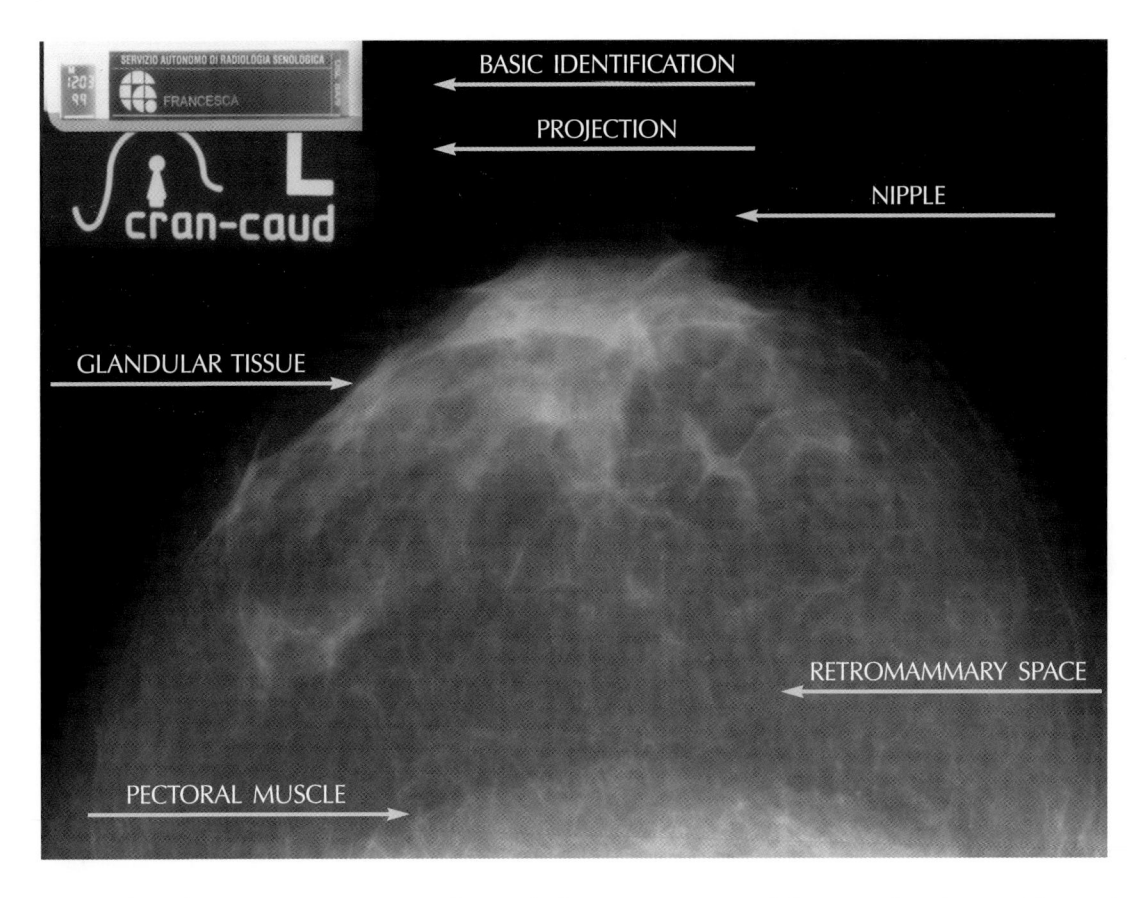

Preliminary information basically includes the patient's name, date of the mammographic examination, side and quadrant(s) examined, and projection used. These are all important for follow-up.

The technical parameters by which the correct execution of the mammogram is assessed relate both to the breast to be examined and to the image acquired.

The breast

– correct positioning

– correct compression

– absence of skinfolds and artefacts

The image

– identification visible

– breast positioned centrally on the film

– retromammary area visible

– pectoralis muscle included

– nipple in line

– even darkening

– submammary groove visible

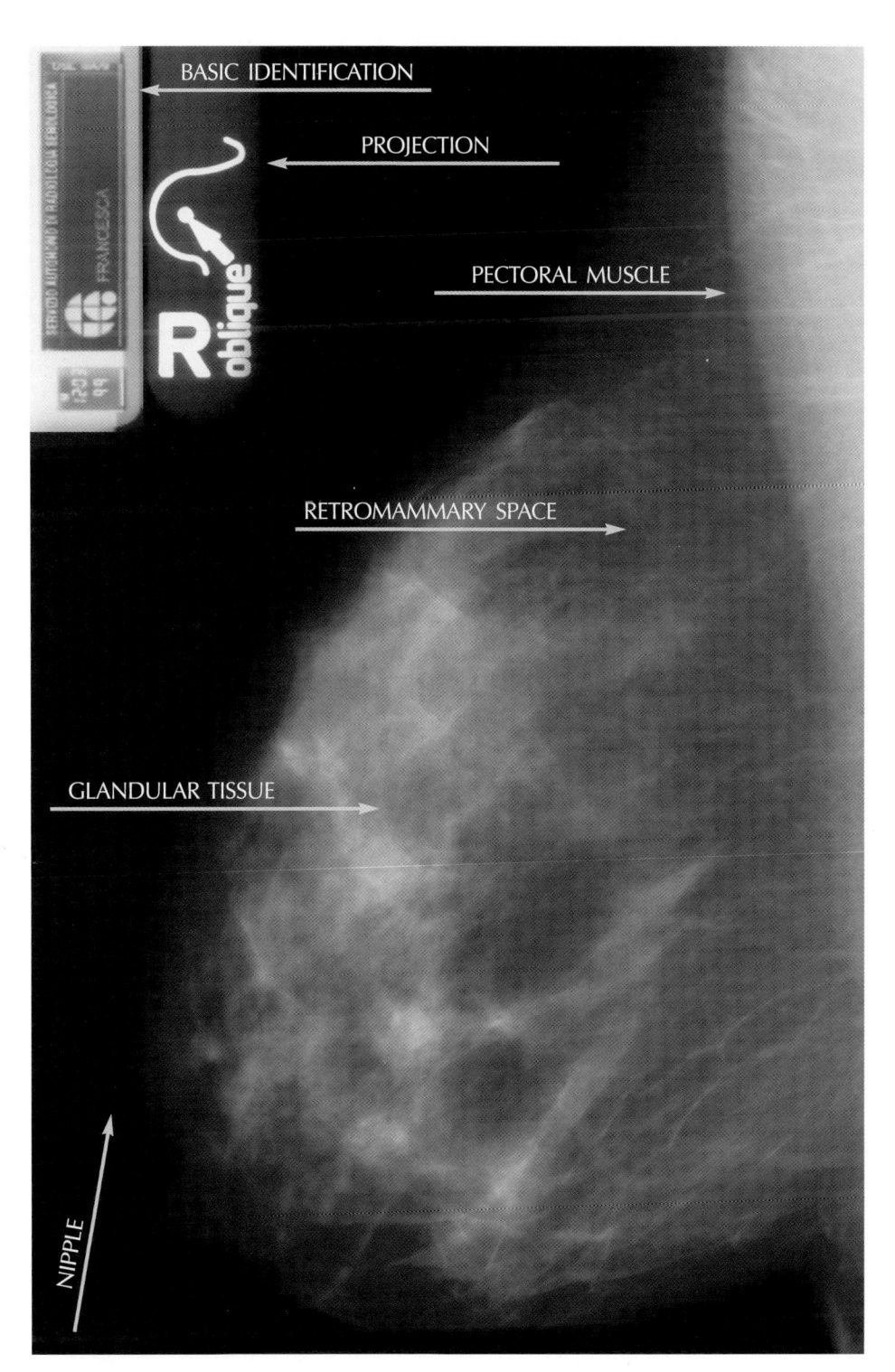

INTERPRETING AND REPORTING

b) Detection

Systematic comparison of right and left mammograms is fundamental.
Sequential examination of limited areas of the mammograms using the horizontal and oblique masking method described by Tabar makes it easier to detect subtle lesions and small, asymmetric opacities within the breast and along its contours.

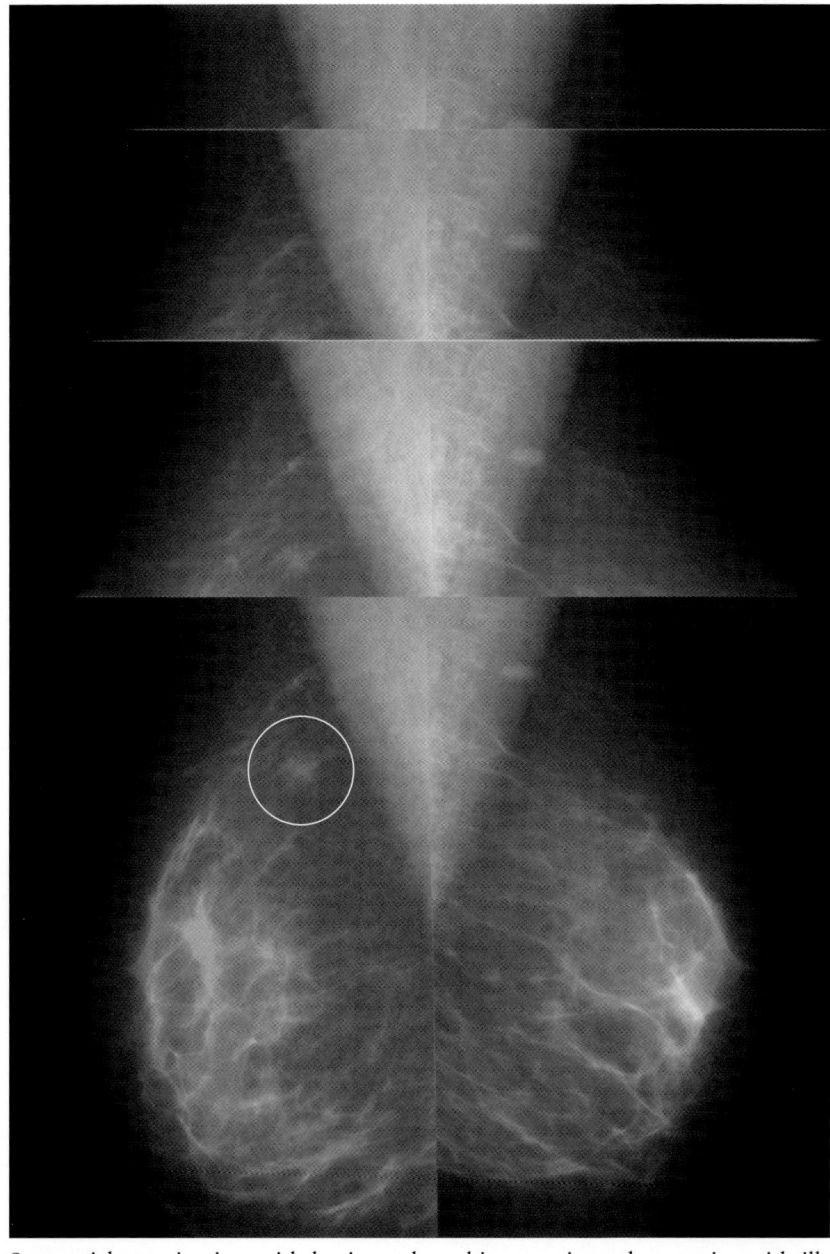

Sequential examination with horizontal masking: an irregular opacity with ill-defined margins is evident in the left breast close to the axilla.

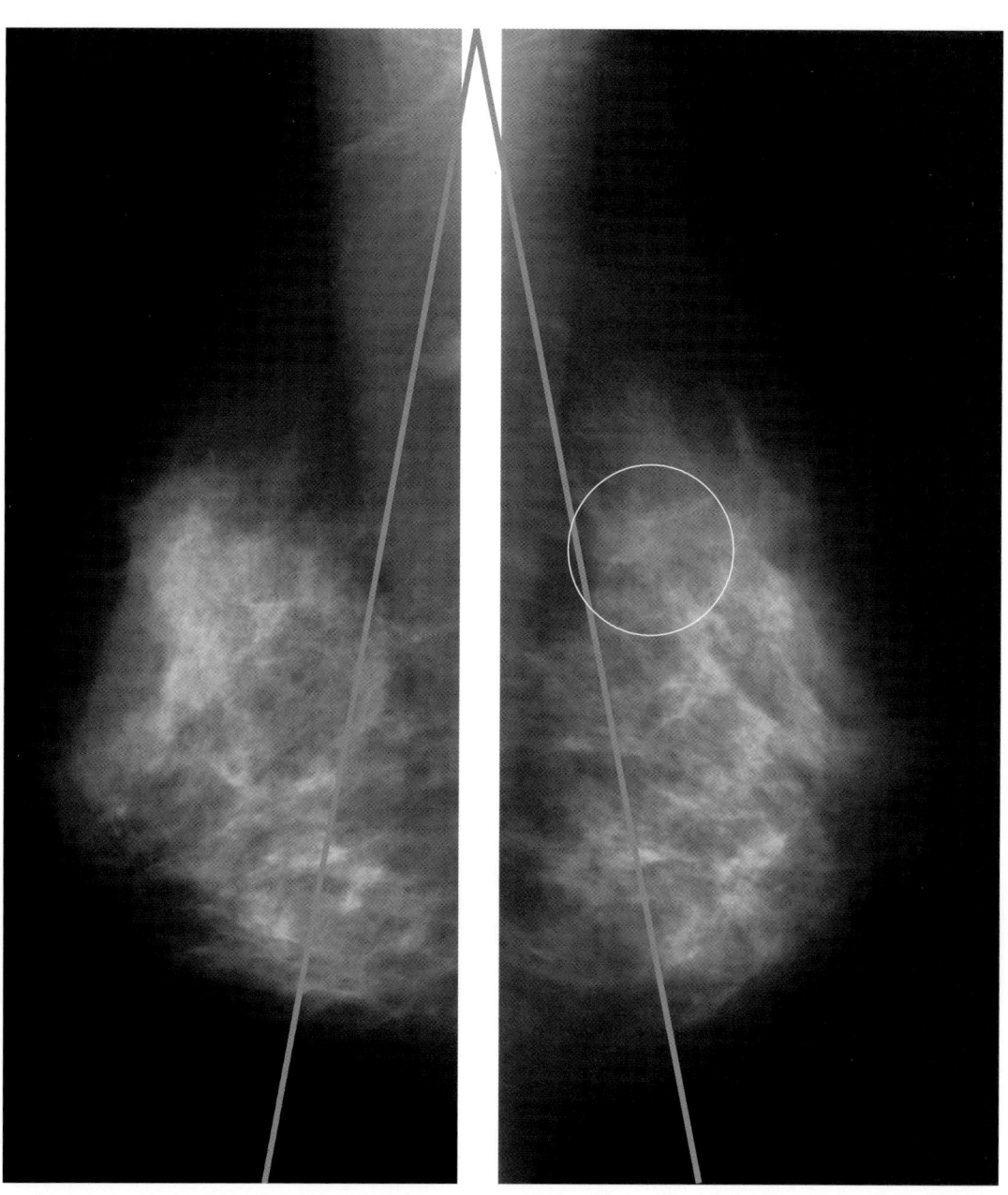

Sequential examination in oblique masking. Marginal deep distortion of the parenchyma in the right breast.

Once you have found one lesion, there is still the rest of the breast and the other, contralateral one to be carefully examined. Bear in mind that there may be multiple or bilateral lesions; detecting a benign lesion may sometimes have the effect of dangerously lowering one's level of attention, which can impair the quality of the final diagnosis.

Asymmetries due to artefacts or overlapping structures must be carefully distinguished. Their significance and location should be assessed in relation to the normal parenchymal and stromal structures in orthogonal projections and with the aid of spot compression views. Comparison with previous films may provide important information, especially if the older mammograms were of the same quality.

c) Analysis

Once an anomaly has been detected, its morphology and structure must be closely analysed and classified on the basis of its elementary signs and characteristics (opacities, distortions, calcifications, etc.).

d) Integration with other diagnostic procedures

In a multimodal diagnostic study of the breast the clinical breast examination findings must be assessed together with the mammograms and the results of any additional examinations (ultrasound, cytology, microhistology) so as to limit the risk of false positives or negatives. Various other factors, such as the patient's age, time of occurrence of the lesion or onset of symptoms, of changes in the lesion or symptoms that may occur spontaneously or be induced by therapy, help orient the diagnosis and distinguish a benign from a malignant lesion. Any clinical difficulties must be described in the mammography report.

e) Synthesis

This part of the report reflects the radiologist's knowledge and skill. It is the most crucial phase of interpretation since it will have an impact on the overall diagnostic conclusion and on the recommendations for further action. These are the elements that reassure a patient of the radiologist's reliability and ability.

The radiologist will clearly state in the diagnostic assessment whether the case is normal, benign, suspicious or malignant, since this will influence further clinical decisions. Recommendations may include periodic follow-up examinations when no breast pathology has been detected (in accordance with the guidelines), or short-interval follow-up for lesions identified as benign, with – as appropriate suggestions as to the medical therapy.

INTERPRETING AND REPORTING

COMMUNICATION AND LANGUAGE

The language used to convey the radiologist's interpretation in the report should be semantically correct, succinct, clear and to the point. Careful choice of the right words, when describing the signs identified through the different diagnostic procedures used, is key to prompt understanding by the reader of a report. Avoid unnecessary preliminary considerations or verbose circumlocutions to describe findings, especially when they are normal. Describe only the signs of the pathology at hand.

In short, the typical report should comprise:
- a very brief description of the breast structure (adipose, fibroglandular, dense)
- a clear, short description of the signs found
- an assessment of the significance of the basic semiologic findings
- recommendations on what action might be taken next.

The terminology used should be logical and consistent throughout the description, clinical impression, diagnostic assessment of findings and recommendations suggested in the report, which should answer some essential questions while providing fundamental information.

QUESTIONS TO ANSWER

Are there clinical and mammographic signs of a lesion?

If findings indicate a normal breast once the clinical and mammographic examinations have been conducted properly and the results of any other investigation have been carefully scrutinized and taken into account, then the case may be classified as normal or negative. The patient should be immediately informed so that she may be reassured and relieved of the anxiety generated by the examination.

Do the signs definitely suggest a benign lesion?

There are not many situations in which a breast examination reveals a definitely benign pattern with no room for doubt. However, should this be the case the patient should be expressly informed. No further examinations are warranted and over-zealous follow-up is of no clinical value and will only constitute a source of anxiety for the patient.

Do the signs suggest or indicate a malignancy?

When the findings raise suspicion or are clearly indicative of a malignancy, the patient should be informed not only in the written report but also in person, with tact and thoughtfulness. A calm talk about what therapeutic options lie ahead will not only confirm the radiologist's professionalism but will also provide considerable reassurance and support to the patient.

Does the lesion require histological confirmation?
When irregular opacities or calcifications are present and whenever the clinical, mammographic or cytological findings arouse any suspicion or doubt, histological examination of the lesion is required. Note that not even negative cytology justifies not doing a biopsy when clinical and mammographic examinations arouse suspicion.

Are further investigations necessary?
The radiologist is responsible for the overall diagnostic work-up and flow chart of a case and will therefore suggest any further tests that might be necessary. In line with the professional gold standard, it is best if the radiologist personally takes care of the whole diagnostic procedure.

Is referral necessary?
The radiologist may refer the patient to another specialist should the clinical features of the case call for this.

Are short-interval follow-up or periodic breast examinations for early diagnosis necessary?
If the findings strongly suggest a benign lesion, follow-up at middle-length intervals may be recommended to check that no changes occur in the lesion without undue risks for the patient. This avoids unnecessary biopsies and scar formation which may raise subsequent problems of interpretation.

INFORMATION TO GIVE

Type of mammography structure (ultrasound)
State preliminarily whether the breast tissue pattern is difficult to explore. This may be due to its intrinsic density or to changes in the fibroglandular structure following surgery, radiation therapy or reconstructive surgery. In very dense breast, where the sensitivity of mammography may be limited, it may be appropriate to emphasize that the breast is difficult to explore and encourage the patient to see her physician for periodic breast examinations.

Site of the lesion
Indicate the site of the lesion in the two orthogonal projections and its position with reference to the different quadrants. Specify particular sites, such as the retroareolar area, the deep region over the pectoral muscle fascia, the submammary groove, or axillary tail.

INTERPRETING AND REPORTING

Imaging signs
Briefly describe the basic findings of the breast imaging using the terminology normally employed for the type of test done (opacity, microcalcifications, US mass, etc).

Size of lesion
Give the maximum diameter of the lesion because this information is important for choosing the surgical option. Spicules should be included when measuring stellate opacities; for calcifications, the whole area containing them will be counted in the measurement.

Relationship of the lesion with the skin and deeper layers
Skin infiltrations and any suspicion that the deeper fascia of the pectoralis major muscle may be involved are important when the therapist evaluates the prognosis.

Multifocality and multicentricity
When a lesion is suspicious, carefully check whether it is single and examine all quadrants of the breast to check there are no other lesions. Multicentricity is often a contraindication to conservative surgical management.

Diagnostic feedback
Asking for a copy of the histology report is a simple and effective sign of professional scrupulousness and of the radiologist's determination to improve continuously. Feedback from additional diagnostic tests and awareness of our mistakes are instrumental in establishing the positive predictive value of different diagnostic methods, the costs of bioptic procedures, and the radiologist's overall diagnostic reliability. It may also provide us with an opportunity to improve our working methods.

ESTABLISHING THE LOCATION OF A LESION

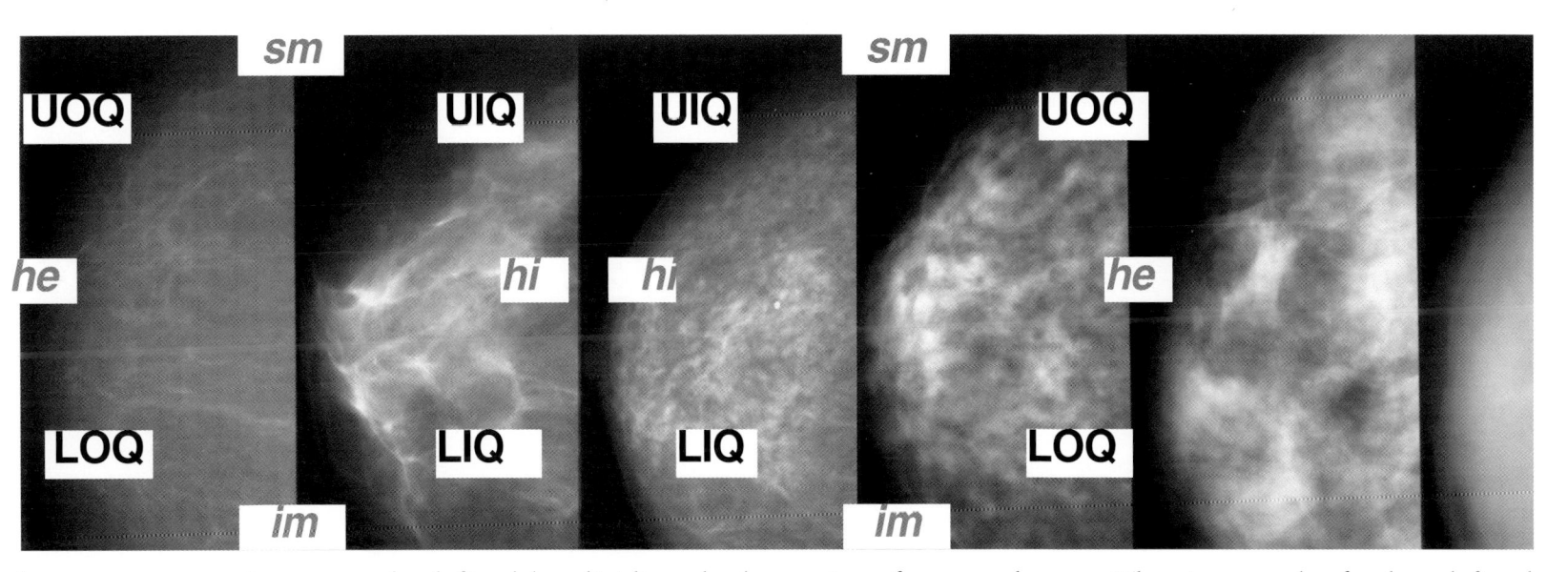

The location of a lesion on the mammogram is commonly defined by dividing the breast into four quadrants. The site may be further defined by reference to the horizontal (internal and external: i, e) and the vertical median plane (super-median and infra-median: s, i).

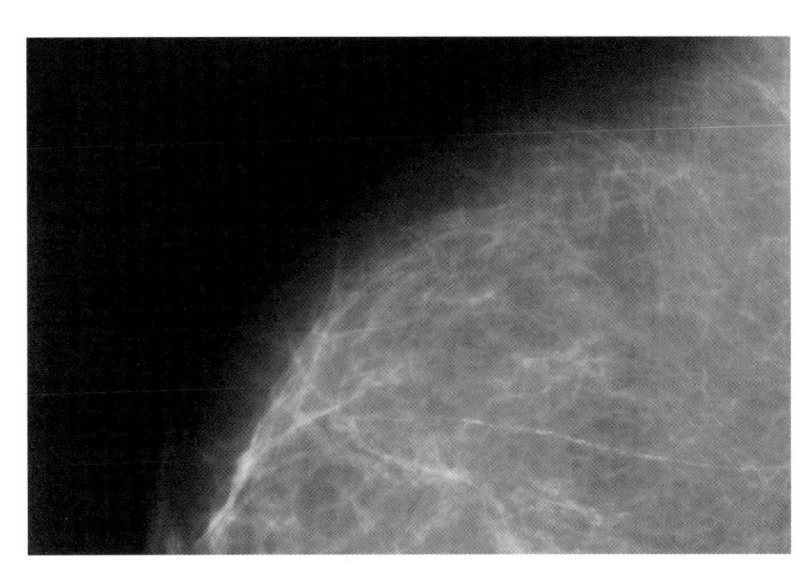

More rarely, but especially when clinical findings are available, the site of a lesion may be defined by referring to a clock face set in front of the observer. Do not forget to indicate which breast is involved (right/left).

INTERPRETING AND REPORTING

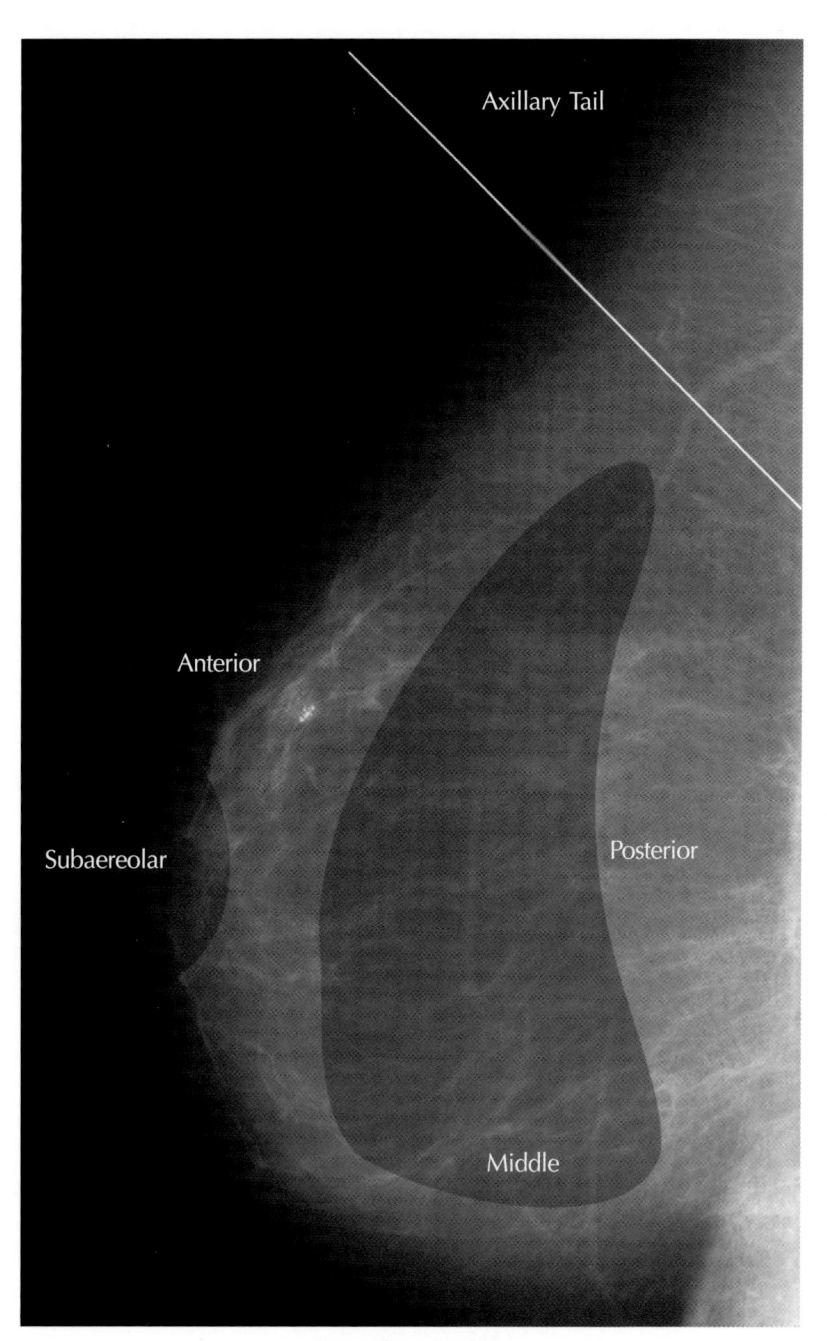

The depth of the breast in craniocaudal and lateral projections can be indicated as subareolar, anterior, central, and posterior.

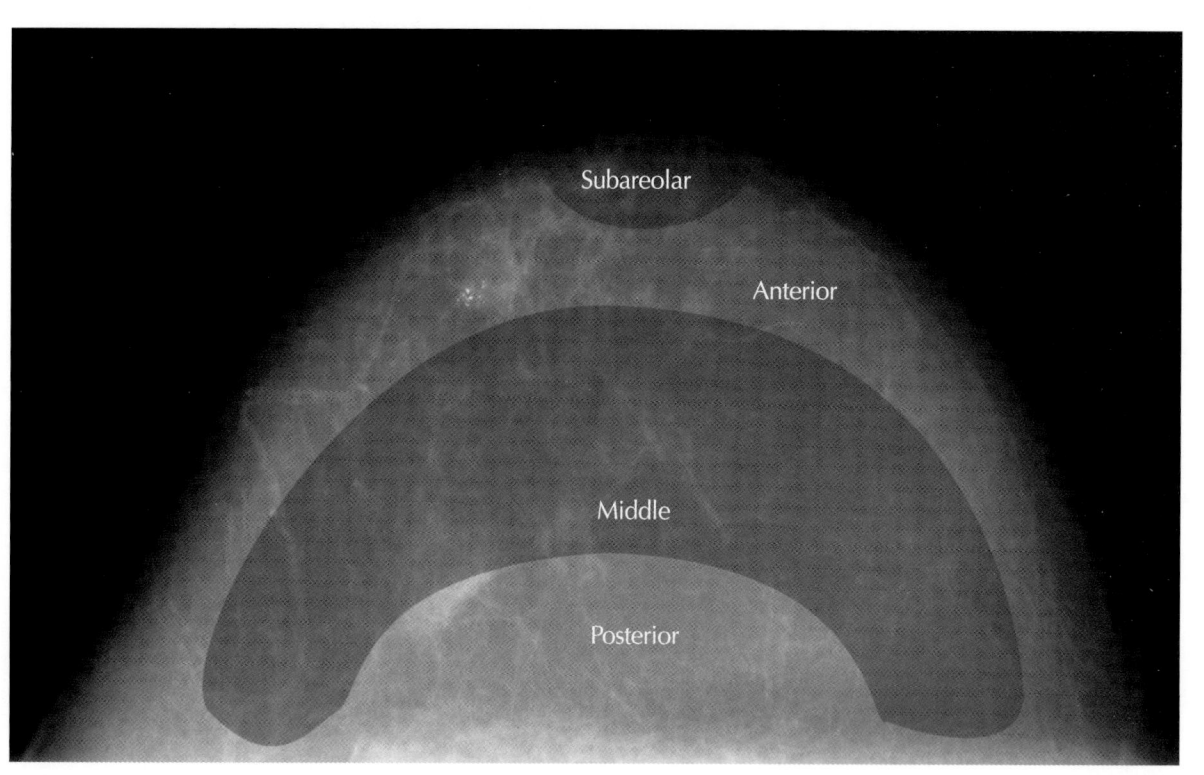

Lateral projection

Craniocaudal projection

THE Re.Co.R.M. DIAGNOSTIC ASSESSMENT CATEGORIES

THE RE.CO.R.M. DIAGNOSTIC ASSESSMENT CATEGORIES

After describing any anomalies found, the radiologist will provide an overall and conclusive assessment of their meaning and then suggest what action should be taken or what should be done in the long run.

The assessment categories proposed in RE.CO.R.M (from the Italian "Reporting and Codifying the Results of Mammography") provide a brief, standardized way of expressing the diagnostic assessment and recommending future decisions:

Category R1
Negative finding
No pathology. When no abnormal finding is detected, *periodic clinical and/or breast imaging examination is recommended*, depending on the patient's age.

Category R2
Benign Findings
When there is no doubt that a lesion is benign, such as calcified fibroadenomas, lipomas, lipid cysts, post-traumatic fat necrosis or large, "patchy" calcifications, vascular calcifications, secretory rod-like calcifications, or "milk-of-calcium" calcifications, *periodic breast examination or a short-interval follow-up after six months is recommended* to assess the clinical evolution. Needle-biopsy cytology is not a routine option and will be resorted to when the radiologist feels it is indicated, on a case-by-case basis.

VPP = < 5%

Benign findings

Category R3
Probably benign findings

This category is the most difficult to define and carries the greatest risk of error. Conceptually, it indicates the presence of lesions that are almost certainly benign but that present some small likelihood of malignancy, owing to the fact that their morphologic features are in some way really very ambiguous to classify as **regular/benign or irregular, ill-defined/malignant,** especially in case of tiny lesions or in particular clinical situations. It is not possible, as a matter of fact, to clearly categorize and avoid assessment subjectivity so that and it must be accepted as a real limit of mammography. An example might be isolated, small, circumscribed opacities, solid at ultrasound, with relatively regular margins. In the vast majority of cases, these are benign lesions, such as fibroadenomas, solitary papillomas or, in a broader sense, dysplastic nodules; more seldom, however, these may be the features of a medullary, mucous, papillary, or infiltrating ductal carcinoma. Similarly, some subtle, low density focal asimmetry or architectural distortion as well as round, punctate or powdery calcifications have no chance to be differentiated as benign or malignant. Difficulties for diagnostic assessment may occur more easily on a baseline mammography, in absence of prior comparable examinations or in case of evolution or changes of the finding of interest over the time.

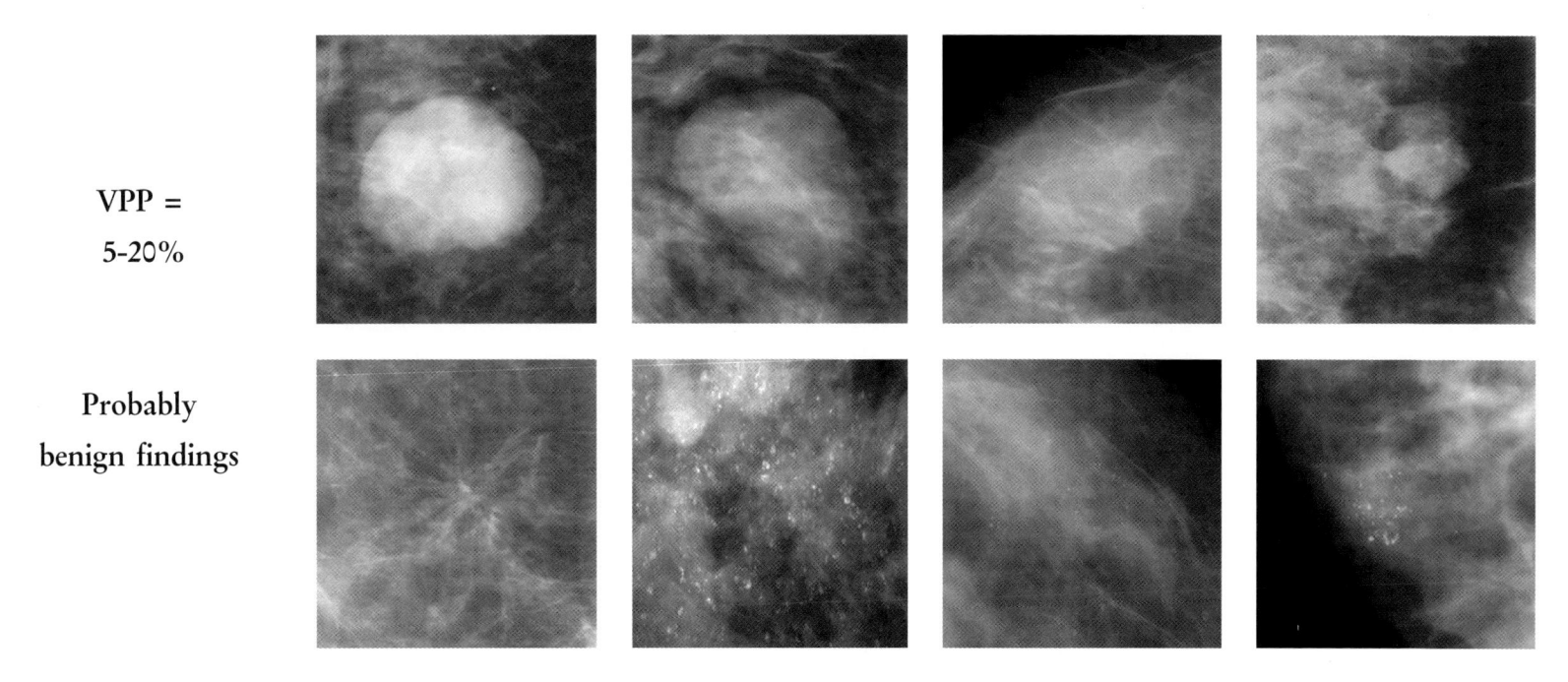

VPP = 5-20%

Probably benign findings

When the overall features are convincingly benign, it is common practice to take a cautious stance and *recommend a six-month follow-up* to evaluate stability of the lesion over the time. Generally, the area of interest is re-examined every six months for two or three years. The rationale derives from a number of clinical, statistical and biological facts. There is a vast literature bearing evidence of how morphological stability is a reliable sign of a benign process in more than 80% of cases, particularly for circumscribed, regular opacity; it is also well known that there are very few chances that a lesion that has remained unchanged over time will prove to be malignant after 6-12 months.

These two considerations warrant short-interval controls as a follow-up for detecting those few small carcinomas with "atypical" benign morphology, without routinely and indiscriminately having to perform invasive procedures such as biopsies. There is also a chance that fine-needle aspiration under ultrasound or mammographic guidance may not sample the correct area or pick up enough material when lesions are very small, less than a centimeter in size. In these cases a control after six months may avoid a false negative result without significantly changing the prognosis if a carcinoma is present.
Further studies and investigations are still needed to boost the reliability of management criteria such as the optimal interval for follow-up and abnormalities eligible for follow-up.

Category R4
Doubtful findings or findings suspicious for malignancy
There are not enough conclusive elements to classify a finding as benign or signs arouse to varying degrees the suspicion of malignancy. The nature of the lesion must be established: *interventional procedures or an excisional biopsy must be recommended*. In principle, a needle biopsy (FNA or Core Biopsy) will be recommended for circumscribed and stellate opacities, or clustered calcifications, especially if they are small, and excisional biopsy will be preferred for distortions of the parenchyma, focal asymmetries, or scattered calcifications.

Category R5
Positive findings for malignancy
When signs with a high positive predictive value for malignancy are present, such as stellate or casting type calcifications, an excisional biopsy is mandatory.

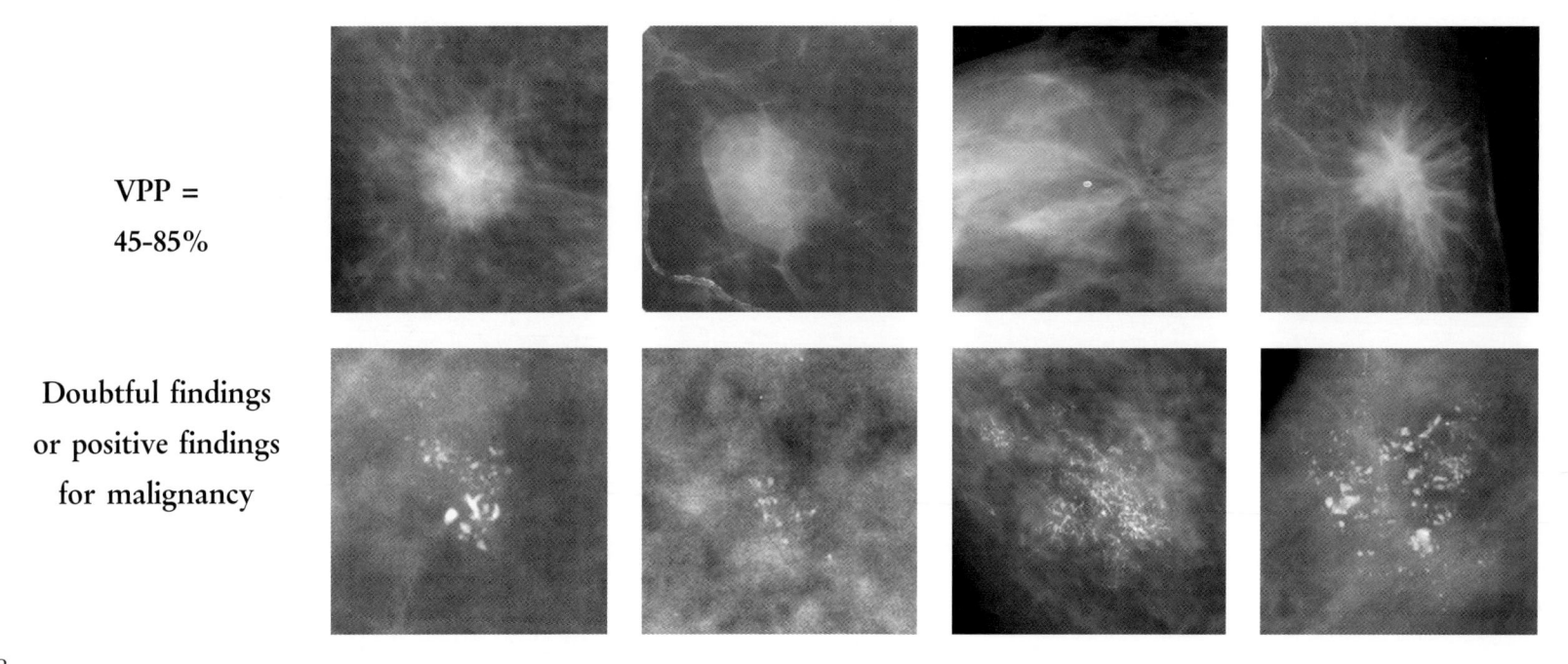

VPP = 45-85%

Doubtful findings or positive findings for malignancy

Part 3

MAMMOGRAPHY AUDIT

MAMMOGRAPHY AUDIT

"Le Cancer c'est une abstraction, les cancers sont une classification, seulement la malade avec le cancer est une realitè" (Ch. M. Gros).

The main purpose of mammography and breast imaging in general is the early detection of breast cancer in the preclinical stage of disease in an asymptomatic and presumably healthy population.

Hence, the fundamental aims of mammography will be:

– to detect the highest possible percentage of breast cancers in a given population

– to rationalize and optimize the diagnostic process, keeping costs and the number of biopsies within reasonable limits

– to detect the highest possible percentage of minimal, lymph node-negative carcinomas, which have a more favourable prognosis.

Attaining these aims ensures the benefits of early detection, permitting conservative management, better quality of life and, especially, lower breast cancer mortality. The highest quality must therefore be guaranteed in the methods and procedures used and in auditing the diagnostic and clinical results.

"The mammography medical audit may be defined as a retrospective evaluation of the appropriateness and accuracy of mammographic image interpretation. It is the distillation of all the Quality Assurance and Quality Control aspects and is the best measure of the interpretative ability of the radiologist as well as the ultimate indicator of mammography performance" (Michael Linver).

Mammography auditing requires feedback information and any other information useful for checking the amount and nature of mistakes made. Acquiring such information is an integral part of the services rendered by a Breast Care Unit.

Detecting and overcoming deficiencies in technique or interpretation meancs refining the knowledge and performance of individual staff members and the unit as a whole, and fostering the professional and cultural growth of the radiologist.

Basic clinical as well as imaging and pathology data have to be collected and standardized before indicators of diagnostic performance procedures can be set up and outcomes determined.

Data to be collected for mammography audit

1. **Dates of when the audit started and ended** (usually yearly) **and total number of examinations performed.**

2. **Epidemiological risk factors:**
   – patient's age;
   – personal or family history of breast cancer (carcinoma during premenopause in first-degree relatives: mother, sister or daughter);
   – previous biopsy for atypical hyperplasia or in situ lobular carcinoma.

3. **Number and type of mammographic examinations:**
   – Indicate examinations on asymptomatic women and examinations to investigate symptoms (if during screening, state whether additional investigations were required after baseline mammography).
   – Short-interval examinations (six months).
   – Indicate number of first examinations, number of scheduled follow-up examinations for prevention, and number of short-interval controls (six months).
   – Indicate number of mammographic examinations according to the Re.Co.R.M classification for diagnostic assessment and decision management on action to be taken:

Category R1: negative	periodic breast examination;
Category R2: benign finding	periodic breast examination or six-month follow-up to evaluate clinical evolution of the case;
Category R3: probably benign finding	six-month follow-up to evaluate clinical evolution of the case or biopsy for histological examination in particular situations on a case-by-case basis according to the individual evaluation;
Category R4: doubtful or suspicious finding for malignancy	interventional procedures needle or excisional biopsy;
Category R5: positive malignancy	excisional biopsy.

4. **Histology reports:**
   Evaluated according to type of biopsy – fine needle, microhistology, excisional.

5. **Data regarding malignancy:**
   Mammographic signs: direct signs (opacities, calcifications, distortions, etc.)
   indirect signs (focal asymmetry, ductal ectasia, etc.)
   absence of mammographic signs.

   Carcinoma is palpable or nonpalpable.
   Carcinoma is visible or not visible with ultrasound.
   Histologic staging of the cancer: histological type, diameter, lymph node status, and grading.

Defining the results

1. **True positives, false positives**, true negatives, false negatives (if possible)

2. **Sensitivity**

3. **Positive predictive value** (calculated on the number of biopsy recommendations)

4. **Specificity**

5. **Percentage of N0 "minimal carcinomas"** detected, broken down into:
   – invasive carcinomas < 1 cm divided into T1a and T1b
   – carcinomas in situ.

6. **Percentage of invasive carcinomas with positive lymph nodes**

7. **Benign/malignant ratio**

8. **Carcinoma detection rate**

9. **Recall rate**

Comments:

True positives (TP): carcinoma diagnosed within one year of a biopsy requested after a mammogram interpreted as positive (Re.Co.R.M. categories 4 and 5).

False positives (FP): no carcinoma detected within one year of a mammogram interpreted as positive, or negative histology for a biopsy taken after a mammography interpreted as positive (Re.Co.R.M. categories 4 and 5).

True negatives (IN): no carcinoma diagnosed within one year of a mammogram interpreted as negative (Re.Co.R.M. categories 1, 2 and 3).

False negatives (TN): carcinoma detected within one year of a mammogram interpreted as negative (Re.Co.R.M. categories 1, 2 and 3).

Sensitivity: the likelihood of detecting a carcinoma in a given population, or the proportion of patients found to have a carcinoma within one year of a mammogram interpreted as suspicious for malignancy (Re.Co.R.M. categories 4 and 5).

$$Sensitivity = TP/(TP + FN)$$

where (TP+FN) is the number of all the carcinomas existing in the population examined, whether properly or improperly investigated. The sensitivity most frequently reported is **85-90%**.

Sensitivity is directly correlated with the overall quality of the mammographic examination (technique, methodology, interpretation) and may vary in relation to the patient's age and the density of the breast tissue. Calculating the "true" sensitivity may be problematic when the exact number of false negatives is lacking and can only be provided by a tumour registry or an organ disease registry. However, false negatives can be calculated among the cases referred for surgery or biopsy by requesting copies of histology reports or other feedback from the pathologist, the patient's physician, or the patient herself.

Positive predictive value (PPV)
This is calculated from the number of biopsies requested after mammograms have been interpreted as suspicious for malignancy (Re.Co.R.M. categories 4 and 5).

$$PPV = TP/\text{number of biopsies} \text{ (or } PPV = TP/TP+FP)$$

MAMMOGRAPHY AUDIT

The range reported in the literature is **25-40%** depending on various factors, such as the age of the population examined, the size of the lesions detected and the sensitivity. The PPV is lower when the population examined is younger and the lesions are smaller.

Specificity: the likelihood of not detecting a carcinoma after a mammogram has been interpreted as negative, or the proportion of patients with no evidence of carcinoma within a year of a mammogram interpreted as negative.

$$\text{Specificity} = TN/(FP + TN)$$

where (FP+TN) is the number of all the normal cases existing in the population examined, whether properly or improperly investigated. The reported average is approximately **90%**.

Percentage of N0 "minimal" carcinomas detected, split into:
- invasive T1 carcinomas
- "minimal" carcinomas divided into T1a, T1b and in situ.

On average these two groups should exceed **50% and 30%,** respectively.

Together with the sensitivity, the percentage of node-positive invasive carcinomas and the ratio of benign to malignant biopsy results, the percentage of N0 minimal carcinomas detected is one of the most important and direct indicators of the effectiveness of early diagnosis in terms of the impact on clinical implications and on mortality.
Currently the mean diameter of lesions detected during clinical examinations is larger than that of lesions detected during screening.

Percentage of node-positive invasive carcinomas
This should be less than **25%**. Reduction of this figure is a priority since positive lymph node status is directly correlated with mortality from breast cancer.

Benign/malignant ratio: The ratio of benign to histologically confirmed malignant lesions is calculated on the total numbers of cases undergoing surgery. Percutaneous biopsies without a surgical specimen for final confirmation and surgical procedures on lesions already diagnosed as benign (for instance, a fibroadenoma that gets bigger) are no counted.
The currently ratio is **0.5** benign lesions to **1** malignant lesion.

Cancer detection rate: this is particularly important in screening programs and comprises:
- the rate of detection at first examinations or prevalent carcinomas: **6-10 cases/1000**
- the rate of detection at follow-up examinations or incident carcinomas: **2-4 cases/1000**
- the rate of detection in relation to age.

It is a reliable indicator of the estimated presence of disease in a given population and is a benchmark for other parameters, such as sensitivity or PPV. A high sensitivity or PPV cannot correspond to a low detection rate, i.e. less than 2 cases/1000.

Recall rate: this is another particularly interesting item in screening programmes since in clinical diagnosis working up mammography is immediately supplemented with additional diagnostic procedures when necessary. It indicates the proportion of further diagnostic imaging methods required to complete mammography (additional projections, magnifications, ultrasound, etc.). It should not exceed 10% of the mammographic examinations done.

MAMMOGRAPHY AUDIT

Table for Calculating sensitivity, specificity and PPV

MAMMOGRAPHY FINDINGS	Results of biopsies	
	Positive Biopsies	Negative Biopsies
Positive (Re.Co.R.M. 4, 5)	TP	FP
Negative (Re.Co.R.M. 1, 2, 3)	FN	TN

Sensitivity = TP/(TP+FN)
Specificity = TN/(TN+FP)
PPV = TP/(TP+FP)

Auditing the results: the objectives

Positive predictive value of biopsy recommendations	**25-40%**
Six-month controls	<10%
Percentage of stage 0 or 1 carcinomas	>50%
Percentage of minimal carcinomas (invasive carcinomas <1 cm or in situ carcinomas)	>30%
Positive lymph nodes	<25%
Sensitivity (if measurable)	>80%
Specificity (if measurable)	>90%
Benign/malignant ratio	0.5/1
Carcinomas detected per 1000 cases (screening)	2-10
Prevalent carcinomas per 1000 first examinations (screening)	6-10
Incident carcinomas per 1000 follow-up examinations (screening)	2-4
Recall rate (screening)	<10%

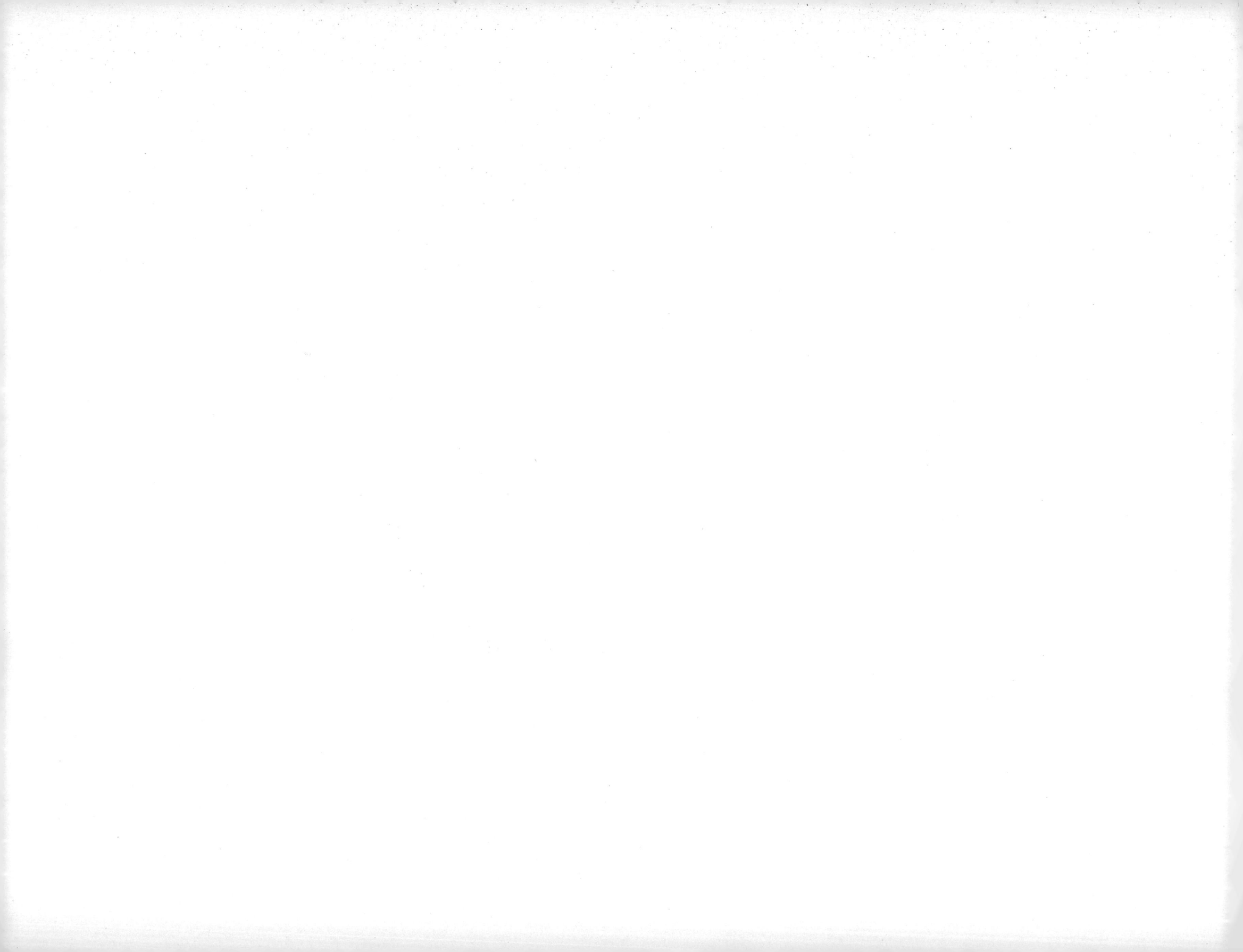